SECTIONAL ANATOMY
for IMAGING PROFESSIONALS

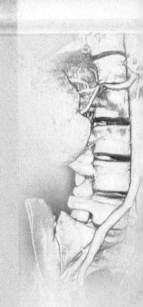

SECTIONAL ANATOMY
for IMAGING
PROFESSIONALS

SECOND EDITION

LORRIE L. KELLEY, MS, RT(R)(MR)(CT)

Associate Professor, CT/MRI Program Director

Boise State University

Boise, Idaho

Connie M. Petersen, MS, RT(R)(CT)

Adjunct Instructor, Radiologic Sciences Program

Boise State University

Boise, Idaho

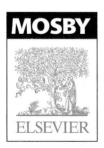

MOSBY

ELSEVIER

11830 Westline Industrial Drive
St. Louis, Missouri 63146

SECTIONAL ANATOMY FOR IMAGING PROFESSIONALS, ed 2

ISBN-13: 978-0-323-02003-9
ISBN-10:   0-323-02003-8

Previous edition copyrighted 1997

ISBN-13: 978-0-323-02003-9
ISBN-10:   0-323-02003-8

Acquisitions Editor: Jeanne Wilke
Developmental Editor: Rebecca Swisher
Book Publishing Manager: Linda McKinley
Publishing Services Manager: Pat Joiner
Design Direction: Teresa McBryan

Printed in the United States of America

Last digit is the print number: 9 8 7 6 5 4

To **James,**
Min beste venn og evig ledsager, jeg smil hver dag på
grunn av deg. You are my favorite.

And to **Kristina, Matthew, Jennifer, John, Michael,
Natalie, Angela,** and **Jamers,** my greatest treasures,
who bless me with their laughter, encourage me with
their unconditional patience and love, and
teach me by their selfless examples.

And to my parents,
Bill and **Darhl Buchanan,**
for teaching me the value of hard work and
sharing their wisdom and encouragement in ways
that strengthen and inspire me.

LLK

To my amazing husband, **Grant,**
for his constant support and unceasing faith in me.
I love the way I am seen through your eyes.

And to **Brady** and **Trinity,**
my shining stars who amaze me with their brilliance every
day and remind me of all that is truly important in life.

To my parents, **Carl** and **Ellen Collins,**
whom I love and admire, Thank you for giving me an
endless abundance of strength, love, and encouragement.

CMP

REVIEWERS

David Hrino, BS, RT(R)(CT)
Operations Manager
Advanced Radiology Services and The Center for
  Women's Well-Being
East Stroudsburg, Pennsylvania

Sherry A. Masotto, MS, RT, R
Program Director
Sharon Regional Health System
School of Radiography
Sharon, Pennsylvania

Rob McLaughlin, MA, RT(R)
Program Director and Associate Professor
Radiologic Technology
Louisiana State University at Eunice
Eunice, Louisiana

Barbara Peck, MBA, RT(R)(QM)
Clinical Coordinator/Assistant Program Director
Programs in Medical Imaging
Emory University
Atlanta, Georgia

Debra Poelhuis, MS, RT(R)(M)
Director
Radiography Program
Montgomery Community College
Pottstown, Pennsylvania

Elizabeth Price, MS, RT(R)(M)(CT)
Director
Radiologic Services
Burlington County College
Pemberton, New Jersey

Ray Winters, MS, RT(R)(CT)
Associate Professor/Chair
Radiologic Sciences Department
Arkansas State University
Jonesboro, Arkansas

Gary Zimmerman, MS, RT(R)(CT)(MR)
Professor
Oregon Institute of Technology
Klamath Falls, Oregon

PREFACE

This text was written to address the needs of today's practicing health professional. As technology in diagnostic imaging advances, so does the need to competently recognize and identify cross-sectional anatomy. Our goal was to create a clear, concise text that would demonstrate in an easy-to-use yet comprehensive format the anatomy the health professional is required to understand to optimize patient care. The text was purposely designed to be used both as a clinical reference manual and as an instructional text, either in a formal classroom environment or as a self-instructional volume.

Included are over 850 high-quality MR and CT images for every feasible plane of anatomy most commonly imaged. An additional 350 anatomic maps and line drawings related to the MR and CT images add to the learner's understanding of the anatomy being studied. In addition, pathology boxes describe common pathologies related to the anatomy presented, assisting the reader in making connections between the images in the text and common pathologies that will be encountered in clinical practice. Tables that summarize muscle group information include points of origin and insertion, as well as functions, for the muscle structures pertinent to the images the reader is studying.

NEW TO THIS EDITION

- Reference drawings with the corresponding scanning planes appear with the actual images so that they are easily referenced. Students will be able to easily make the correlation between the scanning planes and the resulting images.
- Nearly 300 new scans include more 3D and vascular images to better demonstrate current technology.
- A new introductory chapter provides a foundation by teaching the terminology related to sectional anatomy and prepares the reader to make the most of the content of the text.

CONTENT AND ORGANIZATION

The images include identification of vital anatomic structures to assist the health professional in locating and identifying the desired anatomy during actual clinical examinations. The narrative accompanying these images clearly and concisely describes the location and function of the anatomy in a format easily understood by health professionals. The text is divided into chapters by separate portions of the anatomy.

Each chapter of the text contains an outline that provides an overview of the chapter's contents, pathology boxes that briefly describe common pathologies related to the anatomy being presented, tables designed to organize and summarize the anatomy contained in the chapter, and reference illustrations that provide the correct orientation for scanning the anatomy of interest.

ANCILLARIES

A Workbook and an Instructor's Electronic Resource complement the text. When used together, these additional tools create a virtual learning system/reference resource.

Workbook: The Workbook provides practice opportunities for the user to identify specific anatomy. The Workbook includes learning objectives that focus on the key elements of each chapter, a variety of practice items to test the reader's knowledge of key concepts, labeling exercises to test the reader's knowledge of the anatomy, post test questions, and answers to exercises and post tests.

Instructor's Electronic Resource: The Instructor's Electronic Resource may be used in a formal academic setting as desired. This instructor resource on CD-ROM contains lecture outlines, key terms, and suggested readings for each chapter plus an electronic image collection. The IER material may also be accessed by instructors through the accompanying Evolve website at http://evolve.elsevier.com/Kelley/sectionalanatomy/. The Evolve website also provides the instructor with online access to a course-management platform for deployment of course elements online.

Lorrie L. Kelley
Connie M. Petersen

ACKNOWLEDGMENTS

Many provided encouragement as the compilation of this text commenced. Perhaps "persistent prodding" would be a more accurate description. Becky Swisher is our champion; she had the tiresome duty of encouraging us to meet our deadlines and the graceful persistence to ensure that we eventually met our extended deadlines. We are indebted to her for her editorial assistance in seeing this project through to completion.

We wish to extend our gratitude to everyone who thought the first edition had value and to those who took the time to provide constructive criticism and suggestions for further improvements and increased accuracy. And to the many students who were not shy in providing feedback so that we could see the text from many different perspectives.

The following individuals and institutions deserve special acknowledgment:

- The faculty at Boise State University for their support and patience as we faced fast-approaching deadlines.
- Dale Sanger for spending a great number of hours helping to find just the right CT images necessary for this book. Dale made the daunting task of acquiring a very large number of CT images a lot of fun. Thank you so very much for all your help, patience, and humor.
- Gina Bernstrom, Susan Goode, and Lynda Snider for helping to find so many great cases and for taking on extra work to allow Dale Sanger the time to search for and produce the many CT images that we needed. We are so grateful for your help.
- Mary Pullin from Philips Medical Systems for providing some beautiful MR images.
- Dave Arnold and St. Luke's Regional Medical Center for providing the majority of the MR images.
- Intermountain Medical Imaging in Meridian and its employees for providing the majority of the CT images.
- Mercy Medical Center and its employees for allowing us access to obtain some very nice CT images.

We owe a debt of gratitude to Jeanne Robertson, who provided numerous new illustrations and revised many old drawings in record time. Because of her efforts and talent, there is more consistency in the visual presentation of the artwork throughout the text.

Lorrie L. Kelley
Connie M. Petersen

CONTENTS

1 INTRODUCTION TO SECTIONAL ANATOMY, 1

Anatomic Positions and Planes, 2
Terminology and Landmarks, 3
Body Cavities, 5
Abdominal and Pelvic Divisions, 8
Image Display, 11

2 CRANIUM AND FACIAL BONES, 17

Cranium, 18
Facial Bones, 49
Temporomandibular Joint, 59
Paranasal Sinuses, 64
Orbit, 72

3 BRAIN, 85

Meninges, 86
Ventricular System, 89
Cerebrum, 98
Diencephalon, 109
Limbic System, 113
Brainstem, 117
Cerebellum, 124
Cerebral Vascular System, 127
Cranial Nerves, 148

4 SPINE, 163

Vertebral Column, 164
Ligaments, 179
Muscles, 186
Spinal Cord, 193
Plexuses, 204
Vasculature, 219

5 NECK, 225

Organs, 226
Muscles, 260
Vascular Structures, 269

6 THORAX, 275

Bony Thorax, 276
Lungs, 279
Pleural Cavities, 283

Bronchi, 283
Mediastinum, 286
Lymphatic System, 290
Heart and Vasculature, 293
Great Vessels, 304
Coronary Circulation, 323
Azygos Venous System, 329
Muscles, 330
Breast, 335

7 ABDOMEN, 337

Abdominal Cavity, 338
Liver, 351
Gallbladder and Biliary System, 367
Pancreas, 373
Spleen, 376
Adrenal Glands, 378
Urinary System, 382
Stomach, 389
Intestines, 392
Abdominal Aorta and Branches, 401
Inferior Vena Cava and Tributaries, 418
Lymph Nodes, 423
Muscles of the Abdominal Wall, 424

8 PELVIS, 429

Bony Pelvis, 430
Muscles, 438
Viscera, 447
Vasculature, 475
Lymph Nodes, 487

9 UPPER EXTREMITY, 489

Shoulder, 491
Elbow, 523
Wrist and Hand, 540
Neurovasculature, 561

10 LOWER EXTREMITY, 567

Hip, 568
Knee and Lower Leg, 593
Ankle and Foot, 625
Neurovasculature, 655

Credits, 665

SECTIONAL ANATOMY
for IMAGING
PROFESSIONALS

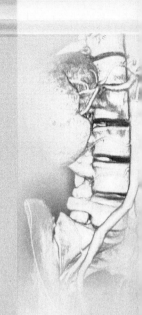

CHAPTER 1

INTRODUCTION TO SECTIONAL ANATOMY

Sectional anatomy has had a long history. Beginning back as early as the sixteenth century, the great anatomist and artist, Leonardo da Vinci, was among the first to represent the body in anatomic sections. In the following centuries, numerous anatomists continued to provide illustrations of various body structures in sectional planes to gain greater understanding of the topographical relationships of the organs. The ability to see inside the body for medical purposes has been around since 1895, when Wilhelm Conrad Roentgen discovered x-rays. Since that time, medical imaging has evolved from the static, 2-dimensional (2D) image of the first x-ray to the 2D cross-section image of computed tomography (CT) and finally to the 3-dimensional (3D) imaging techniques used today. These changes warrant the need for medical professionals to understand and identify human anatomy in both 2D and 3D images.

Sectional anatomy emphasizes the physical relationship between internal structures. Prior knowledge of anatomy from drawings or radiographs may assist in understanding where specific structures are located on a sectional image. For example, it may be difficult to recognize all the internal anatomy of the pelvis in cross section, but by identifying the femoral head on the image, it will be easier to recognize soft tissue structures adjacent to the hip in the general location of the slice (Figure 1.1).

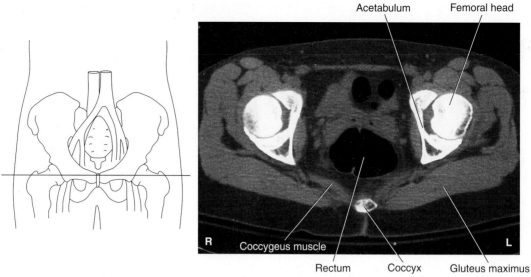

Figure 1.1
Cross-section image of hips.

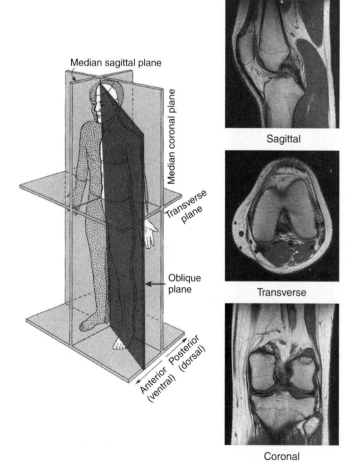

Figure 1.2
Anatomic position and planes of the body.

ANATOMIC POSITIONS AND PLANES

For our purposes, sectional anatomy encompasses all the variations of viewing anatomy as a 2D slice taken from an arbitrary angle through the body while in anatomic position.

In anatomic position the body is standing erect, face and toes pointing forward, and arms at the side with the palms facing forward. Sectional images are acquired and displayed according to one of the four fundamental anatomic planes that pass through the body (Figure 1.2). The four anatomic planes are defined as follows:

1. **Sagittal plane:** a vertical plane that passes through the body, dividing it into right and left portions
2. **Coronal plane:** a vertical plane that passes through the body, dividing it into anterior (ventral) and posterior (dorsal) portions
3. **Axial (transverse) plane:** a horizontal plane that passes through the body, dividing it into superior and inferior portions
4. **Oblique plane:** a plane that passes diagonally between the axes of two other planes

Medical images of sectional anatomy are, by convention, displayed in a specific orientation. Images are viewed with the right side of the image corresponding to the viewer's left side (Figure 1.3).

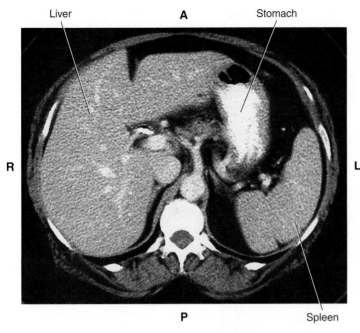

Liver   A   Stomach

R

L

P   Spleen

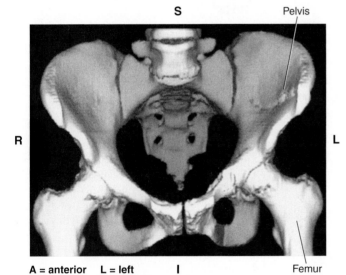

S   Pelvis

R   L

A = anterior   L = left   I
P = posterior   S = superior
R = right   I = inferior

Femur

Figure 1.3
Display orientation.

TABLE 1.1	Directional Terminology
DIRECTION	DEFINITION
Superior	Above; at a higher level
Inferior	Below; at a lower level
Anterior/ventral	Toward the front or anterior surface of the body
Posterior/dorsal	Toward the back or posterior surface of the body
Medial	Toward the midsagittal plane
Lateral	Away from the midsagittal plane
Proximal	Toward a reference point or source within the body
Distal	Away from a reference point or source within the body
Superficial	Near the body surface
Deep	Farther into the body and away from the body surface
Cranial/cephalic	Toward the head
Caudal	Toward the feet
Rostral	Toward the nose
Ipsilateral	On the same side
Contralateral	On the opposite side
Thenar	The fleshy part of the hand at the base of the thumb
Volar	Pertaining to the palm of the hand or flexor surface of wrist
Palmar	The front or palm of the hand
Plantar	The sole of the foot

TABLE 1.2	Regional Terminology
DIRECTION	DEFINITION
Abdominal	Abdomen
Antebrachial	Forearm
Antecubital	Front of elbow
Axillary	Armpit
Brachial	Upper arm
Calf	Lower posterior portion of leg
Carpal	Wrist
Cephalic	Head
Cervical	Neck
Costal	Ribs
Cubital	Posterior surface of elbow area of the arm
Femoral	Thigh
Flank	Side of trunk adjoining the lumbar region
Gluteal	Buttock
Inguinal	Groin
Lumbar	Lower back between the ribs and hips; loin
Mammary	Upper chest or breast
Occipital	Back of the head
Ophthalmic	Eye
Pectoral	Upper chest or breast
Pelvic	Pelvis
Perineal	Perineum
Plantar	Sole of foot
Popliteal	Back of knee
Sacral	Sacrum
Sternal	Sternum
Thigh	Upper portion of leg
Thoracic	Chest
Umbilical	Navel
Vertebral	Spine

TERMINOLOGY AND LANDMARKS

Directional and regional terminology is used to help describe the relative position of specific structures within the body. Directional terms are defined in Table 1.1, and regional terms are defined in Table 1.2 and demonstrated in Figure 1.4.

External Landmarks

External landmarks of the body are helpful to identify the location of many internal structures. The commonly used external landmarks are shown in Figures 1.5 and 1.6.

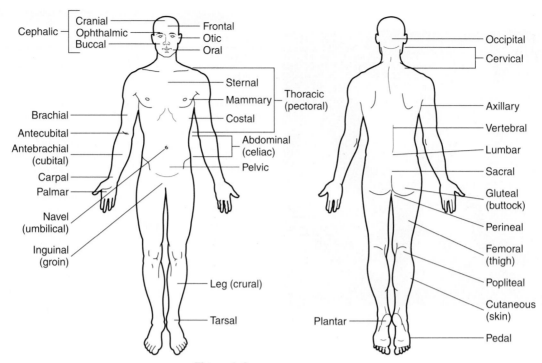

Figure 1.4
Regional terminology of the body.

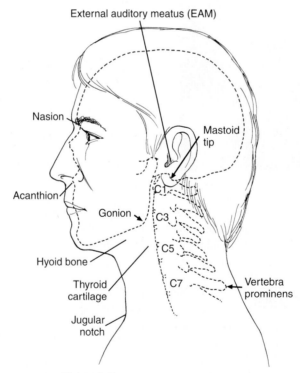

Figure 1.5
Surface landmarks of the head and neck.

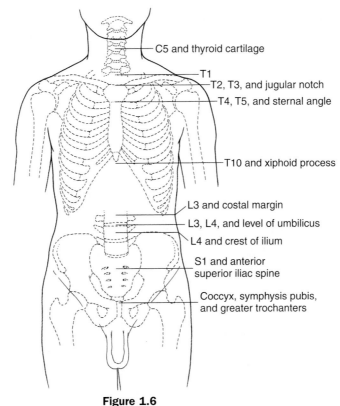

C5 and thyroid cartilage

T1

T2, T3, and jugular notch

T4, T5, and sternal angle

T10 and xiphoid process

L3 and costal margin

L3, L4, and level of umbilicus

L4 and crest of ilium

S1 and anterior superior iliac spine

Coccyx, symphysis pubis, and greater trochanters

Figure 1.6
Surface landmarks of the body.

Internal Landmarks

Internal structures, in particular vascular structures, can be located by referencing them to other identifiable regions or locations such as organs or the skeleton (Figure 1.7 and Table 1.3).

BODY CAVITIES

The body consists of two main cavities: the dorsal and ventral cavities. The dorsal cavity is located posteriorly and includes the cranial and spinal cavities. The ventral cavity, the largest body cavity, is subdivided into the thoracic and abdominopelvic cavities. The thoracic cavity is further subdivided into two lateral pleural cavities and a single, centrally located cavity called the mediastinum. The abdominal cavity can be subdivided into the abdominal and pelvic cavities (Figure 1.8, *A* and *B*). The structures located in each cavity are listed in Table 1.4.

TABLE 1.3   Internal Landmarks

LANDMARK	LOCATION
Aortic arch	2.5 cm below jugular notch
Aortic bifurcation	L4-L5
Carina	T4-T5, sternal angle
Carotid bifurcation	Upper border of thyroid cartilage
Celiac trunk	4 cm above transpyloric plane (Figure 1.10)
Circle of Willis	Suprasellar cistern
Common iliac vein bifurcation	Upper margin of sacroiliac joint
Conus medullaris	T12 to L1, L2
Heart—apex	5th intercostal space, left midclavicular line
Heart—base	Level of 2nd and 3rd costal cartilages behind sternum
Inferior mesenteric artery	4 cm above bifurcation of abdominal aorta
Inferior vena cava	L5
Portal vein	Posterior to pancreatic neck
Renal arteries	Anterior to L1, inferior to superior mesenteric artery
Superior mesenteric artery	2 cm above transpyloric plane
Thyroid gland	Thyroid cartilage
Vocal cords	Midway between superior and inferior border of thyroid cartilage

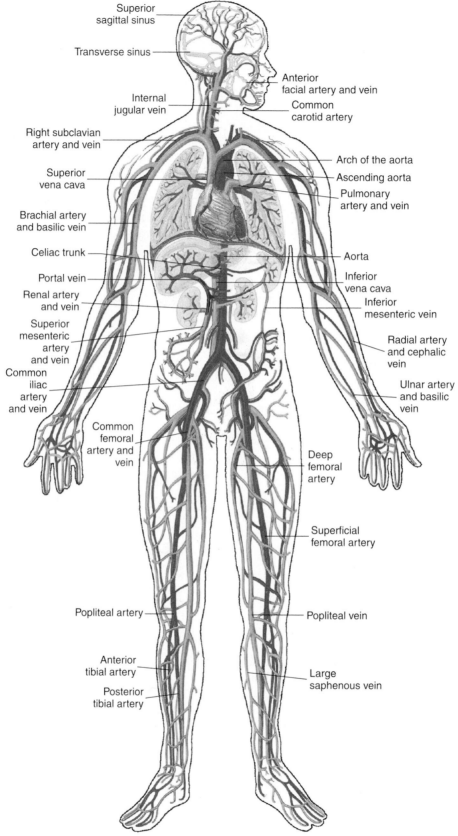

Figure 1.7
Anterior view of major arteries and veins of the body.

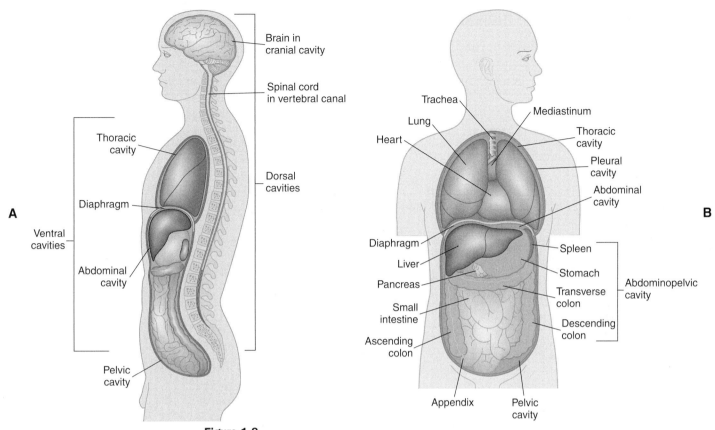

Figure 1.8
A, Sagittal view of body cavities. **B,** Anterior view of body cavities.

TABLE 1.4   Body Cavities

MAIN BODY CAVITIES	CONTENTS
DORSAL	*BRAIN AND SPINAL CORD AND VERTEBRAE*
Ventral	
Thoracic	
• Mediastinum	• Thymus heart, great vessels, trachea, esophagus, and pericardium
• Pleural	• Lungs, pleural membranes
Abdominal and pelvic	
• Abdominal	• Peritoneum, liver, gallbladder, pancreas, spleen, stomach, intestines, kidneys, ureters, and blood vessels
• Pelvic	• Rectum, urinary bladder, male and female reproductive system

ABDOMINAL AND PELVIC DIVISIONS

The abdomen is bordered superiorly by the diaphragm and inferiorly by the superior pelvic aperture (pelvic inlet). The abdomen can be divided into quadrants or regions. These divisions are useful to identify the general location of internal organs and provide descriptive terms for the location of pain or injury from a patient's history.

Quadrants

The midsagittal plane and transverse plane intersect at the umbilicus to divide the abdomen into four quadrants (Figure 1.9, *A*):

> Right upper quadrant (RUQ)
> Right lower quadrant (RLQ)
> Left upper quadrant (LUQ)
> Left lower quadrant (LLQ)

For a description of the structures located within each quadrant, see Table 1.5.

Regions

The abdomen can be further divided by four planes into nine regions. The two horizontal planes are the transpyloric and transtubercular planes. The transpyloric plane is found midway between the xiphisternal joint and the umbilicus, passing through the inferior border of the L1 vertebra. The transtubercular plane passes through the tubercles on the iliac crests, at the level of the L5 vertebral body. The two sagittal planes are the midclavicular lines. Each line runs inferiorly from the midpoint of the clavicle to the midinguinal point (Figure 1.9, *B*). The nine regions can be organized into three groups:

SUPERIOR
- Right upper hypochondrium
- Epigastrium
- Left hypochondrium

MIDDLE
- Right lateral
- Umbilical
- Left lateral

INFERIOR
- Right inguinal
- Hypogastrium
- Left inguinal

TABLE 1.5   **Organs Found within Abdominopelvic Quadrants**

QUADRANT	ORGANS
Right upper quadrant (RUQ)	Right lobe of liver, gallbladder, right kidney, portions of stomach, small and large intestines
Left upper quadrant (LUQ)	Left lobe of liver, stomach, tail of the pancreas, left kidney, spleen, portions of large intestines
Right lower quadrant (RLQ)	Cecum, appendix, portions of small intestine, right ureter, right ovary, right spermatic cord
Left lower quadrant (LLQ)	Most of small intestine, portions of large intestine, left ureter, left ovary, left spermatic cord

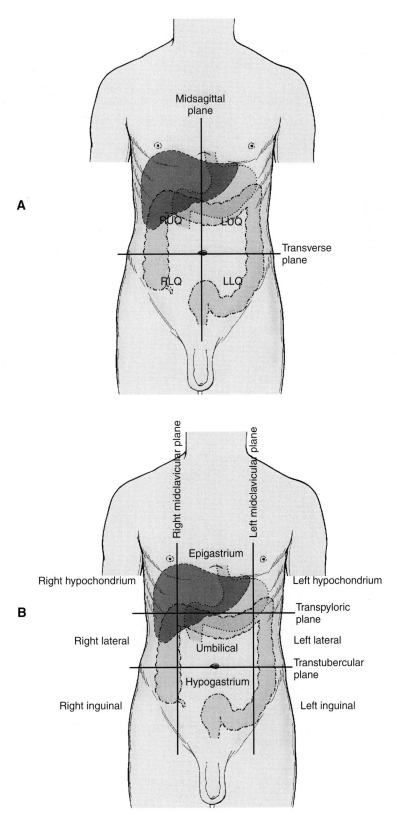

Figure 1.9
A, Four abdominal quadrants. **B,** Nine abdominal regions.

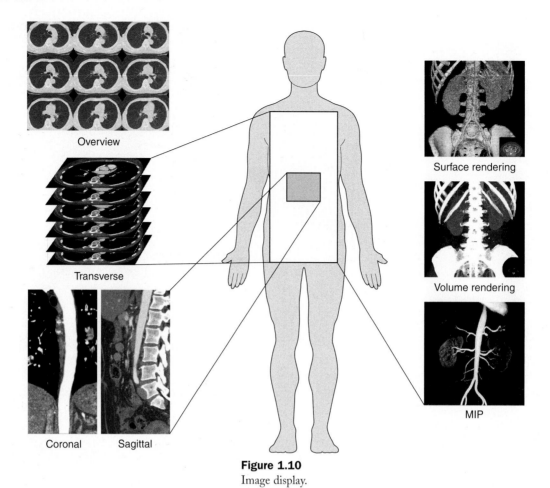

Overview

Transverse

Coronal

Sagittal

Surface rendering

Volume rendering

MIP

Figure 1.10
Image display.

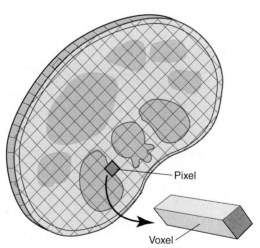

Pixel

Voxel

Figure 1.11
Representation of a pixel and voxel. *MIP,* Maximum intensity projection.

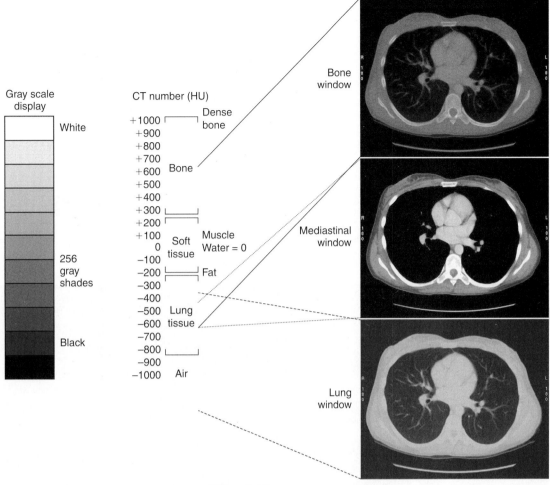

Figure 1.12
CT numbers and windowing.

IMAGE DISPLAY

The following section is intended to introduce the reader to the various methods with which sectional images will be displayed within the text (Figure 1.10). For a more in-depth discussion of the topics, refer to the reference list at the end of the chapter.

Gray Scale

Each digital image can be divided into individual regions called *pixels* or *voxels* that are then assigned a numerical value corresponding to a specific tissue property of the structure being imaged (Figure 1.11). The numerical value of each voxel is assigned a shade of gray for image display. In CT, the numerical value (CT number) is referenced to a Hounsfield unit (HU), which represents the attenuating properties or density of each tissue. Water is used as the reference tissue

and is given a value of zero. Any CT number greater than zero will represent tissue that is denser than water and will appear in progressively lighter shades of gray to white. Tissues with a negative CT number will appear in progressively darker shades of gray to black. In magnetic resonance (MR), the gray scale represents the specific tissue relaxation properties of T1, T2, and relative spin density. The gray scale in MR images can vary greatly because of inherent tissue properties and can appear different with each patient and across series of images.

The appearance of each digital image can be altered to include more or fewer shades of gray by adjusting the gray scale, a process called *windowing*. Windowing is used to optimize visualization of specific tissues or lesions. Window width (WW) is the parameter that allows for the adjustment of the gray scale (number of shades of gray), and window level (WL) basically sets the density of the image (Figures 1.12 and 1.13).

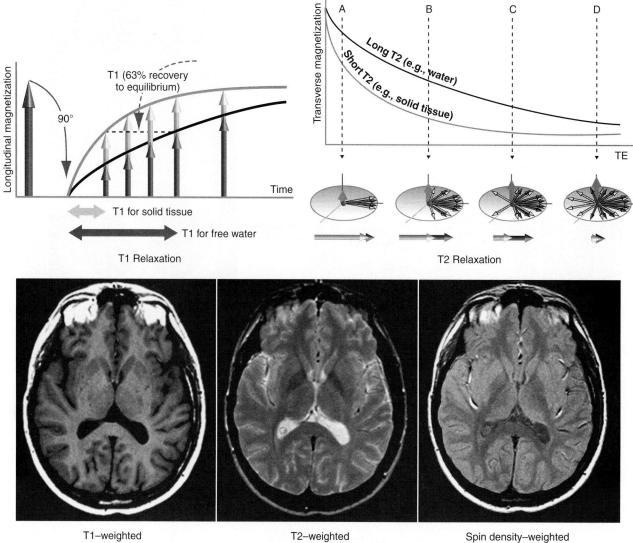

T1 Relaxation

T2 Relaxation

T1–weighted   T2–weighted   Spin density–weighted

Figure 1.13
MR tissue relaxation.

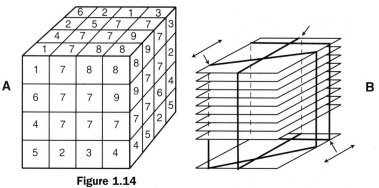

Figure 1.14
A, Digital cube. **B,** Stack of transverse images.

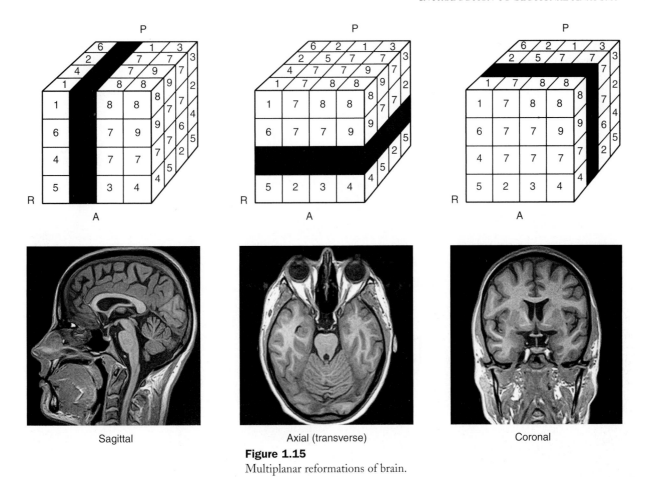

Sagittal

Axial (transverse)

Coronal

Figure 1.15
Multiplanar reformations of brain.

Voxels

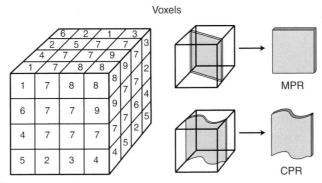

MPR

CPR

Figure 1.16
Curved planar reformation. *MPR*, Multiplanar reformation; *CPR*, curved planar reformation.

Multiplanar Reformation and 3D Imaging

Several postprocessing techniques can be applied to the original 2D digital data that will provide additional 3D information for the physician. All current post-processing techniques depend on creating a stack of digital data from the original 2D images, which then results in a cube of digital information (Figure 1.14, *A* and *B*).

MULTIPLANAR REFORMATION (REFORMAT) (MPR) Images reconstructed from data obtained along any projection through the cube result in a sagittal, coronal, transverse, or oblique image (see Figure 1.10; Figure 1.15).

CURVED PLANAR REFORMATION (REFORMAT) (CPR) Images are reconstructed from data obtained along an arbitrary curved projection through the cube (Figure 1.16). All 3D algorithms use the principle of ray tracing in which imaginary rays are sent out from a camera viewpoint. The data are then rotated on an arbitrary axis, and the imaginary ray is passed through the data in specific increments. Depending on the method of reconstruction, unique information is projected onto the viewing plane (Figure 1.17).

SHADED SURFACE DISPLAY (SSD) A ray from the camera's viewpoint is directed to stop at a particular user-defined threshold value. With this method, every voxel with a value greater than the selected threshold is rendered opaque, creating a surface. That value is then projected onto the viewing screen (see Figure 1.10; Figure 1.18).

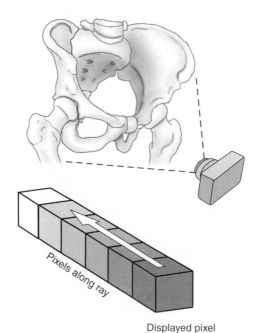

Figure 1.17
Ray tracing.

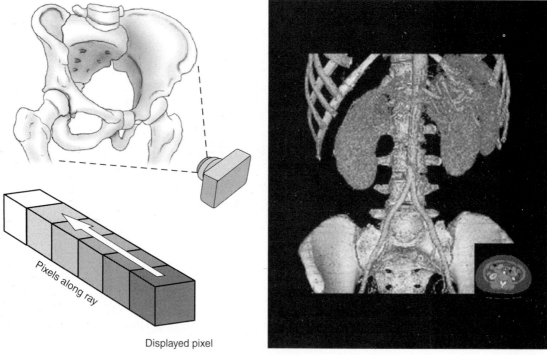

Figure 1.18
Shaded surface display (SSD).

MAXIMUM INTENSITY PROJECTION (MIP)   A ray from the camera's viewpoint is directed to stop at the maximum voxel value. With this method, only the brightest voxels will be mapped into the final image (Figure 1.19).

VOLUME RENDERING (VR)   The contributions of each voxel are summed along the course of the ray from the camera's viewpoint. The process is repeated numerous times in order to determine each pixel value that will be displayed in the final image (Figure 1.20).

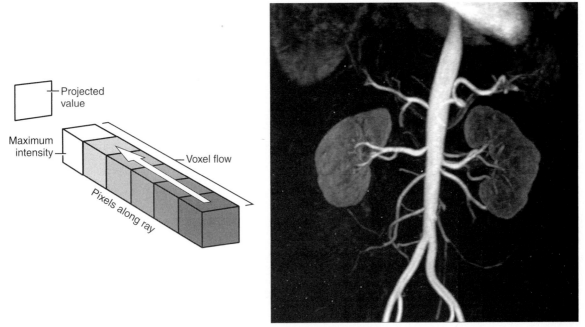

Figure 1.19
Maximum intensity projection (MIP).

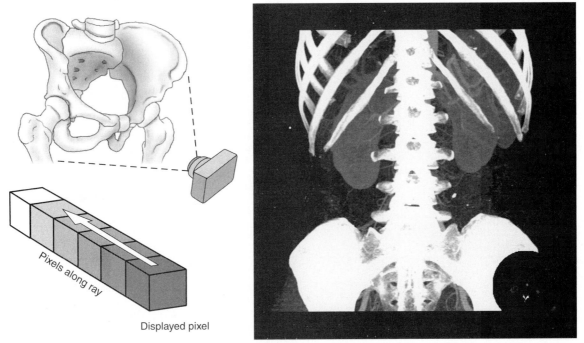

Figure 1.20
Volume rendering (VR).

References

Ballinger PW: *Radiographic positions and radiologic procedures,* ed 10, St. Louis, 2003, Mosby.

Benson HJ, Gunstream SE, et al: *Anatomy and physiology laboratory textbook,* ed 4, Dubuque, IA, 1988, Wm. C. Brown.

Calhoun PS, Kuszyk BS, Heath DG, et al: Three-dimensional volume rendering of spiral CT data: Theory and method, *RadioGraphics* 19:745, 1999.

Curry RA, Tempkin BB: *Ultrasonography: An introduction to normal structure and functional anatomy,* ed 2, St. Louis, 2004, Saunders.

Hofer M: *CT teaching manual,* New York, 2000, Thieme Medical Publishers.

Moore KL: *Clinically oriented anatomy,* ed 3, Baltimore, 1992, Williams & Williams.

Seeram E: *Computed tomography; physical principle, clinical applications, and quality control,* ed 2, Philadelphia, 2001, Saunders.

Todd EM: *The neuroanatomy of Leonardo da Vinci,* Park Ridge, IL, 1991, American Association of Neurological Surgeons.

Udupa JK: Three-dimensional visualization and analysis methodologies: A current perspective, *RadioGraphics* 19:783, 1999.

White M: *Leonardo: the first scientist,* New York, 2000, St. Martin's Press.

CRANIUM AND FACIAL BONES

Gentlemen, damn the sphenoid bone!

OLIVER WENDELL HOLMES (1809-1894)
Opening of anatomy lectures at Harvard Medical School

The complex anatomy of the cranium and facial bones can be intimidating. However, with three-dimensional (3D) and multiple imaging planes (Figure 2.1), the task of learning these structures can be simplified. It is important to understand normal sectional anatomy of the cranium and facial bones to identify pathologic disorders and injuries that may occur within this area. This chapter demonstrates the sectional anatomy of the following structures:

CRANIUM
Parietal Bone
Frontal Bone
Ethmoid Bone
Sphenoid Bone
Occipital Bone
Temporal Bone
Structures of the External, Middle, and Inner Ear
Sutures
Fontanels

FACIAL BONES
Nasal Bone, Lacrimal Bone, Maxilla, Palatine Bone, and Zygoma
Inferior Nasal Conchae and Vomer
Mandible

TEMPOROMANDIBULAR JOINT
Bony Anatomy
Articular Disk and Ligaments
Muscles

PARANASAL SINUSES
Ethmoid
Maxillary
Sphenoid
Frontal
Osteomeatal Complex

ORBIT
Bony Orbit
Soft Tissue Structures
Lacrimal Apparatus
Muscles of the Eye
Optic Nerve

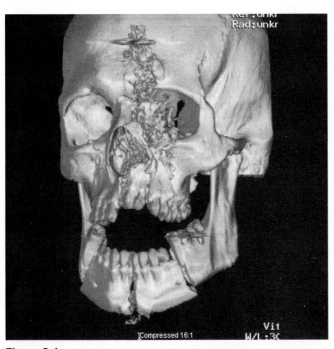

Figure 2.1
3D CT reconstruction of skull. Trauma resulting from a gunshot wound.

CRANIUM

The **cranium** is composed of eight bones that surround and protect the brain. These bones include the occipital (1), temporal (2), sphenoid (1), ethmoid (1), parietal (2), and frontal (1) bones (Figures 2.2 through 2.5). The base of the cranium houses three fossae called the *anterior, middle,* and *posterior cranial fossae*. The **anterior cranial fossa** (frontal fossa) is composed primarily of the frontal bone, ethmoid bone, and lesser wing of the sphenoid bone and contains the frontal lobes of the brain. The **middle cranial fossa** (temporal fossa) is formed primarily by the body of the sphenoid and temporal bones and houses the pituitary gland, hypothalamus, and temporal lobes of the brain. The **posterior cranial fossa** (infratentorial fossa) is formed by the occipital and temporal bones and contains the cerebellum and brainstem (Figure 2.6). For additional detail of the contents found within the cranial fossa, see Table 2.1. Each cranial bone is structurally unique, which can make identification of the physical components challenging.

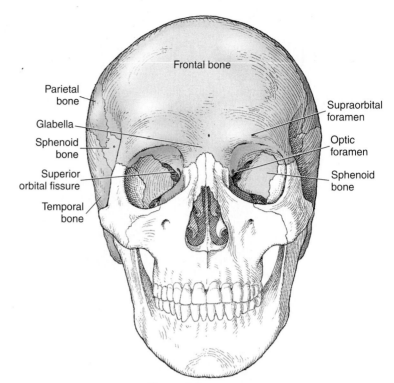

Figure 2.2
Anterior view of skull.

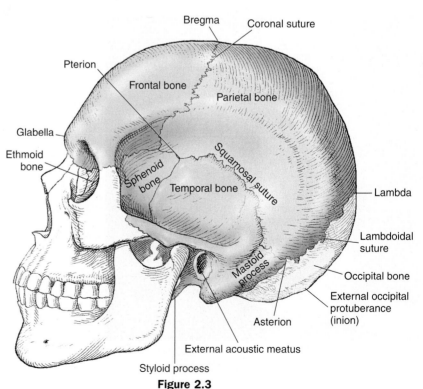

Figure 2.3
Lateral view of skull.

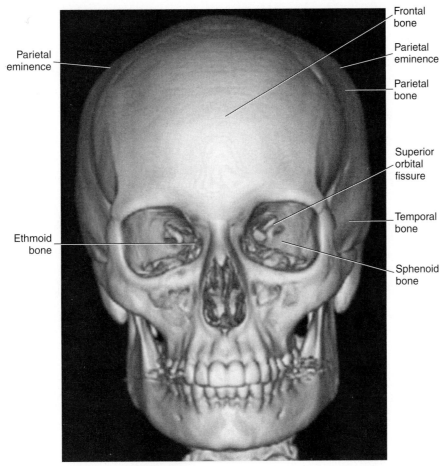

Parietal eminence

Frontal bone

Parietal eminence

Parietal bone

Superior orbital fissure

Temporal bone

Sphenoid bone

Ethmoid bone

Figure 2.4
3D CT reconstruction of anterior skull.

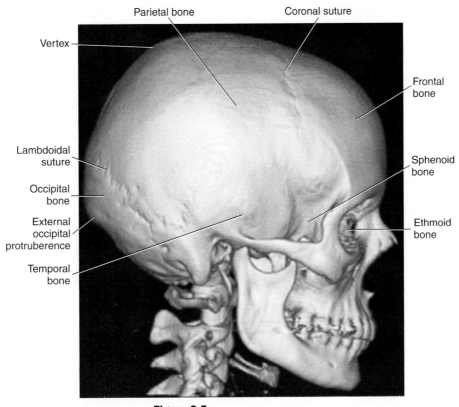

Parietal bone

Coronal suture

Vertex

Frontal bone

Lambdoidal suture

Sphenoid bone

Occipital bone

Ethmoid bone

External occipital protruberence

Temporal bone

Figure 2.5
3D CT reconstruction of lateral skull.

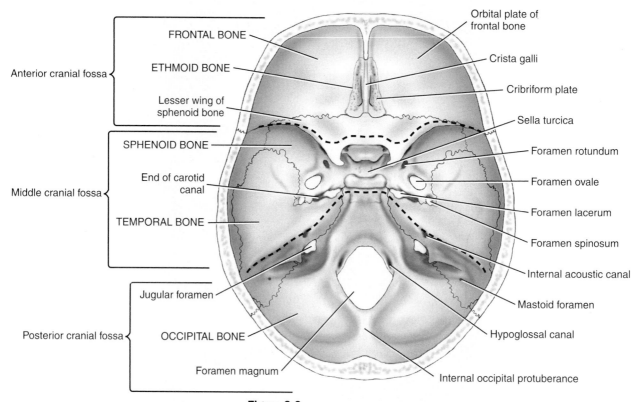

Figure 2.6
Superior view of cranial fossae.

TABLE 2-1   Contents of the Cranial Fossae

FOSSA	CONTENTS
Anterior cranial fossa	Frontal lobes of cerebrum; olfactory bulbs
Middle cranial fossa	Temporal lobes of cerebrum, pituitary gland, optic nerves and chiasm, cavernous sinus, trigeminal ganglion, internal carotid artery, hypothalamus and the following cranial nerves: trigeminal, oculomotor, trochlear, abducent, and ophthalmic
Posterior cranial fossa	Cerebellum, pons, medulla oblongata, midbrain, and the following cranial nerves: facial, vestibulocochlear, glossopharyngeal, vagus, accessory, hypoglossal

Parietal Bone

The two **parietal bones** form a large portion of the sides of the cranium. Prominent markings and grooves that are found within the inner surface of the cranium are formed by corresponding meningeal vessels and cerebral gyri and sulci (Figure 2.7). The parietal bones articulate with the frontal, occipital, temporal, and sphenoid bones. The superior point between the parietal bones is the **vertex,** which is the highest point of the cranium (Figure 2.8). Each parietal bone has a central prominent bulge on its outer surface termed the **parietal eminence.** The width of the cranium can be determined by measuring the distance between the two parietal eminences (Figure 2.4).

KEY: **CS,** Coronal suture; **SS,** sagittal suture; **LS,** lambdoidal suture; **0,** occipital bone.

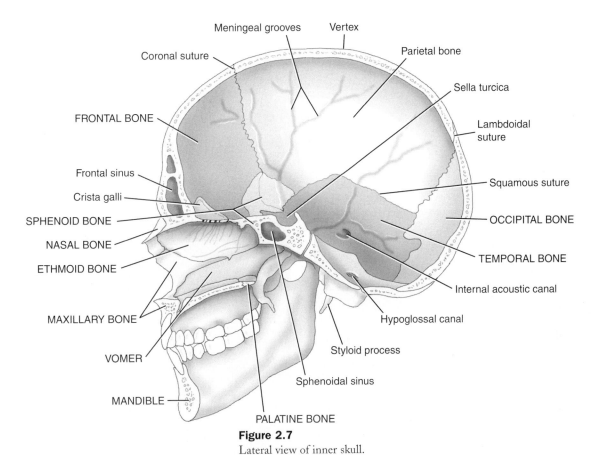

Figure 2.7
Lateral view of inner skull.

Figure 2.8
3D CT reconstruction of lateral surface of cranium.

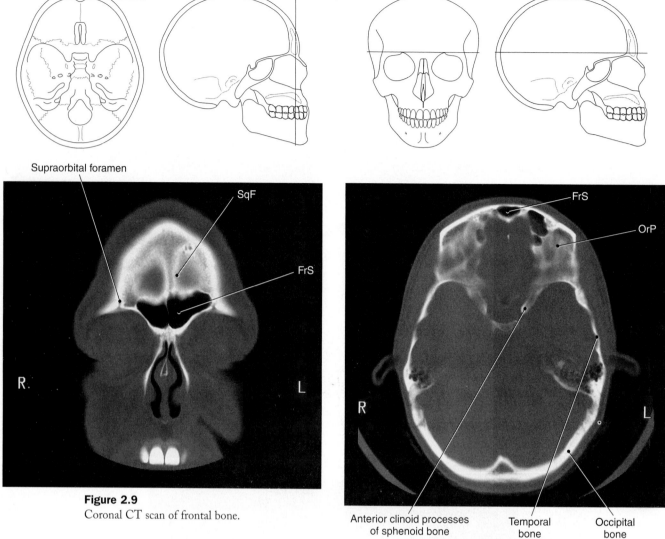

Figure 2.9
Coronal CT scan of frontal bone.

Figure 2.10
Axial CT scan of orbital plates.

KEY: SqF, Squamous portion of frontal bone; **FrS,** frontal sinus; **OrP,** orbital plane of frontal bone.

Frontal Bone

The **frontal bone** consists of a vertical and a horizontal portion. The **vertical** or **squamous portion** forms the forehead and anterior vault of the cranium (Figures 2.2 through 2.5). The vertical portion contains the frontal sinuses, which lie on either side of the midsagittal plane (Figures 2.7 and Figure 2.9). The **horizontal portion** forms the roof over each orbit termed the **orbital plate** and the majority of the anterior cranial fossa (Figures 2.6 and 2.10). Located in the superior portion of each orbit is the **supraorbital notch,** or foramen, which exists for the passage of nerves and arteries (Figures 2.2 and 2.9). Between the orbital plates is an area termed the **ethmoid notch,** which receives the cribriform plate of the ethmoid bone (Figure 2.6).

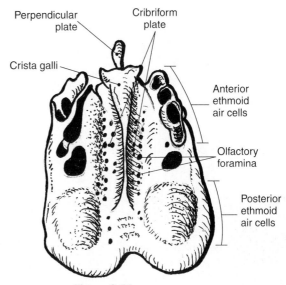

Figure 2.11
Superior view of ethmoid bone.

KEY: **EtB,** Ethmoid bulla; **CrP,** cribriform plate; **Per,** perpendicular plate of ethmoid bone.

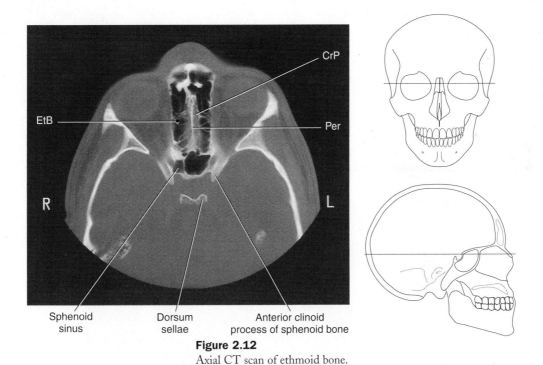

Figure 2.12
Axial CT scan of ethmoid bone.

Ethmoid Bone

The **ethmoid bone** is the smallest of the cranial bones and is situated in the anterior cranial fossa. This cube-shaped bone can be divided into four parts: horizontal portion, vertical portion, and two lateral masses (labyrinths) (Figures 2.11 and 2.12). The **horizontal portion,** called the **cribriform plate,** fits into the ethmoidal notch of the frontal bone (Figure 2.6). This plate contains many foramina for the passage of olfactory nerves. The **crista galli,** a bony projection stemming from the midline of the cribriform plate, projects superiorly to act as an attachment for the falx cerebri, which is the connective tissue that anchors the brain to the anterior cranial fossa (Figures 2.13 and 2.14). The **vertical portion** of the ethmoid bone, called the **perpendicular plate,** projects inferiorly from the cribriform plate to form a portion of the bony nasal septum. The **lateral masses** incorporate thin-walled **orbital plates** that create a portion of the medial orbit. Contained within the lateral masses are many ethmoid air cells **(ethmoid sinuses),** one of the largest being the **ethmoid bulla.** Projecting from the lateral masses are two scroll-shaped processes called the **superior** and **middle nasal conchae** (turbinates), and the **uncinate process.** Between the uncinate process and ethmoid bulla is a narrow groove called the **infundibulum,** which is an important landmark of the paranasal sinuses (Figures 2.13 and 2.14).

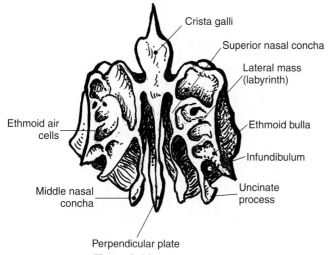

Figure 2.13
Anterior view of ethmoid bone.

KEY: **EtB,** Ethmoid bulla; **Inf,** infundibulum; **Unc,** uncinate process of ethmoid bone; **mME,** middle meatus.

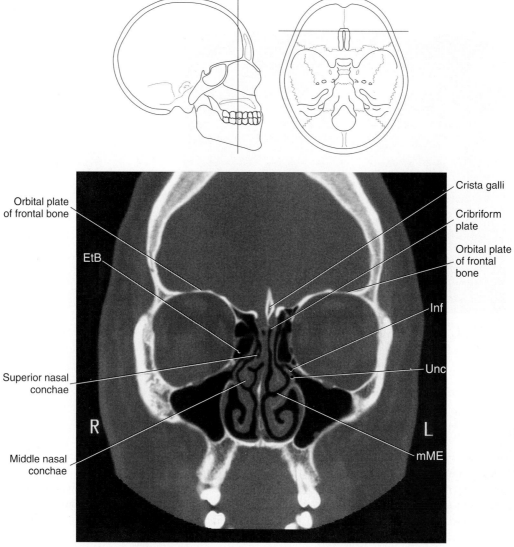

Figure 2.14
Coronal CT scan of ethmoid bone with crista galli.

Sphenoid Bone

The butterfly-shaped **sphenoid bone** extends completely across the floor of the middle cranial fossa. This bone forms the majority of the base of the skull and articulates with the occipital, temporal, parietal, frontal, and ethmoid bones. The main parts of the sphenoid bone are the body, lesser wings (2), and greater wings (2) (Figure 2.15). Located within the **body** of the sphenoid bone is a deep depression called the **sella turcica,** which houses the hypophysis (pituitary gland). Directly below the sella turcica are two air-filled cavities termed **sphenoid sinuses** (Figures 2.12 and 2.16). The anterior portion of the sella turcica is formed by the **tuberculum sellae** and the pos-

terior portion by the **dorsum sellae.** The dorsum sellae gives rise to the **posterior clinoid processes** (Figures 2.17 and 2.18). The triangular-shaped **lesser wings** attach to the superior aspect of the body and form two sharp points called **anterior clinoid processes:** These serve as attachment sites, along with the posterior clinoid processes, for the tentorium cerebelli (Figures 2.15 and 2.19). The **optic canal** is completely contained within the lesser wing and provides passage of the optic nerve and ophthalmic artery (Figure 2.19). The **greater wings** extend laterally from the sides of the body and contain three paired foramina—**rotundum, ovale,** and **spinosum**—through which nerves and blood vessels course (Figures 2.15 and 2.20

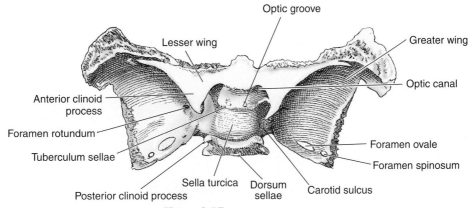

Figure 2.15
Superior view of sphenoid bone.

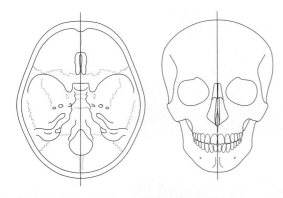

Figure 2.16
Sagittal CT reformat of sella turcica.

KEY: **TS,** Tuberculum sella; **ST,** sella turcica; **SpS,** Sphenoid sinus; **DS,** dorsum sella.

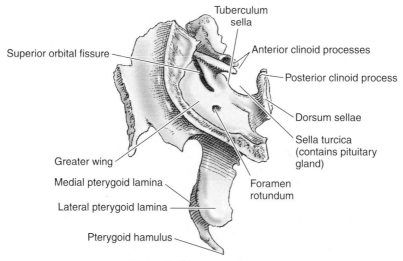

Figure 2.17
Lateral view of sphenoid bone.

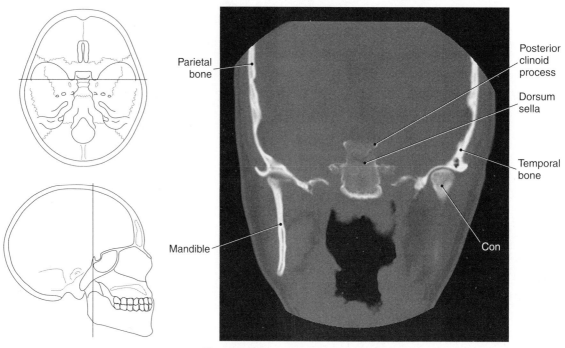

Figure 2.18
Coronal CT scan of dorsum sella.

KEY: Con, Condyloid process of mandible.

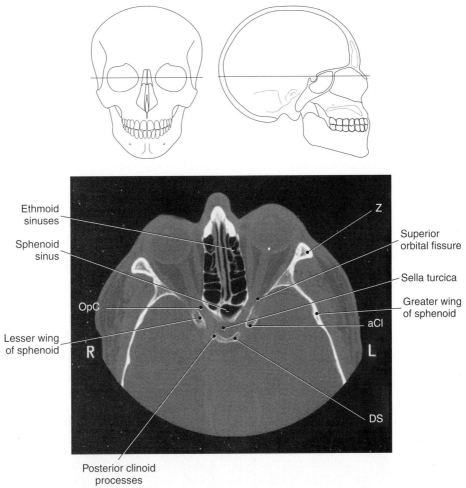

Ethmoid
sinuses

Sphenoid
sinus

OpC

Lesser wing
of sphenoid

R

Z

Superior
orbital fissure

Sella turcica

Greater wing
of sphenoid

aCl

L

DS

Posterior clinoid
processes

Figure 2.19
Axial CT scan of anterior clinoid processes and sphenoid bone.

KEY: **OpC,** Optic canal; **Z,** zygoma; **aCl,** anterior clinoid processes; **DS,** dorsum sella.

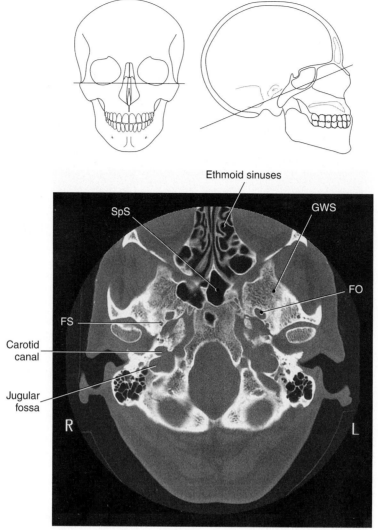

Figure 2.20
Axial CT scan of sphenoid bone with foramina ovale and spinosum.

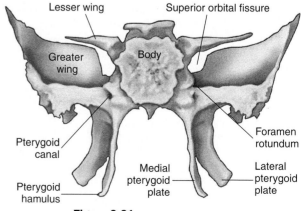

Figure 2.21
Anterior view of sphenoid bone.

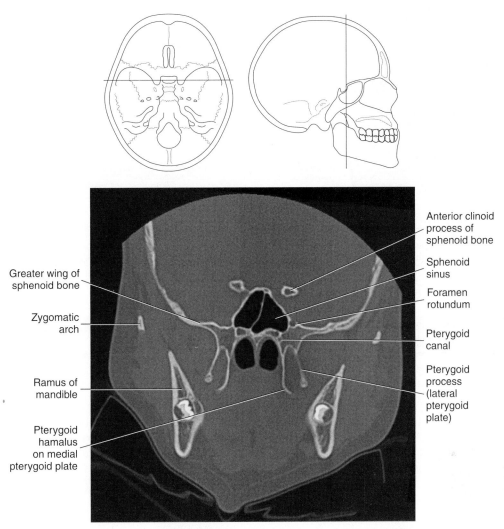

Figure 2.22
Coronal CT scan of sphenoid bone.

through 2.22; Table 2.2). Located between the lesser and greater wings is a triangular opening, for the passage of cranial nerves and vessels, termed the **superior orbital fissure** (Figures 2.2, 2.4, 2.19, and 2.21). The superior orbital fissure transmits the oculomotor, trochlear, abducens, and ophthalmic division of the trigeminal nerves as well as the superior ophthalmic vein. Extending from the inferior surface of each greater wing is a pterygoid process, which is divided into medial and lateral sections (pterygoid plates). The **pterygoid plates** serve as attachment sites for the pterygoid muscles used in movements of the lower jaw. The medial section is longer and has a hook-shaped projection on its inferior end termed the **pterygoid hamulus** that provides an anchor for gliding motion for the muscle responsible for opening the eustachian tube (Figures 2.17, 2.21, and 2.22). At the base of the pterygoid process is the **pterygoid canal,** an opening for the passage of the petrosal nerve (Figures 2.21 and 2.22). The pterygoid processes articulate with the palatine bones and vomer to form part of the nasal cavity.

The sphenoid bone is considered the keystone of the cranial bones because it is the only bone that articulates with all of the other cranial bones.

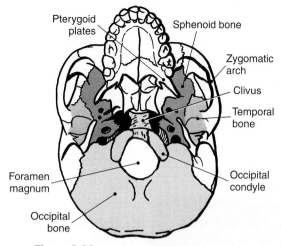

Figure 2.23
Inferior surface of occipital bone and cranium.

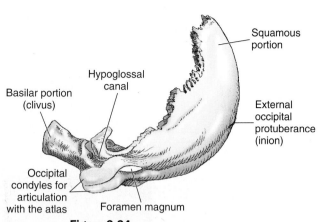

Figure 2.24
Lateroinferior aspect of occipital bone.

TABLE 2-2   Foramina and Fissures of the Skull

BONE	FORAMEN/FISSURE	MAJOR STRUCTURES USING PASSAGEWAY
Frontal	Supraorbital foramen (or notch)	Supraorbital nerve and artery
	Frontal foramen (or notch)	Frontal artery and nerve
Ethmoid	Cribriform plate	Olfactory nerve (I)
Sphenoid	Foramen rotundum	Maxillary branch of trigeminal nerve (V)
	Foramen ovale	Mandibular branch of trigeminal nerve (V)
	Foramen spinosum	Middle meningeal artery
	Pterygoid canal	Petrosal nerve
	Optic canal	Optic nerve and ophthalmic artery
	Superior orbital fissure	Oculomotor nerve (III), trochlear nerve (IV), ophthalmic branch of trigeminal nerve (V), abducens nerve (VI), ophthalmic vein
Sphenoid and maxillary bone	Inferior orbital fissure	Maxillary branch of trigeminal nerve (V)
Occipital	Foramen magnum	Medulla oblongata and accessory nerve (XI)
	Hypoglossal canal	Hypoglossal nerve (XII)
Temporal	Carotid canal	Internal carotid artery
Temporal and occipital bone	Jugular foramen	Internal jugular vein, glossopharyngeal nerve (IX), vagus nerve (X), and accessory nerve (XI)
	External auditory meatus	Air in canal conducts sound to tympanic membrane
	Internal auditory meatus	Vestibulocochlear nerve (VIII) and facial nerve (VII)
Temporal, sphenoid, and occipital bones	Foramen lacerum	Fibrocartilage, internal carotid artery as it leaves carotid canal to enter cranium, nerve of pterygoid canal and a meningeal branch from the ascending pharyngeal artery
	Stylomastoid foramen and facial nerve canal	Facial nerve (VII)
Maxillary	Infraorbital foramen	Infraorbital nerve and maxillary branch of trigeminal nerve (V)
Lacrimal with maxilla	Lacrimal groove, nasolacrimal canal	Lacrimal sac and nasolacrimal duct
Mandible	Mental foramen	Mental artery and nerve

Occipital Bone

The **occipital bone** forms the posterior cranial fossa and the inferoposterior portion of the cranium. On the inferior portion of the occipital bone is a large oval aperture called the **foramen magnum** (Figure 2.23). This opening allows the brainstem to continue as the spinal cord. The occipital bone can be divided into four portions: lateral condyles (2), basilar portion (1),

and squamous portion (1) (Figure 2.24). The **lateral condyles** project inferiorly to articulate with the first cervical vertebra (atlas) at the atlanto-occipital joint (Figures 2.25 and 2.26). Located obliquely at the base of the condyles and anterolateral to the foramen magnum are the **hypoglossal canals** through which the hypoglossal nerve (CN XII) courses (Figures 2.7, 2.24, 2.25, and 2.27; Table 2.2). The **basilar portion** forms the

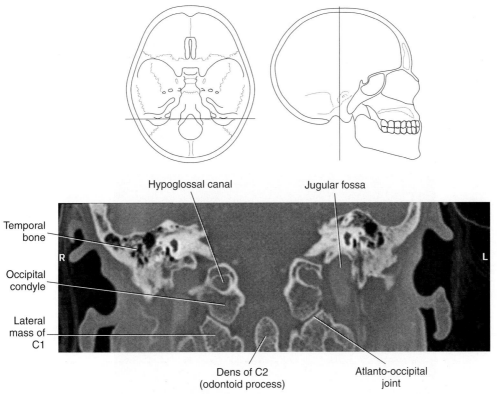

Hypoglossal canal   Jugular fossa

Temporal
bone

R   L

Occipital
condyle

Lateral
mass of
C1

Dens of C2   Atlanto-occipital
(odontoid process)   joint

Figure 2.25
Coronal CT reformat of occipital condyles.

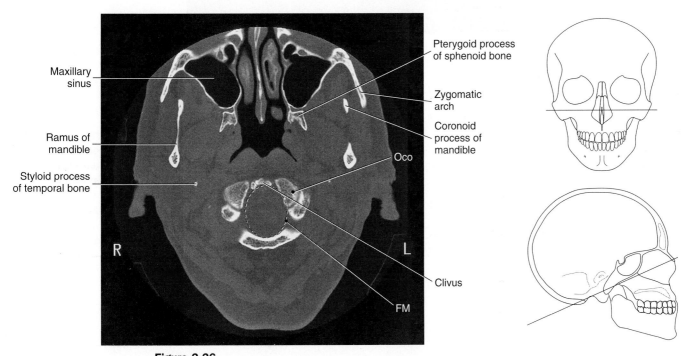

Maxillary
sinus

Pterygoid process
of sphenoid bone

Zygomatic
arch

Coronoid
process of
mandible

Ramus of
mandible

Oco

Styloid process
of temporal bone

R   L

Clivus

FM

Figure 2.26
Axial CT scan of occipital bone at level of foramen magnum and lateral condyles.

KEY: Oco, Occipital condyle; **FM,** foramen magnum.

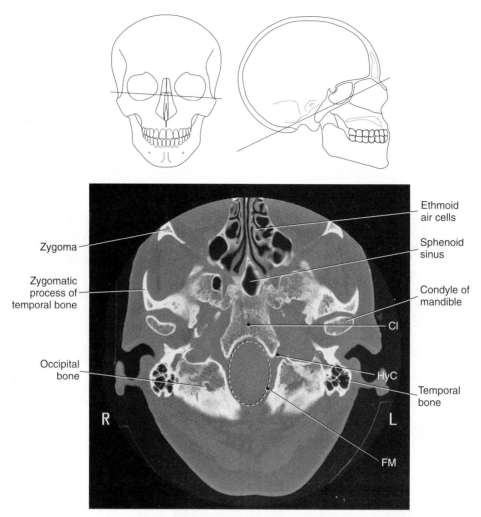

Figure 2.27
Axial CT scan of occipital bone at level of clivus.

anterior margin of the foramen magnum and slopes superiorly and anteriorly to meet with the dorsum sella of the sphenoid bone to form the **clivus** (Figures 2.27 and 2.28). The **squamous portion** curves posterosuperiorly from the foramen magnum to articulate with the parietal and temporal bones (Figure 2.3). Located on the inner surface of the squama is a bony projection termed the **internal occipital protuberance,** which marks the site where the dural venous sinuses converge (Figure 2.29).

> **Pathology in the posterior cranial fossa could result in neurologic deficits related to the 10 cranial nerves exiting the brainstem. These might include changes in level of consciousness due to pressure on the pons and medulla, or motor deficits related to injuries of the cerebellum.**

KEY: CI, Clivus; **HyC,** hypoglossal canal; **FM,** foramen magnum; **ZyP,** zygomatic process; **MF,** mandibular fossa; **JF,** jugular foramen; **FL,** foramen lacerum; **CC,** carotid canal; **EAM,** external auditory meatus; **Mac,** mastoid air cells.

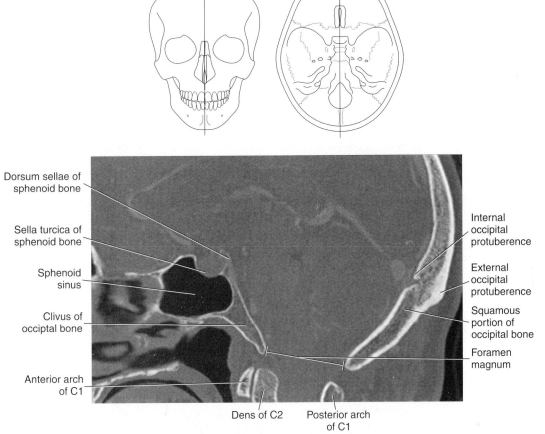

Dorsum sellae of sphenoid bone

Sella turcica of sphenoid bone

Sphenoid sinus

Clivus of occiptal bone

Anterior arch of C1

Internal occipital protuberence

External occipital protuberence

Squamous portion of occipital bone

Foramen magnum

Dens of C2   Posterior arch of C1

Figure 2.28
Sagittal CT reformat of occipital bone.

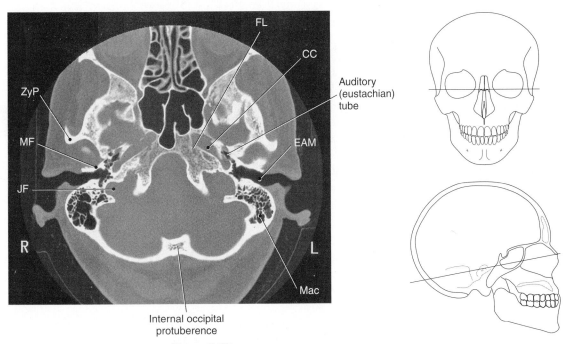

FL

CC

Auditory (eustachian) tube

ZyP

MF

JF

EAM

R   L

Mac

Internal occipital protuberence

Figure 2.29
Axial CT scan of internal occipital protuberance.

Temporal Bone

The two **temporal bones** contain many complex and important structures. They form part of the sides and base of the cranium and together with the sphenoid bone create the middle cranial fossa (Figures 2.3 and 2.6). The temporal bone can be divided into four portions: squamous, tympanic, mastoid, and petrous (Figures 2.30 and 2.31). The thin **squamous portion** projects upward to form part of the sidewalls of the cranium (Figure 2.3). Extending from the squamous portion is the **zygomatic process,** which projects anteriorly to the zygoma of the face to form the **zygomatic arch** (Figures 2.22, 2.27, 2.30, and 2.32). At the base of the zygomatic process is a bony eminence termed the **articular tubercle** that forms the anterior boundary of the **mandibular fossa.** The mandibular fossa is the depression that articulates with the condyloid process of the mandible, creating the temporomandibular joint (Figures 2.30 and 2.33). The **tympanic portion** lies below the squama and forms the majority of the **external auditory meatus** (Figures 2.29, 2.30,

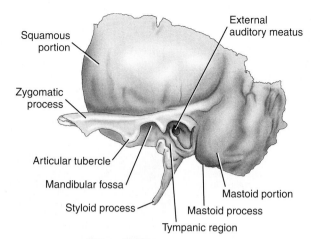

Figure 2.30
Sagittal view of temporal bone.

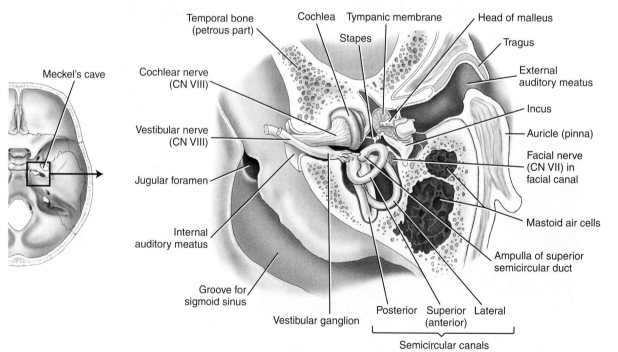

Figure 2.31
Superior view of petrous portion of temporal bone with middle and inner ears.

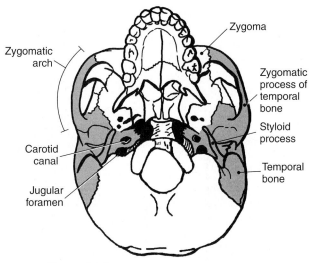

Figure 2.32
Inferior surface of temporal bone and cranium.

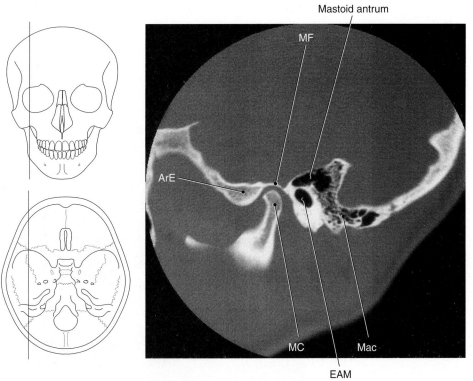

Figure 2.33
Sagittal CT reformat of temporal bone.

KEY: MF, Mandibular fossa; **ArE,** articular tubercle; **MC,** mandibular condyle; **EAM,** external auditory meatus; **Mac,** mastoid air cells.

and 2.33). Just posterior to the tympanic portion is the **mastoid portion,** which has a prominent conical region termed the **mastoid process** (Figures 2.30, 2.33, 2.34, and 2.35). The mastoid process encloses the mastoid air cells and mastoid antrum. The **mastoid antrum** is located on the anterosuperior portion of the mastoid process. It is an air-filled cavity that communicates with the middle ear (tympanic cavity) (Figures 2.33 and 2.34). The **petrous portion** of the temporal bone is pyramidal in shape and situated at an angle between the sphenoid and occipital bones (Figure 2.31). The posterior surface of the petrous pyramid forms the anterior bony limit of the posterior fossa. Near the center of this surface is the opening to the **internal auditory canal,** which transmits the seventh and eighth cranial nerves (Figures 2.31 and 2.35). Other openings associated with the posterior surface of the petrous pyramid are the **jugular foramen** and the **carotid canal,** which provide passage for the internal jugular vein and the internal carotid artery (Table 2.2). An enlargement of the jugular foramen is the **jugular fossa** (Figures 2.32, 2.36, and 2.38). The carotid canal courses superiorly at its lower segment then changes direction and is seen coursing posterior to anterior (Figures 2.29

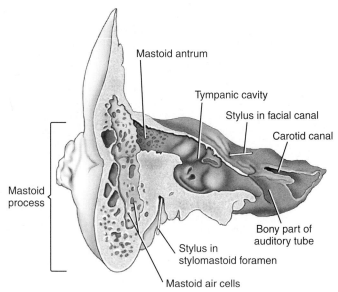

Figure 2.34
Coronal view of temporal bone.

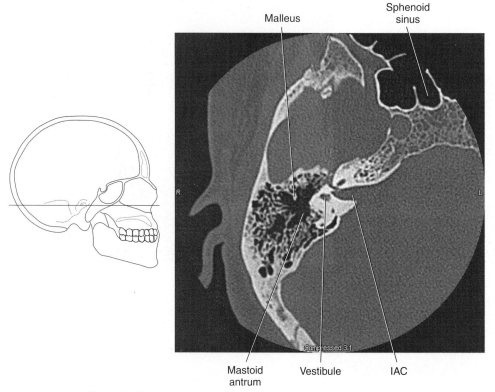

Figure 2.35
Axial CT scan of temporal bone with internal auditory canal (IAC).

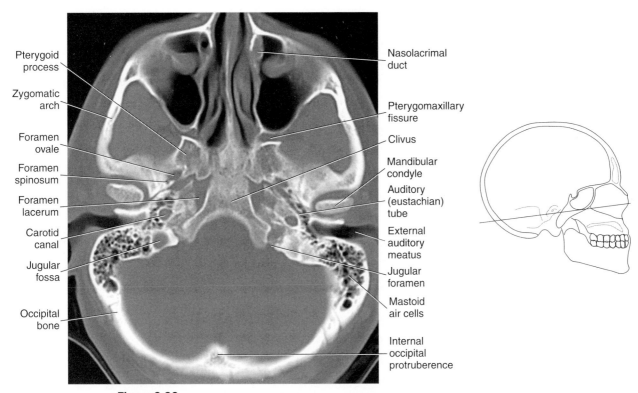

Pterygoid process

Zygomatic arch

Foramen ovale

Foramen spinosum

Foramen lacerum

Carotid canal

Jugular fossa

Occipital bone

Nasolacrimal duct

Pterygomaxillary fissure

Clivus

Mandibular condyle

Auditory (eustachian) tube

External auditory meatus

Jugular foramen

Mastoid air cells

Internal occipital protruberence

Figure 2.36
Axial CT scan of temporal bone with foramen lacerum, jugular fossa, and carotid canal.

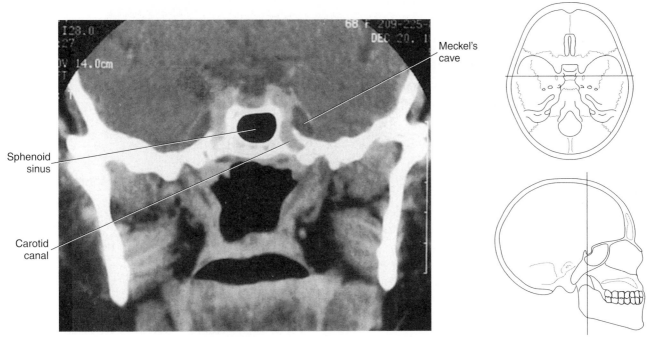

Meckel's cave

Sphenoid sinus

Carotid canal

Figure 2.37
Coronal CT scan of temporal bone with Meckel's cave.

and 2.37). Superior to the carotid canal is an indentation on the petrous portion called **Meckel's cave** (Figures 2.31 and 2.37). Also known as the *trigeminal cave,* Meckel's cave is located between two layers of dura and encloses the trigeminal ganglion. Between the apex of the petrous pyramid, the body of the sphenoid bone and the basilar portion of the occipital bone is a jagged slit termed the **foramen lacerum,** which contains cartilage and allows the internal carotid artery to enter the cranium, providing small arteries that supply the inner surface of the cranium (Figures 2.29 and 2.36 and Table 2.2). The inferior surface of the petrous pyramid gives rise to the long slender **styloid process** that is attached to several muscles of the tongue and ligaments of the hyoid bone (Figures 2.26, 2.30, and 2.38). The **stylomastoid foramen** is situated between the mastoid process and the styloid process. This foramen constitutes the end of the **facial nerve canal** (facial canal) (Figures 2.34 and 2.38 and Table 2.2). The interior of the petrous pyramid houses the delicate middle and inner ear structures.

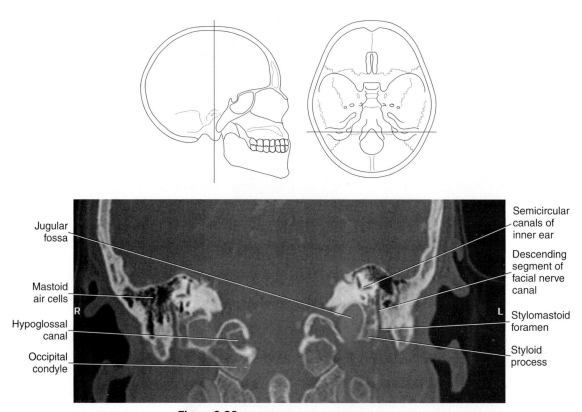

Jugular fossa

Mastoid air cells

Hypoglossal canal

Occipital condyle

Semicircular canals of inner ear

Descending segment of facial nerve canal

Stylomastoid foramen

Styloid process

Figure 2.38
Coronal CT reformat of stylomastoid foramen.

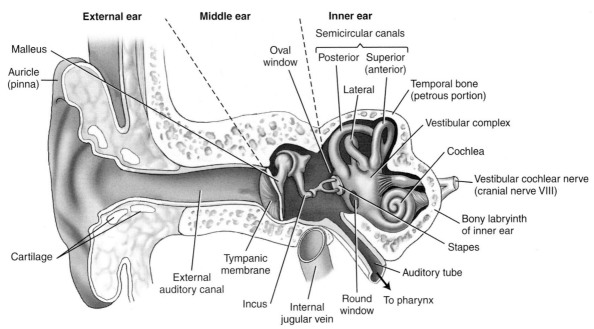

Figure 2.39
Orientation of the external, middle, and inner ear in coronal view.

Structures of the External, Middle, and Inner Ear

The structures of the ear can be divided into three main portions: external, middle, and inner (Figure 2.39 through 2.54).

The **external ear** consists of the **auricle** and the **external auditory meatus.** The external auditory meatus is a sound-conducting canal that terminates at the tympanic membrane of the middle ear (Figure 2.36). The air-containing **middle ear,** or **tympanic cavity,** communicates with both the mastoid antrum and the nasopharynx. Air is conveyed from the naso-pharynx to the tympanic cavity through the **auditory tube (eustachian tube)** (Figures 2.36 and 2.39). The middle ear con-sists of the **tympanic membrane** and three **auditory ossicles (malleus, incus,** and **stapes)** (Figure 2.39). The tympanic membrane transmits sound vibrations to the auditory ossicles. The auditory ossicles, which are suspended in the middle ear, conduct sound vibrations from the tympanic membrane to the oval window of the inner ear (Figures 2.45 through 2.54).

The **inner ear,** or **bony labyrinth,** contains the **vestibule** and **semicircular canals,** which control equilibrium and balance, and the **cochlea,** which is responsible for hearing (Figures 2.39 through 2.42). The vestibule is a small compartment located between the semicircular canals and the cochlea. Two openings of the vestibule are the **oval window** (Figure 2.40) for the foot-plate of the stapes and the **vestibular aqueduct,** which contains the endolymphatic duct (Figure 2.43). The semicircular canals are continuous with the vestibule and are easily identified because of their three separate passages (superior [anterior], posterior, and lateral) that are at right angles to each other (Figures 2.38, 2.39, and 2.40). The cochlea is a conical struc-ture with a base that lies on the **internal auditory canal** (Figure 2.41). Located within the basilar turn of the cochlea is

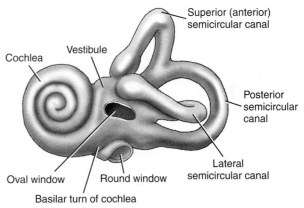

Figure 2.40
Bony labyrinth.

the **round window,** which allows the fluid of the inner ear to move slightly for propagation of sound waves (Figures 2.40 and 2.43). Within the bony labyrinth is a complicated system of ducts called the **membranous labyrinth.** The membranous labyrinth is filled with **endolymph,** a fluid that helps with the propagation of sound waves. Extending from the vestibule is a slender **endolymphatic duct** that terminates as the **endo-lymphatic sac,** which is located between two dural layers on the posterior wall of the petrous pyramid (Figures 2.43 and 2.44). The endolymphatic duct and sac are thought to be responsible for the reabsorption of endolymph and may contribute to vestibular dysfunction. Figures 2.45 through 2.54 provide sequential computed tomography (CT) images through the external, middle, and inner ear in the axial and coronal planes, respectively.

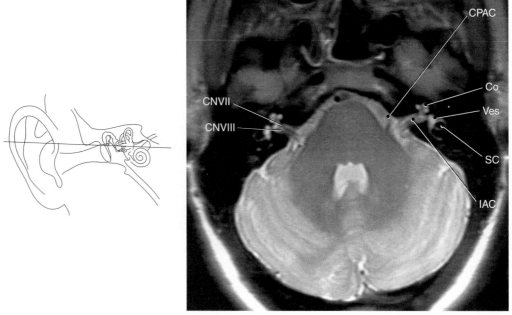

Figure 2.41
Axial, T2-weighted MR scan of inner ear.

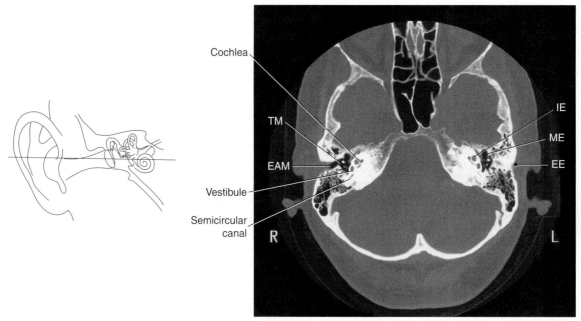

Figure 2.42
Axial CT scan of petrous portion at level of external auditory meatus.

KEY: **CNVII,** Facial nerve; **CNVIII,** vestibulocochlear nerve; **CPAC,** cerebellopontine angle cistern; **Co,** cochlea; **Ves,** vestibule; **SC,** semicircular canal; **IAC,** internal auditory canal; **TM,** tympanic membrane; **EAM,** external auditory meatus; **IE,** inner ear; **ME,** middle ear; **EE,** external ear.

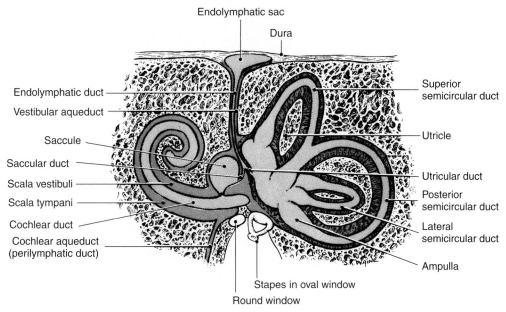

Endolymphatic sac

Dura

Endolymphatic duct

Vestibular aqueduct

Saccule

Saccular duct

Scala vestibuli

Scala tympani

Cochlear duct

Cochlear aqueduct
(perilymphatic duct)

Superior
semicircular duct

Utricle

Utricular duct

Posterior
semicircular duct

Lateral
semicircular duct

Ampulla

Stapes in oval window

Round window

Figure 2.43
Membranous labyrinth.

Endolymphatic sac

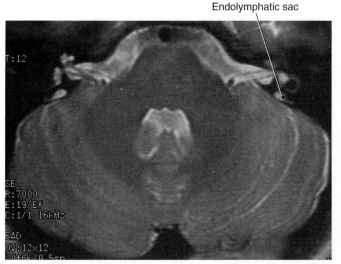

Figure 2.44
Axial, T2-weighted MR scan with enlarged endolymphatic sac.

Meniere's disease is a disorder of the membranous labyrinth that results from a failure of the mechanism controlling the production and elimination of endolymph. In advanced cases there is an increased accumulation of endolymph volume, resulting in an abnormal distention of the membranous labyrinth (endolymphatic hydrops). Meniere's disease is most common in middle age and may become bilateral in up to 50% of affected patients. Symptoms include episodic vertigo accompanied by nausea, fluctuating hearing loss, and a feeling of fullness in the affected ears. The success of surgical intervention in relieving Meniere's disease depends a great deal on the ability to image and evaluate the vestibular aqueduct and endolymphatic duct and sac.

Cholesteatomas are epidermoid cysts of the middle ear that can be acquired or congenital. The lumen of the cyst is filled with debris. As a cholesteatoma enlarges it destroys the ossicles and adjacent bony structures. They are usually associated with chronic infection, aural discharge, and conductive or mixed deafness.

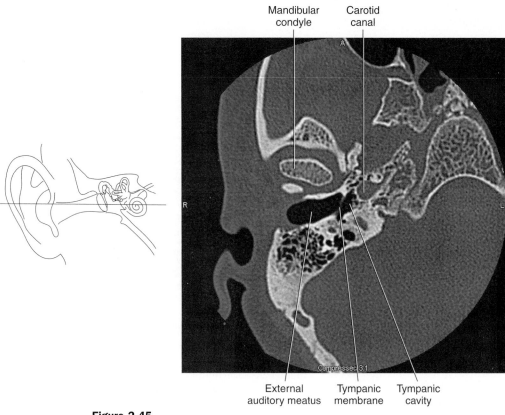

Mandibular condyle   Carotid canal

External auditory meatus   Tympanic membrane   Tympanic cavity

Compressed 3:1

Figure 2.45
Axial CT scan of external auditory meatus and tympanic membrane.

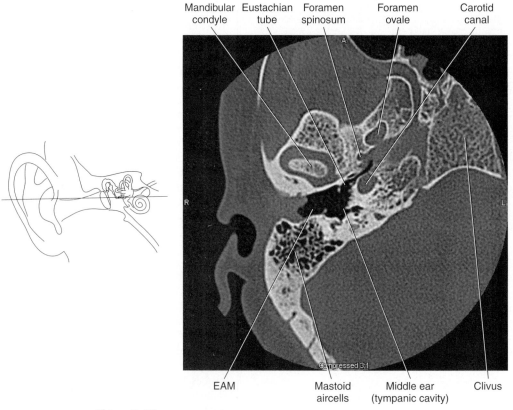

Mandibular condyle   Eustachian tube   Foramen spinosum   Foramen ovale   Carotid canal

EAM   Mastoid aircells   Middle ear (tympanic cavity)   Clivus

Compressed 3:1

Figure 2.46
Axial CT scan of eustachian tube. *EAM,* External auditory meatus.

43

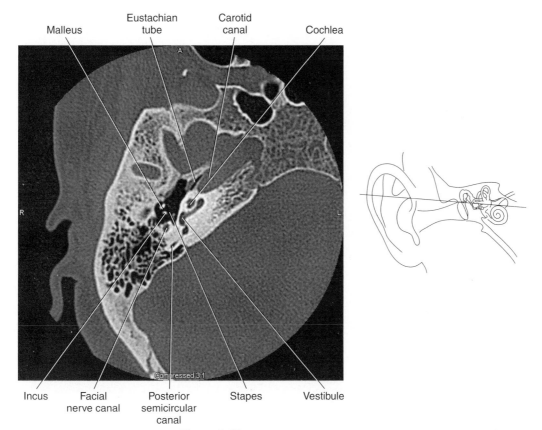

Figure 2.47
Axial CT scan of middle and inner ear.

Malleus · Eustachian tube · Carotid canal · Cochlea

Incus · Facial nerve canal · Posterior semicircular canal · Stapes · Vestibule

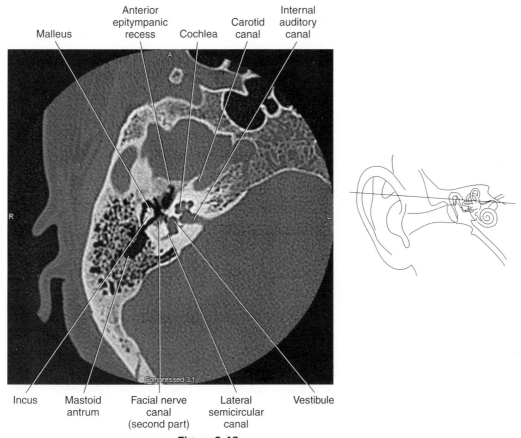

Figure 2.48
Axial CT scan of malleus and incus.

Malleus · Anterior epitympanic recess · Cochlea · Carotid canal · Internal auditory canal

Incus · Mastoid antrum · Facial nerve canal (second part) · Lateral semicircular canal · Vestibule

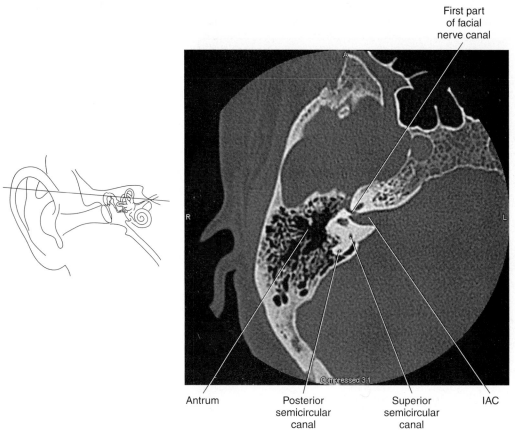

First part
of facial
nerve canal

Antrum   Posterior   Superior   IAC
          semicircular   semicircular
          canal   canal

Figure 2.49
Axial CT scan of internal auditory canal (IAC).

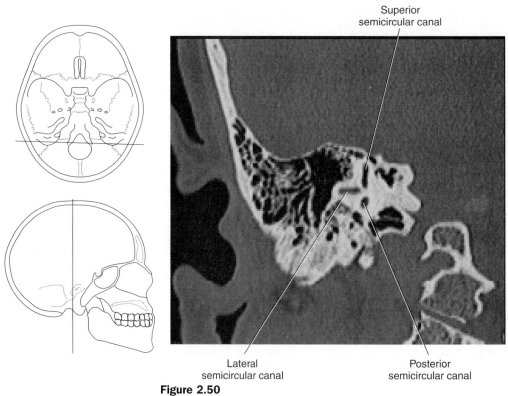

Superior
semicircular canal

Lateral   Posterior
semicircular canal   semicircular
                           canal

Figure 2.50
Coronal CT scan of semicircular canals.

45

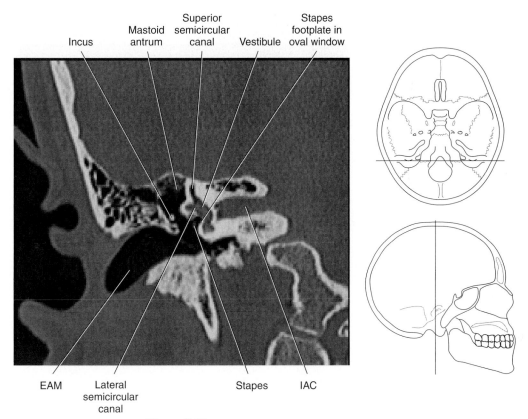

Figure 2.51
Coronal CT scan of internal auditory canal (IAC).

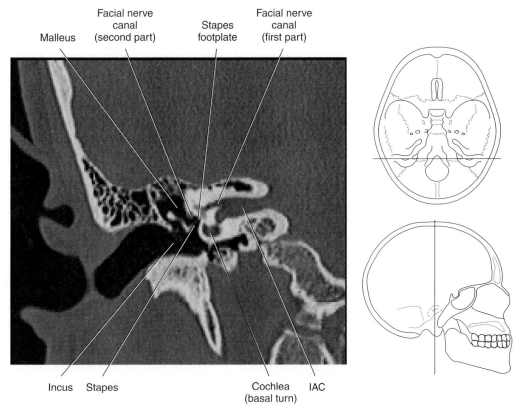

Figure 2.52
Coronal CT scan of ossicles. *IAC,* Internal auditory canal.

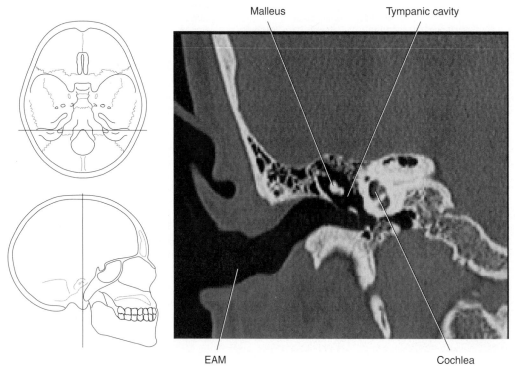

Figure 2.53
Coronal CT scan of external auditory meatus (EAM).

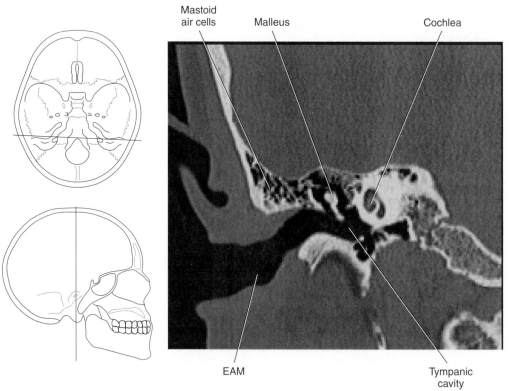

Figure 2.54
Coronal CT scan of cochlea. *EAM*, External auditory meatus.

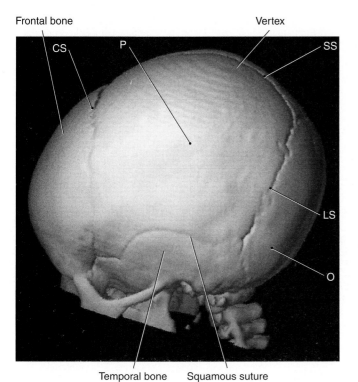

Frontal bone

CS

P

Vertex

SS

LS

O

Temporal bone   Squamous suture

Figure 2.55
3D CT reconstruction of lateral surface of cranium.

Sutures

The cranial bones are joined by four main articulations termed **sutures.** The **squamous suture,** which is located on the side of the cranium, joins the squamous portion of the temporal bone to the parietal bone. The **coronal suture** runs transversely across the top of the cranium and is the articulation between the frontal and parietal bones. The **sagittal suture** provides the articulation between the parietal bones along the midsagittal plane. The **lambdoidal suture** is located posterior in the cranium and joins the occipital and parietal bones (Figures 2.3, 2.55, and 2.56).

> The sutures in neonates are not fully closed, allowing for growth of the head after birth. Craniosynostosis is the result of the premature ossification of one or more of the cranial sutures, which causes abnormal growth of the cranium and could limit the growth of the brain.

KEY: **CS,** Coronal suture; **P,** parietal bone; **SS,** sagittal suture; **LS,** lambdoidal suture; **O,** occipital bone.

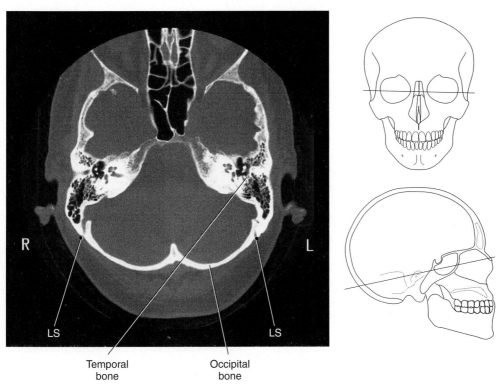

R

L

LS

LS

Temporal bone   Occipital bone

Figure 2.56
Axial CT scan of lambdoidal suture.

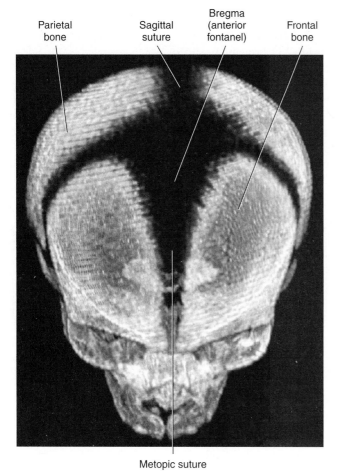

Parietal bone · Sagittal suture · Bregma (anterior fontanel) · Frontal bone · Metopic suture

Figure 2.57
3D CT reconstruction of fetal cranium, superior view.

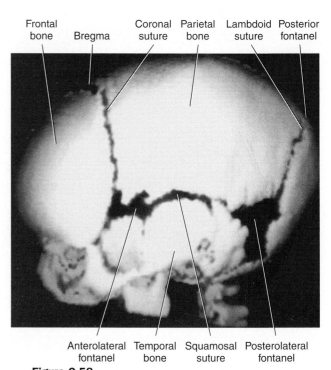

Frontal bone · Bregma · Coronal suture · Parietal bone · Lambdoid suture · Posterior fontanel · Anterolateral fontanel · Temporal bone · Squamosal suture · Posterolateral fontanel

Figure 2.58
3D CT reconstruction of newborn cranium with sutures.

Fontanels

In the newborn cranium are six areas of incomplete ossification called **fontanels.** The largest is the **anterior fontanel** located at the junction of the upper parietal and frontal bones termed the **bregma** (Figure 2.57). This fontanel remains open until the age of 2. Located at the **lambda,** the junction of the parietal and occipital bones is the **posterior fontanel** (Figure 2.58). The posterior fontanels typically close between the first and third months after birth. On the sides of the cranium are four additional fontanels, two **anterolateral (sphenoid)** and two **posterolateral (mastoid)** (Figure 2.58). The anterolateral fontanels are located between the parietal and greater wing of the sphenoid bones. The posterolaterals are located between the junction of the occipital, temporal, and parietal bones. The anterior and posterolateral ossify approximately at 2 years of age, whereas the posterior and anterolateral close between 1 and 3 months after birth (Figure 2.59).

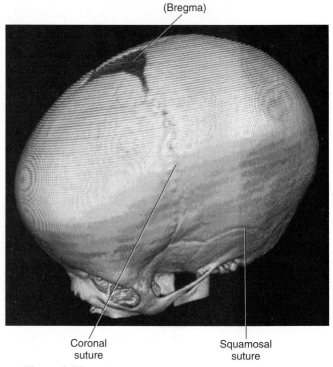

Anterior fontanel (Bregma) · Coronal suture · Squamosal suture

Figure 2.59
3D CT reconstruction of 1-year-old cranium with fontanels.

FACIAL BONES

The face is made up of 14 facial bones. The facial bones can be difficult to differentiate because of their relatively small size and irregular shape. They consist of the nasal (2), lacrimal (2), maxilla (2), palatine (2), zygoma (2), inferior nasal conchae (2), vomer (1), and mandible (1) (Figures 2.60 and 2.61).

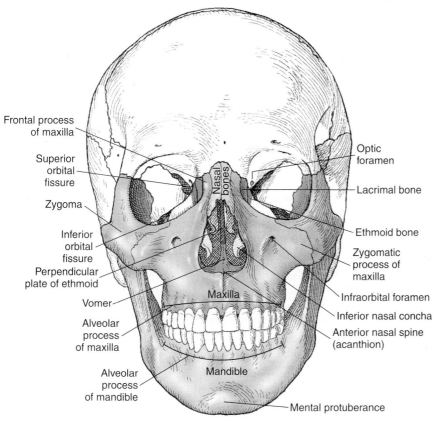

Frontal process of maxilla
Superior orbital fissure
Zygoma
Inferior orbital fissure
Perpendicular plate of ethmoid
Vomer
Alveolar process of maxilla
Alveolar process of mandible

Nasal bones

Optic foramen
Lacrimal bone
Ethmoid bone
Zygomatic process of maxilla
Infraorbital foramen
Inferior nasal concha
Anterior nasal spine (acanthion)

Maxilla
Mandible
Mental protuberance

Figure 2.60
Anterior view of facial bones.

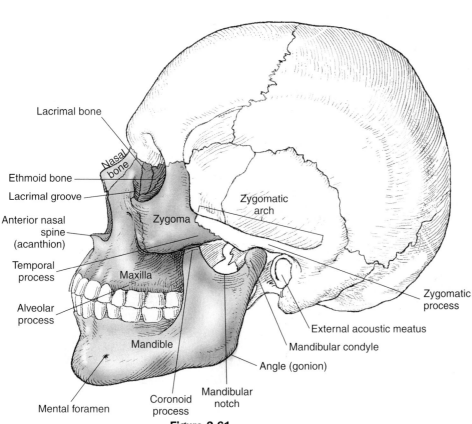

Lacrimal bone
Ethmoid bone
Lacrimal groove
Anterior nasal spine (acanthion)
Temporal process
Alveolar process
Mental foramen

Nasal bone
Zygoma
Maxilla
Mandible
Coronoid process
Mandibular notch

Zygomatic arch
Zygomatic process
External acoustic meatus
Mandibular condyle
Angle (gonion)

Figure 2.61
Sagittal view of facial bones.

Nasal Bone, Lacrimal Bone, Maxilla, Palatine Bone, and Zygoma

The two **nasal bones** form the bony bridge of the nose. Posterior to the nasal bones and maxilla are the **lacrimal bones,** which are situated on the medial wall of each orbit (Figure 2.62). The junction of the lacrimal bones to the maxillae forms the **lacrimal groove,** which accommodates the **lacrimal sacs** that are part of the drainage route for excess lacrimal fluid (tears) (Figures 2.61, 2.62, and 2.63). The largest immovable facial bones are the **maxillary bones,** which fuse at the midline to form a pointed process termed the **anterior nasal spine** (Figures 2.61 through 2.63). An opening on the anterior aspect of the maxilla is the **infraorbital foramen,** which transmits the infraorbital nerve and blood vessels (Figures 2.60 and 2.64). The maxillary bones contain the large **maxillary sinuses** and four processes: frontal process, zygomatic process, alveolar process, and the palatine process (Figures 2.60 and 2.64 through 2.67). The **frontal** and **zygomatic processes** project to articulate with the frontal bones of the cranium and the zygoma bones of the face (Figures 2.64 and 2.65). The inferior border of the maxilla has several depressions that form the **alveolar process,** which accepts the roots of the teeth (Figures 2.60, 2.63, 2.67, and 2.68). The **palatine process** of the maxilla extends posteriorly to form three fourths of the **hard palate.** The posterior one fourth of the hard palate is created by the horizontal portion of the **palatine bones** (Figures 2.66 and 2.67). The palatine bones also extend vertically to form part of the nasal cavity (Figure 2.62). The **zygoma** (malar bone) creates the prominence of the cheek and contributes to the lateral portion of the bony orbit (Figures 2.60, 2.61, 2.63, 2.64, 2.69, and 2.70). The temporal process of the zygoma extends posteriorly to join with the zygomatic process of the temporal bone to form the **zygomatic arch** (Figures 2.61, 2.63, 2.66, and 2.69).

> Le Fort fractures are a result of direct anterior facial injuries. They are classified into three groups according to which facial bones are traumatized. Type I: the alveolar process of the maxilla and the hard palate are separated from the superior part of the skull. Type II: The alveolar, zygomatic and frontal processes of the maxilla along with the nasal bones are separated from the frontal and zygomatic bones. Type III: Virtually the entire facial skeleton, including the maxillae, nasal bones, and zygomatic bones, are separated from the frontal bone above it.

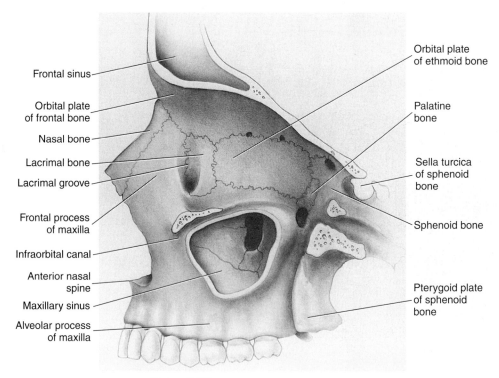

Figure 2.62
Sagittal view of orbit and maxillary region.

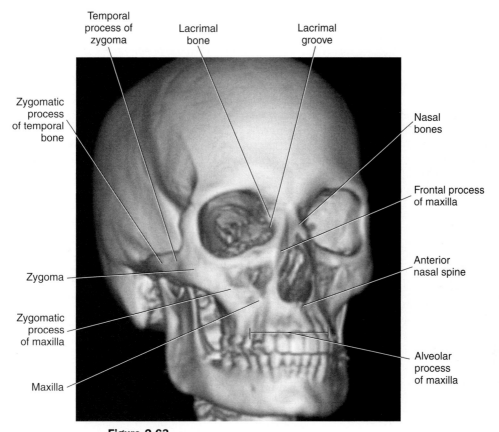

Figure 2.63
3D CT reconstruction of oblique aspect of facial bones.

Temporal process of zygoma

Lacrimal bone

Lacrimal groove

Zygomatic process of temporal bone

Nasal bones

Frontal process of maxilla

Zygoma

Anterior nasal spine

Zygomatic process of maxilla

Maxilla

Alveolar process of maxilla

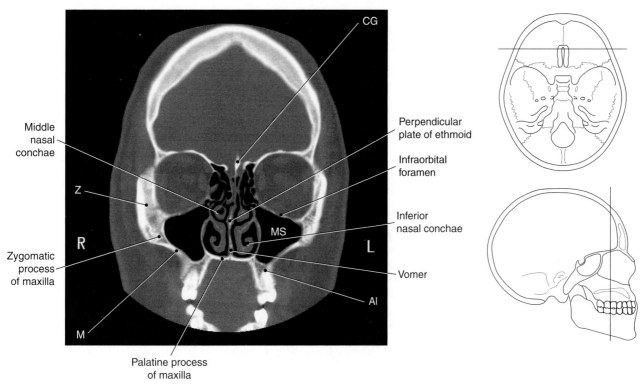

Figure 2.64
Coronal CT scan of maxilla and zygoma.

CG

Middle nasal conchae

Perpendicular plate of ethmoid

Infraorbital foramen

Z

Inferior nasal conchae

R

MS

L

Zygomatic process of maxilla

Vomer

M

Al

Palatine process of maxilla

KEY: Z, Zygoma; **M,** maxilla; **CG,** crista galli; **MS,** maxillary sinus; **Al,** alveolar process of maxilla.

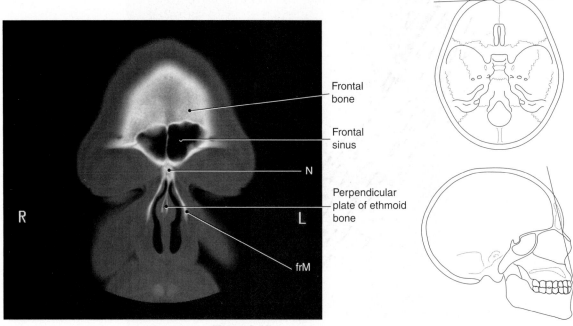

Figure 2.65
Coronal CT scan of nasal bones.

KEY: **N,** nasal bone; **frM,** frontal process of maxilla.

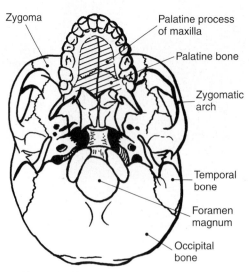

Figure 2.66
Inferior view of facial bones and hard palate.

Alveolar process
of maxilla

Pal

PPS

Hor

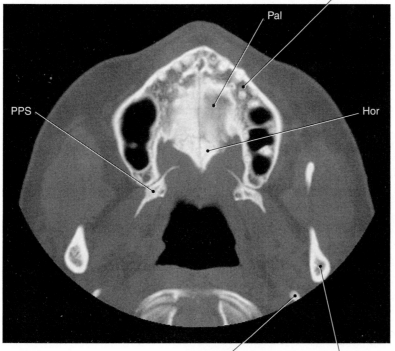
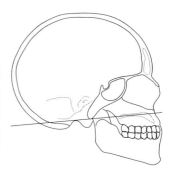

Styloid process
of temporal bone

Mandible

Figure 2.67
Axial CT scan of hard palate.

KEY: **PPS,** Pterygoid process of sphenoid
bone; **Pal,** palatine process of maxilla;
Hor, horizontal portion of palatine bone.

Alveolar process
of maxilla

Ramus of
mandible

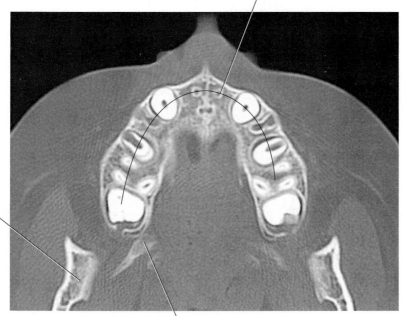
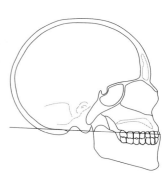

Pterygoid process of
sphenoid bone

Figure 2.68
Axial CT scan of alveolar process of maxilla.

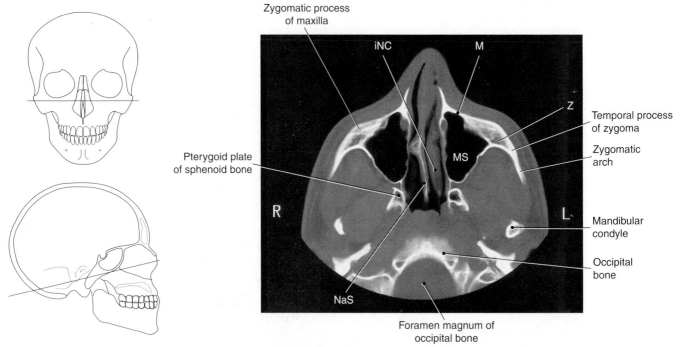

Figure 2.69
Axial CT scan of facial bones.

KEY: iNC, Inferior nasal conchae; **M,** maxilla; **Z,** zygoma; **MS,** maxillary sinus; **NaS,** nasal septum; **N,** nasal bone; **frM,** frontal process of maxilla; **L,** lacrimal bone; **mEt,** middle ethmoid sinuses; **pEt,** posterior ethmoid sinuses; **SpS,** sphenoid sinus; **aEt,** anterior ethmoid sinuses.

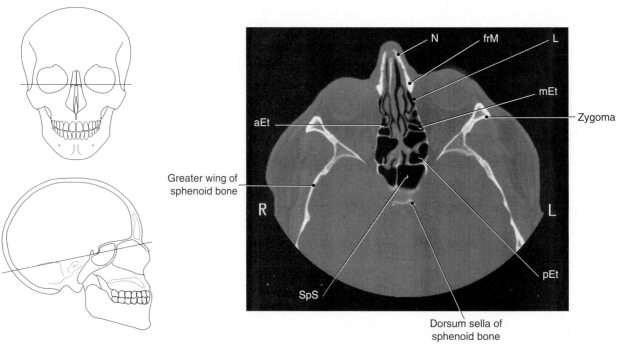

Figure 2.70
Axial CT scan of facial bones and ethmoid sinuses.

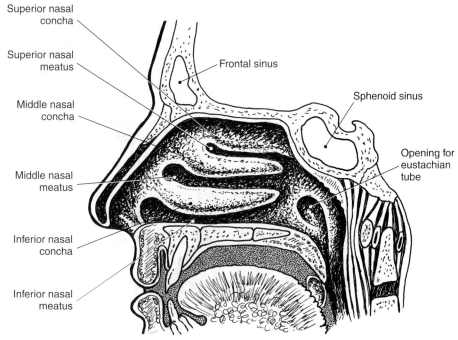

Superior nasal
concha

Superior nasal
meatus

Middle nasal
concha

Middle nasal
meatus

Inferior nasal
concha

Inferior nasal
meatus

Frontal sinus

Sphenoid sinus

Opening for
eustachian
tube

Figure 2.71
Sagittal view of nasal meati.

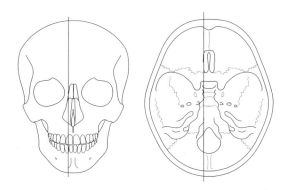

Inferior Nasal Conchae and Vomer

The **inferior nasal conchae** project medially and inferiorly
along the nasal cavity (Figures 2.60, 2.64, and 2.69). They can
be identified by their scroll-like appearance. These conchae,
in conjunction with superior and middle nasal conchae of the
ethmoid bone, divide the nasal cavity into **superior, middle,**
and **inferior meati** (Figures 2.71 and 2.72). The **vomer**
projects superiorly from the base of the nasal cavity to form the
inferior portion of the bony **nasal septum** (Figures 2.60, 2.64,
and 2.69).

KEY: F, Frontal sinus; **s,** sphenoethmoidal sinus; **E,** ethmoid sinus;
S, sphenoid sinus; **Mid Turb,** middle nasal conchae; **Inf turb,** inferior
nasal conchae; **NP,** nasopharynx.

Superior nasal meatus

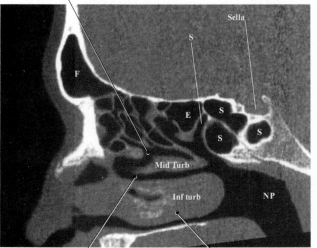

Middle nasal meatus   Inferior nasal meatus

Figure 2.72
Sagittal CT reformat of nasal meati.

Mandible

The largest facial bone is the **mandible.** This bone is composed primarily of horizontal and vertical portions (Figures 2.73 and 2.74). The angle created by the junction of these two portions is termed the **gonion.** The curved horizontal portion, called the *body*, contains an alveolar process (similar to the maxilla) that receives the roots of the teeth of the lower jaw. The **mental foramina** extend through the body of the mandible and allow passage for the mental artery and nerve. The vertical portion of the mandible is called the **ramus** (Figure 2.75). Each ramus has two processes at its superior portion: **coronoid process** and **condyloid process** (**condyle**) (Figures 2.73, 2.74, 2.76, and 2.77). They are separated by a concave surface called the **mandibular notch.** The coronoid process serves as an attachment site for the temporalis and masseter muscles, whereas the condyloid process articulates with the mandibular fossa of the temporal bone to form the **temporomandibular joint (TMJ)** (Figure 2.78).

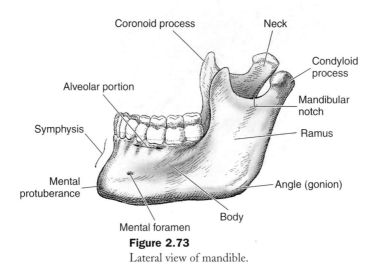

Figure 2.73
Lateral view of mandible.

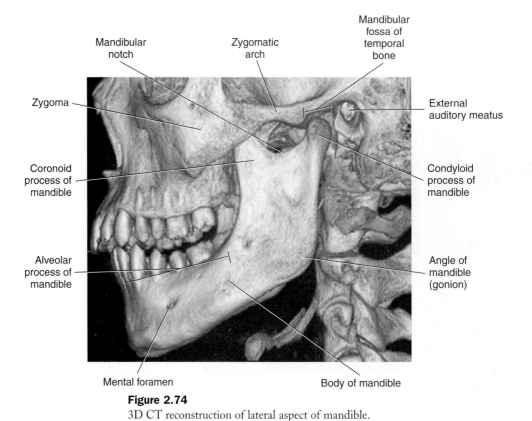

Figure 2.74
3D CT reconstruction of lateral aspect of mandible.

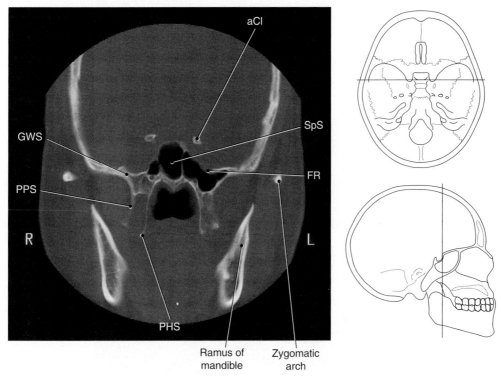

Figure 2.75
Coronal CT scan of mandibular rami.

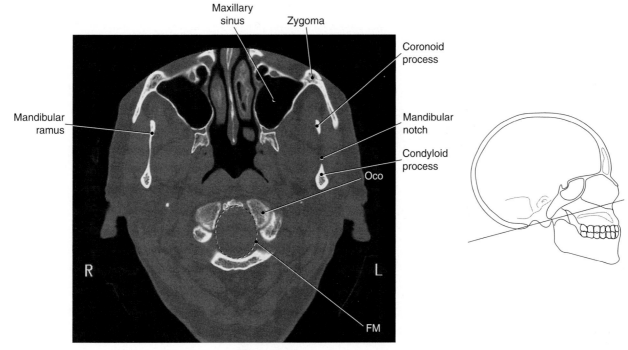

Figure 2.76
Axial CT scan of mandibular rami.

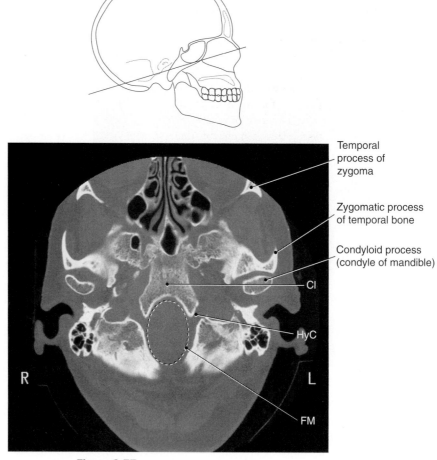

Figure 2.77
Axial CT scan of mandibular condyles.

KEY: **Cl,** Clivus; **HyC,** hypoglossal canal; **FM,** foramen magnum.

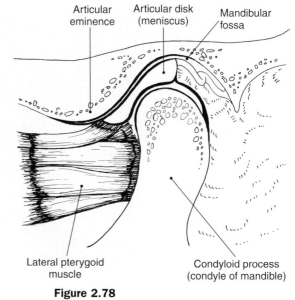

Figure 2.78
Lateral view of temporomandibular joint.

TEMPOROMANDIBULAR JOINT

The temporomandibular joint (TMJ) is a modified hinge joint that allows for the necessary motions of mastication.

Bony Anatomy

The **mandibular fossa** and **articular eminence** of the temporal bone form the superior articulating surface for the mandibular condyle. The articular eminence creates the anterior boundary of the joint, preventing the forward displacement of the mandibular condyle (Figures 2.78 and 2.79).

KEY: **ArE,** Articular eminence; **MF,** mandibular fossa; **EAM,** external auditory meatus; **Mac,** mastoid air cells; **MC,** mandibular condyle.

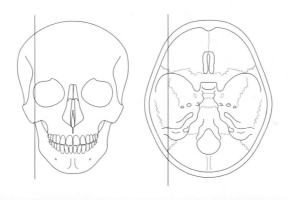

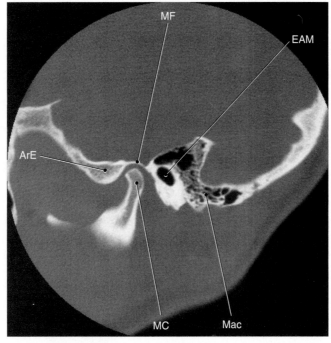

Figure 2.79
Sagittal CT reformat of temporomandibular joint.

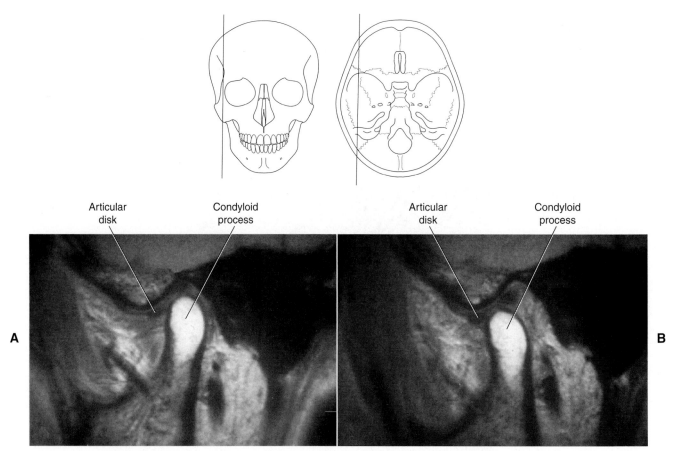

Articular   Condyloid
disk   process

Articular   Condyloid
disk   process

A   B

Figure 2.80
Sagittal, T1-weighted MR scan of temporomandibular joint and articular disk; **(A)** open, **(B)** closed.

Articular Disk and Ligaments

The **articular disk,** frequently called the **meniscus,** is shaped like a bowtie and is interposed between the mandibular condyle and fossa to act as a shock absorber during jaw movement (Figures 2.78 and 2.80). The anterior surface attaches to the lateral pterygoid muscle and is secured posteriorly with fibrous connections to both the temporal bone and the posterior aspect of the condyle. The articular disk is not tightly bound to the fossa, but moves anteriorly with the condyle. Several ligaments help maintain the position of the articular disk. The articular disk is attached to the medial and lateral surfaces of the condyle by the **collateral ligaments** (Figures 2.81 and 2.82). Lateral stability is provided by the **temporomandibular ligament (lateral ligament),** which extends from the articular eminence and zygomatic process to the posterior aspect of the articular disk and the condylar head and neck (Figure 2.83). Additionally, this ligament restricts the posterior movement of the condyle and articular disk.

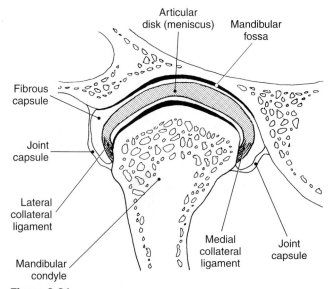

Articular
disk (meniscus)   Mandibular
fossa

Fibrous
capsule

Joint
capsule

Lateral
collateral
ligament

Medial
collateral
ligament

Joint
capsule

Mandibular
condyle

Figure 2.81
Coronal view of temporomandibular joint and collateral ligaments.

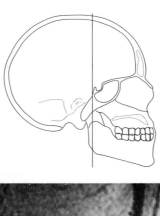

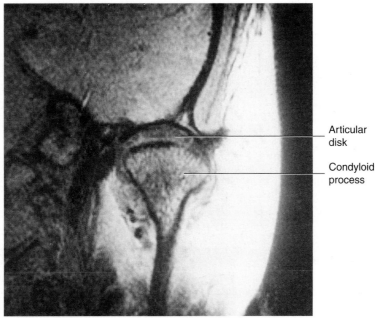

Articular
disk

Condyloid
process

Figure 2.82
Coronal, T1-weighted MR scan of temporomandibular joint.

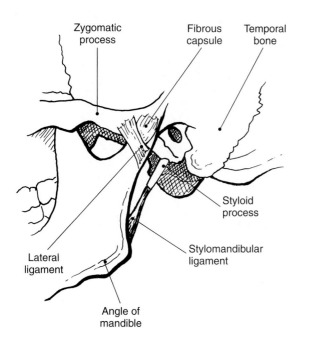

Zygomatic
process

Fibrous
capsule

Temporal
bone

Styloid
process

Stylomandibular
ligament

Lateral
ligament

Angle of
mandible

Figure 2.83
Sagittal view of temporomandibular joint and lateral ligament.

Muscles

The cooperative actions of four muscles located on each side of the TMJ provide the movement of the mandible and are collectively referred to as the **muscles of mastication** (Figure 2.84). The fan-shaped **temporalis muscle** originates on the temporal fossa, inserts on the coronoid process of the mandible, and elevates the mandible. The **masseter muscle** is the strongest muscle of the jaw, arising from the zygomatic arch and inserting on the ramus and angle of the mandible. Its actions include elevation of the mandible (Figures 2.84 and 2.85). The pterygoid muscles (medial and lateral) originate from the pterygoid processes of the sphenoid bone and insert on the angle of the mandible and condylar process, respectively. The **medial pterygoid muscle** acts to close the jaw, whereas the **lateral pterygoid muscle** opens the jaw as well as protrudes and moves the mandible from side to side (Figures 2.86 and 2.87).

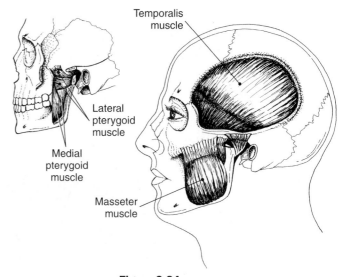

Figure 2.84
Muscles of mastication.

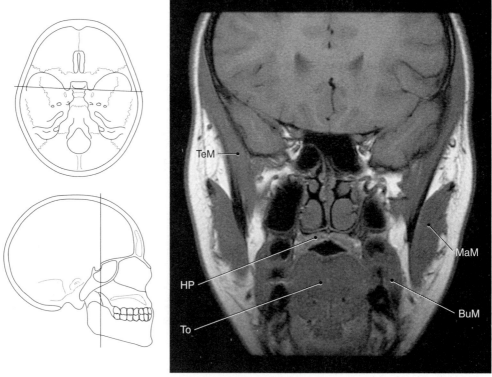

Figure 2.85
Coronal, T1-weighted MR scan of muscles of mastication.

KEY: **TeM,** Temporalis muscle; **HP,** hard palate; **To,** tongue; **MaM,** masseter muscle; **BuM,** buccinator muscle.

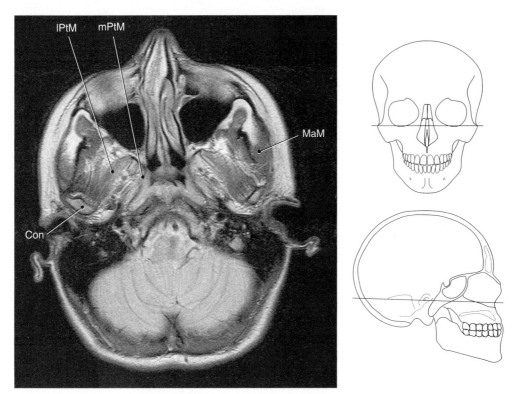

Figure 2.86
Axial, T1-weighted MR scan of pterygoid muscles.

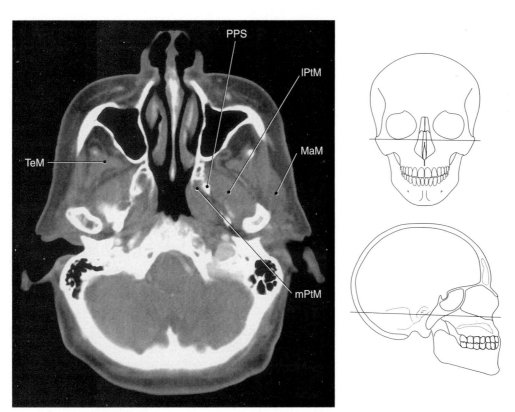

Figure 2.87
Axial CT scan of temporomandibular joint and muscles of mastication.

KEY: **lPtM,** Lateral pterygoid muscle; **mPtM,** medial pterygoid muscle; **MaM,** masseter muscle; **Con,** mandibular condyle; **TeM,** temporalis muscle; **PPS,** pterygoid process of sphenoid bone.

PARANASAL SINUSES

The **paranasal sinuses** are air-containing cavities within the facial bones and skull that communicate with the nasal cavity. The nasal cavity is responsible for filtering airborne particles as it warms and humidifies air going into the lungs. The sinuses are named after the bones in which they originate: **ethmoid, maxillary, sphenoid, frontal.** There is great variance in the size, shape, and development of these sinuses within each individual (Figures 2.88 and 2.89).

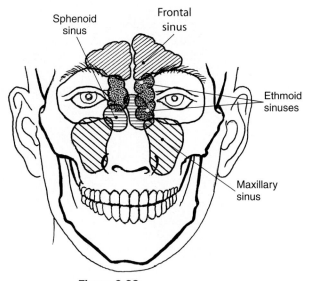

Figure 2.88
Coronal view of paranasal sinuses.

Figure 2.89
Sagittal view of paranasal sinuses.

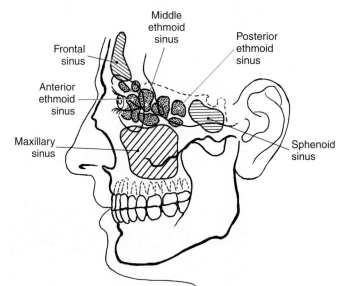

Ethmoid

The **ethmoid** sinuses are contained within the **lateral masses (labyrinths)** of the ethmoid bone. They are present at birth and continue to grow and honeycomb into a varying number of air cells that can be divided into three groups: **anterior, middle,** and **posterior.** The anterior and middle groups drain into the **middle nasal meatus** and the posterior group drains into the **superior nasal meatus** (Figures 2.89 through 2.92 and Table 2.3).

TABLE 2-3   Paranasal Sinus Drainage Location

SINUS	DRAINAGE LOCATION
Ethmoid: anterior and middle	Middle nasal meatus
Ethmoid: posterior	Superior nasal meatus
Maxillary	Middle nasal meatus
Sphenoid	Sphenoethmoidal recess
Frontal	Middle nasal meatus

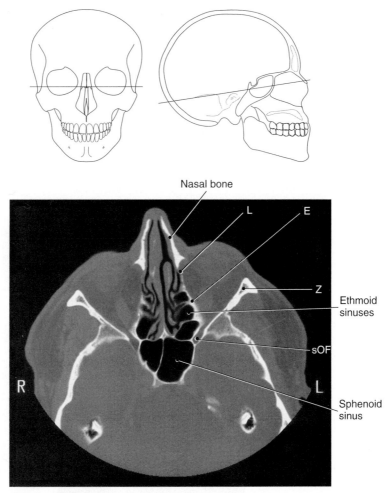

Nasal bone

Figure 2.90
Axial CT scan of sphenoid and ethmoid sinuses.

KEY: L, Lacrimal bone; **E,** ethmoid bone; **Z,** zygoma; **sOF,** superior orbital fissure.

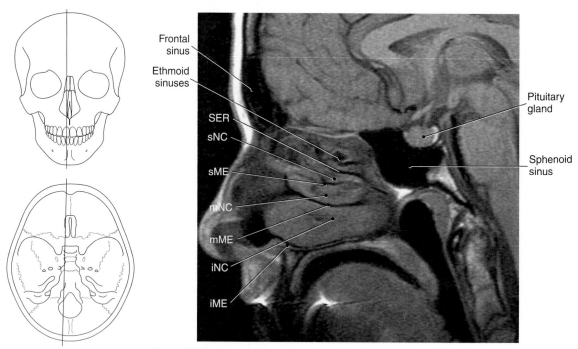

Figure 2.91
Sagittal, T1-weighted MR scan of sphenoid sinuses.

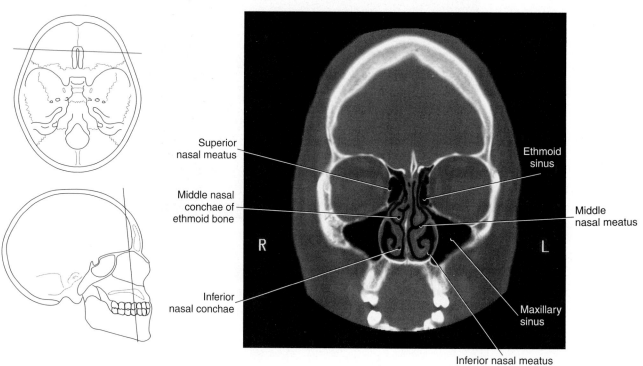

Figure 2.92
Coronal CT scan of ethmoid and maxillary sinuses.

KEY: **SER,** Sphenoethmoidal recess; **sNC,** superior nasal conchae; **sME,** superior nasal meatus; **mNC,** middle nasal conchae; **mME,** middle nasal meatus; **iNC,** inferior nasal conchae; **iME,** inferior nasal meatus; **EtS,** ethmoid sinus.

Maxillary

The paired **maxillary sinuses (antrum of Highmore)** are located within the body of the maxilla, below the orbit and lateral to the nose. These triangular cavities are the largest of the paranasal sinuses in adults but are just small cavities at birth. Their growth stops at approximately the age of 15. The roots of the teeth and the maxillary sinuses are separated by a very thin layer of bone. Often it is difficult to differentiate between the symptoms of sinusitis and infection of the teeth. The maxillary sinuses drain into the middle nasal meatus (Figures 2.88, 2.89, 2.92 and 2.93 and Table 2.3).

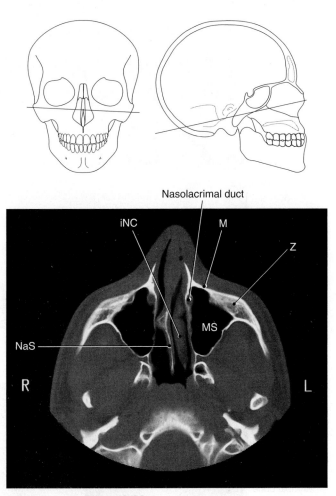

Figure 2.93
Axial CT scan of maxillary sinuses.

KEY: **NaS,** Nasal septum; **iNC,** inferior nasal conchae; **M,** maxilla; **Z,** zygoma; **MS,** maxillary sinus.

Sphenoid

The **sphenoid** sinuses are present at birth but continue to grow until 10 to 12 years of age. They are normally paired and occupy the body of the sphenoid bone just below the **sella turcica.** Each sphenoid sinus opens into the **sphenoethmoidal recess** directly above the **superior concha** and drains into the superior nasal meatus (Figures 2.89 through 2.91, 2.94, and 2.95, and Table 2.3).

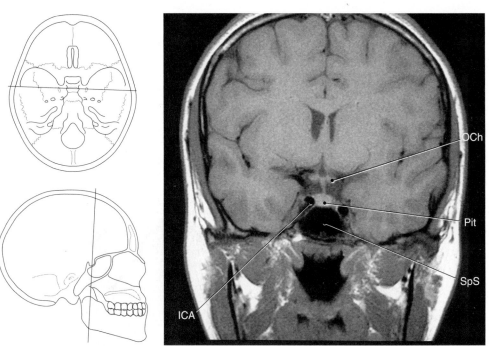

Figure 2.94
Coronal, T1-weighted MR scan of sphenoid sinuses.

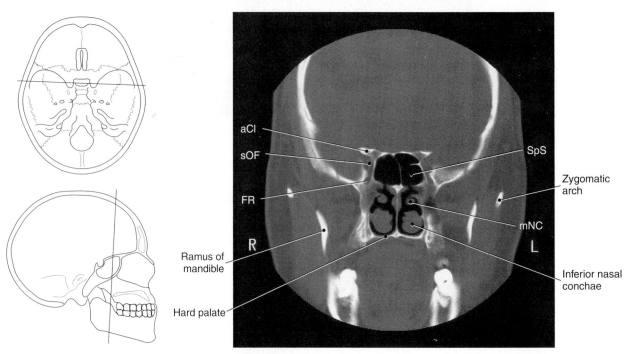

Figure 2.95
Coronal CT scan of sphenoid sinuses.

Frontal

The **frontal** sinuses are located within the **vertical portion** of the frontal bone (Figures 2.89 and 2.91). These sinuses are typically paired and are separated along the sagittal plane by a **septum** (Figure 2.96). The frontal sinuses are rarely symmetric, vary greatly in size, and can contain numerous septa. These sinuses do not form or become aerated in the frontal bone until approximately the age of 6, making them the only paranasal sinuses that are absent at birth. The frontal sinuses drain into the middle nasal meatus (Figures 2.91 and 2.96 and Table 2.3). The inferior meatus only receives drainage from the naso-lacrimal duct.

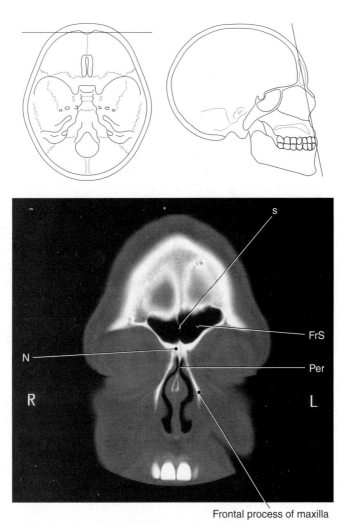

Figure 2.96
Coronal CT scan of frontal sinuses.

KEY: N, Nasal bone; **s,** septum; **FrS,** frontal sinus; **Per,** perpendicular plane of ethmoid bone.

Osteomeatal Complex

Drainage of the paranasal sinuses occurs through various openings or **ostia.** The major drainage pathways and structures of these osteomeatal channels form the **osteomeatal complex (OMC)** (Figures 2.97 through 2.99). There are two osteomeatal channels; the anterior OMC and posterior OMC. The **anterior OMC** includes the ostia for the frontal and maxillary sinuses, frontal recess, infundibulum, and middle meatus. The anterior OMC provides communication between the frontal, anterior and middle ethmoid, and maxillary sinuses. The **posterior OMC** consists of the sphenoethmoidal recess and the superior nasal meatus. The sphenoethmoidal recess lies just lateral to the nasal septum, above the superior nasal concha, and drains the sphenoid sinuses. Key structures to identify of the OMC include the infundibulum, middle meatus, uncinate process, semilunar hiatus, and ethmoid bulla. The **infundibulum** is a narrow oblong canal that serves as the primary drainage pathway from the maxillary sinuses into the middle meatus. The medial wall of the infundibulum is created by the **uncinate process.** The uncinate process is a thin, hook-shaped bony plate that arises from the floor of the anterior ethmoid sinuses and projects posteriorly and inferiorly, ending in a free edge. The free edge of the uncinate process forms the **semilunar hiatus,** which opens directly into the middle meatus. The semilunar hiatus is a gap located between the ethmoid bulla and uncinate process that forms the opening of the infundibulum. Also draining into the middle meatus is the ethmoid bulla, located superior and posterior to the infundibulum, which receives drainage from the anterior and middle ethmoid air cells (Figures 2.98 and 2.99). CT imaging in a direct coronal plane with a bony algorithm will provide the best demonstration of these structures.

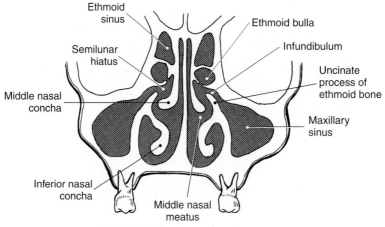

Figure 2.97
Coronal view of osteomeatal complex.

CRANIUM AND FACIAL BONES

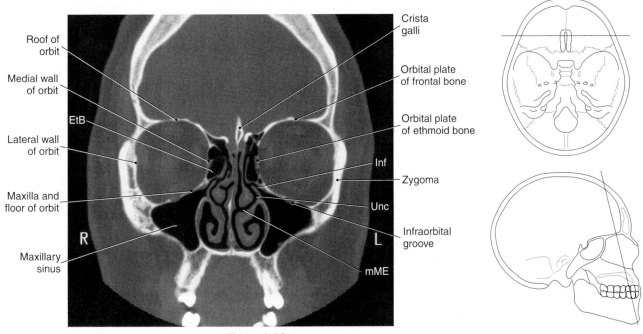

Roof of orbit
Medial wall of orbit
EtB
Lateral wall of orbit
Maxilla and floor of orbit
Maxillary sinus
R
Crista galli
Orbital plate of frontal bone
Orbital plate of ethmoid bone
Inf
Zygoma
Unc
L
Infraorbital groove
mME

Figure 2.98
Coronal CT scan of osteomeatal complex.

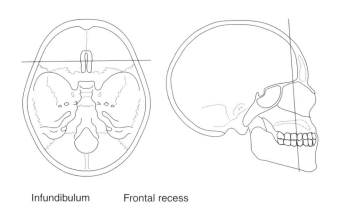

Infundibulum   Frontal recess

Maxillary sinus   Middle nasal meatus   Ethmoid bulla

KEY: **EtB,** Ethmoid bulla; **Inf,** infundibulum; **Unc,** uncinate process; **mME,** middle meatus.

Figure 2.99
Coronal CT scan of frontal recess.

ORBIT

Bony Orbit

The bony **orbits** are cone-shaped recesses that contain the globes, extraocular muscles, blood vessels, nerves, adipose and connective tissues, and most of the lacrimal apparatus. The junction of the frontal, sphenoid, and ethmoid bones of the cranium and the lacrimal, maxillary, palatine, and zygomatic bones of the face form the orbit (Figures 2.100 and 2.101). Each orbit presents a roof, floor, medial wall, lateral wall, and an apex. The **roof** of the orbit is composed of the orbital plate of the frontal bone and most of the lesser wing of the sphenoid bone. On the anterolateral surface of the roof is the **lacrimal fossa** in which lies the lacrimal gland (Figure 2.100). The **medial wall** is exceedingly thin and is formed by a portion of the frontal process of the maxilla, the lacrimal bone, ethmoid bone, and body of the sphenoid bone (Figures 2.98, 2.102, and 2.103). On the anterior surface of the medial wall is the **lacrimal groove** for the lacrimal sac (Figures 2.100 through 2.102). The **lacrimal groove** is contained within the lacrimal bone and communicates below with the inferior meatus of the nasal cavity through the nasolacrimal canal. The **floor** of the orbit, which is also the roof of the maxillary sinus, is made up of the maxilla, zygoma, and palatine bone. The **lateral wall** is the thickest wall and is formed by the greater wing of the sphenoid bone and the zygoma (Figures 2.98, 2.100, and

2.103). The posterior portion of the orbit or the apex is basically formed by the optic canal (optic foramen) and the superior orbital fissure. The **optic canal** and the superior and inferior orbital fissures allow various structures to enter and exit the orbit and establish communication between the orbit and middle cranial fossa. The optic canal forms an angle of about 37 degrees with the sagittal plane of the head; it is bounded medially by the body of the sphenoid bone, superiorly by the lesser wing of the sphenoid, and inferiorly and laterally by the **inferior root (optic strut)** of the lesser wing of the sphenoid bone (Figures 2.100 through 2.104). Coursing through the optic canal are the ophthalmic artery and optic nerve. The **superior orbital fissure** is a triangular opening located between the greater and lesser wings of the sphenoid bone that allows for the cranial nerves, oculomotor (III), trochlear (IV), ophthalmic branch of the trigeminal (V), and abducens (VI) to course as well as the ophthalmic veins (Figures 2.100, 2.103, and 2.104). At the orbital apex, the inferior and lateral walls of the orbit are separated by the **inferior orbital fissure** through which the maxillary branch of the trigeminal nerve (V) courses (Figures 2.100, 2.104, and 2.105). The medial lip of the inferior orbital fissure is notched by the **infraorbital groove,** which passes forward in the orbital floor to become the **infraorbital canal** that opens on the anterior surface of the maxilla as the **infraorbital foramen** (Figures 2.98, 2.100, and 2.102).

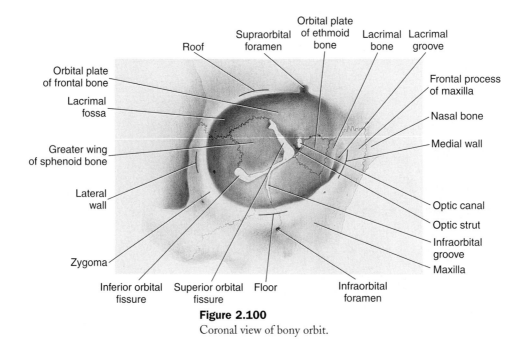

Figure 2.100

Coronal view of bony orbit.

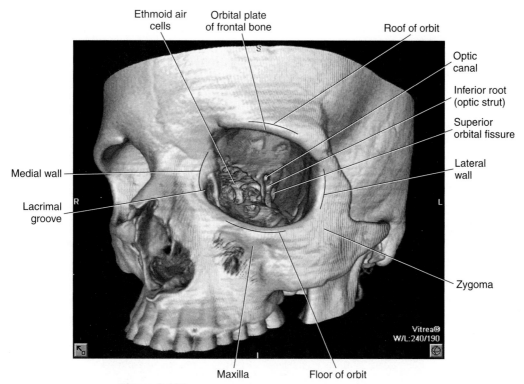

Ethmoid air cells

Orbital plate of frontal bone

Roof of orbit

Optic canal

Inferior root (optic strut)

Superior orbital fissure

Lateral wall

Medial wall

Lacrimal groove

Zygoma

Maxilla

Floor of orbit

Figure 2.101
Oblique 3D CT reconstruction of bony orbit and optic canal.

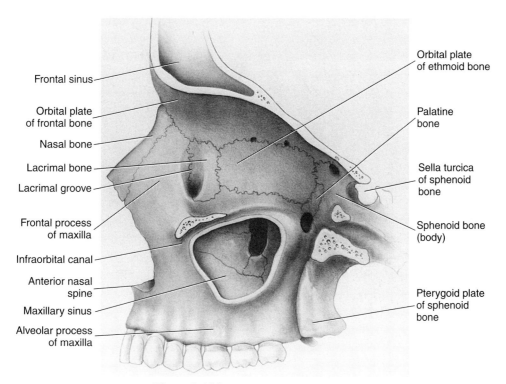

Frontal sinus

Orbital plate of frontal bone

Nasal bone

Lacrimal bone

Lacrimal groove

Frontal process of maxilla

Infraorbital canal

Anterior nasal spine

Maxillary sinus

Alveolar process of maxilla

Orbital plate of ethmoid bone

Palatine bone

Sella turcica of sphenoid bone

Sphenoid bone (body)

Pterygoid plate of sphenoid bone

Figure 2.102
Sagittal view of orbit and maxillary region.

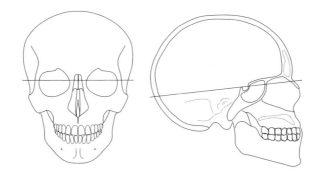

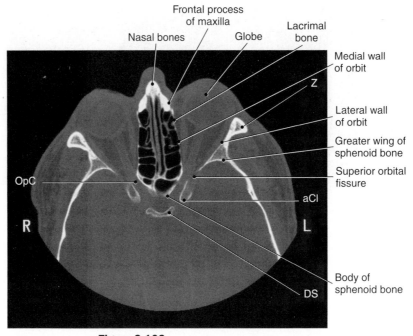

Figure 2.103
Axial CT scan of optic canal.

KEY: **OpC,** Optic canal; **Z,** zygoma; **aCl,** anterior clinoid process; **DS,** dorsum sella.

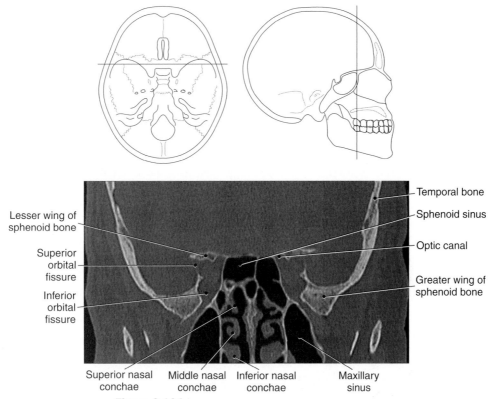

Figure 2.104
Coronal CT reformat of orbital fissures and optic canal.

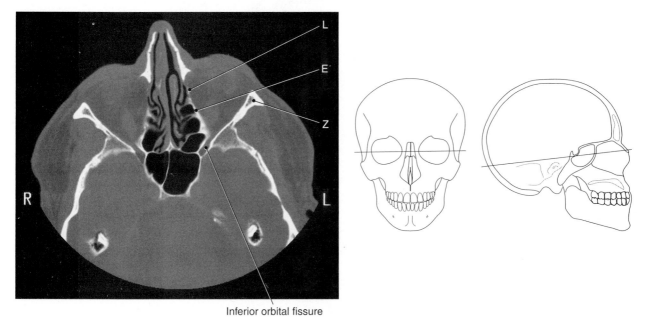

Inferior orbital fissure

Figure 2.105
Axial CT scan of inferior orbital fissure.

KEY: L, lacrimal bone; **E,** ethmoid bone; **Z,** zygoma.

Soft Tissue Structures

GLOBE   The globe of the eye has an irregular, spherical shape and sits in the socket of the bony orbit. The **globe** is divided into **anterior** and **posterior compartments** (Figure 2.106). The anterior compartment is a small cavity located anterior to the **lens.** It contains the **cornea** and **iris** and is filled with **aqueous humor** that helps maintain intraorbital pressure. The larger posterior compartment is located behind the lens and is surrounded by the **retina.** The retina consists of layers of tissue that include the photoreceptors responsible for vision. The posterior chamber contains a jelly like substance called the **vitreous humor** that helps maintain the shape of the eyeball (Figures 2.106 through 2.108). Located in the superolateral portion of the orbit is the **lacrimal gland,** which produces tears (Figures 2.109 through 2.111).

> Direct trauma to the globe will commonly result in a blowout fracture of the orbit. These fractures most commonly involve the floor of the orbit causing herniation of the orbital contents, which results in diplopia. A medial blowout fracture involving the orbital plate of the ethmoid bone is much less common but may cause open communication between the frontal and ethmoid sinuses and the orbit. Coronal imaging best demonstrates the floor of the orbit.

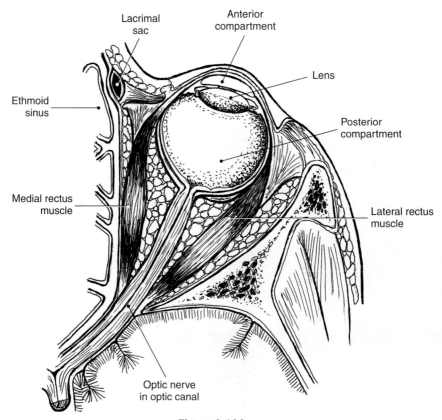

Figure 2.106
Axial view of orbit.

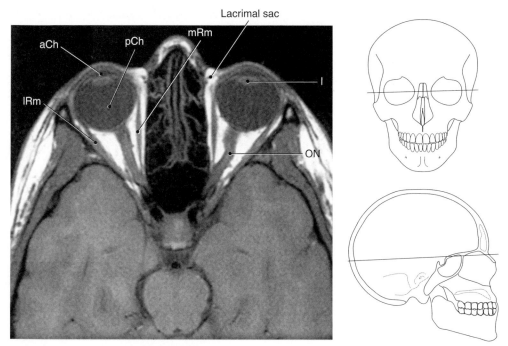

Figure 2.107
Axial, T1-weighted, MR scan of orbit at midglobe.

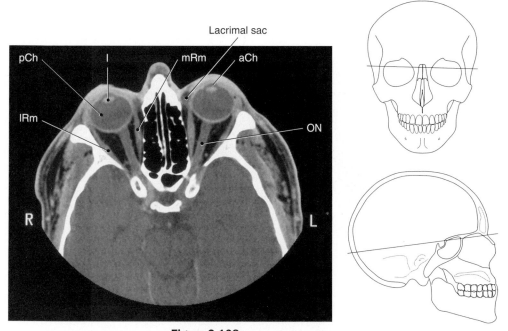

Figure 2.108
Axial CT scan of orbit at midglobe.

KEY: lRm, Lateral rectus muscle; **aCh,** anterior chamber; **pCh,** posterior chamber; **mRm,** medial rectus muscle; **l,** lens; **ON,** optic nerve.

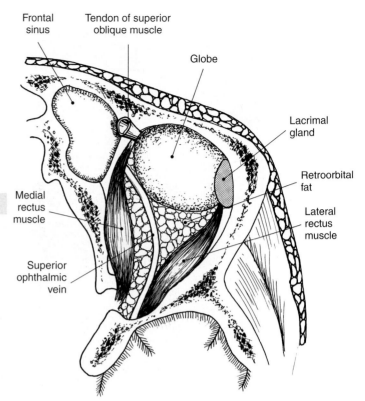

Frontal sinus

Tendon of superior oblique muscle

Globe

Lacrimal gland

Retroorbital fat

Lateral rectus muscle

Medial rectus muscle

Superior ophthalmic vein

KEY: LG, Lacrimal gland; **G,** globe; **SOV,** superior ophthalmic vein.

Figure 2.109
Axial view of orbit with lacrimal gland.

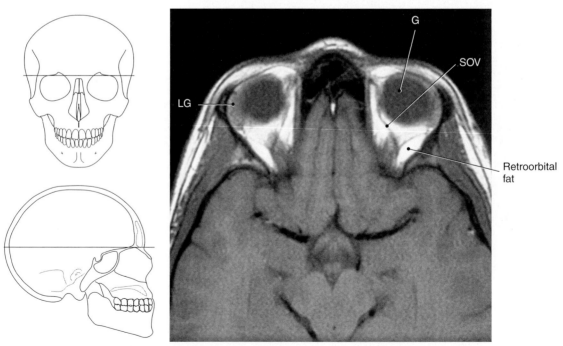

G

SOV

LG

Retroorbital fat

Figure 2.110
Axial, T1-weighted MR scan of orbit with lacrimal gland and superior ophthalmic vein.

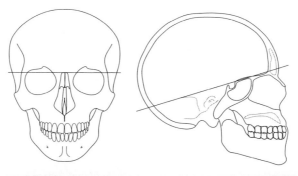

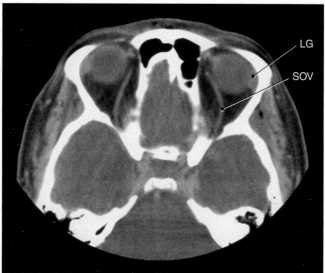

Figure 2.111
Axial CT scan of orbit with lacrimal gland and superior ophthalmic vein.

KEY: LG, Lacrimal gland; **SOV,** superior ophthalmic vein.

Lacrimal Apparatus

Each lacrimal apparatus consists of a lacrimal gland, lacrimal canaliculi, lacrimal sac, and nasolacrimal duct and is responsible for the production and distribution of tears. Tears are important in keeping the eye moist and clean, removing waste, preventing bacterial infections, and providing nutrients and oxygen to portions of the eye. The almond-shaped **lacrimal gland** is found nestled in the lacrimal groove, superior and lateral to the globe, where it provides most of the tear volume.

On blinking, the tears will collect in the area of the medial canthus and then empty into small canals termed **lacrimal canaliculi** that lead to the lacrimal sac. The **lacrimal sac,** found within the lacrimal groove of the orbit, continues inferiorly to form the **nasolacrimal duct** that passes through the nasolacrimal canal of the maxillary and lacrimal bones to empty into the inferior nasal meatus (Figures 2.108, 2.112, and 2.113).

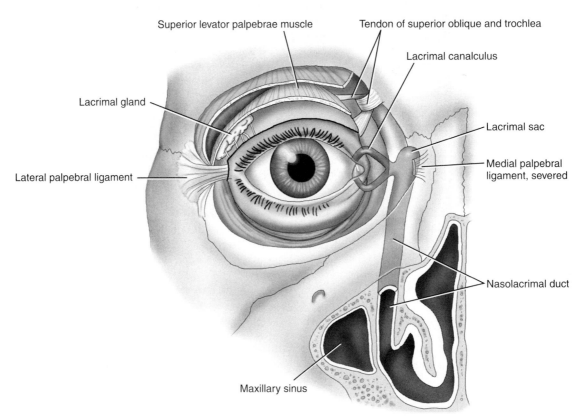

Figure 2.112
Coronal view of lacrimal apparatus.

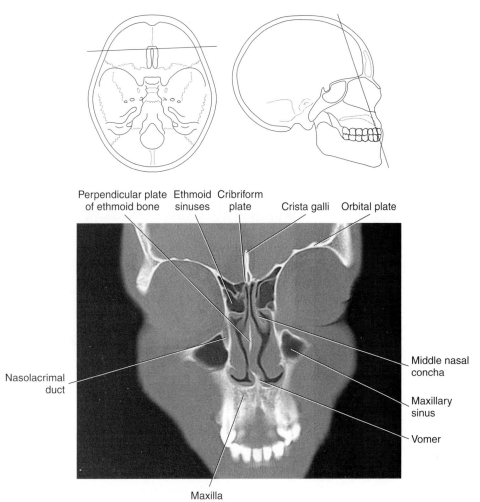

Perpendicular plate of ethmoid bone   Ethmoid sinuses   Cribriform plate   Crista galli   Orbital plate

Nasolacrimal duct

Middle nasal concha

Maxillary sinus

Vomer

Maxilla

Figure 2.113
Coronal CT scan with nasolacrimal canal.

Muscles of the Eye

Six major muscles work together to control the movement of the eye. The **rectus muscle group** consists of four muscles that arise from a common tendinous ring that surrounds the optic nerve and is located at the medial portion of the superior orbital fissure. The **superior, inferior, medial,** and **lateral rectus muscles** act to abduct and adduct the eyeball (Figures 2.106 through 2.108 and 2.114 through 2.119). Two **oblique muscles, superior** and **inferior,** abduct and rotate the eyeball. The superior oblique is located medial to the superior rectus muscle, and the inferior oblique lies below and anterior to the inferior rectus muscle (Figures 2.114 through 2.119).

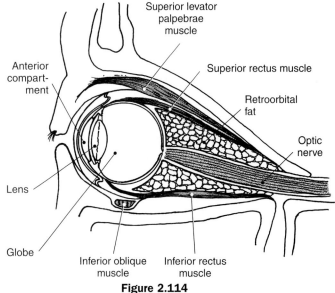

Superior levator palpebrae muscle

Superior rectus muscle

Retroorbital fat

Optic nerve

Anterior compartment

Lens

Globe

Inferior oblique muscle

Inferior rectus muscle

Figure 2.114
Sagittal view of orbit.

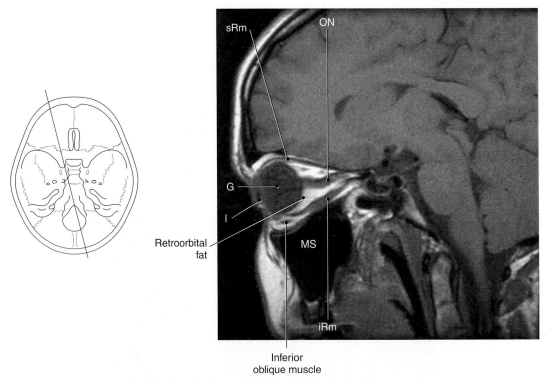

Figure 2.115
Sagittal oblique, T1-weighted MR scan of orbit and optic nerve.

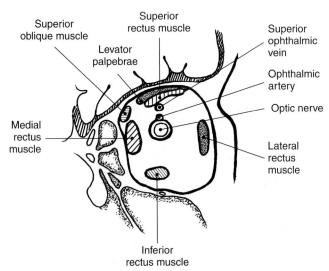

Figure 2.116
Coronal view of orbit and optic nerve.

Optic Nerve

The **optic nerve** is the nerve of sight. It commences at the posterior surface of the globe and courses posteromedially to exit the orbit through the optic canal and is entirely surrounded by dura mater from the meninges of the brain (Figures 2.106 through 2.108). The ophthalmic artery courses adjacent to the optic nerves as they exit through the optic canal. The **superior ophthalmic vein** is easily recognized as it originates from the medial orbit and courses below the superior rectus muscle (Figures 2.109 through 2.111). **Retro-orbital fat** surrounds the muscular and vascular structures within the orbit, which allows for better visualization of the structures in cross-sectional imaging (Figures 2.114, 2.115, 2.117, and 2.118).

KEY: **sRm,** Superior rectus muscle; **ON,** optic nerve; **G,** globe; **I,** lens; **MS,** maxillary sinus; **iRm,** inferior rectus muscle; **sOm,** superior oblique muscle; **sRm,** superior rectus muscle; **OpA,** ophthalmic artery; **mRm,** medial rectus muscle; **iRm,** inferior rectus muscle; **SOV,** superior ophthalmic vein; **lRm,** lateral rectus muscle; **ON,** optic nerve.

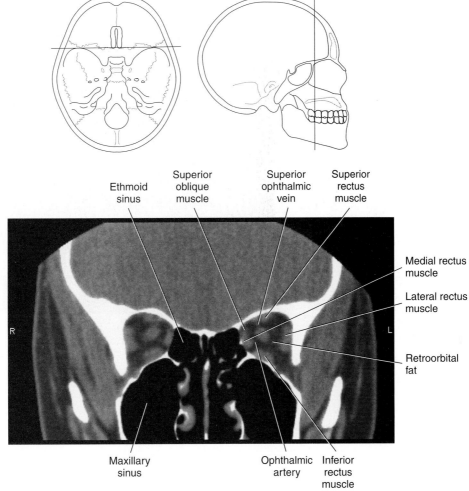

Figure 2.117

Coronal CT scan of orbit with optic nerve and vessels.

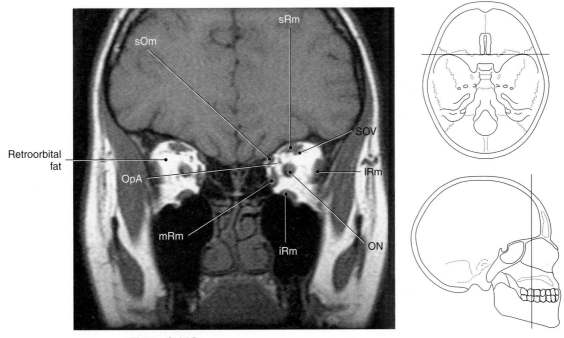

Figure 2.118

Coronal, T1-weighted MR scan of orbit with rectus muscle group.

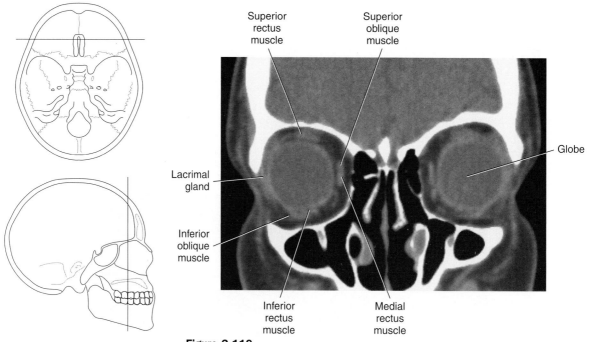

Figure 2.119
Coronal CT scan of globe and lacrimal gland.

REFERENCES

Abrahams PH, Marks SC Jr, Hutchings RT: *McMinn's color atlas of human anatomy,* ed 5, St. Louis, 2003, Mosby.

Agur AM: *Grant's atlas of anatomy,* Baltimore, 1996, Williams & Wilkins.

Ballinger PW: *Merrill's atlas of radiographic positions and radiologic procedures,* ed 10, St. Louis, 2003, Mosby.

Gray H: *Gray's anatomy,* ed 15, New York, 1995, Barnes & Noble.

Harnsberger HR: *Handbook of head and neck imaging,* ed 2, St. Louis, 1995, Mosby.

Leblanc A: *Atlas of hearing and balance organs,* New York, 1999, Springer-Verlag.

Mancuso AA: *Workbook for MRI and CT of the head and neck,* ed 2, Baltimore, 1989, Williams & Wilkins.

Marieb EN: *Human anatomy and physiology,* ed 6, New York, 2004, Benjamin Cummings.

Martini FH: *Fundamentals of anatomy and physiology,* ed 3, Englewood Cliffs, NJ, 1995, Prentice-Hall.

Mosby's dictionary of medicine, nursing, and health professions, ed 7, St. Louis, 2006, Mosby.

Seidel HM, Ball JW, Dains JE, et al: *Mosby's guide to physical examination,* ed 6, St. Louis, 2006, Mosby.

Som PM, Curtin HD: *Head and neck imaging,* ed 4, St. Louis, 2003, Mosby.

Valvassori GE, Mahmood FM, Carter BL: *Imaging of the head and neck,* New York, 1995, Thieme Medical Publishers.

Weir J: *Imaging atlas of human anatomy,* ed 3, St. Louis, 2003, Mosby.

CHAPTER 3

BRAIN

From the brain, and from the brain only, arise our pleasures, joys, laughter and jests, as well as our sorrows, pains, griefs, and tears.

HIPPOCRATES (460?-377? BC)
The Sacred Disease

The brain regulates and coordinates many critical functions, from thought processes to bodily movements. For this reason, it is important to identify the anatomy of the brain (Figure 3.1).

MENINGES

VENTRICULAR SYSTEM
Ventricles
Cisterns

CEREBRUM
Gray and White Matter
   Organization
Cerebral Lobes
Basal Nuclei

DIENCEPHALON
Thalamus
Hypothalamus
Epithalamus

LIMBIC SYSTEM

BRAINSTEM
Midbrain
Pons
Medulla Oblongata

CEREBELLUM

CEREBRAL VASCULAR SYSTEM
Arterial Supply
Dural Sinuses
Superficial Cortical and Deep
   Veins

CRANIAL NERVES
Olfactory Nerve (CN I)
Optic Nerve (CN II)
Oculomotor Nerve (CN III)
Trochlear Nerve (CN IV)
Trigeminal Nerve (CN V)
Abducens Nerve (CN VI)
Facial Nerve (CN VII)
Vestibulocochlear Nerve
   (CN VIII)
Glossopharyngeal Nerve (CN IX)
Vagus Nerve (CN X)
Accessory Nerve (CN XI)
Hypoglossal Nerve (CN XII)

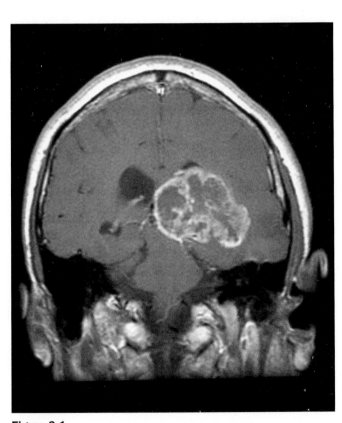

Figure 3.1
Coronal, T1-weighted MR scan of abnormal brain with contrast enhancement.

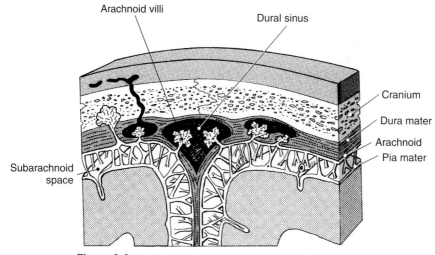

Figure 3.2
Coronal cross section of meninges and subarachnoid space.

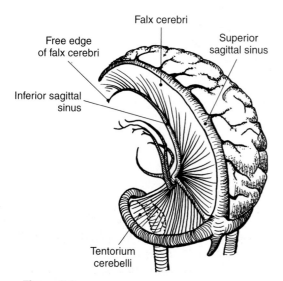

Figure 3.3
Sagittal view of falx cerebri and tentorium cerebelli.

MENINGES

The brain is a delicate organ that is surrounded and protected by three membranes called the **meninges** (Figure 3.2). The outermost membrane, the **dura mater** (tough mother), is the strongest. This double-layered membrane is continuous with the periosteum of the cranium. Located between the two layers of dura mater are the meningeal arteries and the dural sinuses. The dural sinuses provide venous drainage from the brain. Folds of dura mater help to separate the structures of the brain and provide additional cushioning and support. The dural folds include the falx cerebri, tentorium cerebelli, and the falx cerebelli. The **falx cerebri** separates the cerebral hemispheres, whereas the **tentorium cerebelli,** which spreads out like a tent, forms a partition between the cerebrum and cerebellum (Figures 3.3 through 3.6).

> **Tic douloureux (trigeminal neuralgia) is a neurologic syndrome involving the trigeminal nerve. Usually occurring in middle age, this syndrome is characterized by short stabbing pains along the distribution of the trigeminal nerve.**

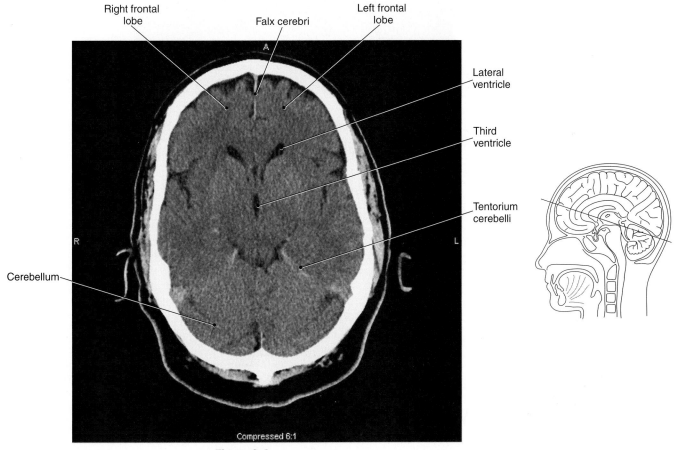

Right frontal
lobe

Falx cerebri

Left frontal
lobe

Lateral
ventricle

Third
ventricle

Tentorium
cerebelli

Cerebellum

Compressed 6:1

Figure 3.4
Axial CT scan of falx cerebri and tentorium cerebelli.

The **falx cerebelli** separates the two cerebellar hemispheres. The middle membrane, known as the *arachnoid membrane* (spiderlike), is a delicate, transparent membrane that is separated from the dura mater by a potential space called the **subdural space.** The arachnoid membrane follows the contour of the dura mater. The inner layer, or **pia mater** (delicate, tender mother), is a highly vascular layer that adheres closely to the contours of the brain. The **subarachnoid space** separates the pia mater from the arachnoid mater. This space contains cerebrospinal fluid that circulates around the brain and spinal cord and provides further protection to the central nervous system (CNS) (Figure 3.2).

> **Skull fractures with rupture of the meningeal arteries can cause a life-threatening condition known as an *epidural hematoma.***

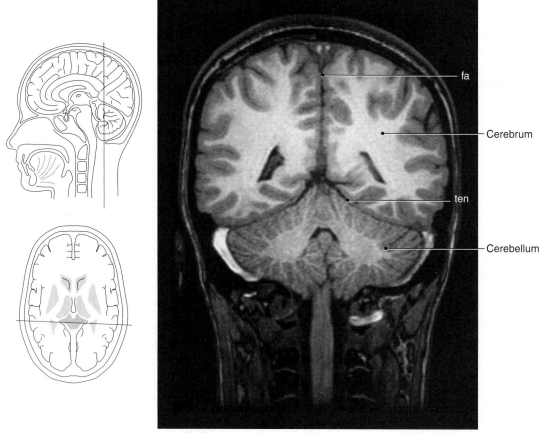

Figure 3.5
Coronal, T1-weighted MR scan of falx cerebri and tentorium cerebelli.

Cerebrum

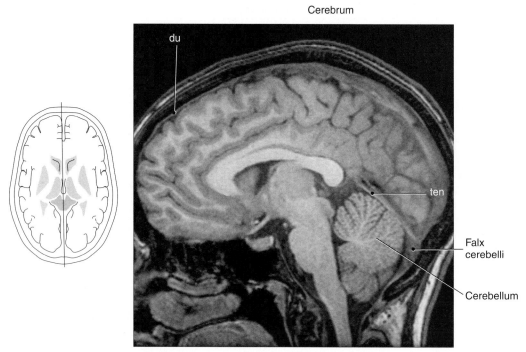

Figure 3.6
Sagittal, T1-weighted MR scan of tentorium cerebelli.

KEY: **fa,** Falx cerebri; **ten,** tentorium cerebelli.

VENTRICULAR SYSTEM

Ventricles

The **ventricular system** provides a pathway for the circulation of the cerebral spinal fluid (CSF) throughout the CNS. A major portion of the ventricular system is composed of four fluid-filled cavities **(ventricles)** located deep within the brain (Figures 3.7 and 3.8). The two most superior cavities are the **right** and **left lateral ventricles** (Figure 3.9). These ventricles lie within each cerebral hemisphere and are separated at the midline by a thin partition known as the **septum pellucidum** (Figures 3.10 and 3.11). The lateral ventricles consist of a central portion called the *body* and three extensions: the **frontal (anterior), occipital (posterior),** and **temporal (inferior) horns** (Figures 3.9 through 3.16). The junction of the body and the occipital and temporal horns form the triangular area termed the **trigone (atria).** The lateral ventricles open downward into the third ventricle through

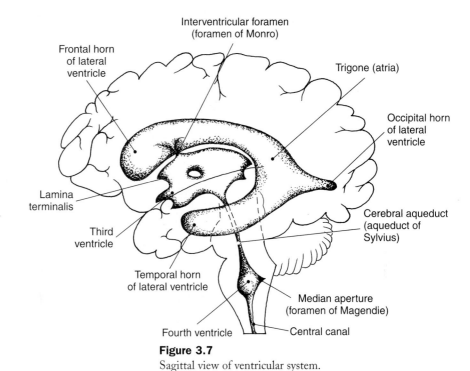

Figure 3.7
Sagittal view of ventricular system.

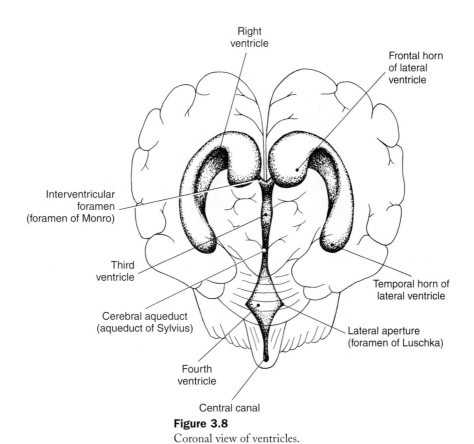

Figure 3.8
Coronal view of ventricles.

KEY: FMo, Foramen of Monroe; **3V,** third ventricle; **LVah,** lateral ventricle, anterior horn; **LVoh,** lateral ventricle, occipital horn; **chp,** choroid plexus; **Sep,** septum pellucidum.

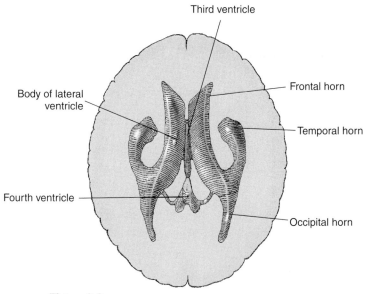

Figure 3.9
Superior view of ventricles in relation to surface of brain.

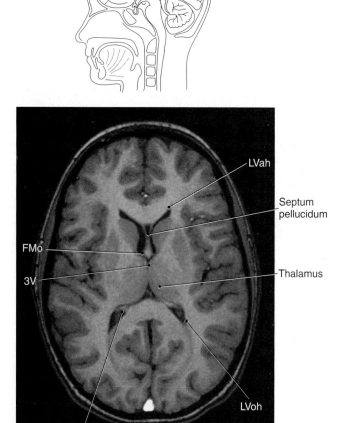

Figure 3.10
Axial, T1-weighted MR scan of lateral and third ventricles.

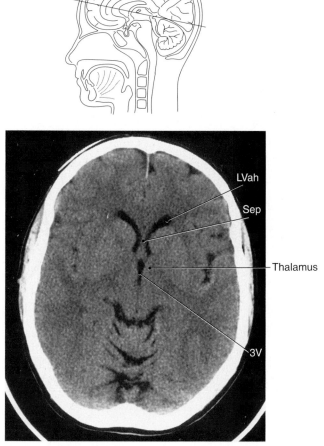

Figure 3.11
Axial CT scan of lateral and third ventricles.

the paired **interventricular foramen (foramen of Monro)** (Figures 3.8 and 3.10). The **third ventricle** is a thin slitlike structure, located midline just inferior to the lateral ventricles (Figures 3.7 through 3.11). The anterior wall of the third ventricle is formed by a thin membrane termed the **lamina terminalis,** and the lateral walls are formed by the thalamus. The third ventricle communicates with the fourth ventricle via a long, narrow passageway termed the **cerebral aqueduct (aqueduct of Sylvius).** The cerebral aqueduct reaches the fourth ventricle by traversing the posterior portion of the midbrain (Figures 3.7, 3.8 and 3.13). The **fourth ventricle** is a diamond-shaped cavity located anterior to the cerebellum and posterior to the pons (Figures 3.13, 3.14, and 3.16). Separating the fourth ventricle from the cerebellum is a thin membrane forming the **superior** and **inferior medullary velum** (Figure 3.13). CSF exits the ventricular system through foramina in the fourth ventricle to communicate with the basal cisterns. The major exit route for CSF passage is the **foramen of Magendie,** located on the posterior wall of the fourth ventricle, which allows communication with the cisterna magna. There are two lateral apertures termed the **foramen of Luschka** (Figures 3.8 and 3.17). The apertures allow for the passage of CSF between the ventricles and the subarachnoid space.

> The septum pellucidum is frequently used as a landmark to determine if the midline of the brain has shifted as a result of trauma or pressure.

KEY: LV, Lateral ventricle; **3V,** third ventricle; **aque,** cerebral aqueduct; **smed,** superior medullary velum; **4V,** fourth ventricle.

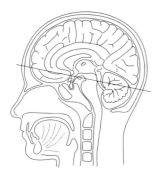

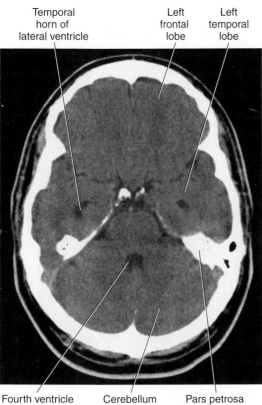

Temporal horn of lateral ventricle   Left frontal lobe   Left temporal lobe

Fourth ventricle   Cerebellum   Pars petrosa of temporal bone

Figure 3.12
Axial CT scan of temporal horns of the lateral ventricles.

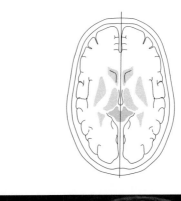

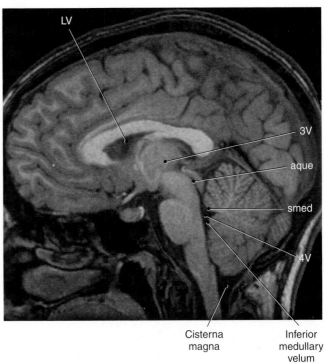

LV

3V

aque

smed

4V

Cisterna magna   Inferior medullary velum

Figure 3.13
Sagittal, T1-weighted MR scan of ventricular system.

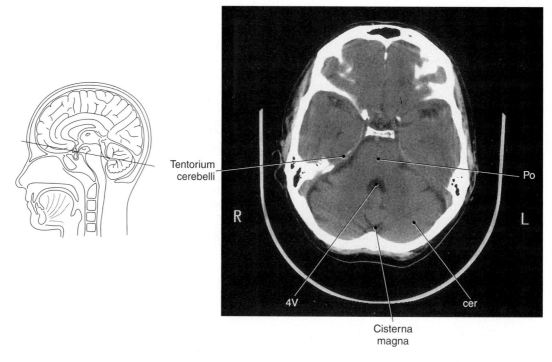

Tentorium
cerebelli

Po

R

L

4V

cer

Cisterna
magna

Figure 3.14
Axial CT scan of fourth ventricle.

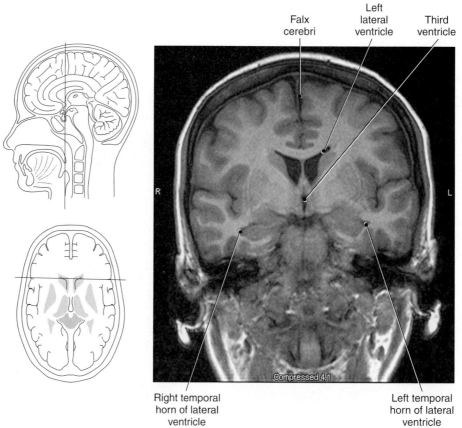

Falx
cerebri

Left
lateral
ventricle

Third
ventricle

R

L

Compressed 4:1

Right temporal
horn of lateral
ventricle

Left temporal
horn of lateral
ventricle

Figure 3.15
Coronal, T1-weighted MR scan of temporal horns of the lateral ventricles.

KEY: Po, Pons; **4V,** fourth ventricle; **cer,** cerebellum.

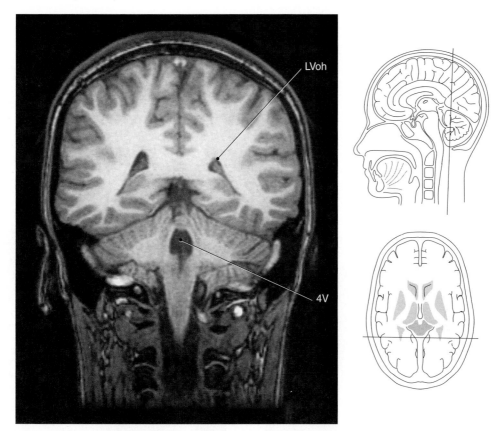

LVoh

4V

Figure 3.16
Coronal, T1-weighted MR scan of lateral and fourth ventricles.

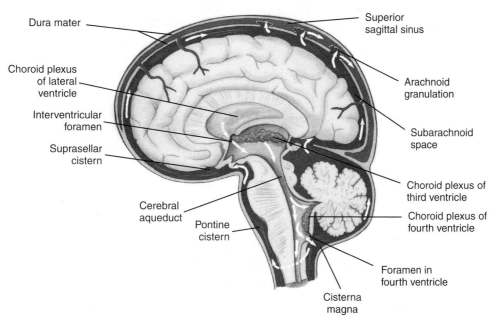

Dura mater

Choroid plexus
of lateral
ventricle

Interventricular
foramen

Suprasellar
cistern

Cerebral
aqueduct

Pontine
cistern

Cisterna
magna

Superior
sagittal sinus

Arachnoid
granulation

Subarachnoid
space

Choroid plexus of
third ventricle

Choroid plexus of
fourth ventricle

Foramen in
fourth ventricle

Figure 3.17
Sagittal view of choroid plexus and flow of CSF through the ventricular system.

KEY: **LVoh,** Lateral ventricle, occipital horn; **4V,** fourth ventricle.

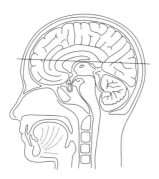

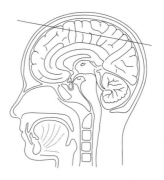

Pitting from
arachnoid
granulations

Septum
pellucidum

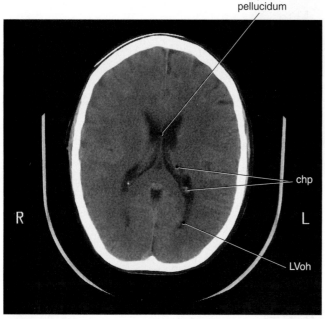

R

L

chp

LVoh

Figure 3.18
Axial CT scan of lateral ventricles with calcified choroid plexus.

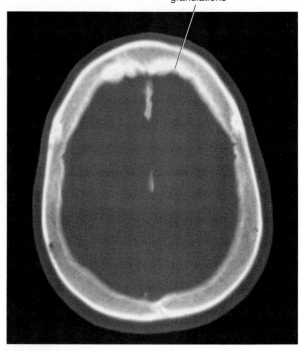

Figure 3.19
Axial CT scan at vertex with arachnoid granulations.

Located within the ventricular system is a network of blood vessels termed the **choroid plexus,** which produces CSF. The choroid plexus lines the floor of the lateral ventricles, roof of the third ventricle, and inferior medullary velum of the fourth ventricle (Figure 3.17). Frequently the choroid plexus is partially calcified, making it more noticeable on computed tomography (CT) scans (Figure 3.18). There exists a continuous circulation of CSF in and around the brain. Excess CSF is reabsorbed in the dural sinuses by way of **arachnoid villi.** These villi are berrylike projections of arachnoid that penetrate the dura mater (Figure 3.2). Enlargements of the arachnoid villi are termed *granulations*. Within the calvaria these granulations can cause pitting or depressions that are variations of normal anatomy (Figure 3.19).

KEY: **chp,** Choroid plexus; **LVoh,** lateral ventricle, occipital horn.

Cisterns

The **subarachnoid space** is a relatively narrow fluid-filled space surrounding the brain and spinal cord. There are locations, primarily around the base of the brain, where the subarachnoid space becomes widened (Figure 3.17). The combined term for these widened areas or pools of CSF is the **basal (subarachnoidal) cisterns** (Figure 3.20). Each cistern is generally named after the brain structure it borders. It is important to recognize the location of these cisterns so they are not misinterpreted as abnormalities.

KEY: **SuC,** Suprasellar cistern; **InC,** interpeduncular cistern; **AmC,** ambient cistern; **QuC,** quadrigeminal cistern.

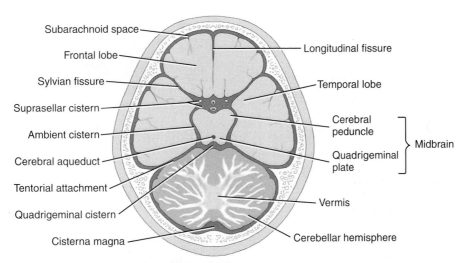

Figure 3.20
Axial view of basal cisterns.

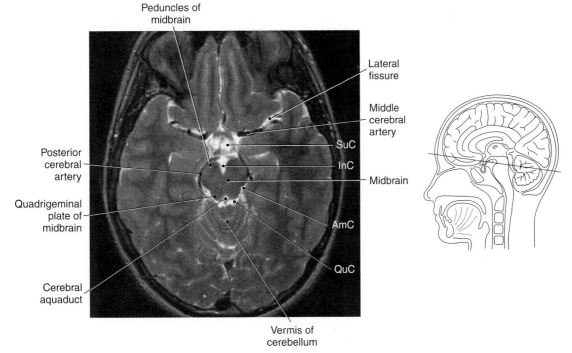

Figure 3.21
Axial, T2-weighted MR scan of ambient, suprasellar, and interpeduncular cisterns.

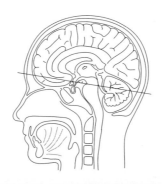

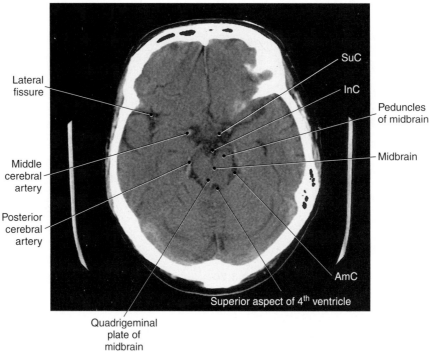

Figure 3.22
Axial CT scan of ambient, suprasellar, and interpeduncular cisterns.

One of the largest cisterns is the **cisterna magna.** It is located in the lower posterior fossa between the medulla oblongata, cerebellar hemispheres, and occipital bone. It is continuous with the subarachnoid space of the spinal canal (Figures 3.13, 3.14, and 3.17). The **interpeduncular cistern** is located between the peduncles of the midbrain and communicates inferiorly with the pontine cistern (Figures 3.21 and 3.22). The **pontine cistern** is located just anterior and inferior to the pons and communicates laterally with the **cerebellopontine angle (CPA) cistern** (Figures 3.17, 3.23, and 3.24). Important structures located within the cerebellopontine angle cistern include cranial nerves V, VII, and VIII, and the superior and anterior inferior cerebellar arteries. The **ambient cistern** courses around the lateral surface of the midbrain, connecting the interpeduncular cistern with the quadrigeminal (superior) cistern (Figures 3.20 through 3.22). The **quadrigeminal cistern** lies between the splenium of the corpus callosum and the superior surface of the cerebellum just posterior to the colliculi of the midbrain or the quadrigeminal plate (Figures 3.20 through 3.22). Located above the sella is the **suprasellar (chiasmatic) cistern,** which contains the optic chiasm and the circle of Willis (Figures 3.20 through 3.22).

***KEY:* SuC,** Suprasellar cistern; **InC,** interpeduncular cistern; **AmC,** ambient cistern.

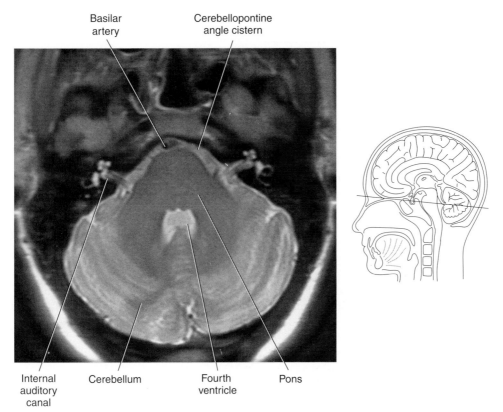

Basilar
artery

Cerebellopontine
angle cistern

Internal
auditory
canal

Cerebellum

Fourth
ventricle

Pons

Figure 3.23
Axial, T2-weighted MR scan of cerebellopontine angle cistern.

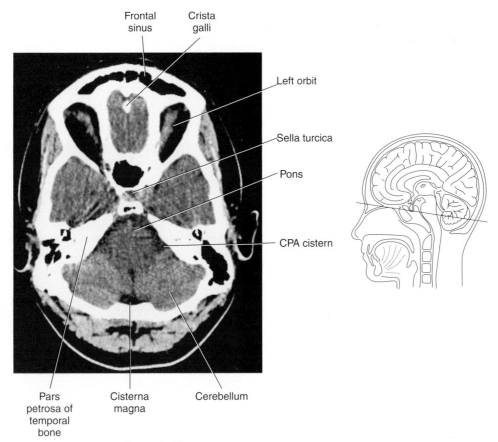

Frontal
sinus

Crista
galli

Left orbit

Sella turcica

Pons

CPA cistern

Pars
petrosa of
temporal
bone

Cisterna
magna

Cerebellum

Figure 3.24
Axial CT scan of cerebellopontine angle (CPA) cistern.

CEREBRUM

The **cerebrum** is the largest portion of the brain and is divided into **left** and **right cerebral hemispheres.** Each hemisphere contains neural tissue arranged in numerous folds called **gyri.** The gyri are separated by shallow grooves called **sulci** and by deeper grooves called **fissures.** The main sulcus that can be identified on CT and magnetic resonance (MR) images of the brain is the **central sulcus,** which divides the **precentral gyrus** of the frontal lobe and **postcentral gyrus** of the parietal lobe (Figures 3.25 and 3.26). These gyri are important to identify because the precentral gyrus is considered the motor strip of the brain and the postcentral gyrus is considered the sensory strip of the brain. Other gyri important for imaging include the cingulate, parahippocampal, and auditory (transverse gyri of Heschl) gyri (see Limbic System and Temporal Lobe). The two main fissures of the cerebrum are the **longitudinal fissure** and the **lateral fissure (Sylvian fissure)** (Figures 3.27 and 3.28). The longitudinal fissure is a long, deep furrow that divides the left and right cerebral hemispheres. Located in this fissure is the falx cerebri and superior sagittal sinus. The lateral fissure is a deep furrow that separates the frontal and parietal lobes from the temporal lobe. Numerous blood vessels, primarily branches of the middle cerebral artery, follow the course of the lateral fissure (Figures 3.21 and 3.22).

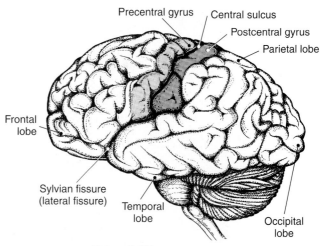

Figure 3.25
Sagittal view of central sulcus.

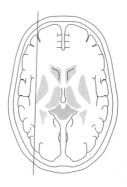

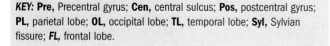

KEY: Pre, Precentral gyrus; **Cen,** central sulcus; **Pos,** postcentral gyrus; **PL,** parietal lobe; **OL,** occipital lobe; **TL,** temporal lobe; **Syl,** Sylvian fissure; **FL,** frontal lobe.

Figure 3.26
Sagittal, T1-weighted MR scan of cerebral lobes and central sulcus.

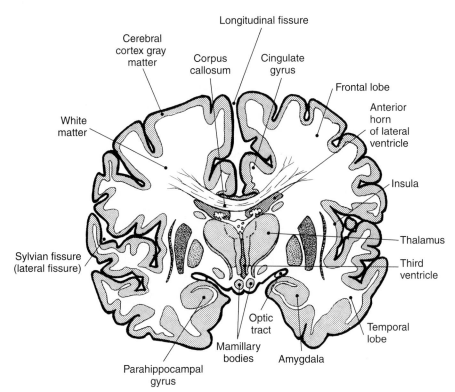

Figure 3.27
Coronal view of cerebrum.

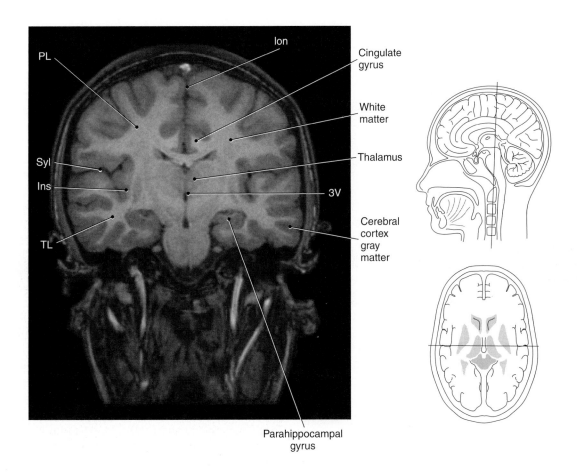

Figure 3.28
Coronal, T1-weighted MR scan of cerebrum.

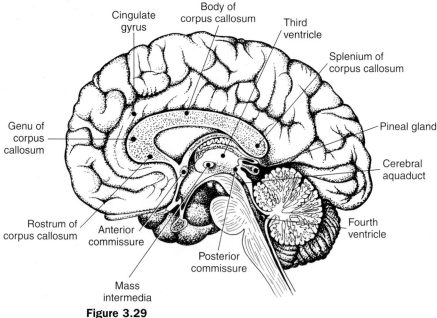

Figure 3.29
Midsagittal view of cerebral cortex and corpus callosum.

Figure 3.30
Midsagittal, T1-weighted MR scan of cerebral cortex and corpus callosum.

Gray and White Matter Organization

The cerebrum as a whole has many critically important functions, including thought, judgment, memory, and discrimination. The cerebrum consists of **gray matter** (neuron cell bodies) and **white matter** (myelinated axons) (Figures 3.27 and 3.28). The **cerebral cortex,** the outermost portion of the cerebrum, is composed of gray matter approximately 3 to 5 mm thick. The cortex not only receives sensory input but also sends instructions to the muscles and glands for control of bodily movement and activity. Deep to the cortex is the white matter, which contains fibers that create pathways for the transmission of nerve impulses to and from the cortex. The largest and densest bundle of white matter fibers within the cerebrum is the **corpus callosum.** This midline structure forms the roof of the lateral ventricles and connects the right and left cerebral hemispheres. The four parts to the corpus callosum, from anteroinferior to posterior, are the **rostrum, genu, body, and splenium** (Figures 3.29 through 3.32).

Two other important bundles of white matter fibers are the anterior and posterior commissures (Figure 3.29). The **anterior commissure** crosses the midline within the lamina terminalis and connects the anterior portions of each temporal lobe (Figures 3.33 and 3.34). The **posterior commissure** is a pathway made of several fibers that transmit nerve impulses for pupillary (consensual) light reflexes. This pathway crosses the midline posterior to the third ventricle, immediately above the cerebral aqueduct and inferior to the pineal gland (Figure 3.34).

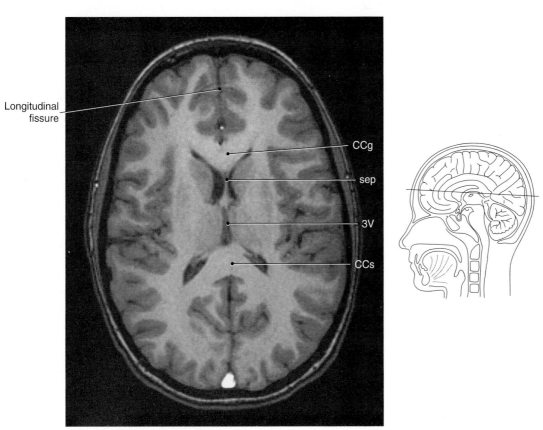

Figure 3.31
Axial, T1-weighted MR scan of corpus callosum.

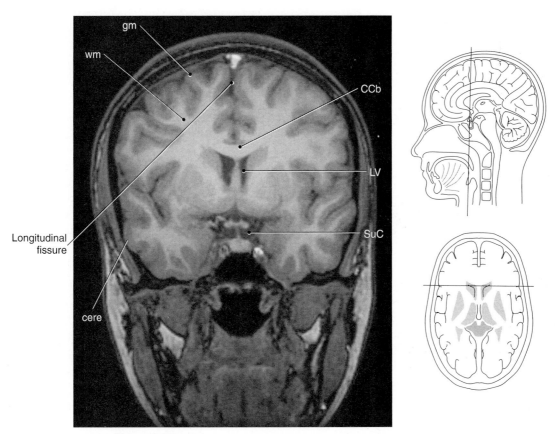

Figure 3.32
Coronal, T1-weighted MR scan of cerebral cortex and corpus callosum.

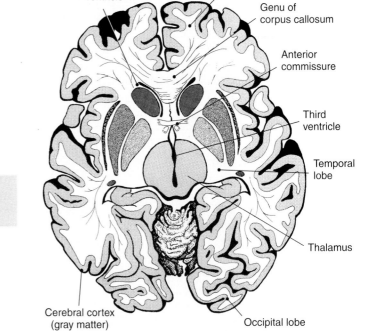

Figure 3.33
Axial view of cerebral cortex and corpus callosum.

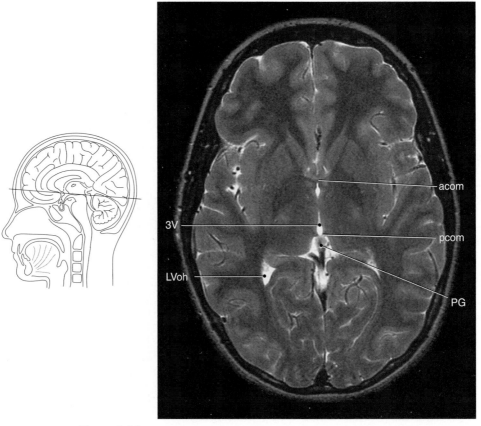

Figure 3.34
Axial, T2-weighted MR scan of anterior and posterior commissures.

BRAIN *103*

Cerebral Lobes

The cerebral cortex of each hemisphere can be divided into four individual lobes: frontal, parietal, occipital, and temporal (Figure 3.35). These four lobes correspond in location to the cranial bones with the same name. Each lobe has critical regions, which are associated with specific functions. The **frontal lobe** is the most anterior lobe of the brain. The boundaries of the frontal lobe are the central sulcus, which separates it from the parietal lobe, and the lateral fissure, which separates it from the temporal lobe (Figure 3.36). The frontal lobe mediates a wide variety of functions such as reasoning, judgment, emotional response, planning and execution of complex actions, and control of voluntary muscle movement. The frontal lobe is also involved with the production of speech and contains the motor speech (language) center, **Broca's area.** Broca's area lies unilaterally on the inferior surface of the frontal lobe dominant for language, typically in the left frontal gyrus (Figure 3.35). This area is involved in the coordination or programming of motor movements for the production of speech sounds. The **parietal lobe** is located in the middle portion of each cerebral hemisphere just posterior to the central sulcus. The horizontal portion of the lateral fissure separates the parietal lobe from the temporal lobe (Figure 3.35). The parietal lobe is associated with the perception of temperature, touch, pressure, vibration, pain, and taste and is involved in writing and in some aspects

of reading. The most posterior lobe, the **occipital lobe,** is separated from the parietal lobe by the parieto-occipital fissure. This lobe is involved in the conscious perception of visual stimuli. The **primary visual area** receives input from the optic tract via the optic radiations extending from the thalamus (Figure 3.36). The **temporal lobe** is anterior to the occipital lobe and is separated from the parietal lobe by the lateral fissure (Figure 3.37). Conscious perceptions of auditory and olfactory stimuli are functions of the temporal lobe as well as dominance for language. Memory processing occurs via the amygdala and hippocampus, clusters of gray matter located in the **parahippocampal gyrus** of the temporal lobe (Figures 3.27 and 3.28). Located on the **superior temporal gyrus** is the auditory cortex, which can be divided into the primary and secondary auditory areas. The primary auditory area, **Heschl's gyrus,** receives the major auditory sensory information from the bilateral cochlea, whereas the secondary auditory area, **Wernicke's area,** is the center for the comprehension and formulation of speech (Figure 3.35). Deep to the temporal lobe is another area of cortical gray matter termed the **insula** (island of Reil), often referred to as the *fifth lobe.* The insula is separated from the temporal lobe by the lateral fissure and is thought to mediate the motor and sensory functions of the viscera (Figures 3.36 and 3.38).

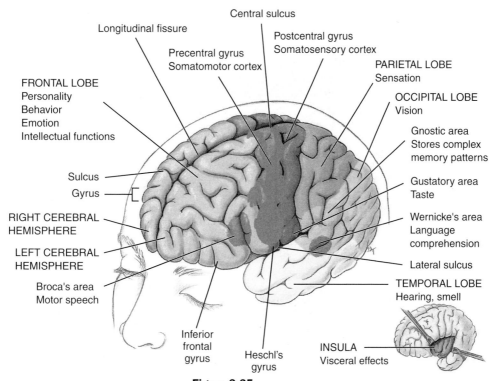

Figure 3.35
Sagittal view of cerebral lobes.

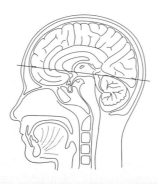

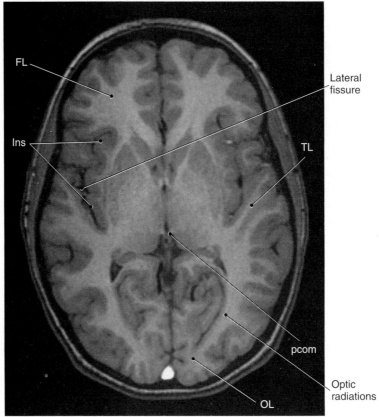

Figure 3.36
Axial, T1-weighted MR scan of cerebral lobes.

KEY: **Ins,** Insula; **FL,** frontal lobe; **TL,** temporal lobe; **pcom,** posterior commissure; **OL,** occipital lobe.

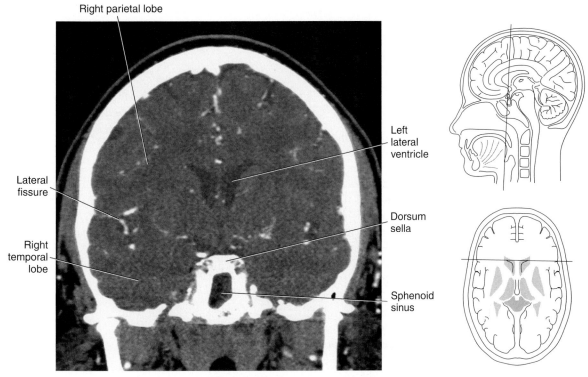

Right parietal lobe

Lateral fissure

Right temporal lobe

Left lateral ventricle

Dorsum sella

Sphenoid sinus

Figure 3.37
Coronal CT reformat of cerebral lobes.

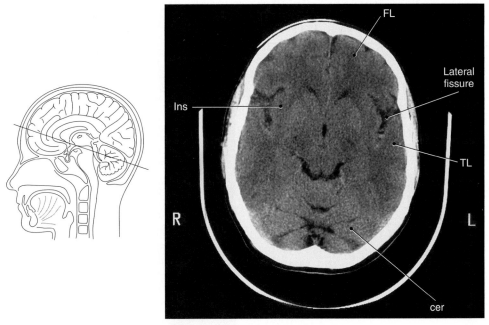

FL

Lateral fissure

Ins

TL

R

L

cer

Figure 3.38
Axial CT scan of cerebral lobes.

KEY: **Ins,** Insula; **FL,** frontal lobe; **TL,** temporal lobe; **cer,** cerebellum.

Basal Nuclei

The **basal nuclei (ganglia)** are a collection of subcortical gray matter consisting of the caudate nucleus, lentiform nucleus, and claustrum (Figures 3.39 and 3.40). Collectively, they contribute to the planning and programming of muscle action and movement. The largest basal nuclei are the caudate nucleus and lentiform nucleus. Both nuclei serve as relay stations between the thalamus and the cerebral cortex of the same side. The **caudate nucleus** parallels the lateral ventricle and consists of a head, body, and tail. The **head** causes an indentation to the frontal horns of the lateral ventricles, and the **tail** terminates at the amygdala in the temporal lobe (Figures 3.41 through 3.43). The **lentiform nucleus** is a biconvex lens–shaped mass of gray matter located between the insula, caudate nucleus, and thalamus. The lentiform nucleus can be further divided into the **globus pallidus** and the **putamen.** The **claustrum** is a thin linear layer of gray matter lying between the insula and the lentiform nucleus and is thought to be involved with the mediation of visual attention (Figures 3.41 through 3.44). Tracts of white matter separate the basal nuclei and transmit electrical impulses throughout the brain. The **internal capsule** is shaped like a boomerang and separates the thalamus and caudate nucleus from the lentiform nucleus. The **external capsule** is a thin layer of white matter that separates the claustrum from the lentiform nucleus. Another thin layer of white matter located between the claustrum and insular cortex is the **extreme capsule** (Figures 3.41 through 3.44).

It is the control of the basal nuclei that allows for the unconscious coordination for swinging our arms with our legs as we walk.

KEY: LVah, lateral ventricle, anterior horn; **Amy,** amygdala; **Hip,** hippocampus.

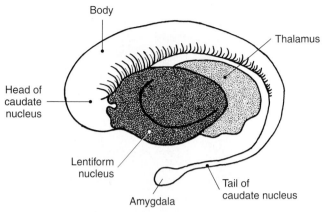

Figure 3.39
Sagittal view of basal nuclei.

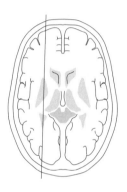

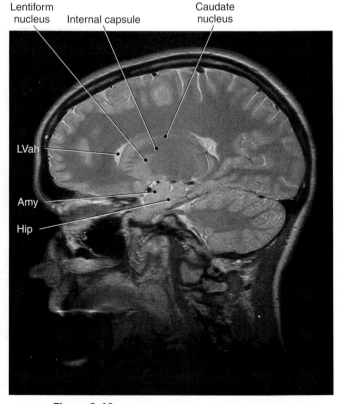

Figure 3.40
Sagittal, T2-weighted MR scan with basal nuclei.

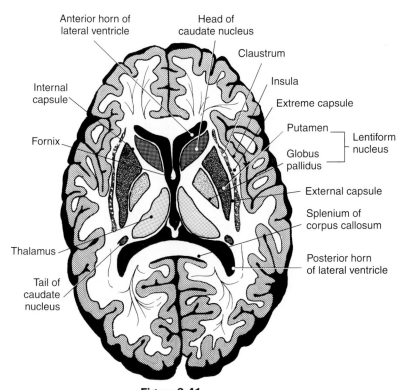

Figure 3.41
Axial view of basal nuclei.

KEY: **inc,** Internal capsule; **exc,** external capsule; **cl,** claustrum; **th,** thalamus; **hcn,** head of caudate nucleus; **ln,** lentiform nucleus; **Ins,** insula; **pu,** putamen; **gl,** globus pallidus.

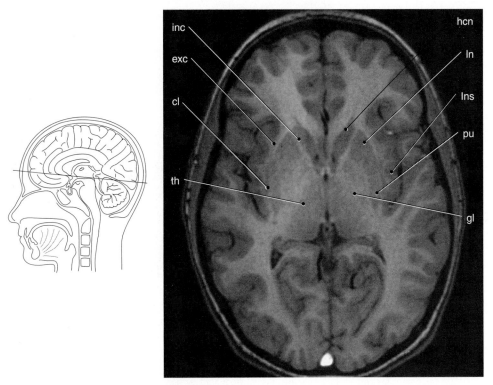

Figure 3.42
Axial, T1-weighted MR scan of basal nuclei.

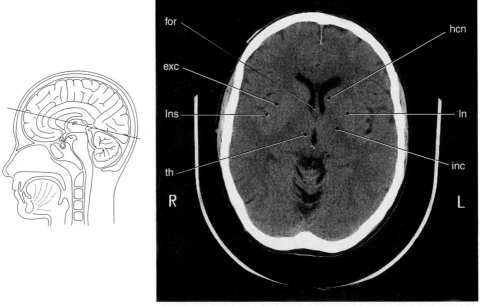

Figure 3.43
Axial CT scan of basal nuclei.

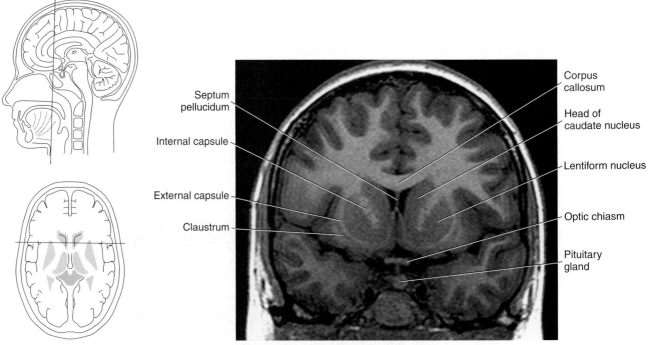

Figure 3.44
Coronal, T1-weighted MR scan of basal nuclei.

KEY: **for,** Fornix; **exc,** external capsule; **Ins,** insula; **th,** thalamus; **hcn,** head of caudate nucleus; **ln,** lentiform nucleus; **inc,** internal capsule.

DIENCEPHALON

Thalamus

The **thalamus** consists of a pair of large oval gray masses that are interconnected with most regions of the brain and spinal cord via a vast number of fiber tracts. The thalamus makes up a portion of the walls of the third ventricle and connects through the middle of the third ventricle by adhesions known as the **massa intermedia.** The thalamus serves as a relay station to and from the cerebral cortex for all sensory stimuli with the exception of the olfactory nerves (Figures 3.27, 3.28, 3.39, and 3.41 through 3.43).

Hypothalamus

The **hypothalamus** consists of a cluster of small but critical nuclei located below the thalamus just posterior to the optic chiasm and forming the floor of the third ventricle. Anatomically it includes the optic chiasm, mammillary bodies, infundibulum, and pituitary gland (Figures 3.45 and 3.46).

The hypothalamus functions to integrate the activities of the autonomic, endocrine, and limbic systems by helping to maintain homeostasis as it controls activities such as the regulation of temperature, appetite, sexual drive, and sleep patterns. In addition, the hypothalamus modulates the activities of the anterior and posterior lobes of the pituitary gland through the release of neurohormones that stimulate or inhibit the release of pituitary hormones.

The **pituitary gland (hypophysis)** is an endocrine gland connected to the hypothalamus by the infundibulum. The **infundibulum** is a slender stalk located between the optic chiasm and the mammillary bodies (Figures 3.45 and 3.46). The pituitary gland is nestled in the sella turcica at the base of the brain (Figures 3.47 through 3.49). The protected location of this gland suggests its importance. It is sometimes called the *master gland* because it controls and regulates the functions of many other glands through the action of its six major types of hormones. The pituitary gland can be broken down into an **anterior lobe (adenohypophysis)** and a **posterior lobe (neurohypophysis).**

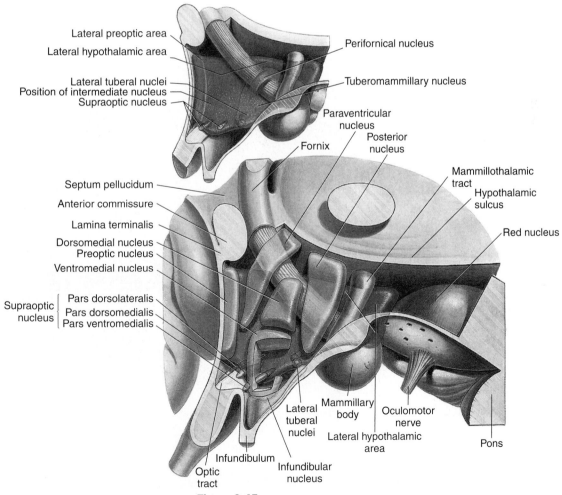

Figure 3.45
Sagittal view of hypothalamic nuclei.

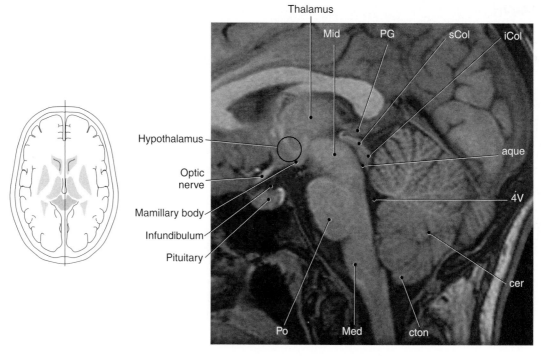

Figure 3.46
Midsagittal, T1-weighted MR scan of brainstem.

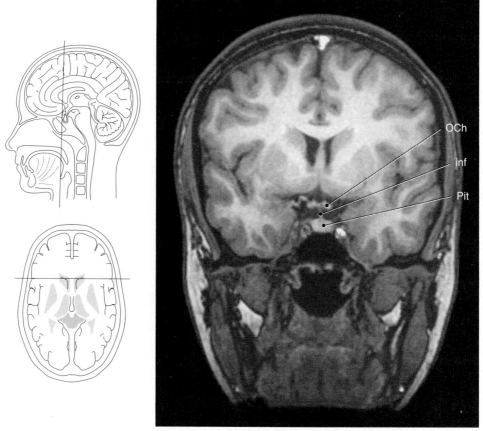

Figure 3.47
Coronal, T1-weighted MR scan of pituitary gland and optic chiasm.

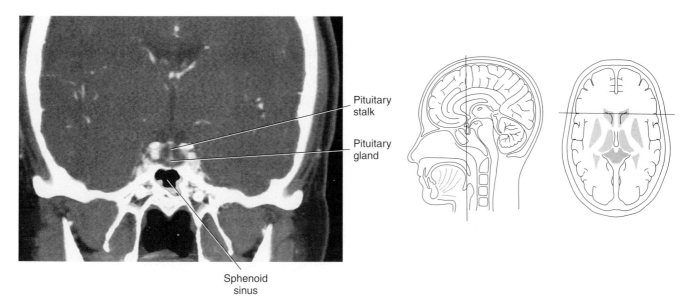

Figure 3.48
Coronal CT scan of pituitary gland.

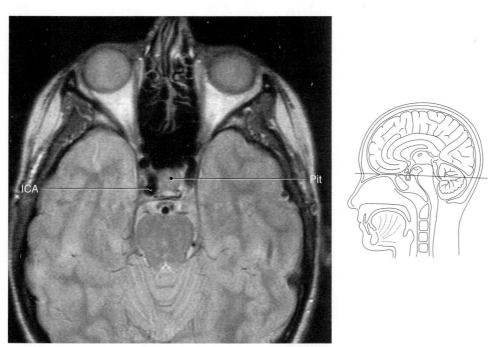

Figure 3.49
Axial, spin density–weighted MR scan of pituitary gland.

KEY: **Mid,** Midbrain; **PG,** pineal gland; **sCol,** superior colliculi; **iCol,** inferior colliculi; **aque,** cerebral aqueduct; **4V,** fourth ventricle; **cer,** cerebellum; **cton,** cerebellar tonsils; **Med,** medulla oblongata; **Po,** pons; **OCh,** optic chiasm; **inf,** infundibulum; **Pit,** pituitary gland; **ICA,** internal carotid artery.

Epithalamus

The **pineal gland,** an endocrine structure, secretes the hormone melatonin that aids in the regulation of day-night cycles and reproductive functions. The pineal gland sits on the roof of the midbrain just posterior to the third ventricle and below the splenium of the corpus callosum. It is sometimes calcified, which aids in its detection on CT scans and lateral radiographs of the cranium (Figures 3.46, 3.50, and 3.51).

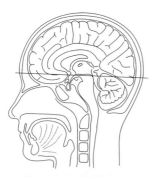

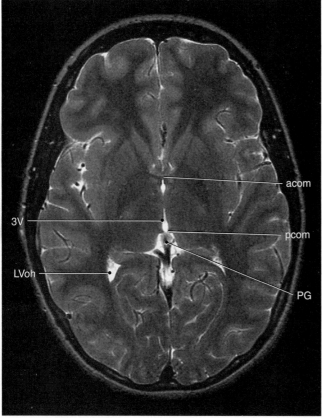

Figure 3.50
Axial, T2-weighted MR scan of pineal gland.

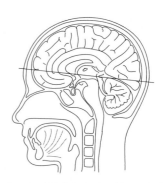

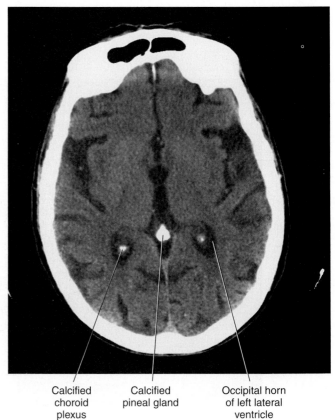

Calcified choroid plexus   Calcified pineal gland   Occipital horn of left lateral ventricle

Figure 3.51
Axial CT scan with calcified pineal gland.

LIMBIC SYSTEM

The **limbic system** is a complex group of interconnected brain structures and fiber tracts located within and adjacent to the medial surface of the temporal lobes. They contain critical connecting pathways that extend to other areas deep within the midbrain, basal nuclei, and cerebral hemispheres (Figure 3.52). These structures have a common functional role in the emotional aspects of behavior. Particularly, the limbic system is involved in aggression, submissive and sexual behavior, memory, learning, and general emotional responses. Structures of the limbic system include the **hippocampus, amygdala, olfactory tracts, fornix, cingulate gyrus,** and **mammillary bodies** (Figure 3.52). The **parahippocampal gyrus** is the inrolled medial border of the temporal lobe that resembles the shape of a seahorse when viewed in the coronal plane. Contained within this gyrus are the hippocampus and amygdala, prominent structures involved with memory and emotion. The **hippocampus** is an important structure that has a strong role in the transition of memory from short-term to long-term memory. The **amygdala** is an almond-shaped mass of gray matter located deep within the parahippocampal gyrus, medial to the hypothalamus and adjacent to the hippocampus (Figures 3.53 through 3.55). The amygdala coordinates the actions of the autonomic and endocrine systems and is concerned with olfactory reflexes and aggressive and sexual behavior. The **olfactory tracts** run underneath the frontal lobes and connect to the amygdala to bring information on the sense of smell to the limbic system (Figures 3.52 and 3.56). The limbic system is integrated with other important structures of the brain via limbic fiber tracts. The most frequently identified limbic tract is the fornix. The **fornix** is an arch-shaped structure that lies below the splenium of the corpus callosum and makes up the inferior margin of the septum pellucidum. It serves specifically to integrate the hippocampus with other functional areas of the brain (Figures 3.52, 3.55, and 3.57). The **cingulate gyrus** is a prominent gyrus located on the medial border of each cerebral hemisphere just superior to the corpus callosum (Figures 3.52, 3.55, and 3.57). The cingulate cortex is considered to be the brain's emotional control center, so it plays an important role in the limbic system. The **mammillary bodies** are two small rounded bodies in the floor of the posterior hypothalamus responsible for memory and motivation. They receive direct input from the hippocampus via the fornix and give rise to fibers that terminate in the periaqueductal gray matter of the midbrain and anterior thalamus (Figures 3.46, 3.52, and 3.53).

> Damage to the hippocampus may result in the loss of memory. High-resolution MR images of the hippocampus are useful in evaluating patients with dementia or seizures associated with hippocampal sclerosis.

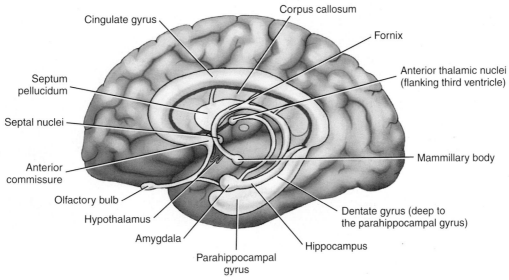

Figure 3.52
Sagittal view of limbic system within the brain.

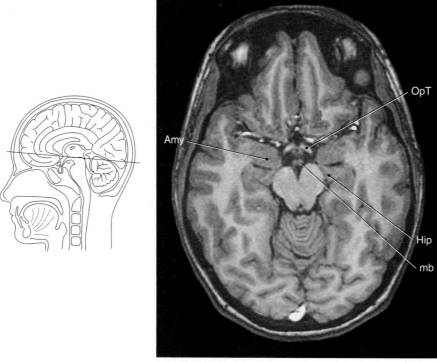

Figure 3.53
Axial, T1-weighted MR scan of hippocampus and amygdale.

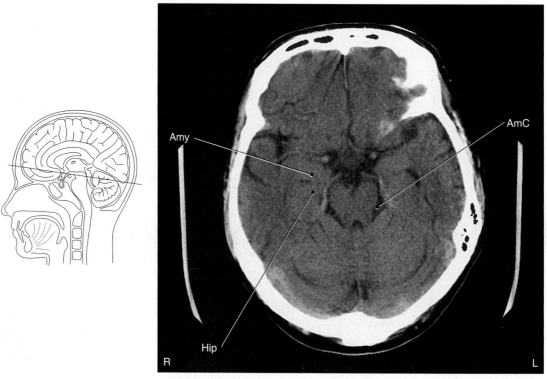

Figure 3.54
Axial CT scan of hippocampus and amygdala.

KEY: **Amy,** Amygdala; **OpT,** optic tract; **Hip,** hippocampus; **mb,** mamillary body; **AmC,** ambient cistern.

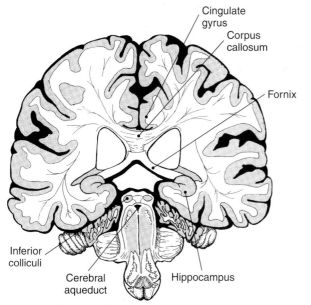

Figure 3.55
Coronal view of hippocampus and fornix.

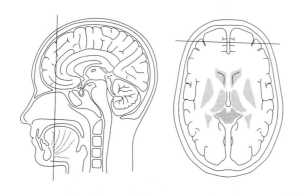

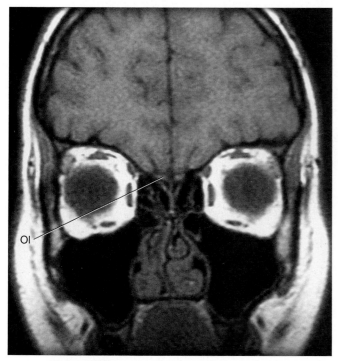

Figure 3.56
Coronal, T1-weighted MR scan of olfactory tracts.

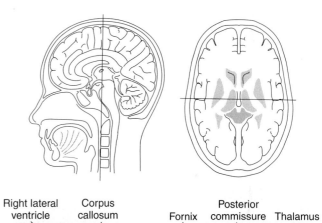

Right lateral ventricle · Corpus callosum · Fornix · Posterior commissure · Thalamus

Hippocampus · Third ventricle · Pons

Figure 3.57
Coronal, T2-weighted MR scan of fornix and the cingulate and parahippocampal gyri.

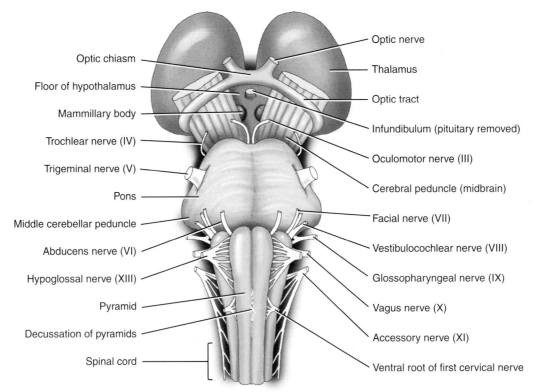

Optic chiasm

Floor of hypothalamus

Mammillary body

Trochlear nerve (IV)

Trigeminal nerve (V)

Pons

Middle cerebellar peduncle

Abducens nerve (VI)

Hypoglossal nerve (XIII)

Pyramid

Decussation of pyramids

Spinal cord

Optic nerve

Thalamus

Optic tract

Infundibulum (pituitary removed)

Oculomotor nerve (III)

Cerebral peduncle (midbrain)

Facial nerve (VII)

Vestibulocochlear nerve (VIII)

Glossopharyngeal nerve (IX)

Vagus nerve (X)

Accessory nerve (XI)

Ventral root of first cervical nerve

Figure 3.58
Coronal view of brainstem and cranial nerves.

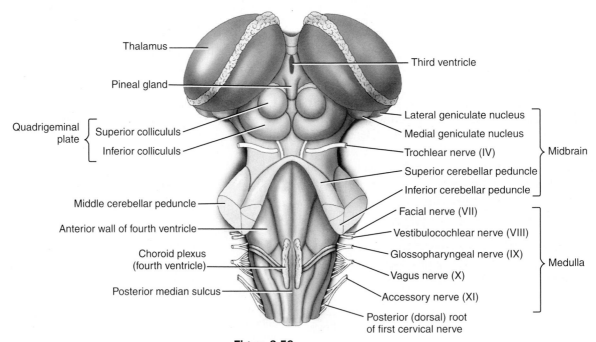

Thalamus

Pineal gland

Quadrigeminal plate
- Superior collicululs
- Inferior collicululs

Middle cerebellar peduncle

Anterior wall of fourth ventricle

Choroid plexus (fourth ventricle)

Posterior median sulcus

Third ventricle

Lateral geniculate nucleus

Medial geniculate nucleus

Trochlear nerve (IV)

Superior cerebellar peduncle

Inferior cerebellar peduncle

Midbrain

Facial nerve (VII)

Vestibulocochlear nerve (VIII)

Glossopharyngeal nerve (IX)

Vagus nerve (X)

Accessory nerve (XI)

Posterior (dorsal) root of first cervical nerve

Medulla

Figure 3.59
Posterior view of brainstem.

BRAINSTEM

The **brainstem** is a relatively small mass of tissue packed with motor and sensory nuclei, making it vital for normal brain function. Ten of the 12 cranial nerves originate from nuclei located in the brainstem. Its major segments are the midbrain, pons, and medulla oblongata (Figures 3.46, 3.58, and 3.59). Located within the central portion of the brainstem and common to all three segments is the **tegmentum,** an area that provides integrative functions such as complex motor patterns, aspects of respiratory and cardiovascular activity, and regulation of consciousness (Figure 3.60). The central core of the tegmentum contains the **reticular formation,** an area containing the cranial nerve nuclei and ascending and descending tracts to and from the brain. The brainstem as a whole acts as a conduit between the cerebral cortex, cerebellum, and spinal cord (Figure 3.61).

> The thalamostriate branches of the middle cerebral artery are located within the internal capsule, causing this area to be the most frequent site of strokes.

Midbrain

The **midbrain** (mesencephalon), which is located above the pons at the junction of the middle and posterior cranial fossae, is the smallest portion of the brainstem. The midbrain is composed primarily of massive bundles of nerve fiber tracts and can be divided into two major segments: **cerebral peduncles** and the **tectum** (colliculi). The midbrain surrounds the cerebral aqueduct, which contains cerebrospinal fluid (CSF) and connects the third and fourth ventricles. Posterior to the cerebral aqueduct is the tectum, or **quadrigeminal plate,** which makes up the roof or dorsal surface of the midbrain (Figure 3.59). The tectum consists of four rounded protuberances termed **colliculi.** The upper pair, **superior colliculi,** is a center for visual reflexes that coordinate movements of the eyes with those of the head and neck. The lower pair, **inferior colliculi,** acts as a relay station for the auditory pathway, providing auditory information to the thalamus (Figures 3.46 and 3.59 through 3.62). Anterior to the cerebral aqueduct are the two large **cerebral peduncles** (Figure 3.63). These ropelike bundles, composed predominantly of axons that are a direct extension of the fibers of the internal capsule, extend from the cerebral cortex to the spinal cord (Figures 3.63 through 3.65). The cerebral peduncles are made more noticeable by the presence of the darkly pigmented **substantia nigra,** a broad layer of cells that contain melanin. The substantia nigra is involved with the production of dopamine, a neurotransmitter in the brain that functions in the control of muscular reflexes. Within the tegmentum of the midbrain, at the level of the superior colliculi, is the red nucleus. The **red nucleus** is composed of a tract of motor nerve fibers and serves as a relay station between the cerebellum and the cerebral hemispheres. The red nucleus

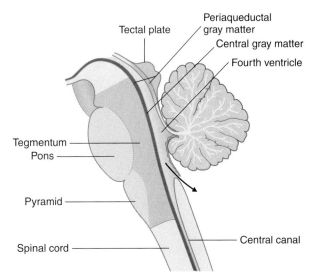

Figure 3.60
Sagittal view of midbrain with tegmentum.

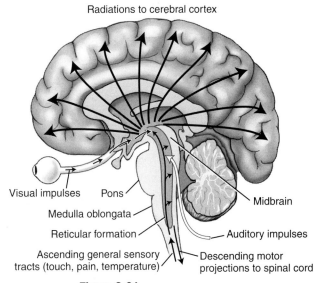

Figure 3.61
Sagittal view of reticular formation.

contributes to the coordination of movements and to the sense of balance. Another portion of the tegmentum is the **periaqueductal gray matter,** which surrounds the cerebral aqueduct. This area receives sensory input that conveys pain and temperature to the brain (Figures 3.63, 3.64, and 3.66).

> If neurons in the substantia nigra are damaged, dopamine production is decreased, leading to the increased muscle spasticity commonly seen in Parkinson's disease.

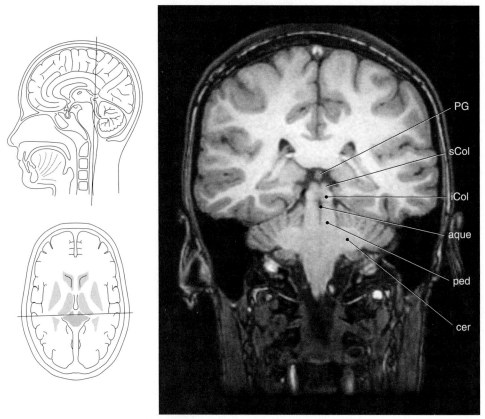

Figure 3.62
Coronal, T1-weighted MR scan of midbrain.

KEY: **PG,** pineal gland; **sCol,** superior colliculi; **iCol,** inferior colliculi; **aque,** cerebral aqueduct; **ped,** cerebral peduncle; **cer,** cerebellum.

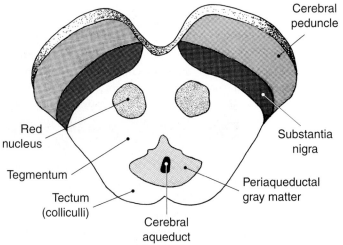

Figure 3.63
Axial view of cerebral peduncles.

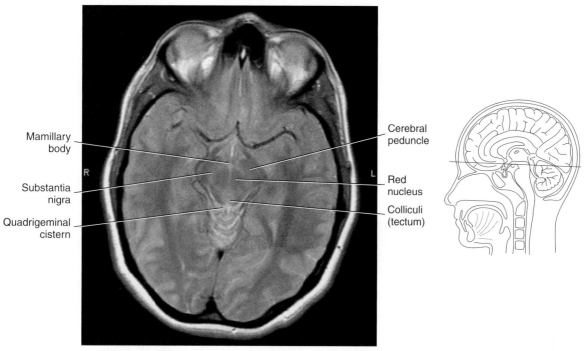

Figure 3.64
Axial, spin density–weighted MR scan of cerebral peduncles and red nucleus.

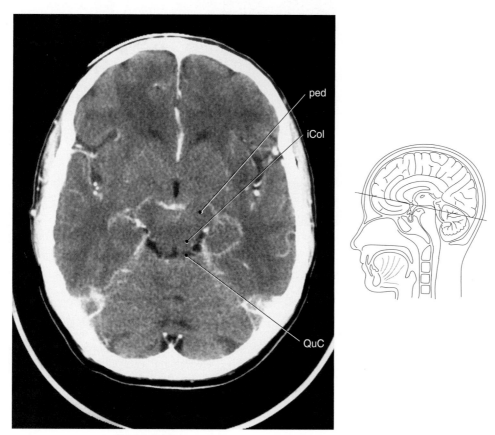

Figure 3.65
Axial CT scan of cerebral peduncles and inferior colliculi.

KEY: ped, Cerebral peduncle; **iCol,** inferior colliculi; **QuC,** quadrigeminal cistern.

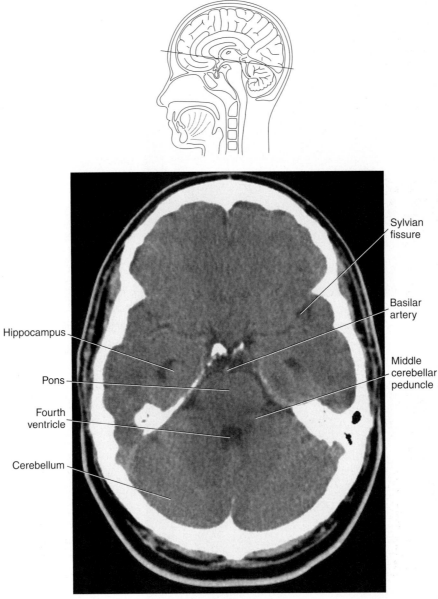

Figure 3.66
Axial CT scan of pons.

Pons

The **pons** is the large oval-shaped expansion of the brainstem centrally located between the midbrain and medulla oblongata. The pons creates a prominent bulge as it lies just posterior to the clivus and anterior to the cerebellum. The term *pons* literally means bridge. This definition is appropriate because the pontine fibers relay signals between the spinal cord and the cerebral and cerebellar cortices (Figures 3.46 and 3.67 through 3.69).

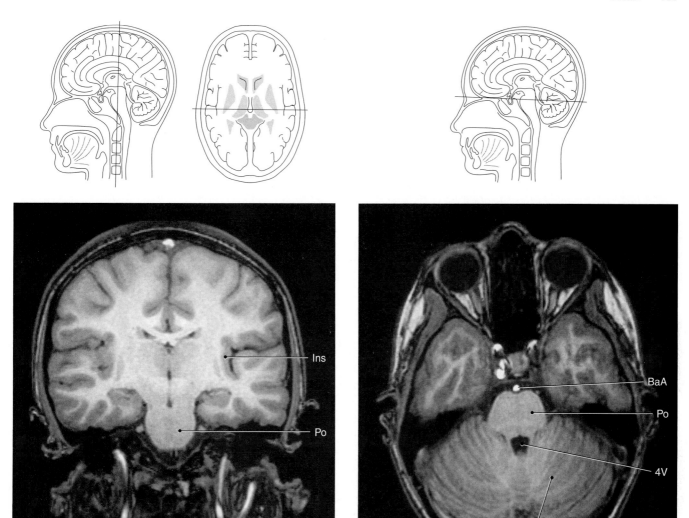

Figure 3.67
Coronal, T1-weighted MR scan of pons.

Figure 3.68
Axial, T1-weighted MR scan of pons and cerebellum.

KEY: **Ins,** Insula; **Po,** pons; **BaA,** basilar artery; **4V,** fourth ventricle.

Medulla Oblongata

The **medulla oblongata** extends from the pons to the foramen magnum, where it continues as the spinal cord (Figure 3.46). The medulla oblongata contains all fiber tracts between the brain and spinal cord, as well as vital centers that regulate internal activities of the body. These centers are involved in the control of heart rate, respiratory rhythm, and blood pressure. The center of the anterior and posterior surfaces of the medulla oblongata is marked by the **anterior** and **posterior median fissures.** These two fissures divide the medulla oblongata into two symmetric halves. Located on either side of the anterior median fissure are two bundles of nerve fibers called **pyramids** (Figures 3.70 and 3.71). The pyramids contain the nerve tracts that contribute to voluntary motor control. At the lower end of the pyramids, some of the nerve tracts cross over (decussate) to the opposite side. This decussation in part accounts for the fact that each half of the brain controls the opposite half of the body. On each lateral surface of the medulla oblongata is a rounded oval prominence called the **olive.** The olives consist of nuclei that are involved in coordination, balance, and modulation of sound impulses from the inner ear (Figures 3.70 through 3.72).

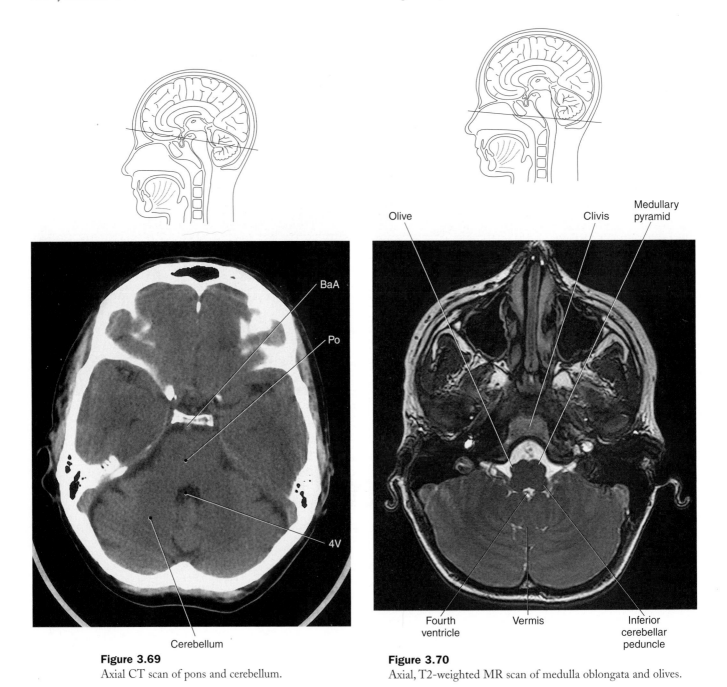

Figure 3.69
Axial CT scan of pons and cerebellum.

Figure 3.70
Axial, T2-weighted MR scan of medulla oblongata and olives.

KEY: **BaA,** Basilar artery; **Po,** pons; **4V,** fourth ventricle.

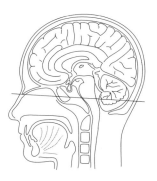

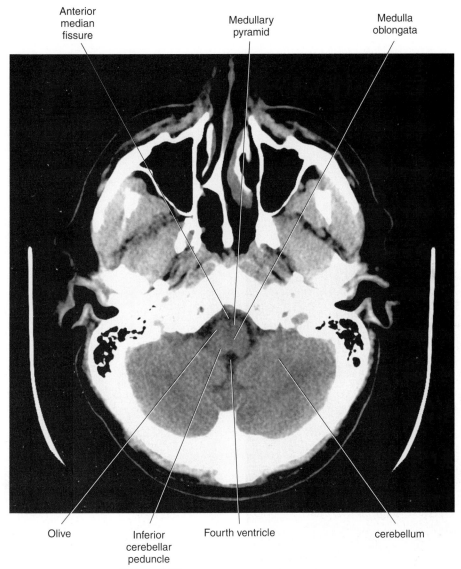

Anterior median fissure

Medullary pyramid

Medulla oblongata

Olive

Inferior cerebellar peduncle

Fourth ventricle

cerebellum

Figure 3.71
Axial CT scan of medulla oblongata and olives.

CEREBELLUM

The **cerebellum,** which is referred to as the "little brain," attaches posteriorly to the brainstem and occupies the posterior cranial fossa (Figure 3.73). The cerebellum is the coordination center for motor functions. Although the cerebellum does not initiate actual motor functions, it uses the brainstem to connect with the cerebrum to execute a variety of movements, including maintenance of muscle tone, posture, and balance, and coordination of movement. The cerebellum consists of two **cerebellar hemispheres** (lateral hemispheres). These hemispheres have an interesting appearance because the folds of gray matter give the appearance of cauliflower. A midline structure called the **vermis** connects the two cerebellar hemispheres (Figure 3.74). On the inferior surface of the cerebellar hemispheres are two rounded prominences called the **cerebellar tonsils** (Figures 3.75 and 3.76). Occasionally, these tonsils can be seen herniating down through the foramen magnum.

A defect involving downward displacement of the brainstem and cerebellum through the foramen magnum is termed *Arnold-Chiari malformation* (deformity) or *tonsillar herniation.*

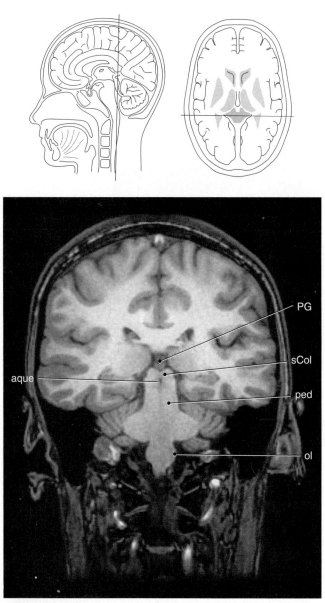

Figure 3.72
Coronal, T1-weighted MR scan of medulla oblongata and olives.

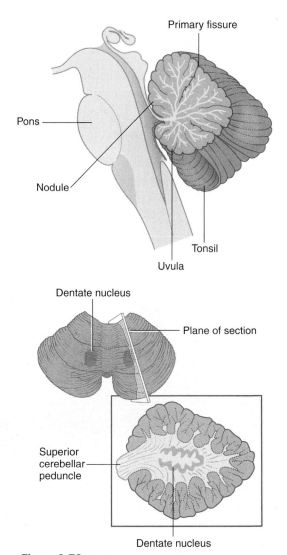

Figure 3.73
Midsagittal view of cerebellum and cerebellar peduncles.

KEY: aque, Cerebral aqueduct; **PG,** pineal gland; **sCol,** superior colliculi; **ped,** cerebral peduncle; **ol,** olive.

Three pairs of nerve fiber tracts, the **cerebellar peduncles,** connect the cerebellum to the brainstem (Figure 3.59). The superior cerebellar peduncles connect the cerebellum to the midbrain. The middle cerebellar peduncles serve as attachments to the pons, and the inferior cerebellar peduncles attach to the medulla oblongata (Figures 3.77 through 3.79). All information traveling to and from the cerebellum is routed through the cerebellar peduncles.

KEY: **Mid,** Midbrain; **ten,** tentorium cerebelli; **cer,** cerebellum; **4V,** fourth ventricle; **cton,** cerebellar tonsils; **StS,** straight sinus; **ver,** vermis; **dn,** dentate nucleus.

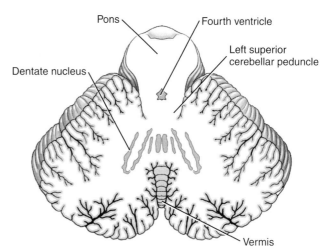

Figure 3.74
Axial section through cerebellum.

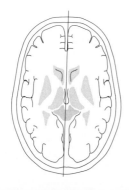

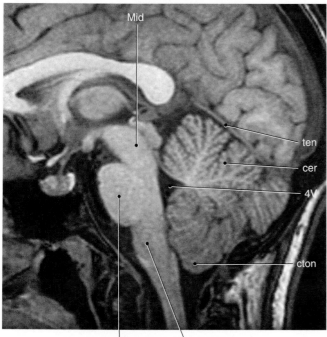

Figure 3.75
Sagittal, T1-weighted MR scan of cerebellum.

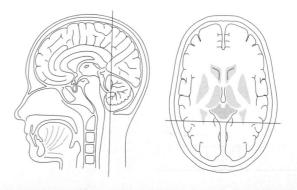

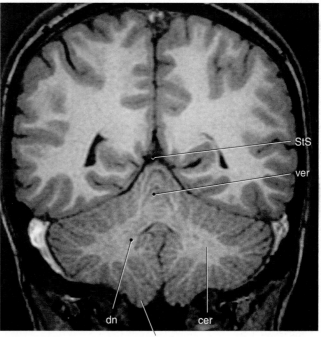

Figure 3.76
Coronal, T1-weighted MR scan of cerebellum and dentate nucleus.

Deep within the center of each cerebellar hemisphere is a collection of nuclei called the **dentate nucleus,** the largest and most lateral of the deep cerebellar nuclei (Figures 3.74 and 3.76). Fibers of the dentate nucleus project to the thalamus via the superior cerebellar peduncles. From here the fibers travel to the motor areas of the cerebral cortex, namely the precentral gyrus, thus influencing motor control.

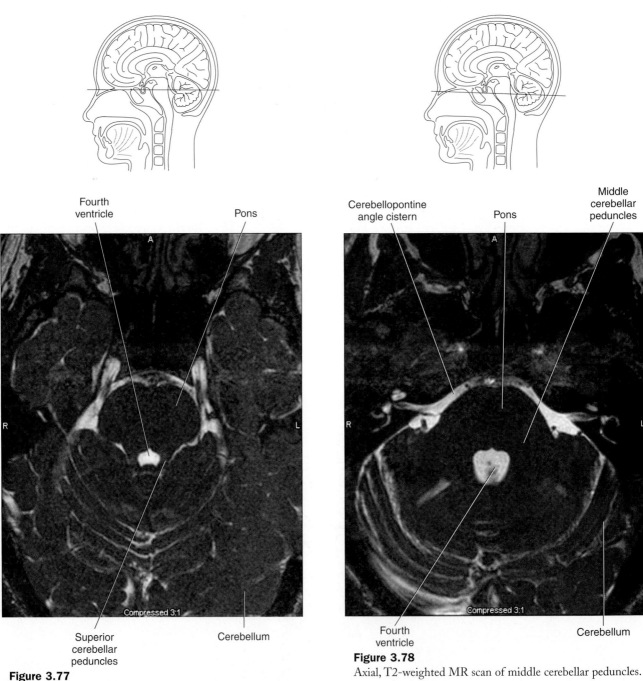

Figure 3.77
Axial, T2-weighted MR scan of superior cerebellar peduncles.

Figure 3.78
Axial, T2-weighted MR scan of middle cerebellar peduncles.

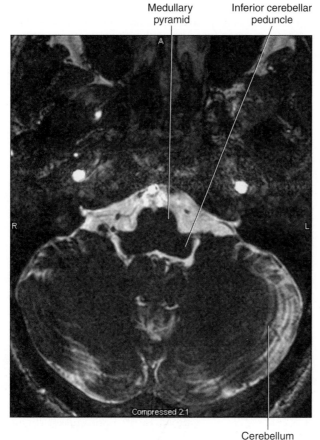

Figure 3.79
Axial, T1-weighted MR scan of inferior cerebellar peduncles.

CEREBRAL VASCULAR SYSTEM

The vascular supply to the brain is unique. In comparison with the arteries in the body, the walls of the arteries in the brain are thin and weak, causing them to be susceptible to aneurysms and strokes. The veins of the brain do not contain valves. This lack of valves allows the blood to flow in either direction, creating a route for blood-borne pathogens to pass from the body to the head and vice versa. The capillaries of the brain are unlike those elsewhere in the body in that they do not allow movement of certain molecules from their vascular compartment into the surrounding brain tissue. This unique quality of impermeability is termed the **blood-brain barrier (BBB).** The presence of a normal BBB prevents large amounts of contrast medium from entering the brain. Pathologic conditions can disrupt the integrity of the BBB, allowing contrast to escape from the vessel into the surrounding tissues.

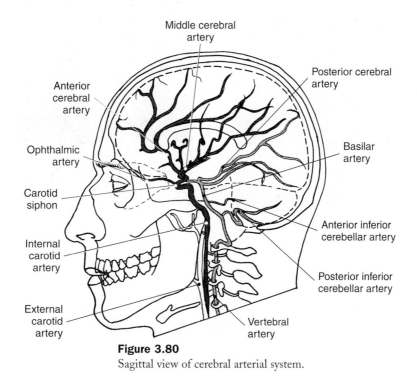

Figure 3.80
Sagittal view of cerebral arterial system.

Arterial Supply

The brain receives arterial blood from two main pair of vessels and their branches, the internal carotid arteries and the vertebral arteries. Many normal variations of the arterial blood supply exist. This section focuses on the most common anatomic findings visualized in cross section (Figures 3.80 and 3.81).

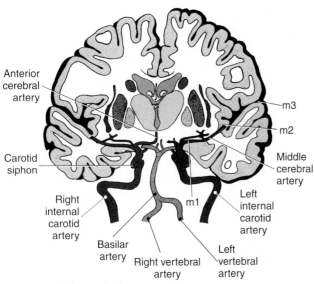

Figure 3.81
Coronal view of cerebral arterial system.

INTERNAL CAROTID ARTERIES The **internal carotid arteries** supply the frontal, parietal, and temporal lobes of the brain and orbital structures. These arteries arise from the bifurcation of the carotid arteries in the neck. They ascend through the base of the skull and enter the carotid canals of the temporal bones (Figures 3.82 and 3.83). The internal carotid artery then turns forward within the cavernous sinus, then up and backward through the dura mater, forming an S shape (which is referred to as the **carotid siphon**) before it reaches the base of the brain (Figures 3.80 and 3.84). As the internal carotid artery exits the cavernous sinus, it branches into the **ophthalmic artery** just inferior to the anterior clinoid process (Figure 3.80). The internal carotid artery then runs lateral to the optic chiasm and branches into the anterior cerebral artery and the larger middle cerebral artery. The **anterior cerebral artery** and its branches supply the anterior frontal lobe and the medial aspect of the parietal lobe (Figure 3.80). The main segments and branches of the anterior cerebral artery are the **horizontal (A1) segment** and the **A2 segment** (Figures 3.84 through 3.86). The horizontal segment extends from the internal carotid artery (ICA) bifurcation and branches into the **medial lenticulostriate arteries** and the **anterior communicating artery.** The medial lenticulostriate arteries supply the head of the caudate nucleus, the anterior limb of the internal capsule, and the anterior globus pallidus. The anterior communicating artery joins the two anterior cerebral arteries just anterior to the optic chiasm (Figure 3.86). The A2 segment

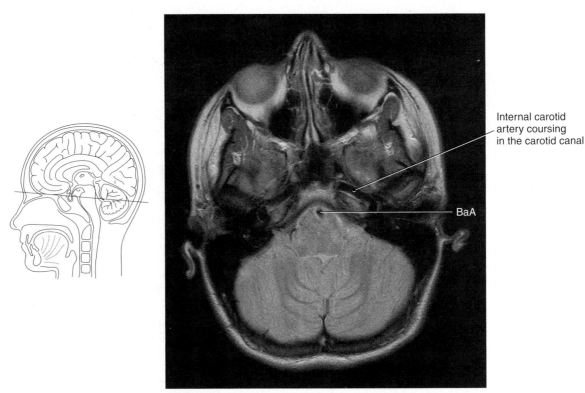

Figure 3.82
Axial, spin density–weighted MR scan with carotid canal.

extends from the anterior communicating artery to course around the genu of the corpus callosum. The major branches of the A2 segment are the **orbitofrontal, frontopolar, pericallosal, callosomarginal, and splenial arteries** (Figure 3.84). The **middle cerebral artery** is by far the largest of the cerebral arteries and is considered a direct continuation of the internal carotid artery. The middle cerebral artery gives off many branches, as it supplies much of the lateral surface of the cerebrum, insula, and anterior and lateral aspects of temporal lobe; nearly all the basal ganglia; and the posterior and anterior

KEY: car, Carotid canal; **BaA,** basilar artery; **EAM,** external auditory meatus; **IAC,** internal auditory canal.

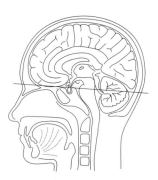

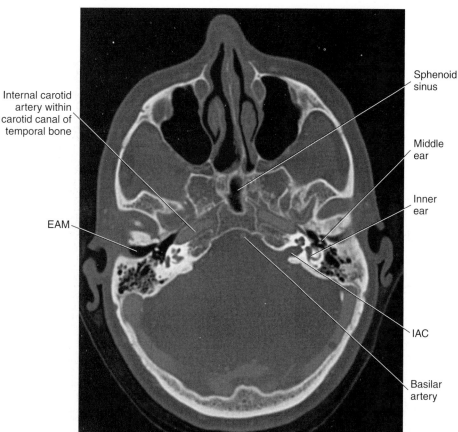

Figure 3.83
Axial CT scan with carotid canal.

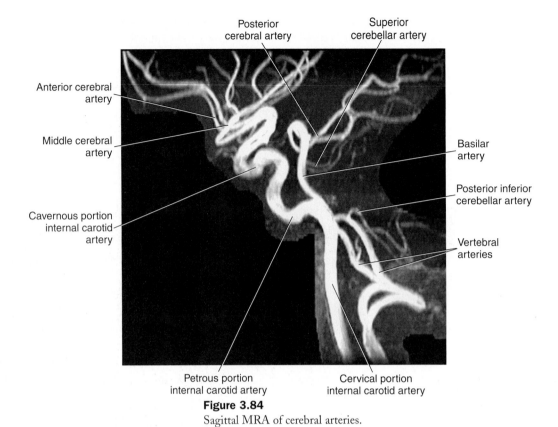

Posterior
cerebral artery

Superior
cerebellar artery

Anterior cerebral
artery

Middle cerebral
artery

Cavernous portion
internal carotid
artery

Basilar
artery

Posterior inferior
cerebellar artery

Vertebral
arteries

Petrous portion
internal carotid artery

Cervical portion
internal carotid artery

Figure 3.84
Sagittal MRA of cerebral arteries.

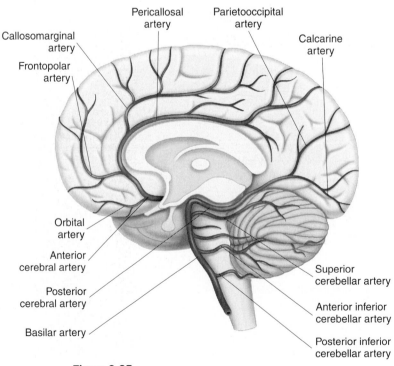

Pericallosal
artery

Parietooccipital
artery

Callosomarginal
artery

Calcarine
artery

Frontopolar
artery

Orbital
artery

Anterior
cerebral artery

Posterior
cerebral artery

Basilar artery

Superior
cerebellar artery

Anterior inferior
cerebellar artery

Posterior inferior
cerebellar artery

Figure 3.85
Sagittal view of anterior cerebral artery and branches.

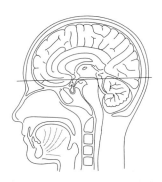

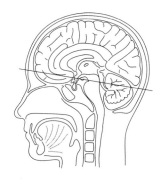

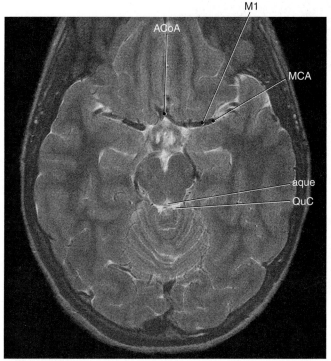

Figure 3.86
Axial, T2-weighted MR scan with anterior communicating and
middle cerebral arteries.

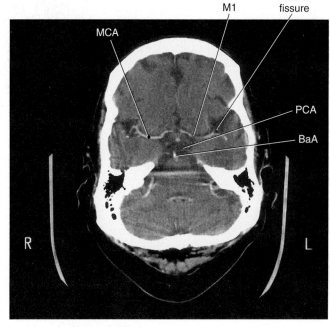

Figure 3.87
Axial CT scan with middle cerebral artery.

internal capsule (Figure 3.80). Three major segments of the
middle cerebral artery are the **horizontal (M1), insular (M2),
and opercular (M3).** The horizontal segment courses from the
origin at the internal carotid artery bifurcation laterally toward
the insula and branches into the **lateral lenticulostriate
arteries.** The insular segment courses along the insula, continuing as the opercular segment that emerges from the
Sylvian fissure at the Sylvian point to split into the superior
and inferior groups of the cortical branches that supply
nearly the entire convex surface of the cerebral hemispheres
(Figures 3.81, 3.86, and 3.87 and Table 3.1).

TABLE 3-1 Internal Carotid Artery Branches

ARTERY	REGION SUPPLIED
Ophthalmic artery	Globe, orbit, frontal scalp, frontal and ethmoid sinuses
Anterior cerebral artery (ACA)	Anterior frontal lobe and medial aspect of parietal lobe, head of caudate nucleus, anterior limb of the internal capsule, and anterior globus pallidus
Middle cerebral artery (MCA)	Lateral surface of the cerebrum, insula, anterior and lateral aspects of temporal lobe, nearly all the basal ganglia, and posterior and anterior internal capsules.

KEY: **MCA,** Middle cerebral artery; **PCA,** posterior cerebral artery; **BaA,** basilar artery; **ACoA,** anterior
communicating artery; **aque,** cerebral aqueduct; **QuC,** quadrigeminal cistern.

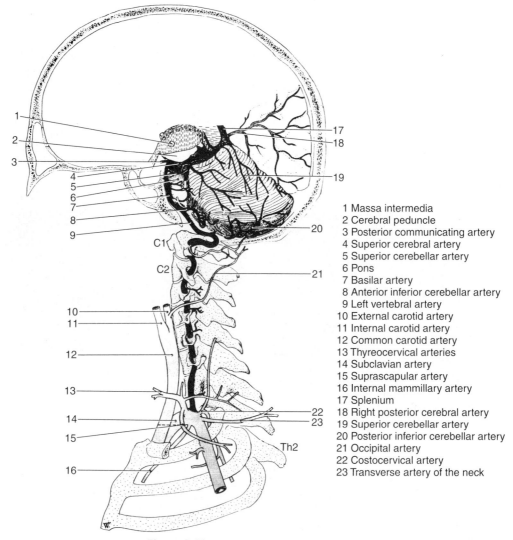

1 Massa intermedia
2 Cerebral peduncle
3 Posterior communicating artery
4 Superior cerebral artery
5 Superior cerebellar artery
6 Pons
7 Basilar artery
8 Anterior inferior cerebellar artery
9 Left vertebral artery
10 External carotid artery
11 Internal carotid artery
12 Common carotid artery
13 Thyreocervical arteries
14 Subclavian artery
15 Suprascapular artery
16 Internal mammillary artery
17 Splenium
18 Right posterior cerebral artery
19 Superior cerebellar artery
20 Posterior inferior cerebellar artery
21 Occipital artery
22 Costocervical artery
23 Transverse artery of the neck

Figure 3.88
Sagittal view of vertebrobasilar arterial system.

VERTEBRAL ARTERIES   The **vertebral arteries** begin in the neck at the subclavian artery and ascend vertically through the transverse foramina of the cervical spine. The vertebral arteries curve around the atlanto-occipital joints to enter the cranium through the foramen magnum (Figure 3.88). The two vertebral arteries course along the medulla oblongata and unite, ventral to the pons, to form the **basilar artery** (Figures 3.81 through 3.82, 3.89, and 3.90). The vertebral and basilar arteries give rise to several pairs of smaller arteries that supply the cerebellum, pons, and inferior and medial surfaces of the temporal and occipital lobes. The four major pairs of arteries are listed in order from inferior to superior: **posterior inferior cerebellar (PICA), anterior inferior cerebellar (AICA), superior cerebellar (SCA),** and **posterior cerebral (PCA)**

(Figures 3.90 through 3.93). Located between the anterior inferior cerebellar artery and superior cerebellar artery are many tiny perforating **pontine vessels. The posterior cerebral arteries** can be divided into three major segments: **precommunicating** or **peduncular (P1), ambient (P2),** and **quadrigeminal (P3)** (Figure 3.90). The precommunicating segment is a short segment that extends laterally from the basilar bifurcation to the posterior communicating artery (Figure 3.93). The **posterior communicating artery** forms a connection between the posterior cerebral artery and the internal carotid artery (Figures 3.94 and 3.95). The ambient segment courses in the ambient cistern from the junction of the posterior communicating artery and the posterior cerebral artery posteriorly around the midbrain, then continues as the quadrigeminal segment

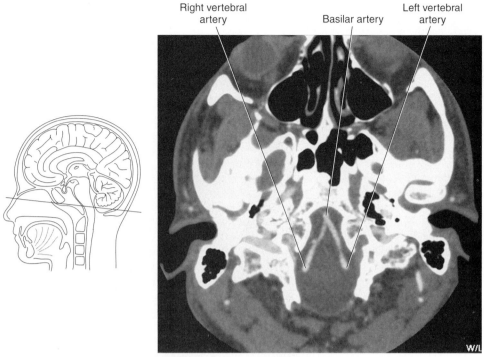

Figure 3.89
Axial CT scan of vertebral and basilar arteries.

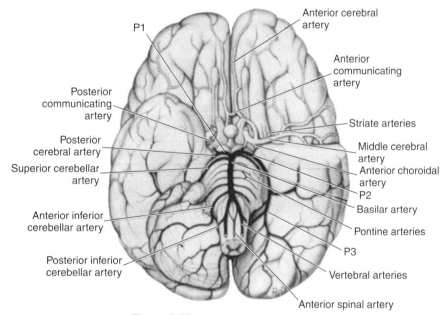

Figure 3.90
Inferior view of brain with basilar artery.

located within the quadrigeminal cistern (Figures 3.96 and 3.97). The quadrigeminal segment frequently divides in the form of a bifurcation or trifurcation to many branches, including several temporal and occipital arteries (Figures 3.96 and 3.97 and Table 3.2).

> AVMs are the most common type of congenital vascular malformation. They consist of a tangle of dilated arteries and veins, usually accompanied by arteriovenous shunting. Approximately 40% of individuals with AVMs will bleed by the age of 40 years.

Posterior   Superior cerebellar   Vertebral
cerebral arteries   artery   arteries

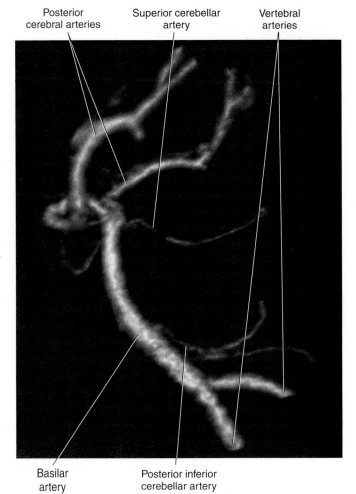

Basilar   Posterior inferior
artery   cerebellar artery

Figure 3.91
Sagittal CTA of vertebral and basilar arteries.

Right vertebral   Basilar artery   Left vertebral
artery   artery

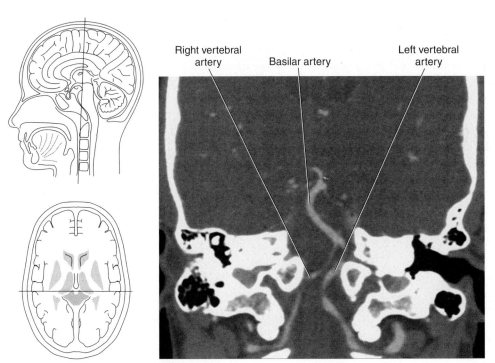

Figure 3.92
Coronal CT reformat of vertebral and basilar arteries.

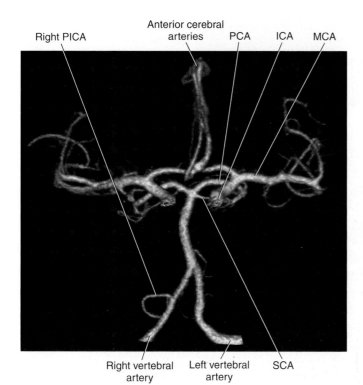

Right PICA

Anterior cerebral arteries   PCA   ICA   MCA

Right vertebral artery   Left vertebral artery   SCA

Figure 3.93
Coronal CTA of circle of Willis.

KEY: **PCA,** Posterior cerebral artery; **ICA,** internal carotid artery; **MCA,** middle cerebral artery; **SCA,** superior cerebellar artery; **ACA,** anterior cerebral artery; **ACoA,** anterior communicating artery; **PCoA,** posterior communicating artery.

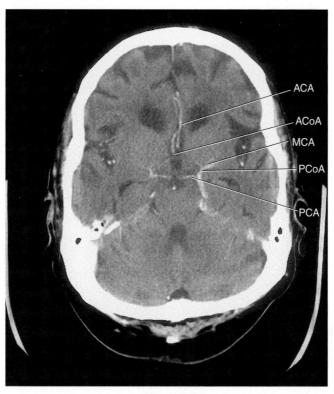

ACA

ACoA

MCA

PCoA

PCA

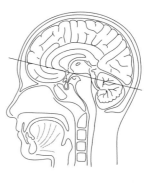

Figure 3.94
Axial CT scan with anterior cerebral artery.

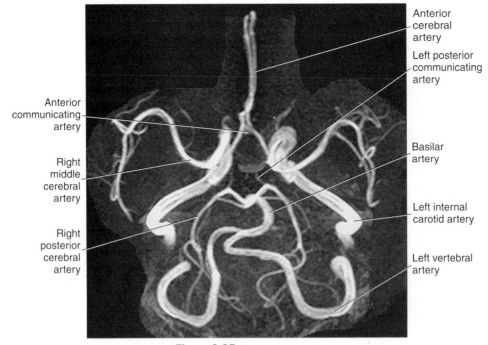

Figure 3.95
Axial MRA of circle of Willis.

KEY: SuC, Suprasellar cistern; **InC,** interpeduncular cistern; **AmC,** ambient cistern; **QuC,** quadrigeminal cistern.

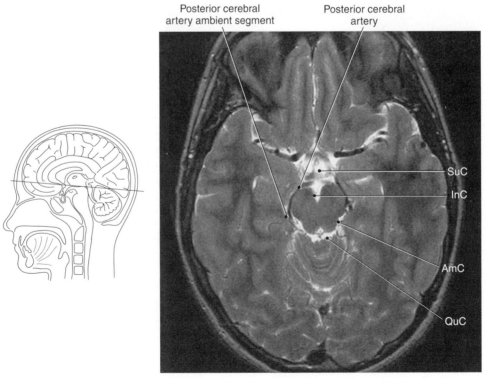

Figure 3.96
Axial, T2-weighted MR scan of middle and posterior cerebral arteries.

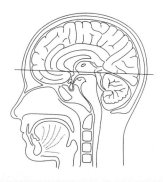

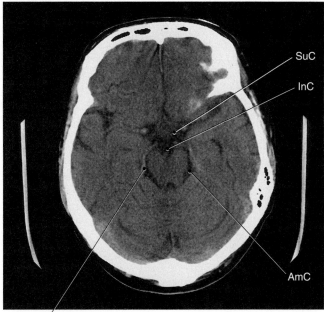

SuC

InC

AmC

Posterior cerebral
artery ambient segment

Figure 3.97
Axial CT scan of posterior cerebral arteries.

TABLE 3-2   **Vertebral and Basilar Artery Branches**

ARTERY	REGION SUPPLIED
Posterior inferior cerebellar (PICA)	Inferior cerebellum
Anterior inferior cerebellar (AICA)	Anterior and inferior cerebellum
Pontine vessels	Pons
Superior cerebellar (SCA)	Superior cerebellum and portions of midbrain and pons
Posterior cerebral artery (PCA)	Occipital and temporal lobes

Pathology involving the cerebrovascular system is the most common cause of cranial neurologic deficits. The brain needs a constant source of oxygen and glucose and is dependent on the vascular system to provide a steady supply. Any injury or disease affecting the cerebrovascular system can result in vascular insufficiency. Vascular interruptions lasting more than a few minutes will result in necrosis of adjacent brain tissue.

KEY: SuC, Suprasellar cistern; **InC,** interpeduncular cistern; **AmC,** ambient cistern.

CIRCLE OF WILLIS   The cerebral arterial circle, or **circle of Willis,** is a critically important anastomosis among the four major arteries (two vertebral and two internal carotid) feeding the brain. The circle of Willis is formed by the anterior and posterior cerebral, anterior and posterior communicating, and the internal carotid arteries. The circle is located mainly in the suprasellar cistern at the base of the brain. Many normal variations of this circle may occur in individuals. The circle of Willis functions as a means of collateral blood flow from one cerebral hemisphere to another in the event of blockage (Figures 3.93, 3.95, and 3.98).

VENOUS DRAINAGE   The venous system of the brain and its coverings is composed primarily of the dural sinuses, superficial cortical veins, and deep veins of the cerebrum.

Dural Sinuses

The **dural sinuses** are very large veins located within the dura mater of the brain. All the veins of the head drain into the dural sinuses and ultimately into the **internal jugular veins** of the neck. The major dural sinuses include superior and inferior sagittal, straight, transverse, sigmoid, cavernous, and petrosal (Figures 3.99 through 3.101). The **superior sagittal sinus** lies in the medial plane between the falx cerebri and the calvaria. It begins at the crista galli, runs the entire length of the falx cerebri, and ends at the internal occipital protuberance of the occipital bone (Figures 3.100 through 3.103). The **inferior sagittal sinus,** which is much smaller than the superior sagittal sinus, runs posteriorly just under the free edge of the falx cerebri (Figures 3.3 and 3.99). The inferior sagittal sinus

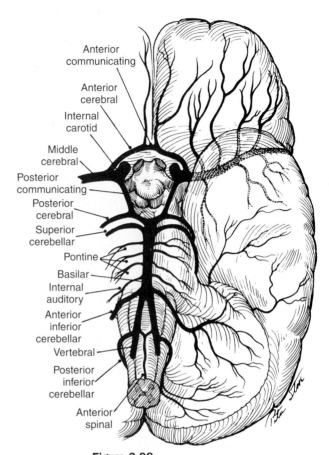

Figure 3.98
Inferior view of circle of Willis.

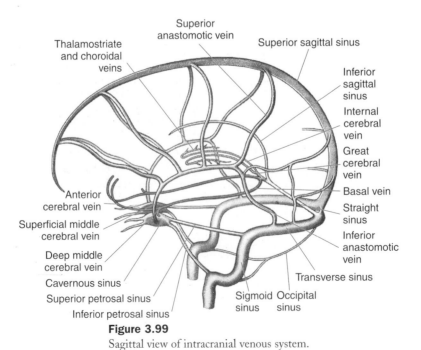

Figure 3.99
Sagittal view of intracranial venous system.

Great cerebral   Superior sagittal   Straight
vein   sinus   sinus

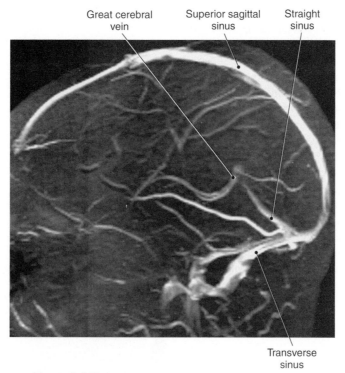

Transverse
sinus

Figure 3.100
Sagittal MR venography (MRV) of cerebral venous system.

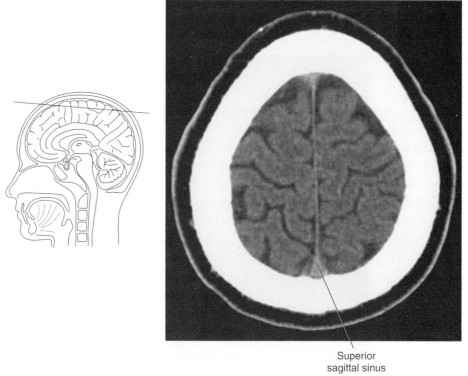

Superior
sagittal sinus

Figure 3.101
Axial CT scan with superior sagittal sinus.

converges with the great cerebral vein (vein of Galen) to form the **straight sinus.** The straight sinus extends along the length of the junction of the falx cerebri and the tentorium cerebelli (Figures 3.102 through 3.104). The junction of the superior sagittal, transverse, and straight sinuses creates the large **confluence of the sinuses** or the **torcular herophili** (Figures 3.104 and 3.105). The **transverse sinuses** extend from the confluence between the attachment of the tentorium and the calvaria. As the transverse sinuses pass through the tentorium cerebelli, they become the **sigmoid sinuses.** The S-shaped sigmoid sinuses continue in the posterior cranial fossa to join the jugular bulbs of the internal jugular veins (Figures 3.106 and 3.107).

The **cavernous sinuses,** located on each side of the sella and body of the sphenoid bone, are formed by numerous interconnected venous channels. They envelop the internal carotid arteries and several cranial nerves. Each cavernous sinus receives blood from the superior and inferior **ophthalmic veins** and communicates with the transverse sinuses by way of the **petrosal sinuses** (Figures 3.99, 3.108 through 3.112).

KEY: SSS, Superior sagittal sinus; **ICV,** internal cerebral vein; **Gal,** vein of Galen; **StS,** straight sinus; **ACA,** anterior cerebral artery.

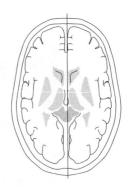

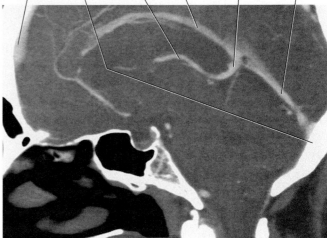

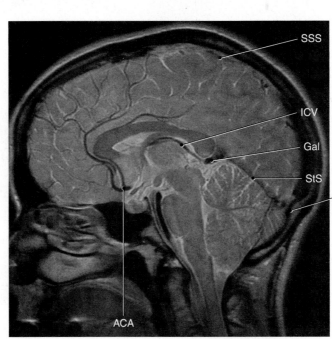

Superior sagittal sinus | Internal occipital protuberance | Internal cerebral vein | Interior sagittal sinus | Great cerebral vein (vein of Galen) | Straight sinus

Figure 3.102
Sagittal CT reformat of inferior sagittal and straight sinuses.

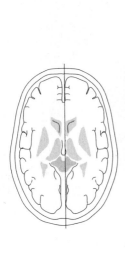

SSS

ICV

Gal

StS

Internal occipital protuberance

ACA

Figure 3.103
Midsagittal, spin density–weighted MR scan with internal cerebral vein.

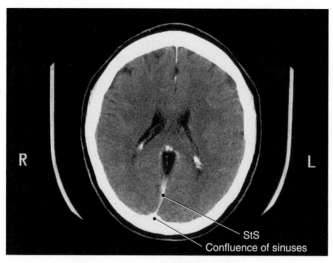
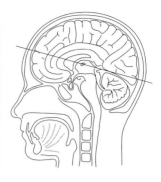

Figure 3.104
Axial CT scan of straight sinus.

StS
Confluence of sinuses

R   L

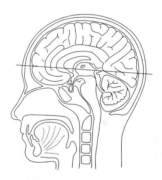

Superior sagittal sinus

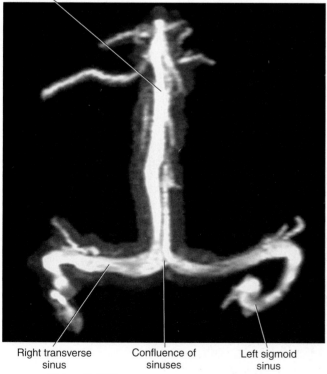

Right transverse sinus   Confluence of sinuses   Left sigmoid sinus

Figure 3.105
Axial MRA with transverse and sigmoid sinuses.

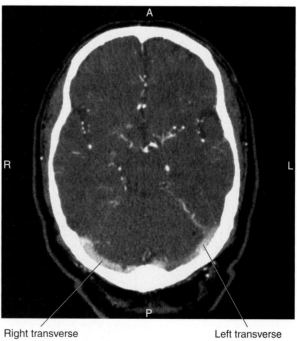

A

R   L

P

Right transverse sinus   Left transverse sinus

Figure 3.106
Axial CT scan of transverse sinus.

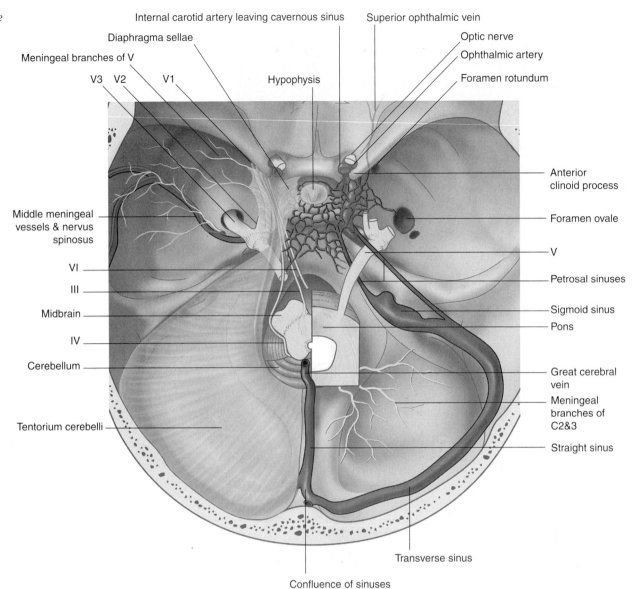

Internal carotid artery leaving cavernous sinus

Diaphragma sellae

Meningeal branches of V

V3 V2 V1

Hypophysis

Superior ophthalmic vein

Optic nerve

Ophthalmic artery

Foramen rotundum

Anterior clinoid process

Foramen ovale

V

Petrosal sinuses

Sigmoid sinus

Pons

Great cerebral vein

Meningeal branches of C2&3

Straight sinus

Middle meningeal vessels & nervus spinosus

VI

III

Midbrain

IV

Cerebellum

Tentorium cerebelli

Transverse sinus

Confluence of sinuses

Figure 3.107

Axial view of dural sinuses.

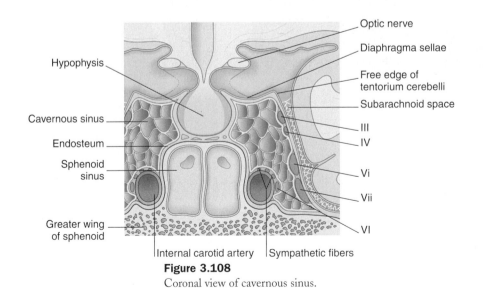

Hypophysis

Cavernous sinus

Endosteum

Sphenoid sinus

Greater wing of sphenoid

Optic nerve

Diaphragma sellae

Free edge of tentorium cerebelli

Subarachnoid space

III

IV

Vi

Vii

VI

Internal carotid artery   Sympathetic fibers

Figure 3.108

Coronal view of cavernous sinus.

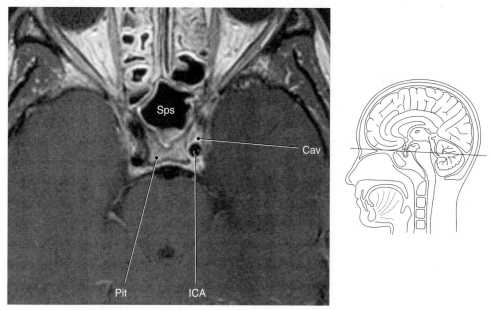

Figure 3.109
Axial, T1-weighted MR scan of cavernous sinus with contrast enhancement.

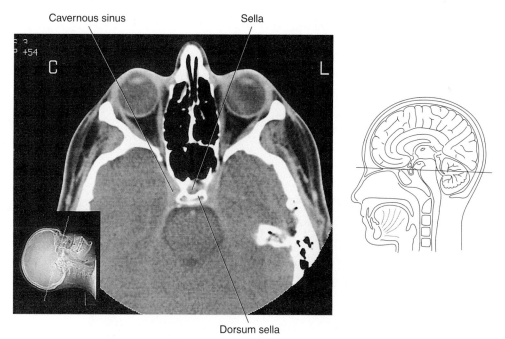

Figure 3.110
Axial CT scan of cavernous sinus with contrast enhancement.

KEY: Sps, Sphenoid sinus; **Cav,** cavernous sinus; **ICA,** internal carotid artery; **Pit,** pituitary gland.

144

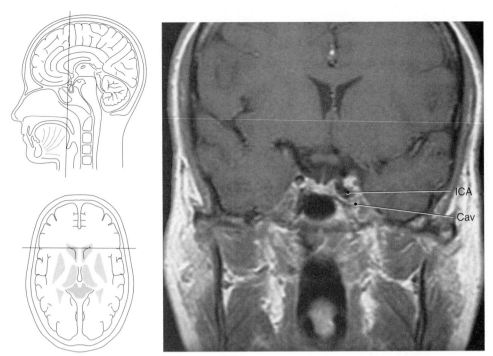

Figure 3.111
Coronal, T1-weighted MR scan of cavernous sinus with contrast enhancement.

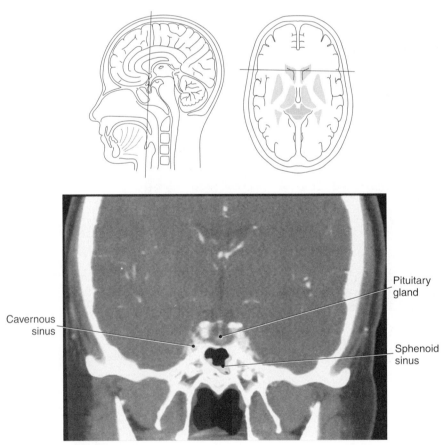

Figure 3.112
Coronal CT scan of cavernous sinus with contrast enhancement.

KEY: **ICA,** Internal carotid artery; **Cav,** cavernous sinus.

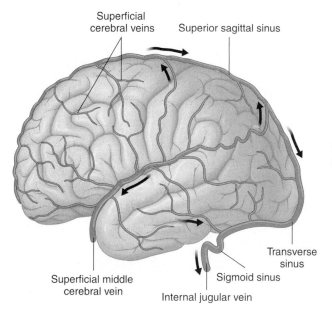

Superficial cerebral veins

Superior sagittal sinus

Superficial middle cerebral vein

Sigmoid sinus

Internal jugular vein

Transverse sinus

Figure 3.113
Sagittal view of superficial cortical veins.

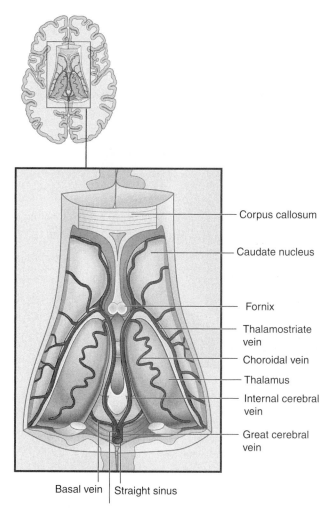

Corpus callosum

Caudate nucleus

Fornix

Thalamostriate vein

Choroidal vein

Thalamus

Internal cerebral vein

Great cerebral vein

Basal vein | Straight sinus

Entry point of inferior sagittal sinus

Figure 3.114
Superior view of deep cerebral veins.

Superficial Cortical and Deep Veins

The **superficial cortical veins** are located along the surface of each cerebral hemisphere and are responsible for draining the cerebral cortex and portions of the white matter. The veins drain into the dural sinuses with numerous anastomoses between the superficial and deep veins (Figure 3.113).

The **deep veins** of the cerebrum drain the white matter and include the thalamostriate, septal, internal cerebral, basal (vein of Rosenthal), and great cerebral vein (vein of Galen) (Figure 3.114). The **thalamostriate vein** runs in a groove between the thalamus and caudate nucleus, where it drains both structures. The **septal vein** runs posteriorly across the septum pellucidum and joins with the thalamostriate veins to create the paired internal cerebral veins at the inferior aspect of the foramen of Monro. The **basal vein of Rosenthal** drains the medial temporal lobe and basal nuclei as it curves posteriorly around the cerebral peduncle and quadrigeminal plate to join with the great cerebral vein. Each **internal cerebral vein** runs posteriorly beneath the third ventricle to meet with the paired basal veins beneath the corpus callosum to form a short trunk, the great cerebral vein. The unpaired **great cerebral vein (vein of Galen)** is a short midline vessel running between the splenium of the corpus callosum and pineal gland, where it joins with the inferior sagittal sinus to form the straight sinus. All cerebral venous output will eventually drain into one of the dural sinuses and ultimately into the internal jugular veins (Figures 3.115 through 3.118).

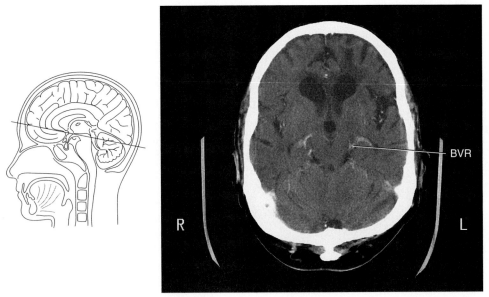

Figure 3.115
Axial CT scan of basal vein of Rosenthal.

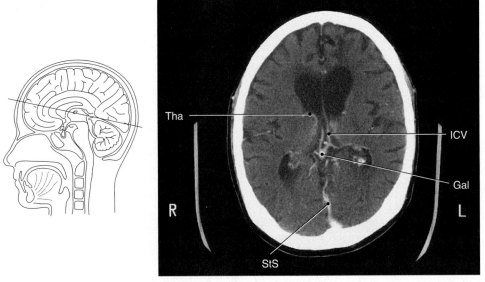

Figure 3.116
Axial CT scan of internal cerebral and thalamostriate veins.

KEY: **BVR,** Basal vein of Rosenthal; **Tha,** thalamostriate; **ICV,** internal cerebral vein; **Gal,** vein of Galen; **StS,** straight sinus.

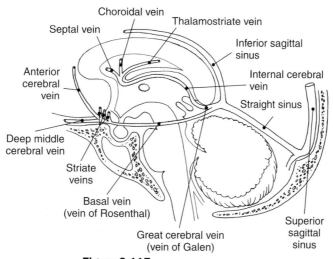

Figure 3.117
Sagittal view of deep cerebral veins.

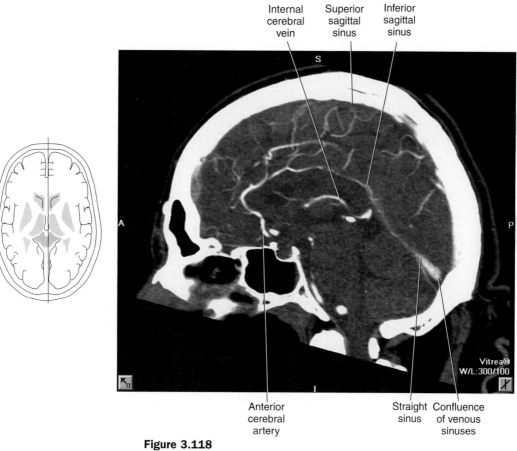

Figure 3.118
Sagittal CT reformat with deep cerebral veins.

CRANIAL NERVES

There are 12 cranial nerves (CNs), numbered from anterior to posterior according to their attachment to the brain. All but the first and second cranial nerves arise from the brain-stem (Figure 3.119). Each of these nerves corresponds to a specific function of the body (Table 3.3). It is important to recognize the adjacent brain structures that act as anatomic landmarks to localize the course of the cranial nerves in the head.

TABLE 3-3   Cranial Nerves

CRANIAL NERVES	TYPE	FORAMEN	FUNCTION
Olfactory (I)	Sensory	Olfactory foramina	Smell
Optic (II)	Sensory	Optic foramen	Vision
Oculomotor (III)	Motor	Superior orbital fissure	Eye movement
Trochlear (IV)	Motor	Superior orbital fissure	Eye movement
Trigeminal (V)	Mixed	Meckel's cave	
Ophthalmic (V_1)	Sensory	Superior orbital fissure	Orbital structures, nasal cavity, forehead
Maxillary (V_2)	Sensory	Foramen rotundum	Cheek, upper jaw, maxillary sinuses
Mandibular (V_3)	Mixed	Foramen ovale	Lower gums, muscles of mastication, tongue
Abducens (VI)	Motor	Superior orbital fissure	Eye movements
Facial (VII)	Mixed	Internal auditory canal, facial canal, stylomastoid foramen	Facial muscles, anterior two thirds of tongue
Vestibulocochlear (VIII)	Sensory	Internal auditory canal	Hearing, equilibrium
Glossopharyngeal (IX)	Mixed	Jugular foramen	Posterior third of tongue, monitors blood pressure, pharynx
Vagus (X)	Mixed	Jugular foramen	Pharynx, larynx, thoracic and abdominal viscera
Accessory (XI)	Motor	Jugular foramen	Pharynx, palate, larynx
Hypoglossal (XII)	Motor	Hypoglossal canal	Tongue muscles

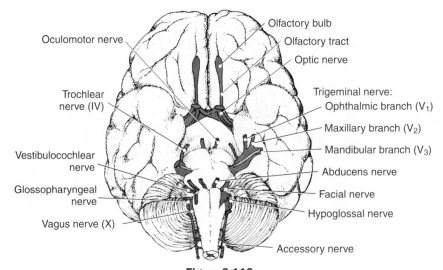

Figure 3.119

Inferior view of brain with cranial nerves.

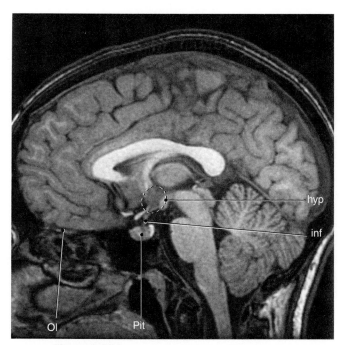

Figure 3.120
Sagittal view of olfactory nerve.

Olfactory Nerve (CN I)

The **olfactory nerve** is the nerve of smell. The olfactory neurosensory cells are located in the covering of the superior nasal concha and the superior part of the nasal septum. The axons of these cells unite to form 18 to 20 small nerve bundles that are known collectively as *olfactory nerve fibers*. The nerve fibers pass through the olfactory foramina in the cribriform plate of the ethmoid bone to synapse with the olfactory bulb in the anterior cranial fossa. The right and left olfactory tracts extend from the olfactory bulbs and run along the inferior surface of the frontal lobes to pass to the lateral hippocampal gyrus and interact with the limbic system (Figures 3.120 through 3.122). Each olfactory nerve is surrounded by the three layers of the cranial meninges.

KEY: **hyp,** Hypothalamus; **inf,** infundibulum; **Pit,** pituitary gland; **Ol,** olfactory nerve.

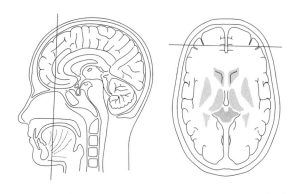

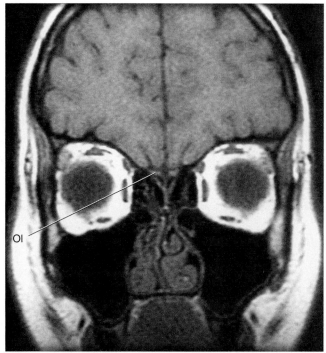

Figure 3.121
Sagittal, T1-weighted MR scan of olfactory nerve.

Figure 3.122
Coronal, T1-weighted MR scan of olfactory tracts.

Damage to the visual system will result in visual losses related to the location of the damage. If the optic nerve is damaged anterior to the optic chiasm, the result will be loss of vision in that eye. At the optic chiasm, damage on the medial aspect will result in loss of peripheral vision, whereas damage on the lateral aspect results in loss of the ipsilateral central (nasal) visual field. If damage occurs posterior to the optic chiasm, the result will be loss of input from the contralateral visual fields of both eyes.

KEY: **OpN,** Optic nerve; **Pit,** pituitary gland.

Optic Nerve (CN II)

The **optic nerve** is the nerve of sight. Sensory nerve cells arise from the retina and converge toward the posterior aspect of the eye. These fibers unite to form the large optic nerve that passes posteromedially through the optic canal into the middle cranial fossa to join its partner at the optic chiasm just anterior to the pituitary stalk. In the optic chiasm, the fibers from the medial side of the retina cross to the opposite side, and the fibers from the lateral aspect remain on the same side (Figures 3.123 through 3.125). This decussation of the medial fibers allows for binocular vision. Posterior to the optic chiasm, the optic nerve extends as optic tracts that continue around the midbrain and terminate in the lateral geniculate bodies of the thalamus. The optic pathway continues posteriorly from the thalamus as nerve axons forming **optic radiations** that are relayed to the visual cortex (Figures 3.125 and 3.126).

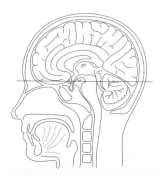

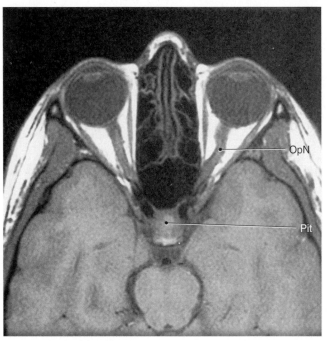

Figure 3.123
Axial, T1-weighted MR scan of optic nerves.

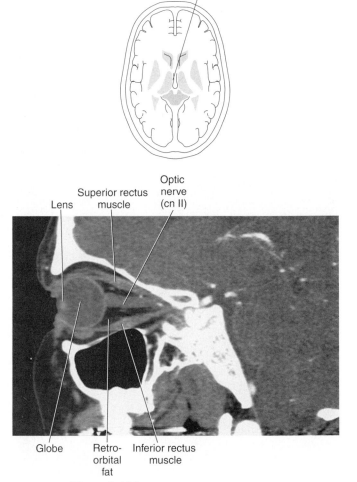

Figure 3.124
Sagittal oblique CT reformat of optic nerve.

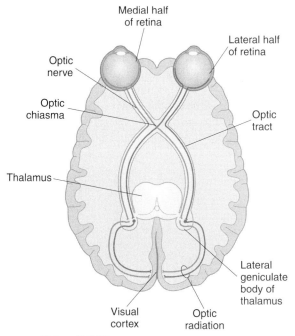

Figure 3.125
Axial view of optic tract and optic radiations.

KEY: **Gal,** vein of Galen; **OpR,** optic radiations.

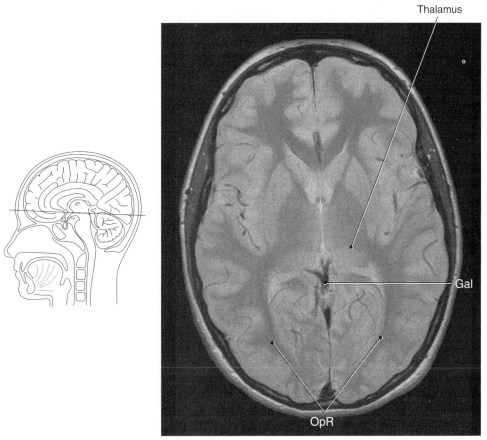

Figure 3.126
Axial, spin density–weighted MR scan with optic radiations.

152   **CHAPTER** 3

Oculomotor Nerve (CN III)

The **oculomotor nerve** moves the eye by supplying fibers to all extraocular muscles of the eye except the superior oblique and lateral rectus muscles. This nerve emerges from the midbrain and passes anteriorly into the interpeduncular cistern. It runs lateral to the posterior communicating artery through the roof of the cavernous sinus and travels in the lateral wall superolateral to the internal carotid artery. The nerve enters the orbit through the superior orbital fissure and then breaks into superior and inferior branches that innervate the superior, medial, and inferior rectus muscles, as well as the inferior oblique and levator palpebrae muscles (Figures 3.127 through 3.129).

Trochlear Nerve (CN IV)

The **trochlear nerve** innervates only the superior oblique muscle of the eye. It is the only cranial nerve that emerges from the posterior surface of the brainstem. The nerve originates in the tegmentum of the midbrain, exits the posterior surface of the midbrain, and travels around the brainstem to enter the cavernous sinus just below the oculomotor nerve. This nerve enters the orbit through the superior orbital fissure, where it finally reaches the superior oblique muscle (Figures 3.127 through 3.129).

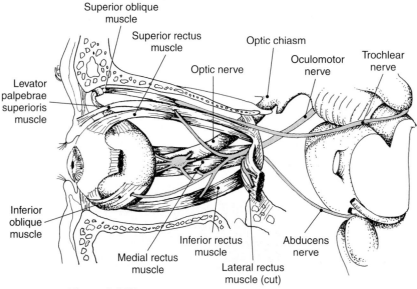

Figure 3.127
Sagittal view of oculomotor, trochlear, and abducens nerves.

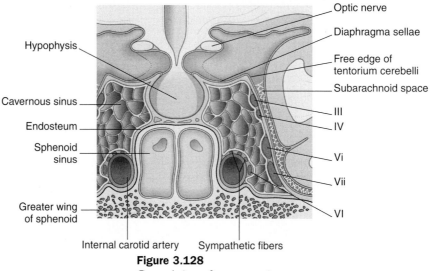

Figure 3.128
Coronal view of cavernous sinus.

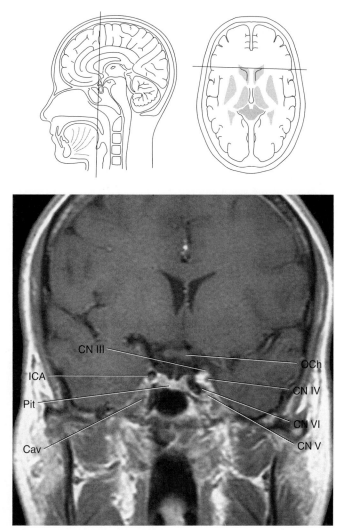

Figure 3.129
Coronal, T1-weighted MR scan of oculomotor and trochlear nerves in cavernous sinus with contrast enhancement.

KEY: **CN III,** Oculomotor nerve; **ICA,** internal carotid artery; **Pit,** pituitary gland; **Cav,** cavernous sinus; **OCh,** optic chiasm; **CN IV,** trochlear nerve; **CN VI,** abducens nerve; **CN V,** trigeminal nerve.

Trigeminal Nerve (CN V)

The **trigeminal nerve,** the largest of the cranial nerves, has three major divisions: ophthalmic, maxillary, and mandibular (Figure 3.130). It is the major sensory nerve of the face and contains motor fibers for the muscles of mastication and sensory fibers from the head. The nerve exits the brain between the pons and the middle cerebellar peduncles. Before trifurcating into three branches, the nerve enters Meckel's cave and forms the gasserian ganglia, where it is covered in dura, resulting in a CSF-filled subarachnoid space referred to as the trigeminal cistern (Figure 3.131). The **ophthalmic branch (V₁)** runs through the lateral wall of the cavernous sinus and enters the orbit through the superior orbital fissure, where it branches again to provide sensation to the lacrimal apparatus, cornea, iris, forehead, ethmoid and frontal sinuses, and nose. The **maxillary branch (V₂)** courses in the lateral wall of the cavernous sinus then exits the skull through the foramen rotundum. Branches of the maxillary nerve continue through the inferior orbital fissure and infraorbital foramen. This branch provides sensation to the cheek, sides of the nose and upper jaw, and maxillary sinuses. The **mandibular branch (V₃)** is considered a "motor" nerve and exits the skull through the foramen ovale. It innervates the muscles of mastication, ear canal, lower jaw and teeth, parotid and sublingual glands, and anterior two thirds of the tongue (Figures 3.131 through 3.133).

Abducens Nerve (CN VI)

The **abducens nerve** supplies motor impulses to the lateral rectus muscle of the eye. It originates near the midline of the lower portion of the pons and ascends through the prepontine cistern to the cavernous sinus. Of all the cranial nerves within the cavernous sinus, the abducens nerve courses most medial. It exits the skull through the superior orbital fissure, where it meets up with the lateral rectus muscle (Figures 3.127 through 3.129).

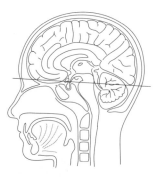

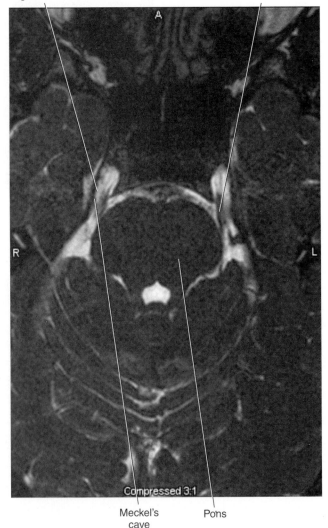

Figure 3.131
Axial, T2-weighted MR scan of trigeminal nerve.

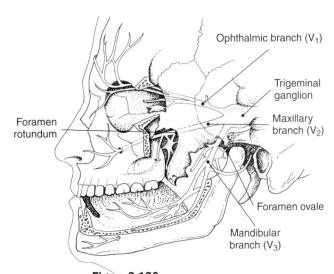

Figure 3.130
Sagittal view of trigeminal nerve.

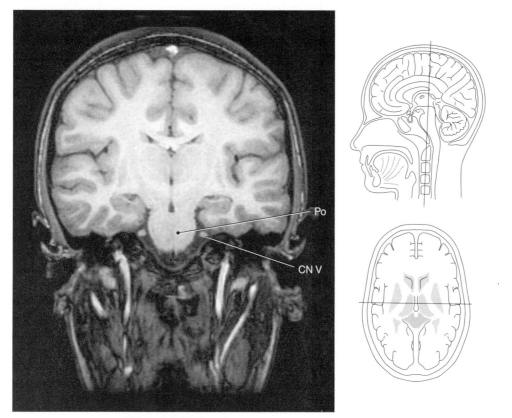

Figure 3.132
Coronal, T1-weighted MR scan of trigeminal nerve.

KEY: **Po,** Pons; **CN V,** trigeminal nerve.

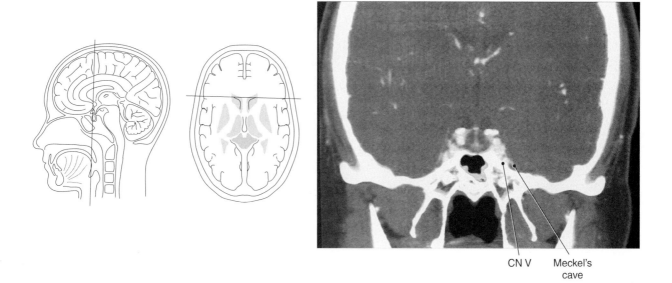

Figure 3.133
Coronal CT scan of Meckel's cave.

Facial Nerve (CN VII)

The **facial nerve** emerges as two distinct roots from the lower portion of the pons in a recess between the olive and inferior cerebellar peduncle and enters the internal auditory canal of the temporal bone. After passing through the temporal bone, the nerve continues along the facial canal, where it finally emerges from the skull through the stylomastoid foramen and runs through the parotid gland. This nerve innervates the facial muscles, lacrimal gland, and sublingual and submandibular glands. In addition, it provides taste sensation to the anterior two thirds of the tongue (Figures 3.134 through 3.138).

Vestibulocochlear Nerve (CN VIII)

The **vestibulocochlear nerve** exits the brainstem at the ponto-medullary junction and enters the internal auditory canal behind the facial nerve. The vestibulocochlear nerve has two distinct components, vestibular and cochlear. The **vestibular branch** picks up impulses from the semicircular canals that aid in the maintenance of equilibrium. The **cochlear branch** receives impulses from the cochlea and separates these impulses into high and low frequencies for the interpretation of sound (Figures 3.135 through 3.138).

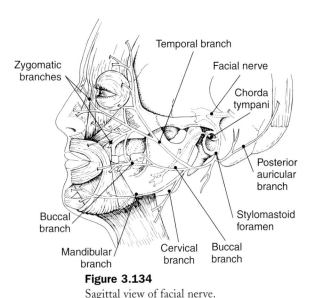

Figure 3.134
Sagittal view of facial nerve.

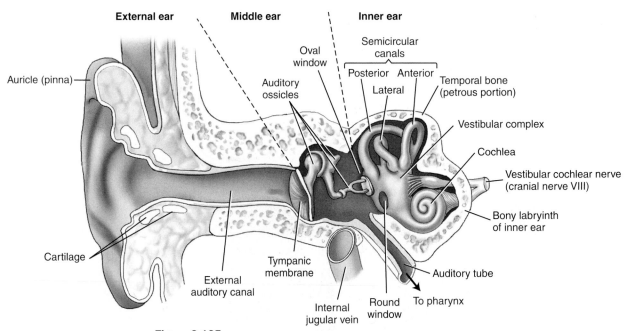

Figure 3.135
Coronal view of facial and vestibulocochlear nerves within inner ear.

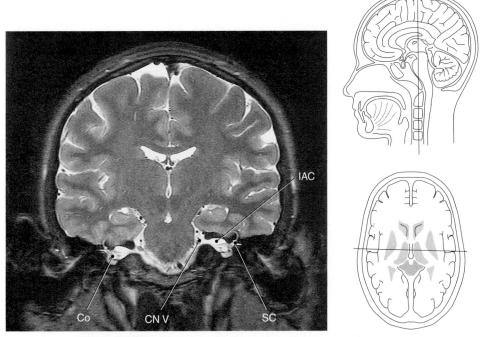

Figure 3.136
Coronal, T2-weighted MR scan of facial and vestibulocochlear nerves.

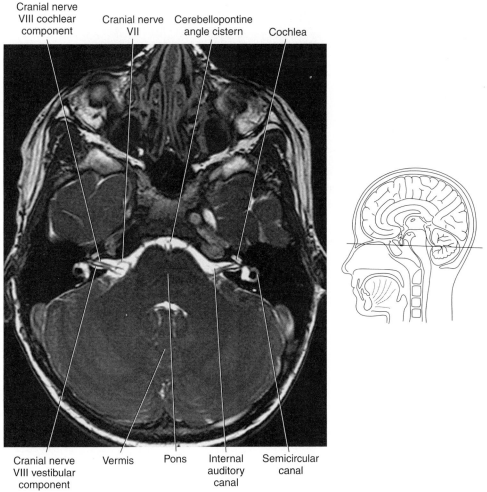

Figure 3.137
Axial, T2-weighted MR scan of facial and vestibulocochlear nerves.

KEY: IAC, Internal auditory canal; **SC,** semicircular canals; **CN V,** trigeminal nerve; **Co,** cochlea.

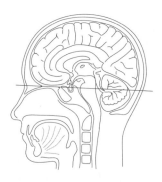

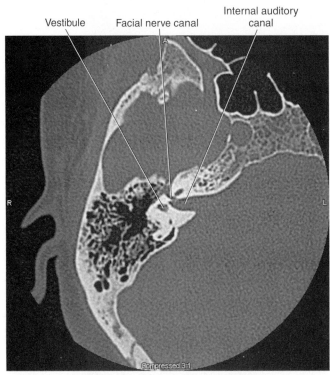

Vestibule   Facial nerve canal   Internal auditory canal

Figure 3.138
Axial CT scan of internal auditory canal.

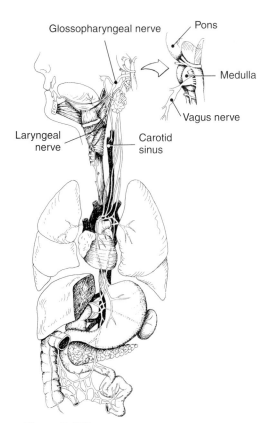

Figure 3.139
Sagittal view of glossopharyngeal and vagus nerves.

Glossopharyngeal Nerve (CN IX)

The **glossopharyngeal nerve** supplies motor impulses to the muscles involved in swallowing. In addition, its sensory component can be divided into three groups: Group 1 innervates the posterior third of the tongue, group 2 provides sensory input of pain and temperature from the middle ear, and group 3 gathers sensory input from the carotid sinus and carotid body, which help control blood pressure and respiration, respectively. The glossopharyngeal nerve emerges as a series of rootlets from the medulla oblongata between the olive and inferior cerebellar peduncles. It exits the cranium through the jugular foramen and courses to the root of the tongue (Figures 3.139 and 3.140).

KEY: ol, Olive; **JF,** jugular foramen; **CN IX,** glossopharyngeal nerve; **CN X,** vagus nerve.

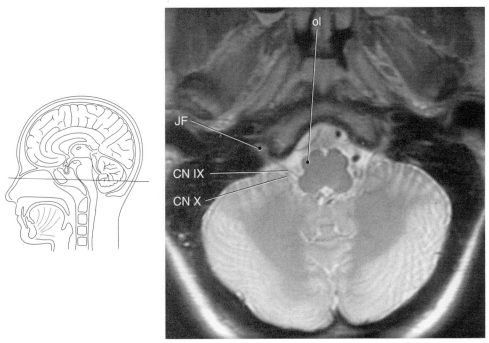

Figure 3.140
Axial, T2-weighted MR scan of jugular foramen and glossopharyngeal and vagus nerves.

Vagus Nerve (CN X)

In Latin, *vagus* means wandering, which the **vagus nerve** does as it "wanders" inferiorly from the brainstem to the splenic flexure in the abdomen. The vagus nerve covers an extensive course to supply areas of the neck, thorax, and abdomen. The vagus nerve arises from the medulla oblongata as 8 to 10 roots between the inferior cerebellar peduncle and the olive eventually converging into two roots that exit the skull through the jugular foramen. It descends through the carotid sheath while in the neck and continues inferiorly to the thorax and abdomen. At the neck, it passes through the superior thoracic aperture between the subclavian artery and brachiocephalic vein, where it continues its course toward the diaphragm behind the respective main bronchi. There are many branches of the vagus nerve that supply such structures as the dura of the posterior fossa, auricle, external auditory meatus, pharynx, soft palate, larynx, heart, stomach, liver, duodenum, and pancreas (Figures 3.139 and 3.140).

Accessory Nerve (CN XI)

The **accessory nerve** has both cranial and spinal roots. These two roots form a common stem before their exit through the jugular foramen. The **cranial root,** an accessory to the vagus nerve, emerges from a series of rootlets arising from the medulla oblongata. These fibers supply the skeletal muscles of the pharynx and palate. The **spinal root** arises from a series of rootlets from the lateral cervical cord to innervate the sternomastoid and trapezius muscles in the neck and back (Figures 3.141 and 3.142).

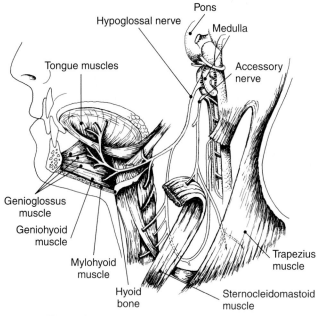

Figure 3.141
Sagittal view of accessory and hypoglossal nerves.

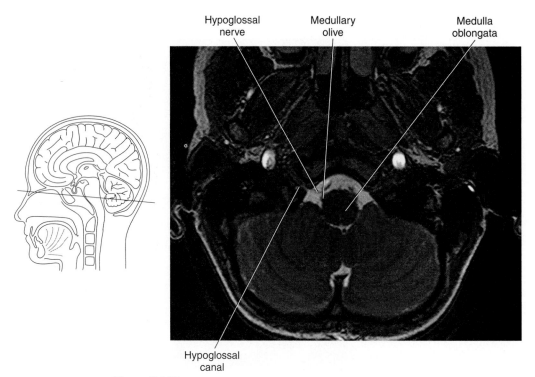

Figure 3.142
Axial, T2-weighted MR scan of accessory and hypoglossal nerves.

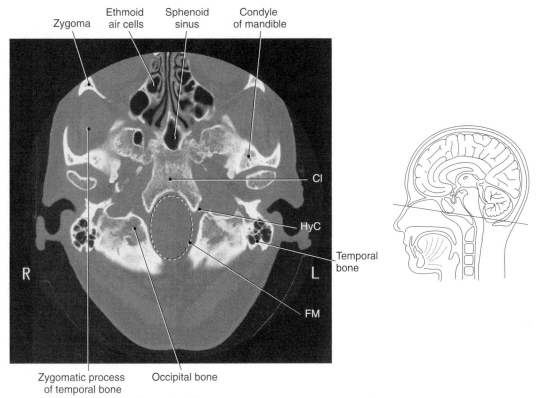

Figure 3.143
Axial CT scan of occipital condyles and hypoglossal canal.

Hypoglossal Nerve (CN XII)

All of the muscles of the tongue with the exception of one are supplied by the **hypoglossal nerve.** Several rootlets arise from the medulla oblongata between the olive and the pyramids. The rootlets unite to form a trunk that passes posterior to the vertebral artery to exit the cranium through the hypoglossal canal of the occipital bone. Inferior to the skull, the hypoglossal nerve crosses lateral to the bifurcation of the common carotid artery to enter the floor of the mouth and innervate the muscles of the tongue (Figures 3.141 through 3.143).

KEY: **CI,** Clivus; **HyC,** hypoglossal canal; **FM,** foramen magnum.

REFERENCES

Agur AM: *Grant's atlas of anatomy,* Baltimore, 1996, Williams & Wilkins.

Ballinger PW: *Merrill's atlas of radiographic positions and radiologic procedures,* St. Louis, 1986, Mosby.

Harnsberger HR: *Handbook of head and neck imaging,* ed 2, St. Louis, 1995, Mosby.

Hayman LA: *Clinical brain imaging: normal structure and functional anatomy,* St. Louis, 1992, Mosby.

Hendelman WJ: *Student's atlas of neuroanatomy,* Philadelphia, 1994, Saunders.

Leblanc A: *Atlas of hearing and balance organs,* New York, 1999, Springer-Verlag.

Mancuso AA: *Workbook for MRI and CT of the head and neck,* ed 2, Baltimore, 1989, Williams & Wilkins.

Martini FH: *Fundamentals of anatomy and physiology,* ed 3, Englewood Cliffs, NJ, 1995, Prentice-Hall.

Osborn AG: *Diagnostic neuroradiology,* St. Louis, 1994, Mosby.

Osborn AG, Tong KA: *Handbook of neuroradiology: brain and skull,* ed 2, St. Louis, 1996, Mosby.

Som PM, Curtin HD: *Head and neck imaging,* ed 3, St. Louis, Mosby, 1996.

Standring S: *Gray's anatomy,* ed 39, Philadelphia, 2005, Churchill Livingstone.

Taveras JM: *Neuroradiology,* ed 3, Baltimore, 1996, Williams & Wilkins.

Valvassori GE, Mahmood FM, Carter BL: *Imaging of the head and neck,* New York, 1995, Thieme Medical Publishers.

Warner JJ: *Atlas of neuroanatomy: with systems organization and case correlations,* Philadelphia, 2001, Butterworth-Heinemann.

CHAPTER 4

SPINE

When you suffer an attack of nerves you're being attacked by the nervous system. What chance has a man got against a system?

RUSSELL HOBAN (1925-)
American writer and illustrator

The spine functions to protect the delicate sensory and motor nerves that allow for peripheral sensations and body movement. Sensory or neurologic loss can be a result of injury or pathologic abnormalities of any of the many areas that compose the normal anatomy of this region (Figure 4.1).

VERTEBRAL COLUMN
   Cervical Vertebrae
   Thoracic Vertebrae
   Lumbar Vertebrae
   Sacrum and Coccyx

LIGAMENTS

MUSCLES
   Superficial Layer
   Intermediate Layer
   Deep Layer

SPINAL CORD
   Spinal Meninges
   Spinal Cord and Nerve Roots

PLEXUSES
   Cervical Plexus
   Brachial Plexus
   Lumbar Plexus
   Sacral Plexus

VASCULATURE
   Spinal Arteries
   Spinal Veins

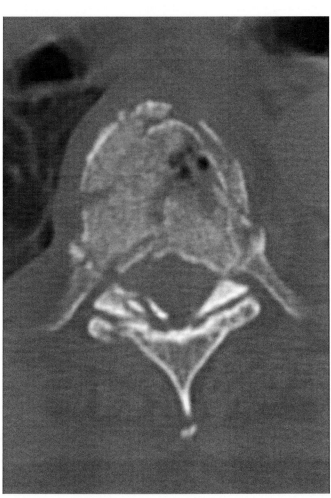

Figure 4.1
Fracture of T-5 body and vertebral arch.

VERTEBRAL COLUMN

The **vertebral column** is a remarkable structure that supports the weight of the body, helps to maintain posture, and protects the delicate spinal cord and nerves. It is made up of 33 vertebrae, which can be separated into cervical, thoracic, lumbar, sacral, and coccygeal sections. Curvatures associated with the vertebral column provide spinal flexibility and distribute compressive forces over the spine. The cervical and lumbar sections convex forward, creating lordotic curves, and the thoracic and sacral sections convex backward, creating kyphotic curves (Figure 4.2).

Vertebrae vary in size and shape from section to section, but a typical vertebra consists of two main parts: the **body (anterior element)** and the **vertebral arch (posterior element)**. The cylindric body is located anteriorly and functions to support body weight (Figures 4.3 and 4.4). The size of the vertebral bodies progressively increases from the superior portion of the vertebral column to the inferior portion of the spine. The compact bone on the superior and inferior surfaces of the body is called the **vertebral end plates.** Located posteriorly is the ringlike arch that attaches to the sides of the body, creating a space called the **vertebral foramen.** The succession of the vertebral foramina forms the **vertebral canal,** which contains and protects the spinal cord. The vertebral arch is formed by pedicles (2), laminae (2), spinous process (1), transverse processes (2), and superior (2) and inferior (2) articular processes (Figures 4.3 through 4.5). The two **pedicles** project from the body to meet with two **laminae** that continue posteriorly and medially to form a **spinous process.** The **transverse processes** project laterally from the approximate junction of the pedicle and lamina (Figures 4.3 and 4.4). On the upper and lower surfaces of the pedicles is a concave surface termed the **vertebral notch** (Figure 4.5). When the superior and inferior notches of adjacent vertebrae meet, they form **intervertebral foramina,** which allow for the transmission of spinal nerves

Figure 4.2
Sagittal view of the spine.

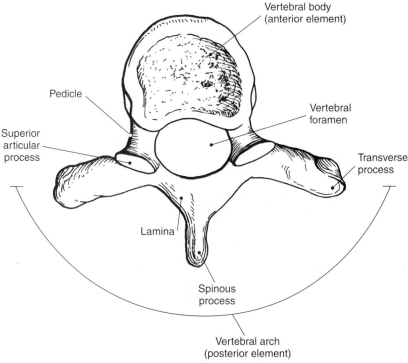

Figure 4.3
Superior view of the typical vertebra.

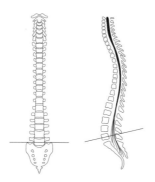

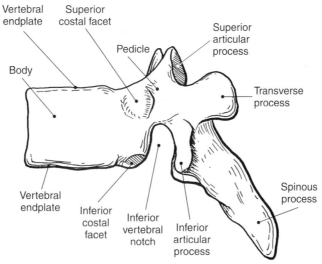

Figure 4.4
Axial CT scan of lumbar vertebra.

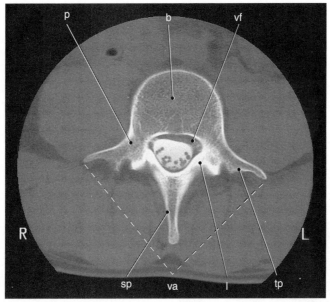

Figure 4.5
Sagittal view of thoracic vertebra.

KEY: p, Pedicle; **b,** body; **vf,** vertebral foramen or canal; **sp,** spinous process; **va,** vertebral arch; **l,** lamina; **tp,** transverse process.

and blood vessels (Figure 4.6). Four **articular processes,** two superior and two inferior, arise from the junctions of the pedicles and laminae to articulate with adjacent vertebrae to form the **zygapophyseal joints (facet joints).** These joints give additional support and allow movement of the vertebral column (Figures 4.7 through 4.10). The vertebral bodies are separated by shock-absorbing cartilaginous **intervertebral disks.** These disks consist of a central mass of soft semigelatinous material called the **nucleus pulposus** and a firm outer portion termed the **annulus fibrosus** (Figures 4.9 through 4.12).

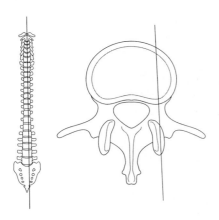

KEY: iarp, Inferior articular process; **d,** disk; **b,** body; **sarp,** superior articular process.

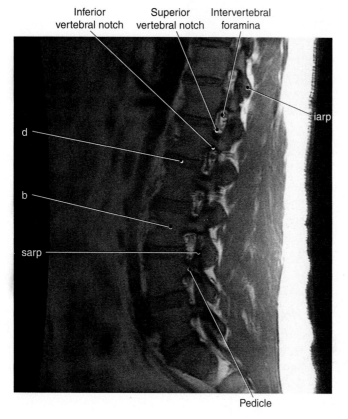

Inferior vertebral notch   Superior vertebral notch   Intervertebral foramina

iarp

d

b

sarp

Pedicle

Figure 4.6
Sagittal, T1-weighted MR scan of lumbar vertebrae.

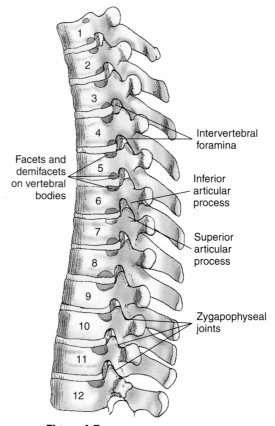

Intervertebral foramina

Facets and demifacets on vertebral bodies

Inferior articular process

Superior articular process

Zygapophyseal joints

Figure 4.7
Sagittal oblique view of thoracic spine.

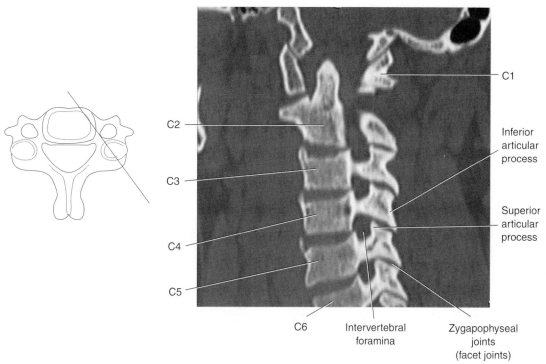

Figure 4.8
Sagittal oblique CT reformat of cervical spine with zygopophyseal joints.

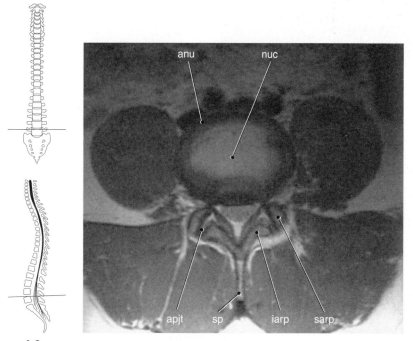

Figure 4.9
Axial, T1-weighted MR scan of lumbar spine with intervertebral disk and zygapophyseal joint.

KEY: anu, Annulus fibrosus; **nuc,** nucleus pulposus; **apjt,** apophyseal joint; **sp,** spinous process; **iarp,** inferior articular process; **sarp,** superior articular process.

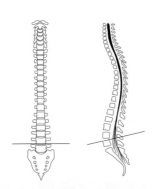

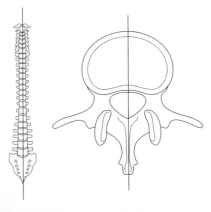

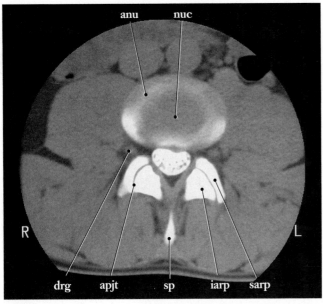

Figure 4.10
Axial CT scan of lumbar spine with intervertebral disk and zygapophyseal joint.

KEY: anu, Annulus fibrosus; **nuc,** nucleus pulposus; **drg,** dorsal root ganglion; **apjt,** apophyseal joint; **sp,** spinous process; **iarp,** inferior articular process; **sarp,** superior articular process.

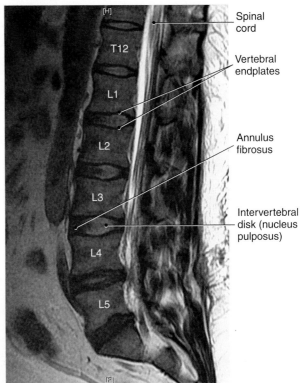

Figure 4.12
Sagittal, T2-weighted MR scan of intervertebral disk.

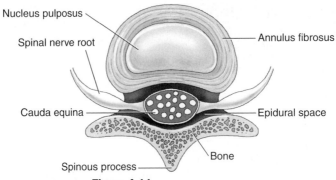

Figure 4.11
Axial view of intervertebral disk.

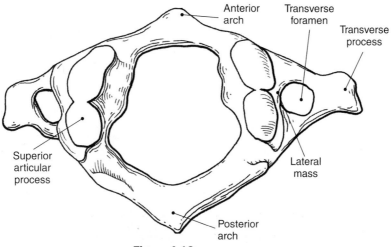

Figure 4.13
Superior view of C1 (atlas).

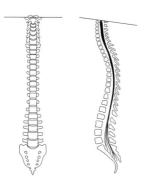

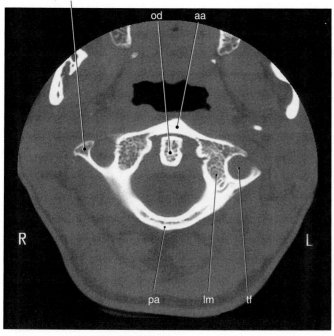

Figure 4.14
Axial CT scan of C1 (atlas).

Cervical Vertebrae

There are seven cervical vertebrae that vary in size and shape to a large degree. Within the transverse process of each cervical vertebra is a **transverse foramen.** These foramina allow passage of the vertebral vessels as they ascend to and descend from the head. The **first cervical vertebra** is termed the **atlas** because it supports the head; its large **superior articular processes** articulate with the occipital condyles of the head to form the **atlantooccipital joint.** The atlas is a ringlike structure that has no body and no spinous process. It consists of an **anterior arch, posterior arch,** and two large **lateral masses** (Figures 4.13 through 4.15). The lateral masses provide the only weight-bearing articulation between the cranium and vertebral column.

The **second cervical vertebra,** the **axis,** has a large **odontoid process (dens)** that projects upward from the superior surface of the body. The odontoid process projects into the anterior ring of the atlas to act as a pivot for rotational movement of the atlas (Figures 4.16 through 4.18). Lateral to the odontoid process on the upper surface of the body are the **superior articular processes,** on which the atlas articulates (Figures 4.19 and 4.20). The spinous process of the axis is the first projection to be felt in the posterior groove of the neck. The cervical vertebrae C3-C6 have a unique configuration with their **bifid spinous process** (Figures 4.21 and 4.22). The seventh cervical vertebra **(vertebra prominens)** has a long spinous process that is typically not bifid. This spinous process is easily palpable posteriorly at the base of the neck (Figures 4.23 through 4.25).

KEY: od, Odontoid process; **aa,** anterior arch; **pa,** posterior arch; **lm,** lateral mass; **tf,** transverse foramen.

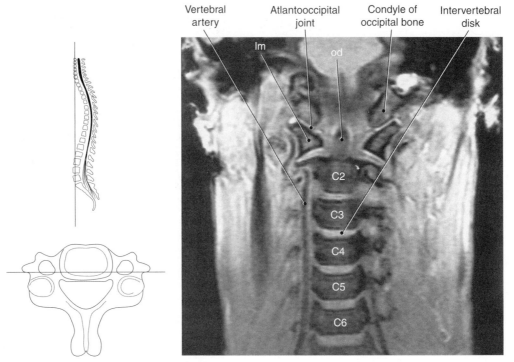

Figure 4.15
Coronal, T1-weighted MR scan of cervical spine.

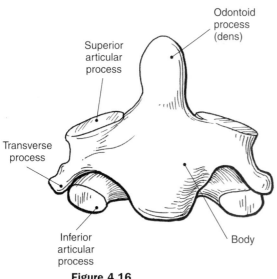

Figure 4.16
Anterior aspect of C2 (axis).

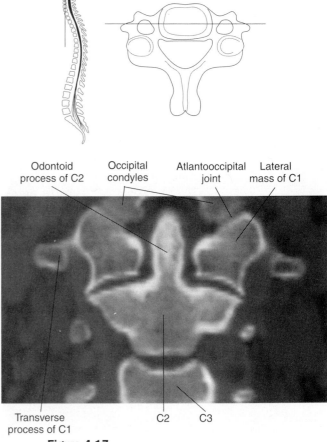

Figure 4.17
Coronal CT reformat of C1 (atlas) and C2 (axis).

KEY: **lm**, Lateral mass; **od**, odontoid process.

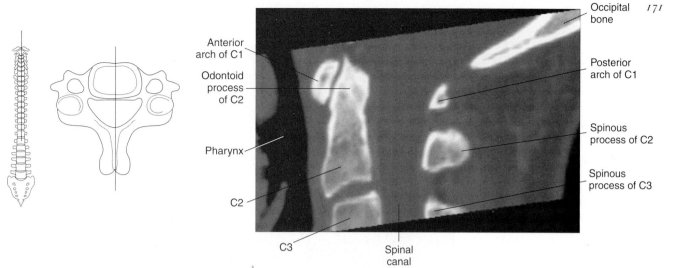

Figure 4.18
Sagittal CT reformat of C1 (atlas) and C2 (axis).

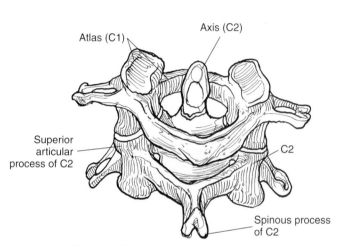

Figure 4.19
Posterosuperior view of cervical vertebrae.

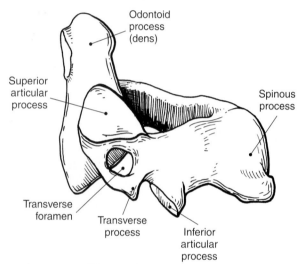

Figure 4.20
Sagittal view of C2 (axis).

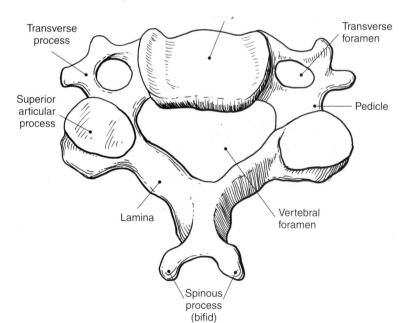

Figure 4.21
Superior aspect of cervical vertebra with bifid spinous process.

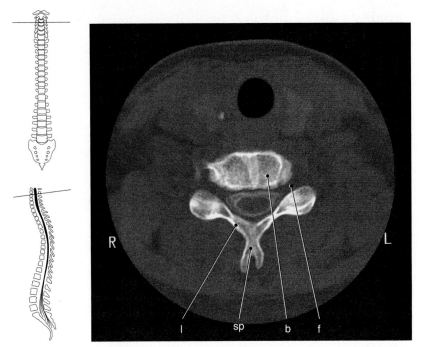

Figure 4.22
Axial CT scan of cervical vertebra with bifid spinous process.

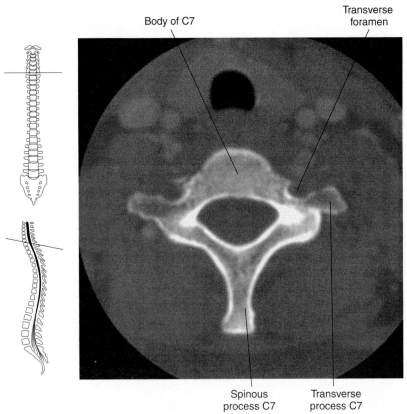

Figure 4.23
Axial CT scan of C7 (vertebral prominens).

KEY: **l,** Lamina; **sp,** spinous process; **b,** body; **f,** intervertebral foramen.

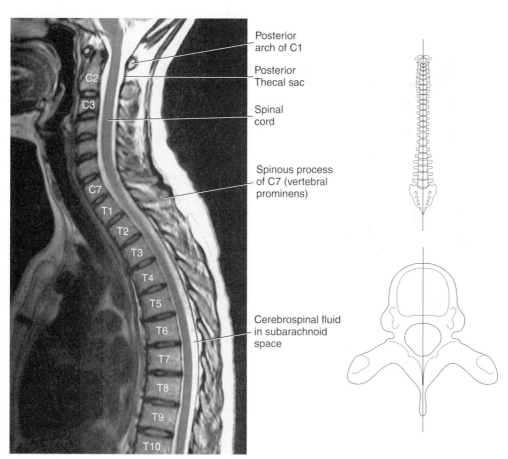

Posterior
arch of C1

Posterior
Thecal sac

Spinal
cord

Spinous process
of C7 (vertebral
prominens)

Cerebrospinal fluid
in subarachnoid
space

C2
C3
C7
T1
T2
T3
T4
T5
T6
T7
T8
T9
T10

Figure 4.24
Midsagittal, T2-weighted MR
scan of cervical and thoracic spine.

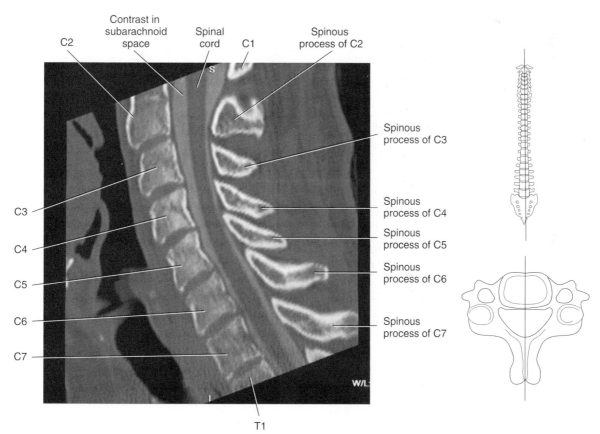

Contrast in
subarachnoid
space

Spinal
cord

C1

Spinous
process of C2

C2

Spinous
process of C3

Spinous
process of C4

Spinous
process of C5

Spinous
process of C6

Spinous
process of C7

C3

C4

C5

C6

C7

T1

S

W/L:

Figure 4.25
Midsagittal CT reformat of cervical spine.

Thoracic Vertebrae

Twelve vertebrae make up the thoracic section. They have typical vertebral configurations except for their characteristic **costal facets (demi facets),** located on the body and transverse process, that articulate with the ribs. The head of the rib articulates with the vertebral bodies at the **costovertebral joints,** whereas the tubercle of the ribs articulates with the transverse processes at the **costotransverse joints.** The spinous processes of the thoracic vertebrae are typically long and slender, projecting inferiorly over the vertebral arches of the vertebrae below (Figures 4.24, 4.26, and 4.27).

KEY: **cvjt,** Costovertebral joint; **b,** body; **p,** pedicle; **r,** rib; **l,** lamina; **sp,** spinous process; **cf,** costal facet; **ctjt,** costotransverse joint.

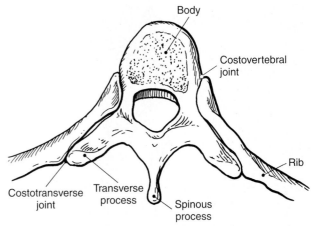

Figure 4.26
Superior view of thoracic vertebra.

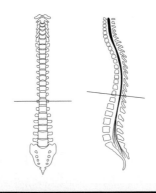

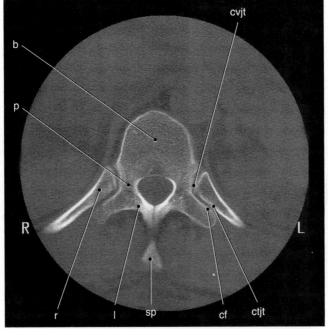

Figure 4.27
Axial CT scan of thoracic vertebra.

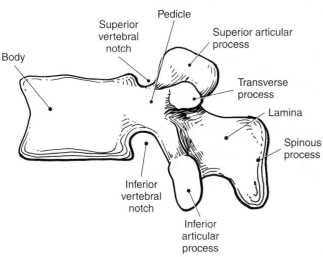

Figure 4.28
3D CT reconstruction of lumbar spine.

Lumbar Vertebrae

The **lumbar** section typically consists of five vertebrae. Their massive bodies increase in size from superior to inferior (Figure 4.28). The largest of the lumbar vertebrae, L5, is characterized by its massive transverse processes. The entire weight of the upper body is transferred from the fifth lumbar vertebra to the base of the sacrum across the L5-S1 disk (Figures 4.29 through 4.32).

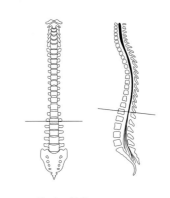

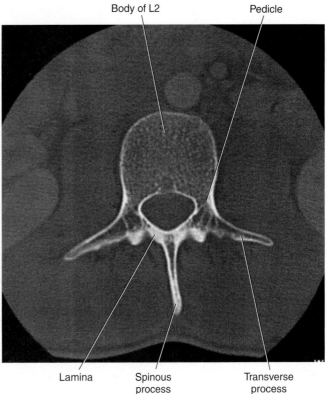

Figure 4.30
Axial CT scan of lumbar vertebra.

Figure 4.29
Sagittal view of lumbar vertebra.

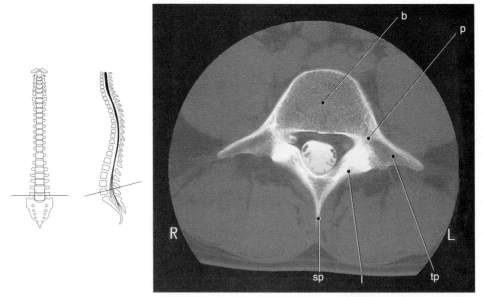

Figure 4.31
Axial CT scan of L5 vertebra (midbody).

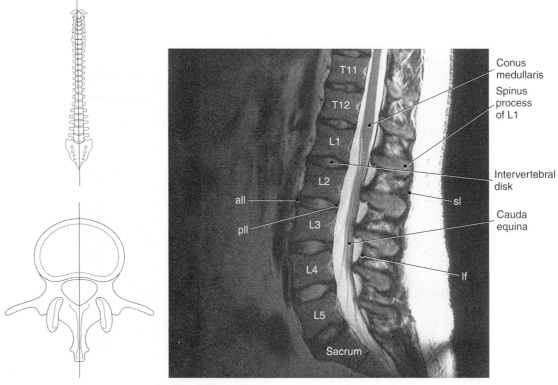

Figure 4.32
Midsagittal, T2-weighted MR scan of lumbar spine.

KEY: **b,** Body; **p,** pedicle; **sp,** spinous process; **l,** lamina; **tp,** transverse process; **all,** anterior longitudinal ligament; **pll,** posterior longitudinal ligament; **lf,** ligamentum flava; **sl,** supraspinous ligament.

Sacrum and Coccyx

The sacral section consists of five vertebrae that fuse to form the **sacrum.** Their transverse processes combine to form the **lateral masses (ala),** which articulate with the pelvic bones at the **sacroiliac joints.** Located within the lateral masses are the **sacral foramina** that allow for the passage of nerves (Figures 4.33 and 4.34). The first sacral segment has a prominent ridge located on the anterior surface of the body termed the **sacral promontory** (Figures 4.35 and 4.36). This bony landmark is used to separate the abdominal cavity from the pelvic cavity. The spinous process of the fifth sacral segment is absent, leaving an opening termed the **sacral hiatus** (Figure 4.2). Located at the sides of the sacral hiatus are the inferior articular processes of the fifth sacral segment that project downward as the **sacral cornu.** Located inferior to the fifth sacral segment is the **coccyx,** which consists of three to five small fused bony segments (Figures 4.33 and 4.35). Superior projections off of the first coccygeal segment, called **cornu,** have ligamentous attachments to the sacral cornu that provide additional stability to the articulation between the sacrum and coccyx. The coccyx represents the most inferior portion of the vertebral column.

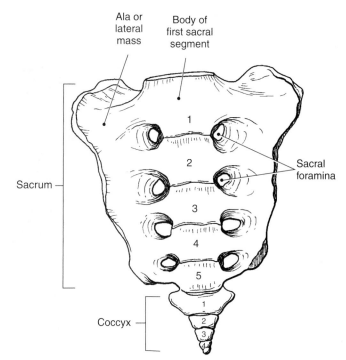

Figure 4.33
Coronal view of sacrum and coccyx.

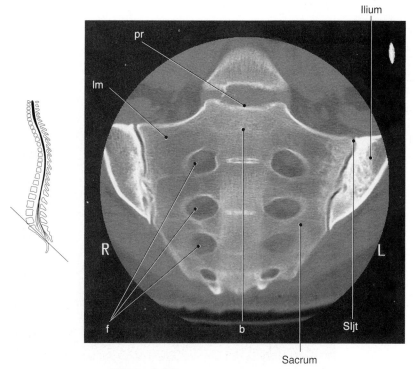

Figure 4.34
Coronal CT scan of sacrum and coccyx.

KEY: **pr,** Sacral promontory; **lm,** lateral mass; **f,** sacral foramina; **b,** body of S1; **Sljt,** sacroiliac joint.

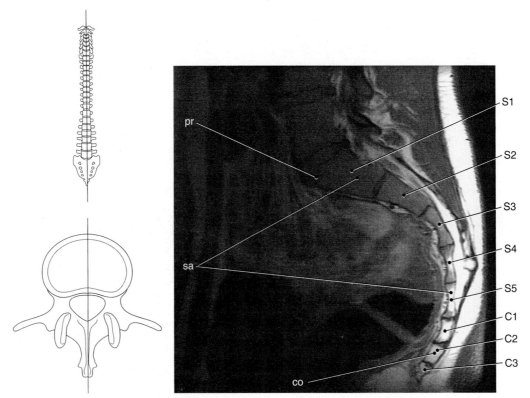

Figure 4.35
Sagittal, T1-weighted MR scan of sacrum and SI joints.

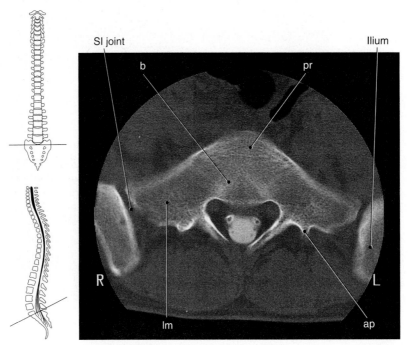

Figure 4.36
Axial CT scan of sacrum and sacroiliac joints.

KEY: pr, Sacral promontory; **sa,** sacrum; **co,** coccyx; **b,** body; **pr,** sacral promontory; **lm,** lateral mass; **ap,** articular process.

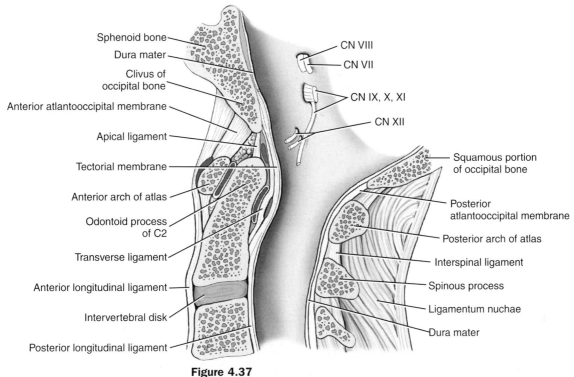

Figure 4.37
Midsagittal view of atlantooccipital joint.

LIGAMENTS

Specific ligaments of the spine serve to connect the cervical vertebrae and the cranium to provide mobility and protection for the head and neck. The **apical ligament** is a midline structure that connects the apex of the odontoid process to the anterior margin of the foramen magnum (Figures 4.37 through 4.39). The **alar ligaments** are two strong bands that extend obliquely from the sides of the odontoid process, upward to the lateral margins of the occipital condyles to limit rotation and flexion of the head (Figures 4.40 and 4.41). The **transverse ligament** extends across the ring of C1 to form a sling over the posterior surface of the odontoid process. It has a small band of longitudinal fibers that ascend to attach to the anterior margin of the foramen magnum and inferiorly to attach to the body of the axis. The transverse ligament functions to hold the odontoid process of C2 against the anterior arch of C1 (Figures 4.40, 4.42, and 4.43). The transverse ligament is sometimes called the **cruciform ligament** because of its crosslike appearance.

Another important ligament of the cervical region is the **ligamentum nuchae,** which serves as an attachment point for muscles. This expansive ligament extends from the external occipital protuberance of the cranium to the spinous processes of the cervical vertebrae (Figures 4.37 through 4.39). The ligamentum nuchae continues inferiorly as the supraspinous ligament. The **supraspinous ligament** is a narrow band of fibers that runs over and connects the tips of the spinous processes

from the seventh cervical vertebra to the lower lumbar vertebrae (Figures 4.44 through 4.46).

In addition to the ligaments listed above, the stability of the suboccipital region of the spine is reinforced with the **atlanto-occipital** and **tectorial membranes.** The atlanto-occipital membrane consists of an anterior and posterior portion that serves to connect the arches of the atlas with the occipital bone. The **anterior atlantooccipital membrane** passes from the anterior arch of the atlas and connects to the anterior margin at the base of the occipital bone. This ligament is the superior extension of the anterior longitudinal ligament. The **posterior atlantooccipital membrane** extends from the posterior margin of the foramen magnum to the posterior arch of the atlas, closing the posterior portion of the vertebral canal between the skull and C1 (Figure 4.37). The **tectorial membrane** is a broad ligament that extends from the clivus of the occipital bone to the posterior body of the axis, covering the dens, transverse, apical, and alar ligaments. The tectorial membrane forms the anterior boundary of the vertebral canal and is continuous with the posterior longitudinal ligament (Figures 4.37 through 4.39).

Several ligaments enclose the vertebral column to help protect the spinal cord and maintain stability of the vertebral column. Two of the larger ligaments are the anterior and posterior longitudinal ligaments (Figure 4.44). The **anterior longitudinal ligament** is a broad fibrous band that extends downward from C1 along the entire anterior surface of the vertebral bodies to the sacrum. This ligament connects the

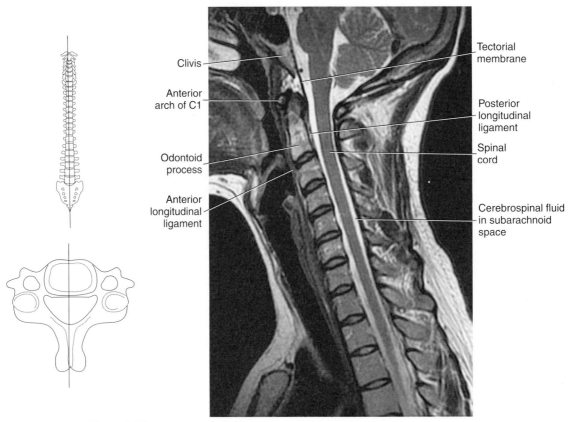

Figure 4.38
Midsagittal, T2-weighted MR scan of cervical spine demonstrating spinal ligaments.

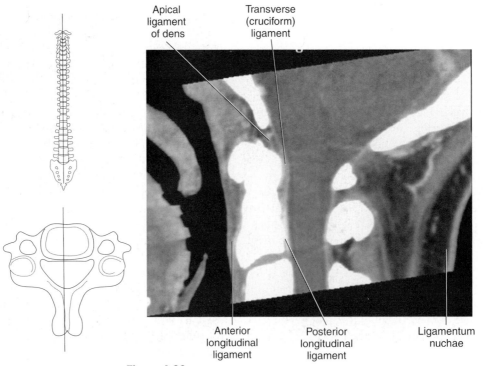

Figure 4.39
Sagittal CT reformat of atlantooccipital joint.

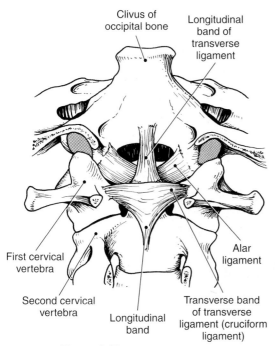

Clivus of occipital bone

Longitudinal band of transverse ligament

First cervical vertebra

Second cervical vertebra

Longitudinal band

Transverse band of transverse ligament (cruciform ligament)

Alar ligament

Figure 4.40
Posterior view of alar ligaments.

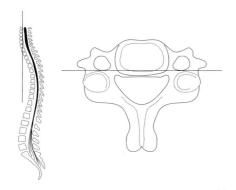

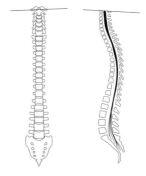

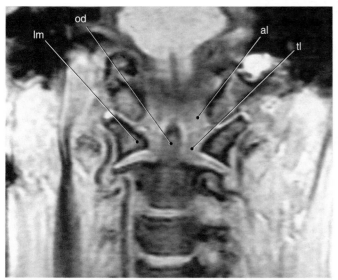

lm

od

al

tl

Figure 4.41
Coronal, T1-weighted MR scan of alar and transverse ligaments.

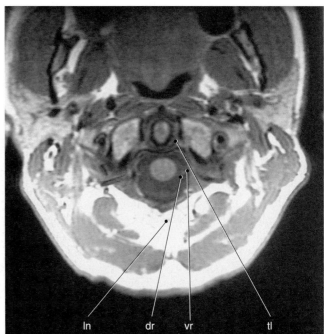

ln

dr

vr

tl

Figure 4.42
Axial, T1-weighted MR scan of cervical vertebra demonstrating spinal ligaments.

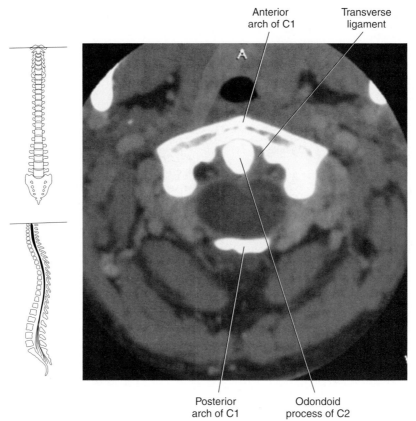

Figure 4.43
Axial CT scan of C1 and C2 demonstrating transverse ligament.

anterior aspects of the vertebral bodies and intervertebral disks to maintain stability of the joints and to help prevent hyperextension of the vertebral column. It is thicker in the thoracic region than in the cervical and lumbar regions, providing additional support to the thoracic spine. The **posterior longitudinal ligament** is narrower and slightly weaker than the anterior longitudinal ligament. It lies inside the vertebral canal and runs along the posterior aspect of the vertebral bodies (Figures 4.44 through 4.49). Unlike the anterior longitudinal ligament, the posterior longitudinal ligament is attached only at the intervertebral disk and adjacent margins. It is separated from the middle of each vertebra by epidural fat that provides passage of the basivertebral veins. The posterior longitudinal ligament runs the entire length of the vertebral column beginning at C2. This ligament helps to prevent posterior protrusion of the nucleus pulposus and hyperflexion of the vertebral column.

The **ligamentum flava** are strong ligaments (consisting of yellow elastic tissue) present on either side of the spinous process. They join the laminae of adjacent vertebral arches, helping to preserve the normal curvature of the spine (Figures 4.44 through 4.49).

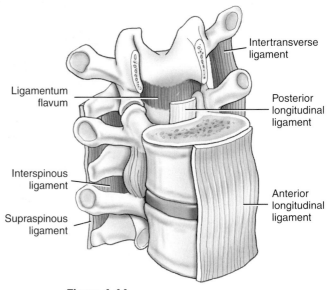

Figure 4.44
Coronal oblique view of spinal ligaments.

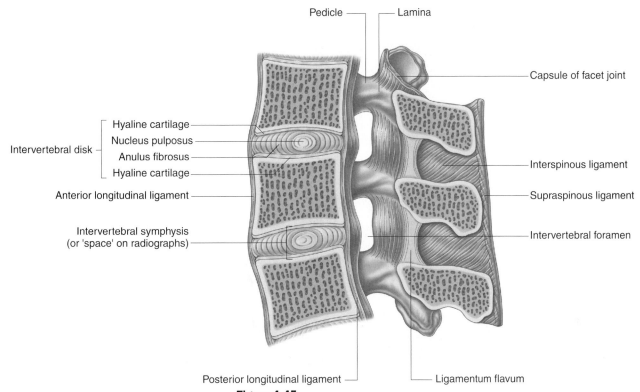

Pedicle — Lamina

Capsule of facet joint

Intervertebral disk —
Hyaline cartilage
Nucleus pulposus
Anulus fibrosus
Hyaline cartilage

Anterior longitudinal ligament

Intervertebral symphysis
(or 'space' on radiographs)

Interspinous ligament

Supraspinous ligament

Intervertebral foramen

Posterior longitudinal ligament — Ligamentum flavum

Figure 4.45
Midsagittal view of spinal ligaments.

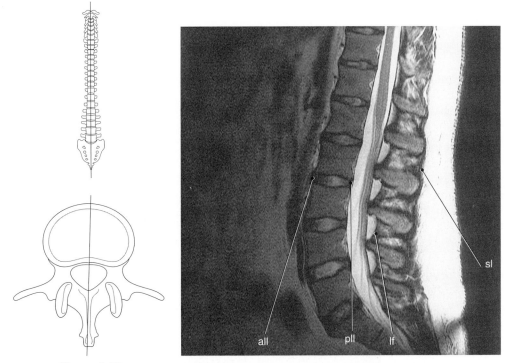

all   pll   lf   sl

Figure 4.46
Midsagittal, T2-weighted MR scan of lumbar spine demonstrating spinal ligaments.

KEY: **all,** Anterior longitudinal ligament; **pll,** posterior longitudinal ligament; **lf,** ligamentum flava; **sl,** supraspinous ligament.

Posterior longitudinal
ligament

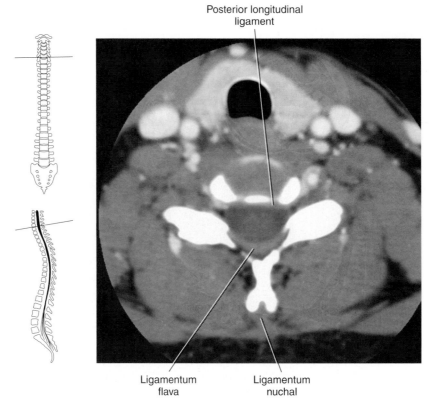

Ligamentum   Ligamentum
flava   nuchal

Figure 4.47
Axial CT scan of cervical vertebra demonstrating spinal ligaments.

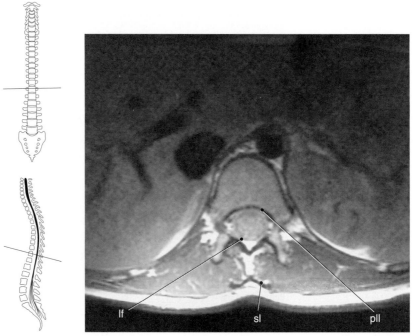

lf   sl   pll

Figure 4.48
Axial, T1-weighted MR scan of thoracic spine demonstrating spinal ligaments.

KEY: **lf,** Ligamentum flava; **sl,** supraspinous ligament; **pll,** posterior longitudinal ligament.

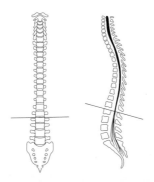

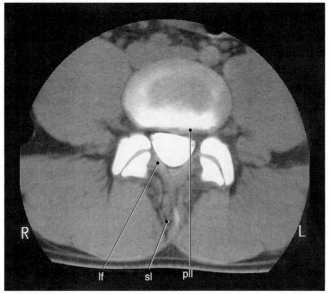

Figure 4.49
Axial CT scan of lumbar vertebra demonstrating spinal ligaments.

KEY: **lf,** Ligamentum flava; **sl,** supraspinous ligament; **pll,** posterior longitudinal ligament.

TABLE 4-1   Spinal Muscles

MUSCLE	ORIGIN	INSERTION
Splenius		
Splenius capitis	Ligamentum nuchae and spinous processes of C7-T3	Mastoid process of temporal bone
Splenius cervicis	Spinous processes of T3-T6	Transverse processes of C1-C4
Erector spinae		
Iliocostalis		
Iliocostalis cervicis	Angles of 4th to 7th ribs	Transverse processes of C4-C6
Iliocostalis thoracis	Angles of 7th to 12th ribs	Angles of ribs 1 to 6; transverse process of C7
Iliocostalis lumborum	Sacrum and iliac crest, spinous processes of lumbar vertebrae	Angles of ribs 7 to 12
Longissimus	Transverse processes of C3-T3	Mastoid process of temporal bone
Longissimus capitis	Transverse processes of T1-T6	Transverse processes of C2-C5
Longissimus cervicis	Transverse processes of lumbar vertebrae	Transverse processes of all thoracic vertebrae, tubercles of inferior 10 ribs
Longissimus thoracis	Fibers blend with semispinalis capitis muscles	Fibers blend with semispinalis capitis muscles
Spinalis		
Spinalis capitis	Lower ligamentum nuchae and spinous process of C7	Spinous process of C2
Spinalis cervicis (inconsistent)	Spinous processes of T11-L2	Spinous processes of T1-T8
Spinalis thoracis		
Transversospinal		
Semispinalis		
Semispinalis capitis	Transverse processes of C7-T6; articular processes of C4-C6	Occipital bone between superior and inferior nuchal lines
Semispinalis cervicis	Transverse processes of T2-T6	Spinous processes of C2-C5
Semispinalis thoracis	Transverse processes of T6-T10	Spinous processes of C6-T4
Multifidus	Transverse processes of thoracic vertebrae and articular processes of four inferior cervical vertebrae, sacrum, and posterior superior iliac spine	Spinous processes of C1-L5
Rotatores	Transverse processes of T2-T12; poorly developed in cervical and lumbar regions	Lamina of T1-T11; poorly developed in cervical and lumbar regions

MUSCLES

Muscles of the back can be separated into three groupings or layers; the superficial layer (splenius muscles), the intermediate layer (erector spinae group), and the deep layer (transversospinal group). The muscle groups that run the length of the spine can be divided into regions according to their location: capitis, cervicis, thoracis, and lumborum (Table 4.1).

Superficial Layer

The **splenius muscles** are located on the lateral and posterior aspect of the cervical and upper thoracic spine. These bandage-like muscles originate on the spinous processes of C7-T6 and the inferior half of the ligamentum nuchae. They are divided into a cranial portion, **splenius capitus,** that inserts on the mastoid process of the temporal bone and a cervical portion, **splenius cervicis,** that inserts on the transverse processes of C1-C4 (Figures 4.50 through 4.53). Together they act to extend the head and neck.

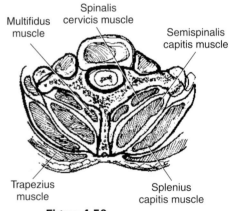

Figure 4.50
Axial view of splenius muscle.

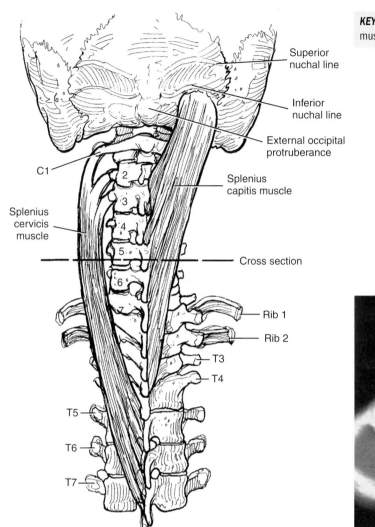

Figure 4.51
Posterior view of splenius muscles.

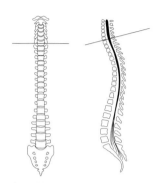

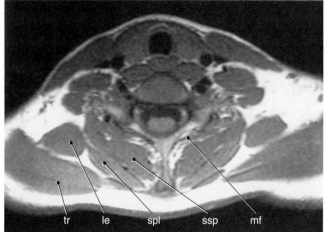

Figure 4.52
Axial, T1-weighted MR scan of cervical vertebra with spinal muscles.

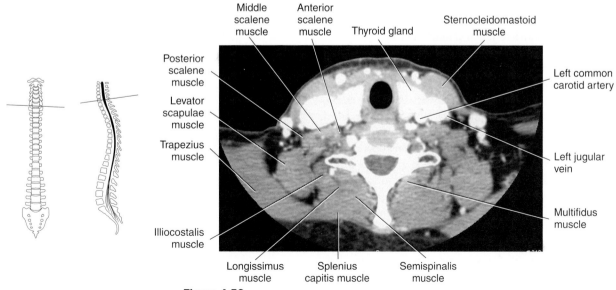

Figure 4.53
Axial CT scan of cervical vertebra with spinal muscles.

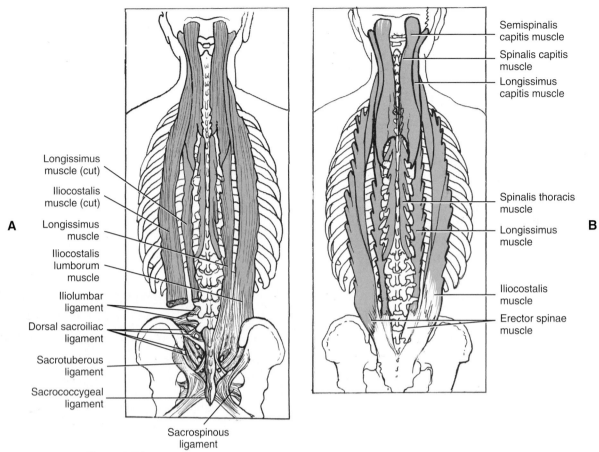

Figure 4.54
A, Posterior view of longissimus and iliocostalis muscles of the erector spinae muscle group.
B, Posterior view of spinalis muscle of the erector spinae muscle group.

Intermediate Layer

The intermediate muscle group, the **erector spinae muscle group,** consists of massive muscles that form a prominent bulge on each side of the vertebral column. The erector spinae muscle group is the chief extensor of the vertebral column and is arranged in three vertical columns, the iliocostalis layer (lateral column), longissimus layer (intermediate column), and the spinalis layer (medial column) (Figures 4.54 and 4.55). This muscle group arises from a common broad tendon from the posterior part of the iliac crest, sacrum, and inferior lumbar spinous processes. The **iliocostalis muscles** run superiorly to attach to the angles of the ribs and transverse processes of C7 to C4. The **longissimus muscles** run superiorly to insert into the tips of the transverse processes of the thoracic and cervical regions, the angles of the ribs, and the mastoid process. The narrow **spinalis muscle group** extends from the spinous processes of the upper lumbar and lower thoracic regions to the spinous processes of the superior thoracic region. The cervicis and capitis portion of the muscle are inseparable from the semispinalis of the transversospinal group (Figures 4.55 through 4.57).

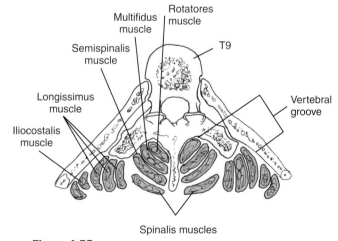

Figure 4.55
Axial view of erector spinae muscle group at thoracic level.

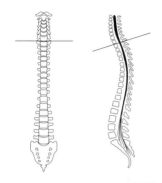

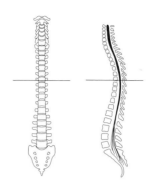

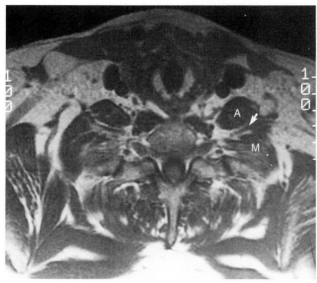

Figure 4.56
Axial, T1-weighted MR scan of thoracic vertebra with spinal muscles. *Arrow,* Brachial plexus.

Brachial plexus · Clavicle · Subclavius muscle · Pectoralis minor muscle · Pectoralis major muscle · Teres major muscle

Levator scapulae muscle · Trapezius muscle · Rhomboid muscle · Erector spinae muscles · Subscapularis muscle · Supraspinatus muscle

Figure 4.57
Axial CT scan of thoracic vertebra with spinal muscles.

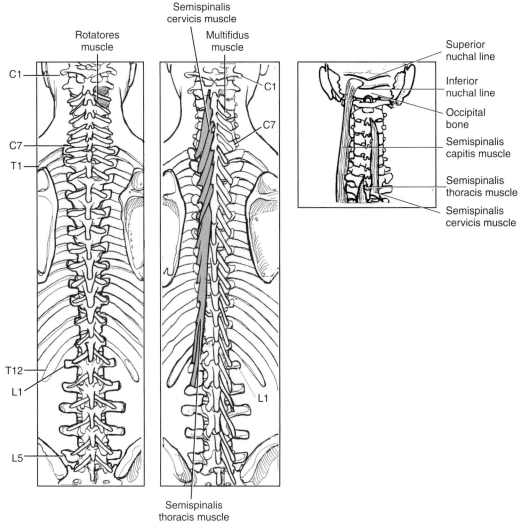

Figure 4.58
Posterior views of transversospinal muscle group.

Deep Layer

The **transversospinal muscles** consist of several short muscles that are located in the groove between the transverse and spinous processes of the vertebrae. They can be separated into the semispinalis, multifidus, and rotatores with a primary function to flex and rotate the vertebral column (Figures 4.55 through 4.58). The **semispinalis** muscles arise from the thoracic and cervical transverse processes and insert on the occipital bone and spinous processes in the thoracic and cervical regions. The semispinalis muscles form the largest muscle mass in the posterior portion of the neck. The **multifidus** muscles consist of many fibrous bundles that extend the full length of the spine and are the most prominent in the lumbar region. The deepest of the transversospinal muscles are the **rotatores,** which connect the lamina of one vertebra to the transverse process of the vertebra below. They are best developed in the thoracic region.

Two additional muscles that are commonly visualized in the lumbar region of the spine are the **quadratus lumborum** and the **psoas** muscles, which are considered abdominal muscles (Figures 4.59 through 4.61). Further information on these muscles can be found in Chapter 7.

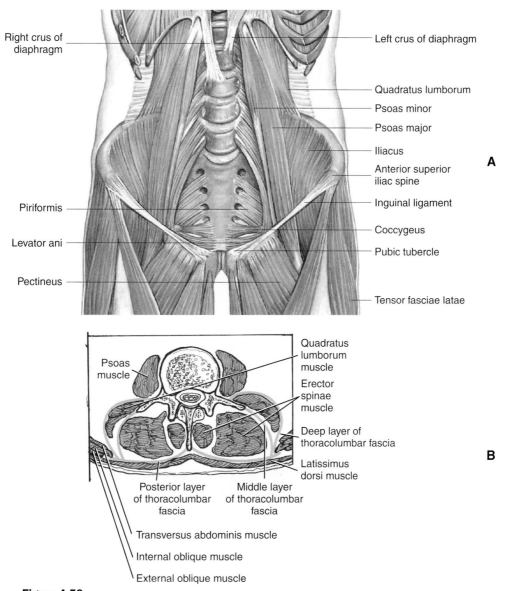

Right crus of diaphragm

Left crus of diaphragm

Quadratus lumborum

Psoas minor

Psoas major

Iliacus

Anterior superior iliac spine

A

Piriformis

Inguinal ligament

Levator ani

Coccygeus

Pectineus

Pubic tubercle

Tensor fasciae latae

Psoas muscle

Quadratus lumborum muscle

Erector spinae muscle

Deep layer of thoracolumbar fascia

Latissimus dorsi muscle

B

Posterior layer of thoracolumbar fascia

Middle layer of thoracolumbar fascia

Transversus abdominis muscle

Internal oblique muscle

External oblique muscle

Figure 4.59
A, Coronal view of quadratus lumborum and psoas muscles. **B,** Axial view of quadratus lumborum and psoas muscles.

Quadiratus lumborum

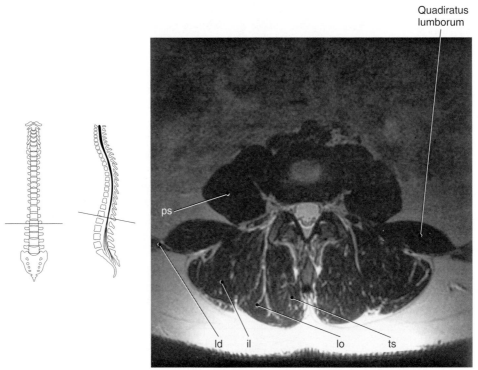

Figure 4.60
Axial, T2-weighted MR scan of lumbar spine with spinal muscles.

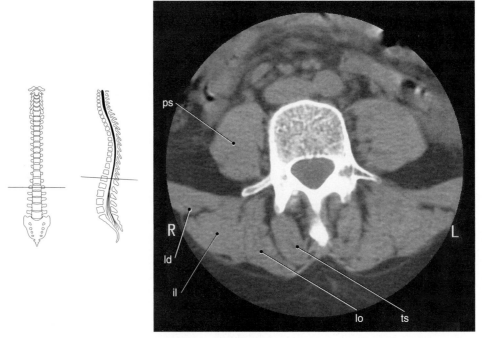

Figure 4.61
Axial CT of lumbar spine with spinal muscles.

KEY: **ps,** Psoas muscle; **ld,** latissimus dorsi muscle; **il,** iliocostalis muscle; **lo,** longissimus muscle; **ts,** transversospinal muscles.

SPINAL CORD

Spinal Meninges

Throughout its length, the delicate spinal cord is surrounded and protected by cerebrospinal fluid, which is contained in the thecal sac formed by the spinal meninges (Figure 4.62). The **spinal meninges** are continuous with the cranial meninges

and can be broken into the same three layers: dura, arachnoid, and pia. The **dura mater** is the tough outer layer that extends to S2, creating the **thecal sac** (Figures 4.63 and 4.64). The spinal dura mater adheres to the posterior longitudinal ligament and is separated from the vertebral column by an **epidural space** that contains fat and vessels. Each spinal nerve is surrounded by dura mater that extends through the intervertebral foramen. The **arachnoid mater** is the thin transparent membrane that is attached to the inner surface of the dura mater. A potential space called the **subdural space** runs between the arachnoid and dura mater. The arachnoid mater is connected to the pia mater by numerous delicate strands creating the spiderlike appearance associated with the arachnoid mater. The space between the arachnoid mater and pia mater is the **subarachnoid space,** which is filled with cerebrospinal fluid and the blood vessels that supply the spinal cord (Figures 4.62, 4.65, and 4.66). The **pia mater** is a highly vascular layer that closely adheres to the spinal cord. At the distal end of the spinal cord, approximately L1, the pia mater continues as a long slender strand called the filum terminale. The **filum terminale** descends through the subarachnoid space to the inferior border of the thecal sac, where it is reinforced by the dura mater. After leaving the thecal sac, it eventually exits

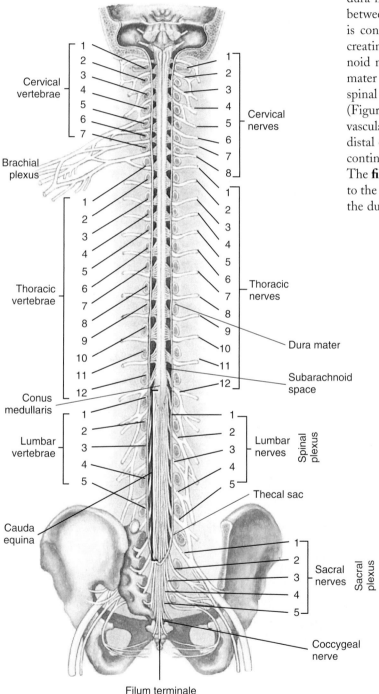

Figure 4.62
Posterior view of spinal meninges, thecal sac, and spinal cord.

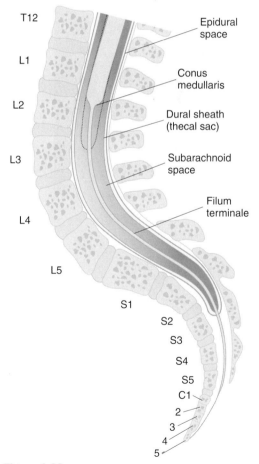

Figure 4.63
Midsagittal view of thecal sac, conus medullaris, and filum terminale.

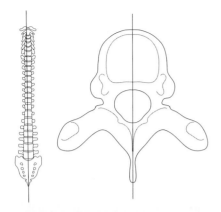

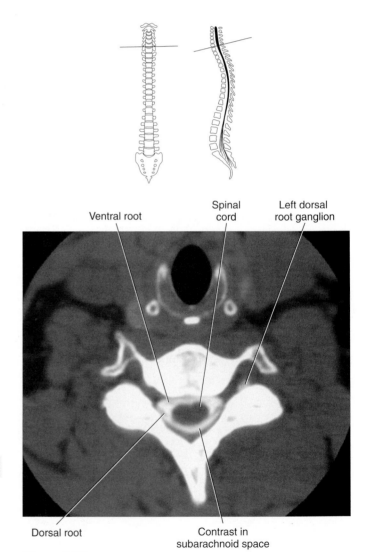

Ventral horn · Body of vertebra · Central canal · Ventral root

Dorsal horn

Dorsal root ganglion

Dorsal root

Bone of vertebra

Subdural space

Epidural space (contains fat)

Subarachnoid space

Dura mater (spinal dural sheath)

Arachnoid

Pia mater

Denticulate ligaments

Spinal meninges

Figure 4.65
Axial view of spinal meninges, dural spaces, and spinal cord.

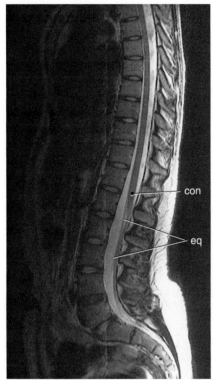

con

eq

Figure 4.64
Midsagittal, T2-weighted MR scan of thecal sac, conus medullaris, and filum terminale.

Ventral root · Spinal cord · Left dorsal root ganglion

Dorsal root

Contrast in subarachnoid space

Figure 4.66
Axial CT scan of cervical spine (postmyelogram) with intrathecal contrast in the subarachnoid space.

KEY: **con,** Conus medullaris; **eq,** cauda equina.

the sacral canal through the sacral hiatus and attaches to the coccyx, providing an anchor between the spinal cord and the coccyx (Figures 4.62 and 4.63). In addition, lateral extensions of the pia mater leave the spinal cord to form 21 pairs of **denticulate ligaments** that attach to the dura, preventing lateral movement of the spinal cord within the thecal sac (Figures 4.65 and 4.67).

> After producing chickenpox, the herpes zoster virus can lie dormant within the ventral horns of the spinal cord for years. When reactivated, the virus attacks the dorsal roots of peripheral nerves, producing a painful rash, with a distribution corresponding to the affected sensory nerve. This condition is termed *shingles*.

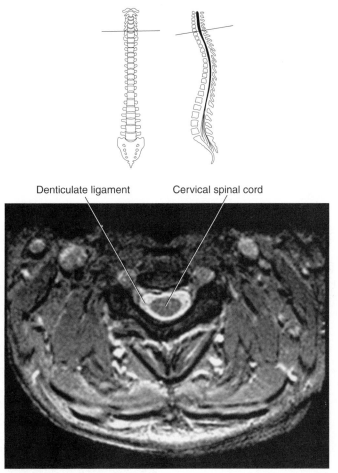

Denticulate ligament   Cervical spinal cord

Figure 4.67
Axial, T2-weighted MR scan of cervical spine with denticulate ligaments.

Spinal Cord and Nerve Roots

The spinal cord functions as a large nerve cable that connects the brain with the body. It begins as a continuation of the medulla at the inferior margin of the brainstem and extends to approximately the first or second lumbar vertebra. The spinal cord tapers into a cone-shaped segment called the **conus medullaris** (Figures 4.62, 4.64, and 4.68 through 4.70). The conus medullaris is the most inferior portion of the spinal cord and is located at approximately the level of the first or second lumbar vertebra. At the termination of the spinal cord, nerves continue inferiorly in bundles. This grouping of nerves has the appearance of a horse's tail and is termed the **cauda equina,** exiting through the lumbosacral foramina (Figures 4.62, 4.68, 4.71, and 4.72).

The spinal cord is composed of white and gray matter. The **white matter** comprises the external borders of the cord and is more abundant. The **gray matter** is composed of nerve cells and runs the entire length of the cord. It is centrally located and surrounds the **central canal,** which contains cerebrospinal fluid and is continuous with the ventricles of the brain (Figures 4.65 and 4.73). In cross section, the gray matter has the appearance of a butterfly. The two posterior projections

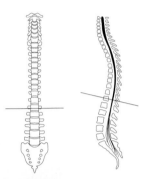

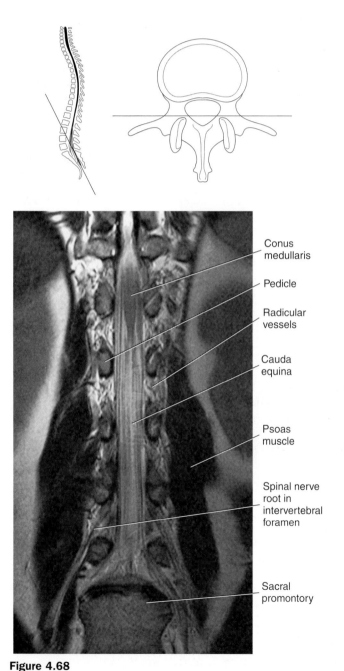

Figure 4.68
Coronal, T2-weighted MR scan of spinal cord with conus medullaris and cauda equina.

Conus medullaris

Pedicle

Radicular vessels

Cauda equina

Psoas muscle

Spinal nerve root in intervertebral foramen

Sacral promontory

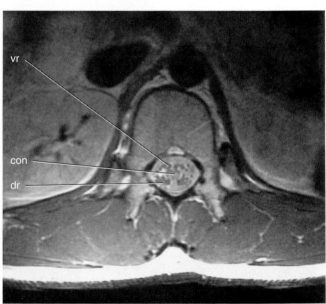

Figure 4.69
Axial, T1-weighted MR scan of conus medullaris.

vr

con

dr

KEY: vr, Ventral root; **con,** conus medullaris; **dr,** dorsal root; **sas,** subarachnoid space; **ef,** epidural fat; **bv,** basivertebral vein; **eq,** cauda equina.

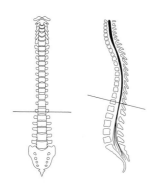

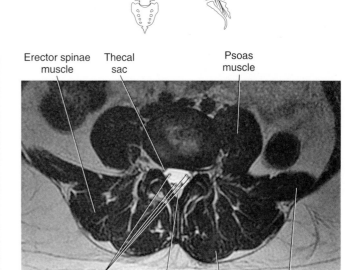

Erector spinae muscle   Thecal sac   Psoas muscle

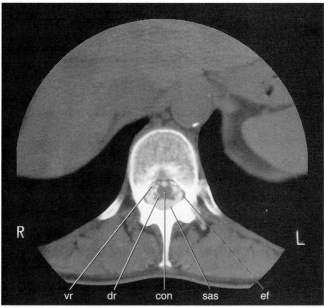

vr   dr   con   sas   ef

Figure 4.70

Axial CT scan of conus medullaris.

Cauda equina   Epidural fat   Multifidus muscle   Quadratus lumborum muscle

Figure 4.71

Axial, T2-weighted MR scan of cauda equina.

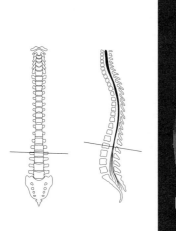

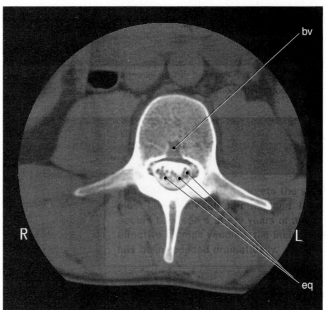

bv

eq

Figure 4.72

Axial CT scan of cauda equina.

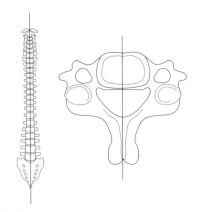

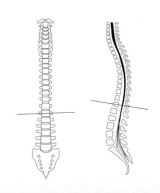

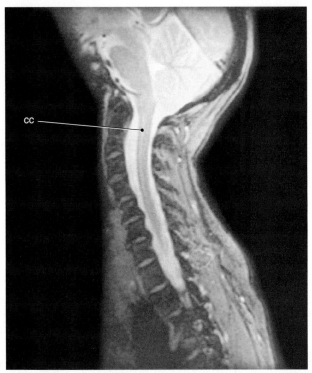

Figure 4.73
Sagittal, T2-weighted MR scan of cervical spine and central canal.

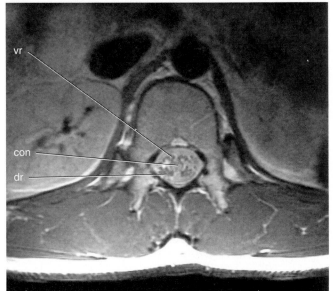

Figure 4.74
Axial, T1-weighted MR scan of spinal cord with ventral and dorsal roots.

KEY: cc, Central canal; **vr,** ventral root; **con,** conus medullaris; **dr,** dorsal root.

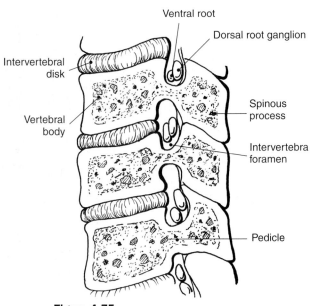

Figure 4.75
Sagittal view of spine with neural foramina.

are the dorsal horns, and the two anterior projections are the ventral horns (Figure 4.65). The **dorsal horns** contain neurons and sensory fibers that enter the cord from the body periphery via the **dorsal roots.** These are called the afferent (sensory) nerve roots (Figures 4.66 and 4.74). The **dorsal root ganglion,** an oval enlargement of the dorsal root that contains the nerve cell bodies of the sensory neurons, is located in the intervertebral foramen (Figures 4.65, 4.66, and 4.75 through 4.79). The **ventral horns** contain the nerve cell bodies of the efferent (motor) neurons. The efferent (motor) nerve roots exit the spinal cord via the ventral root to be distributed throughout the body. Just outside the intervertebral foramina, the ventral and dorsal roots unite to form the 31 pairs of **spinal nerves.**

Eight of these nerve pairs correspond to the cervical region, 12 belong to the thoracic section, 5 correspond to the lumbar region, 5 correspond to the sacrum, and 1 belongs to the coccyx (Figures 4.80 through 4.82). Each spinal nerve provides a specific cutaneous distribution that can be demonstrated on a **dermatome map** (Figure 4.83).

KEY: **drg,** Dorsal root ganglion; **sA,** spinal artery; **eq,** cauda equina; **ps,** psoas muscle.

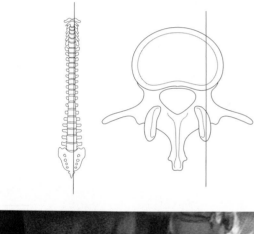

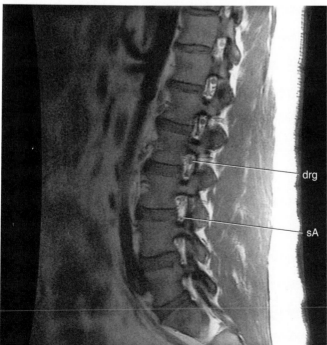

Figure 4.76
Sagittal, T1-weighted MR scan of lumbar spine with neural foramina.

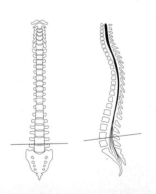

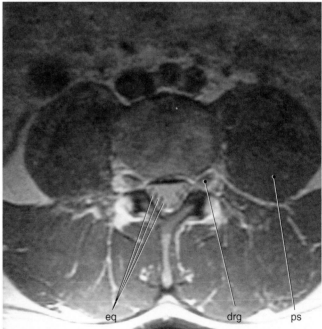

Figure 4.77
Axial, T1-weighted MR scan of lumbar vertebra with dorsal root ganglion.

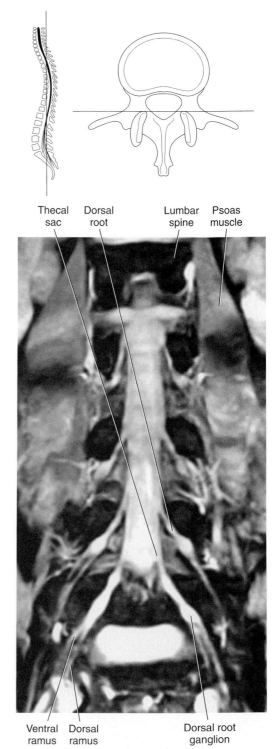

Thecal   Dorsal   Lumbar   Psoas
sac   root   spine   muscle

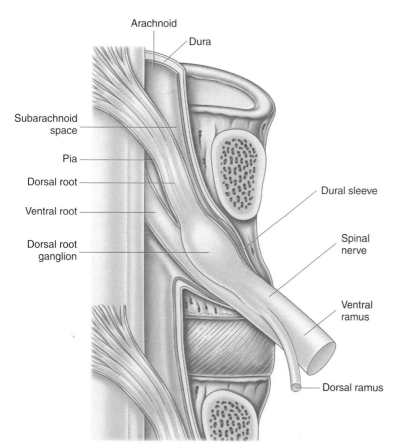

Ventral   Dorsal   Dorsal root
ramus   ramus   ganglion

Figure 4.78
Coronal view of spinal nerve with dorsal and ventral root sleeve.

Figure 4.79
Coronal, T2-weighted MR scan of nerve root sleeve and dorsal ganglion.

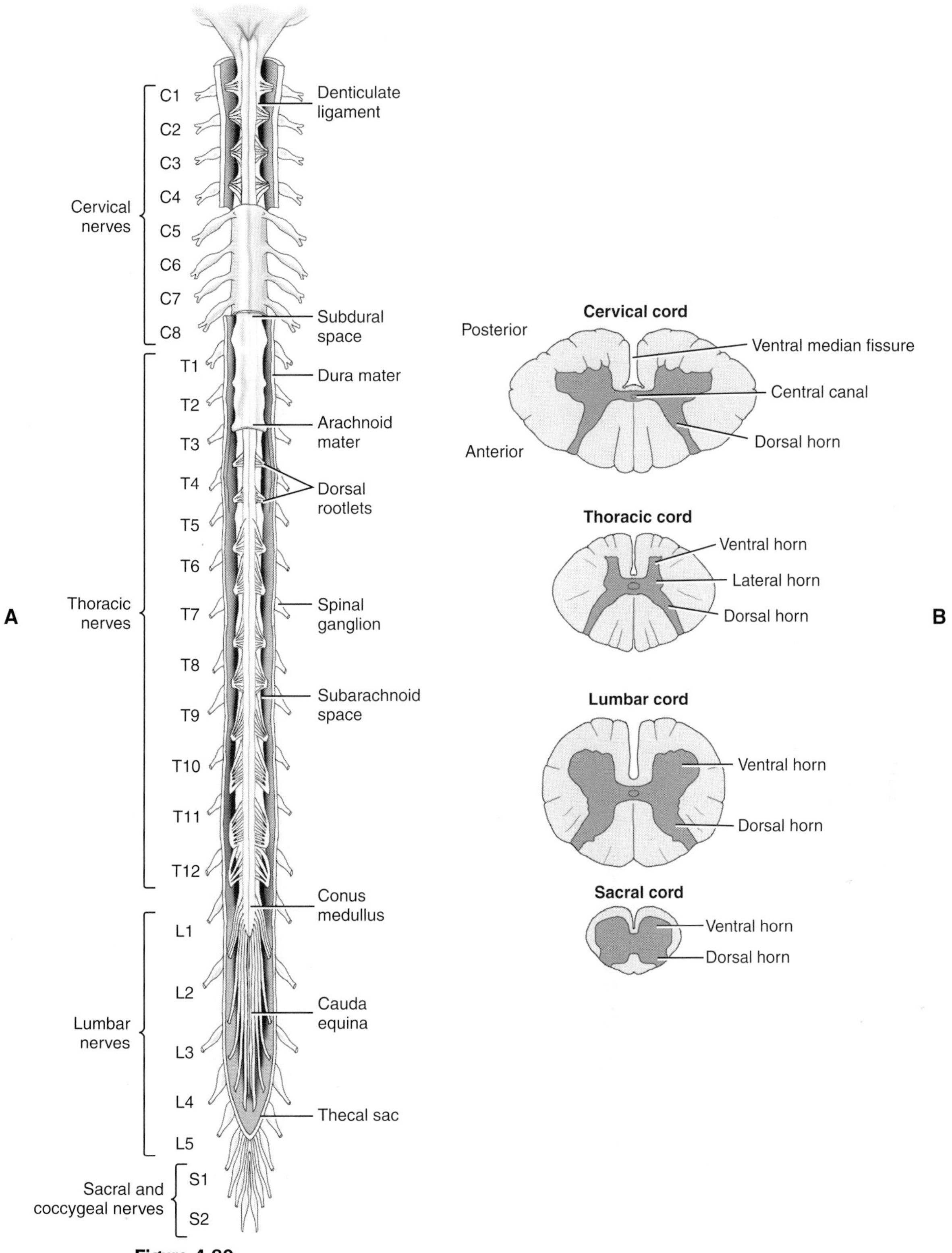

Figure 4.80
A, Posterior view of spinal cord and meninges. **B,** Transverse sections through spinal cord.

Labels in Figure A:
C1, C2, C3, C4, C5, C6, C7, C8 — Cervical nerves
T1, T2, T3, T4, T5, T6, T7, T8, T9, T10, T11, T12 — Thoracic nerves
L1, L2, L3, L4, L5 — Lumbar nerves
S1, S2 — Sacral and coccygeal nerves

Denticulate ligament
Subdural space
Dura mater
Arachnoid mater
Dorsal rootlets
Spinal ganglion
Subarachnoid space
Conus medullus
Cauda equina
Thecal sac

Labels in Figure B:
Cervical cord — Posterior, Anterior, Ventral median fissure, Central canal, Dorsal horn
Thoracic cord — Ventral horn, Lateral horn, Dorsal horn
Lumbar cord — Ventral horn, Dorsal horn
Sacral cord — Ventral horn, Dorsal horn

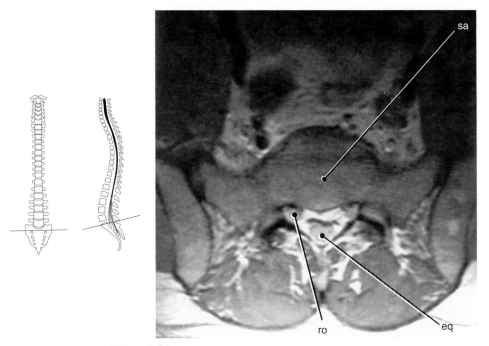

Figure 4.81
Axial, T1-weighted MR scan of sacrum with root sleeve.

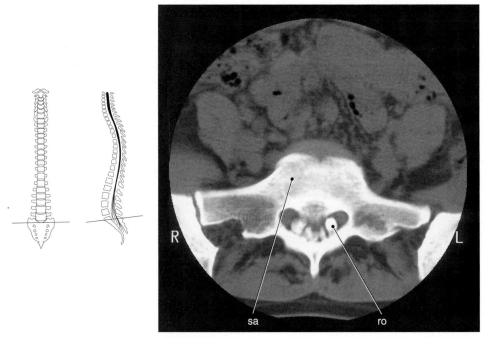

Figure 4.82
Axial CT scan of sacrum with root sleeve.

KEY: **sa,** Sacrum; **eq,** cauda equina; **ro,** root sleeve.

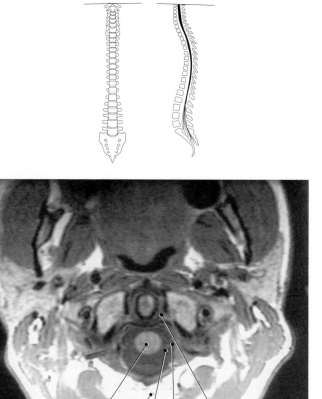

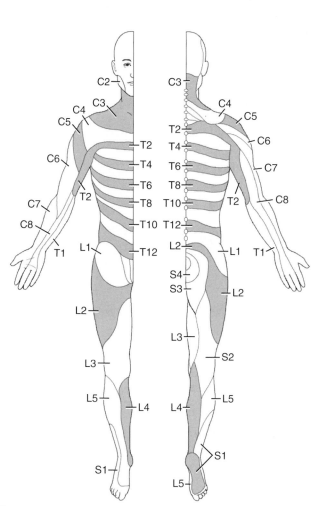

Figure 4.83
Dermatomes. *Left,* Anterior and *Right,* posterior distribution of dermatomes on the surface of the skin.

Cervical spinal cord

Figure 4.84
Axial, T1-weighted MR scan of cervical spinal cord.

KEY: ln, Ligamentum nuchae; **dr,** dorsal root; **vr,** ventral root; **tl,** transverse ligament.

Cervical
spinal cord

Contrast in
subarachnoid space

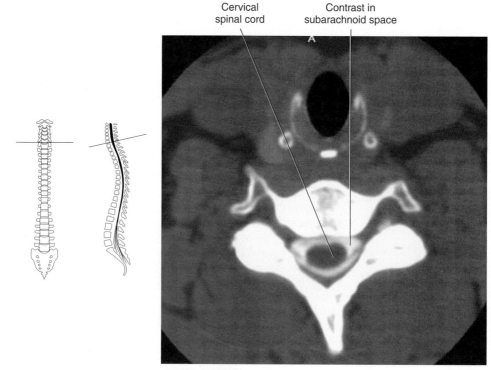

Figure 4.85
Axial CT scan of cervical spinal cord.

PLEXUSES

The spinal cord is enlarged in two regions by the cell bodies of nerves that extend to the extremities. The **cervical enlargement** extends from the vertebral bodies of approximately C3-C7, and the **lumbosacral enlargement** occurs within the lower thoracic region. Cross-section images of the spinal cord at various levels have considerable differences in size and shape because of the changing proportion of gray and white matter (Figures 4.80, and 4.84 through 4.89).

Shortly after emerging from the spinal cord, each nerve divides into **dorsal** and **ventral rami** that contain both motor and sensory fibers (Figure 4.90). The dorsal rami of all spinal nerves extend posteriorly to innervate the skin and muscles of the posterior trunk. The ventral rami of T2-T12 pass anteriorly as the intercostal nerves to supply the skin and muscles of the anterior and lateral trunk. The ventral rami of all other spinal nerves form complex networks of nerves called **plexuses.** These plexuses serve the motor and sensory needs of the muscles and skin of the extremities. The four major nerve plexuses are the cervical, brachial, lumbar, and sacral (Figure 4.91).

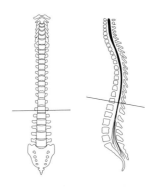

Thoracic spinal cord

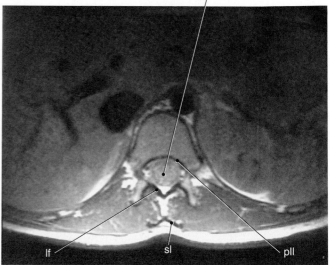

lf   sl   pll

KEY: lf, Ligamentum flava; **sl,** supraspinous ligament; **pll,** posterior longitudinal ligament.

Figure 4.86
Axial, T1-weighted MR scan of thoracic spinal cord.

Vertebral body Thoracic spinal cord Descending aorta

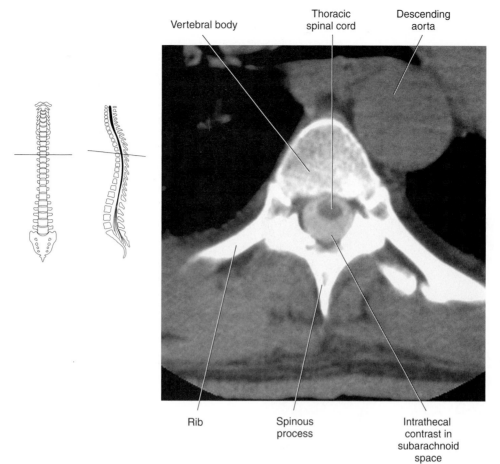

Rib Spinous process Intrathecal contrast in subarachnoid space

Figure 4.87
Axial CT scan of thoracic spinal cord at T-6.

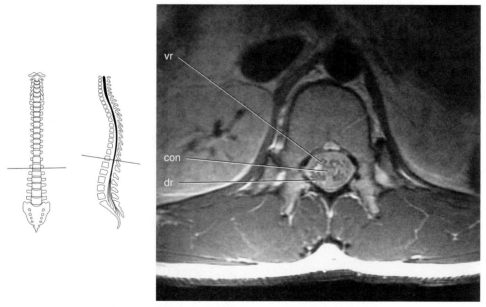

vr con dr

Figure 4.88
Axial, T1-weighted MR scan of spinal cord at conus T-12.

KEY: vr, Ventral root; **con,** conus medullaris; **dr,** dorsal root.

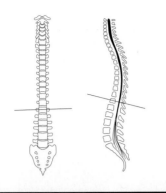

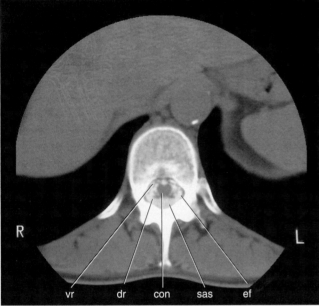

Figure 4.89
Axial CT scan of lumbar spinal cord at conus T-12.

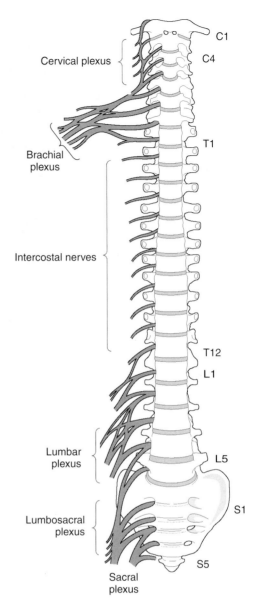

Figure 4.91
Anterior view of major nerve plexuses.

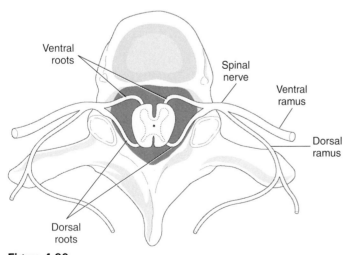

Figure 4.90
Distribution of ventral and dorsal rami in transverse section of spinal cord.

KEY: **vr,** Ventral root; **dr,** dorsal root; **con,** conus medullaris; **sas,** subarachnoid space with contrast; **ef,** epidural fat.

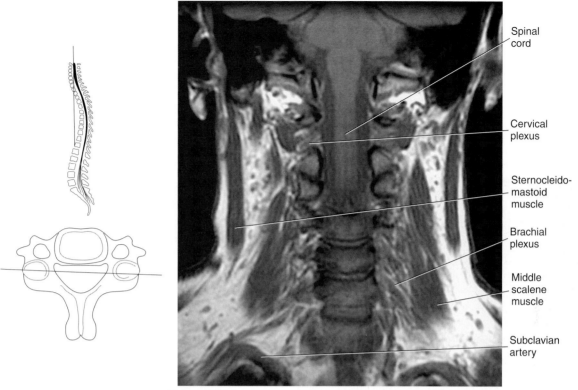

Spinal cord

Cervical plexus

Sternocleido-mastoid muscle

Brachial plexus

Middle scalene muscle

Subclavian artery

Figure 4.92
Coronal, T1-weighted MR scan of cervical plexus.

Cervical Plexus

The **cervical plexus** arises from the upper four ventral rami of C1-C4 to innervate from the neck, lower part of the face and ear, the side of the scalp, and the upper thoracic area. The major motor branch of this plexus is the **phrenic nerve,** which is formed by the branches of C3, C4, and upper division of C5. This nerve descends vertically down the neck and passes into the superior thoracic aperture. The phrenic nerve continues inferiorly to the diaphragm, together with the pericardiophrenic vessels, through the anterior hilum between the mediastinal pleura and the pericardium. The left and right phrenic nerves can be slightly different in lengths. The right phrenic nerve runs along the lateral wall of the superior vena cava and right atrium of the heart. The left phrenic nerve courses lateral to the left ventricle of the heart (Figures 4.91 through 4.94).

> The phrenic nerve, which innervates the diaphragm, is formed by motor fibers from C4-C5. A primary danger of a broken neck is that an injury at or above the level of C4 may result in paralysis of respiratory muscles, resulting in breathing difficulties and impaired speech production.

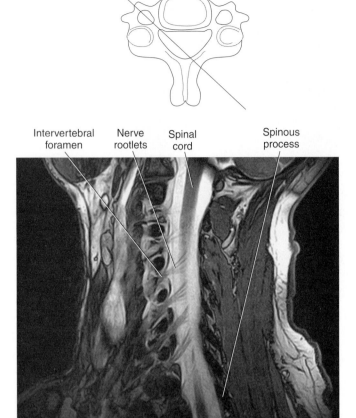

Figure 4.93
Sagittal, T2-weighted MR scan of cervical plexus.

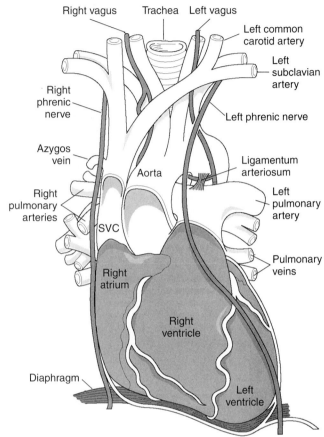

Figure 4.94
Coronal view of phrenic nerve in thoracic cavity. *SVC,* Superior vena cava.

Brachial Plexus

The **brachial plexus** is a large, complex network of nerves arising from the five ventral rami of C5-C8 and T1. The **roots** of the brachial plexus emerge between the anterior and middle scalene muscles, where they continue laterally and inferiorly to divide into three cords just posterior to the clavicle (Figures 4.95 and 4.96). The **cords** extend through the axilla to form five terminal branches: the **musculocutaneous, axillary, median, radial,** and **ulnar** nerves. These nerves provide innervation for the muscles of the upper extremity and shoulder (Figures 4.95 through 4.104).

Herniated intervertebral disks are most common at vertebral levels C5-C6, C6-C7, L4-L5, and L5/S1.

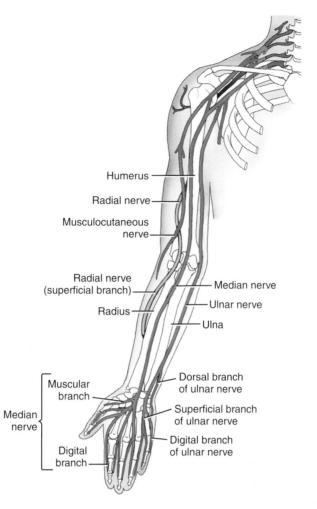

Humerus

Radial nerve

Musculocutaneous nerve

Radial nerve (superficial branch)

Median nerve

Ulnar nerve

Radius

Ulna

Muscular branch

Dorsal branch of ulnar nerve

Superficial branch of ulnar nerve

Median nerve

Digital branch of ulnar nerve

Digital branch

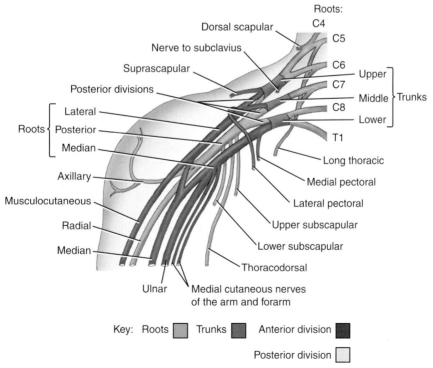

Roots:
C4

Dorsal scapular

C5

Nerve to subclavius

C6

Suprascapular

Upper

C7

Posterior divisions

Middle

Trunks

C8

Lateral

Lower

Roots

Posterior

T1

Median

Long thoracic

Axillary

Medial pectoral

Musculocutaneous

Lateral pectoral

Radial

Upper subscapular

Median

Lower subscapular

Thoracodorsal

Ulnar

Medial cutaneous nerves of the arm and forearm

Key: Roots ☐   Trunks ☐   Anterior division ☐

Posterior division ☐

Figure 4.95

Anterior view of cervical and brachial plexuses.

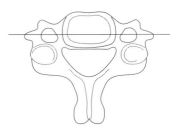

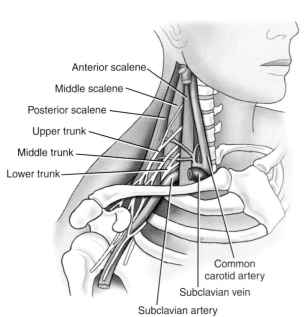

Anterior scalene
Middle scalene
Posterior scalene
Upper trunk
Middle trunk
Lower trunk

Common
carotid artery
Subclavian vein
Subclavian artery

Figure 4.96
Oblique view of brachial plexus.

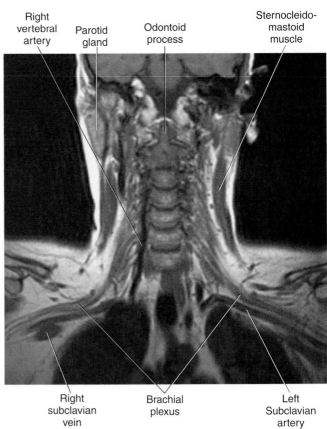

Right
vertebral
artery   Parotid
gland   Odontoid
process   Sternocleido-
mastoid
muscle

Right
subclavian
vein   Brachial
plexus   Left
Subclavian
artery

Figure 4.97
Coronal, T1-weighted MR scan of brachial plexus.

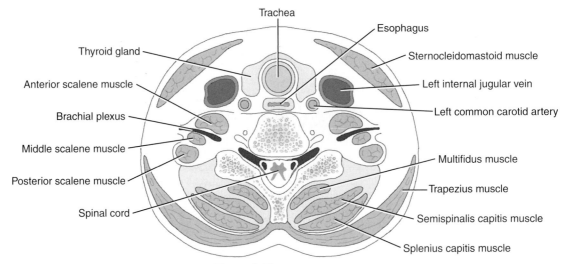

Trachea
Thyroid gland
Anterior scalene muscle
Brachial plexus
Middle scalene muscle
Posterior scalene muscle
Spinal cord

Esophagus
Sternocleidomastoid muscle
Left internal jugular vein
Left common carotid artery
Multifidus muscle
Trapezius muscle
Semispinalis capitis muscle
Splenius capitis muscle

Figure 4.98
Axial view of brachial plexus.

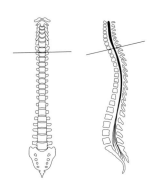

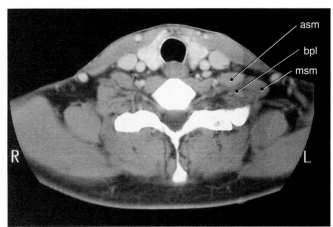

Brachial plexus · Anterior scalene muscle · Middle scalene muscle

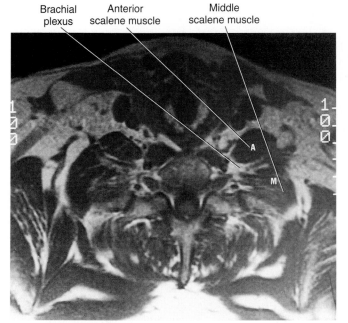

Figure 4.99
Axial, T1-weighted MR scan of brachial plexus.

Figure 4.100
Axial CT scan of brachial plexus.

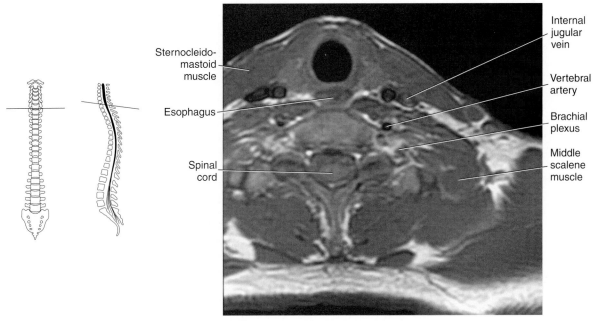

Sternocleido-mastoid muscle

Esophagus

Spinal cord

Internal jugular vein

Vertebral artery

Brachial plexus

Middle scalene muscle

Figure 4.101
Axial, T1-weighted scan of brachial plexus in axillary region.

KEY: asm, Anterior scalene muscle; **bpl,** brachial plexus; **msm,** middle scalene muscle.

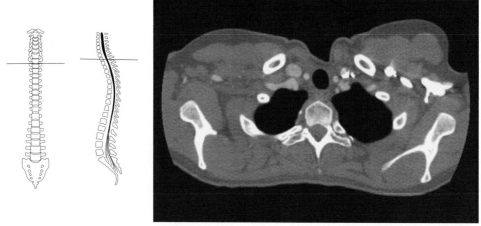

Figure 4.102
Axial CT scan of brachial plexus in axillary region.

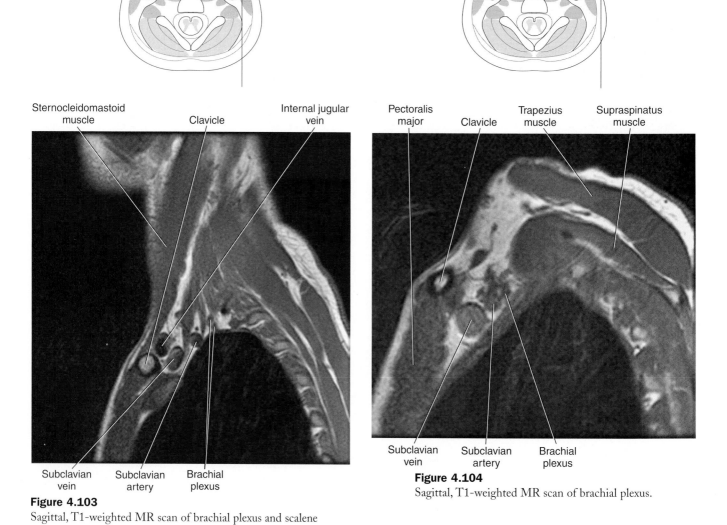

Sternocleidomastoid muscle   Clavicle   Internal jugular vein

Pectoralis major   Clavicle   Trapezius muscle   Supraspinatus muscle

Subclavian vein   Subclavian artery   Brachial plexus

Figure 4.104
Sagittal, T1-weighted MR scan of brachial plexus.

Subclavian vein   Subclavian artery   Brachial plexus

Figure 4.103
Sagittal, T1-weighted MR scan of brachial plexus and scalene muscles.

Lumbar Plexus

The **lumbar plexus** arises from the ventral rami of T12 and L1-L4. The lumbar plexus is situated on the posterior abdominal wall, between the psoas major muscle and the transverse processes of the lumbar vertebrae. In general, it serves the lower abdominopelvic region and anterior and medial muscles of the thigh. The **femoral nerve** is the largest branch of the lumbar plexus descending beneath the inguinal ligament. At the level of the lesser trochanter the femoral nerve divides into several branches, the largest being the **saphenous nerve,** which descends along the medial aspect of the leg to the ankle accompanied by the great saphenous vein. The saphenous nerve innervates the anterior lower leg, some of the ankle, and part of the foot (Figures 4.105 through 4.108).

> **Paraplegia will result from transection of the spinal cord between the cervical and lumbosacral enlargements. Quadriplegia will result if the transection occurs above the level of C3.**

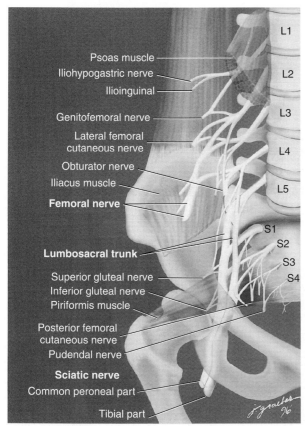

Figure 4.105
Coronal view of lumbar and sacral plexuses.

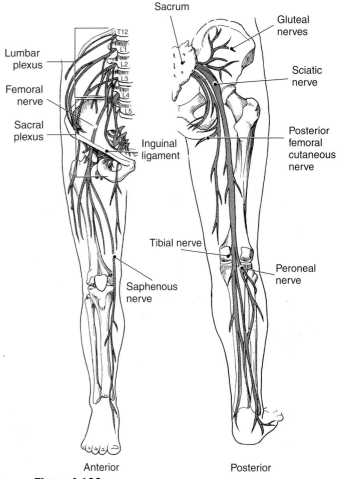

Figure 4.106
Anterior and posterior views of lumbar and sacral plexuses.

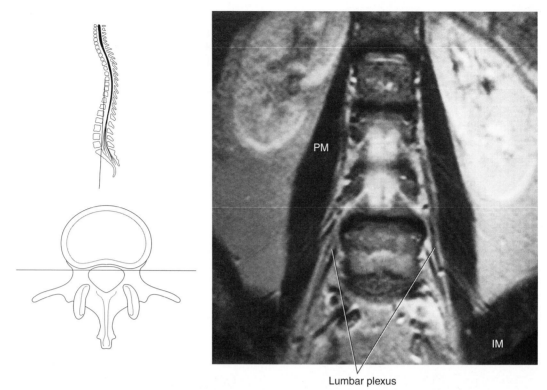

Figure 4.107
Coronal, T1-weighted MR scan of lumbar plexus.

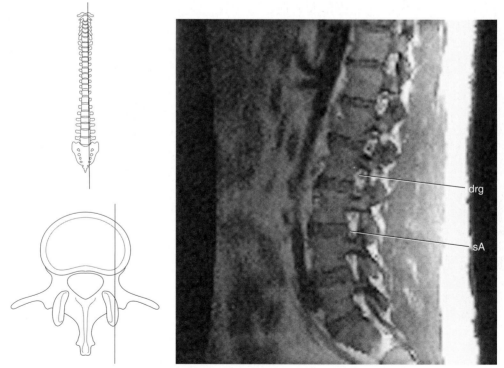

Figure 4.108
Sagittal, T1-weighted MR scan of lumbar plexus.

KEY: PM, Pectoralis major muscle; **IM,** iliacus muscle; **drg,** dorsal root ganglion; **sA,** spinal artery.

Sacral Plexus

Arising from L4-L5 and S1-S4, the nerves of the **sacral plexus** innervate the buttock, posterior thigh, and feet. These nerves converge toward the inferior sacral foramina to unite into a large flattened band. Most of this nerve network continues into the thigh as the **sciatic nerve,** which is the largest nerve in the body. The sciatic nerve exits the pelvis through the greater sciatic foramen and continues to descend vertically along the posterior thigh. In its course it divides into the **tibial** and **peroneal nerves,** which innervate the posterior aspect of the lower extremity. The sacral plexus lies against the posterolateral wall of the pelvis between the piriformis muscle and internal iliac vessels, just anterior to the sacroiliac joint (Figures 4.105, 4.106, and 4.109 through 4.113).

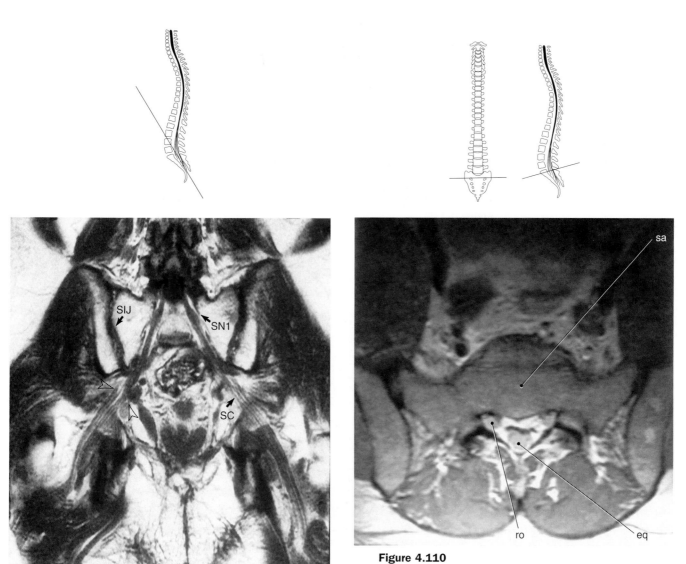

Figure 4.109
Coronal, T1-weighted MR scan of sacroiliac joints and sacral plexus.

Figure 4.110
Axial, T1-weighted MR scan of sacrum and sacral plexus.

KEY: SIJ, Sacroiliac joint; **SN1,** S1 nerve; **SC,** sciatic nerve; **sa,** sacrum; **eq,** cauda equina; **ro,** root sleeve.

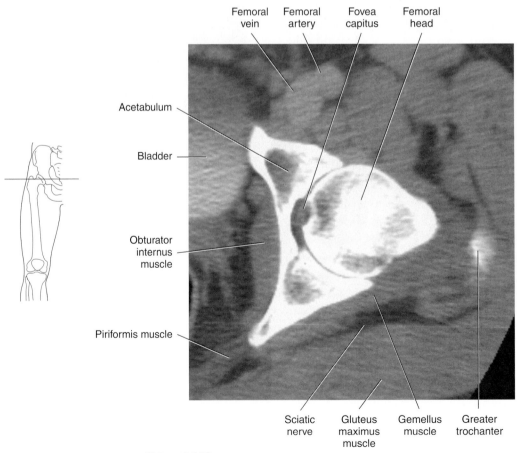

Figure 4.111
Axial, T1-weighted MR scan of femoral head and sciatic nerve.

Figure 4.112
Axial CT scan of femoral head and sciatic nerve.

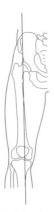

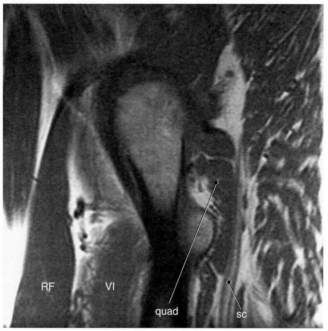

RF   VI

quad   sc

Figure 4.113
Sagittal, T1-weighted MR scan of sciatic nerve.

KEY: FV, Femoral vein; **FA,** femoral artery; **sc,** sciatic nerve; **RF,** rectus femoris; **VI,** vastus intermedius; **quad,** quadratus femoris.

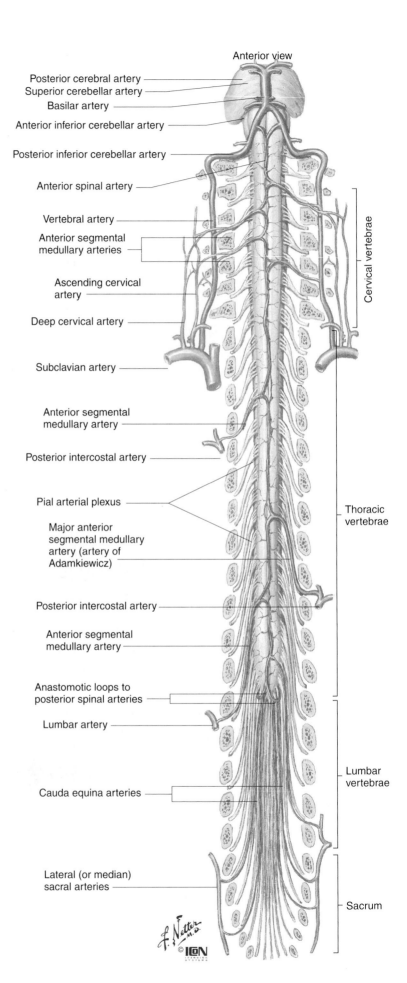

Figure 4.114
Anterior view of anterior spinal artery.

Anterior view

Posterior cerebral artery

Superior cerebellar artery

Basilar artery

Anterior inferior cerebellar artery

Posterior inferior cerebellar artery

Anterior spinal artery

Vertebral artery

Anterior segmental
medullary arteries

Ascending cervical
artery

Deep cervical artery

Subclavian artery

Anterior segmental
medullary artery

Posterior intercostal artery

Pial arterial plexus

Major anterior
segmental medullary
artery (artery of
Adamkiewicz)

Posterior intercostal artery

Anterior segmental
medullary artery

Anastomotic loops to
posterior spinal arteries

Lumbar artery

Cauda equina arteries

Lateral (or median)
sacral arteries

Cervical vertebrae

Thoracic
vertebrae

Lumbar
vertebrae

Sacrum

VASCULATURE

Spinal Arteries

The spinal cord is supplied by a single anterior spinal artery, by a paired posterior spinal arteries, and from a series of spinal branches. The **anterior spinal artery** is formed, just caudal to the basilar artery, by the union of two small branches of the vertebral arteries (Figure 4.114). It runs the entire length of the spinal cord in the anterior median fissure and supplies the anterior two thirds of the spinal cord (Figures 4.115 and 4.116). Although the anterior spinal artery is quite small in diameter, it is widest in the cervical and lumbar enlargements and is much reduced in the thoracic region. The **posterior spinal arteries** arise as small branches of either the vertebral or the posterior inferior cerebellar arteries and descend along the dorsal surface of the spinal cord (Figure 4.117). The posterior one third of the spinal cord is supplied by the posterior spinal arteries. There exist frequent anastomoses joining the two posterior spinal arteries with each other and with the anterior spinal artery. The **spinal branches** arise at various levels from the vertebral, deep cervical, posterior intercostal, lumbar, and

lateral sacral arteries. The spinal branches enter the spinal canal through the intervertebral foramen (Figures 4.117 and 4.118). After giving off an anterior and posterior branch to the wall of the vertebral canal, the spinal branch divides into anterior and posterior radicular arteries that pass along the ventral and dorsal roots into the spinal cord (Figure 4.114). The **anterior radicular arteries** contribute blood to the anterior spinal artery, and the **posterior radicular arteries** contribute blood to the posterior spinal arteries. The largest of the radicular arteries is the **great anterior radicular artery (artery of Adamkiewicz),** which arises in the lower thoracic and upper lumbar region typically between T12 and L3 (Figures 4.114 and 4.116). This vessel makes a major contribution to the anterior spinal artery and provides the main blood supply to the inferior two thirds of the spinal cord.

> **A rupture from an aneurysm of the great radicular artery (artery of Adamkiewicz) may result in paralysis of the lower limbs because the artery provides the main blood supply to the inferior two thirds of the spinal cord.**

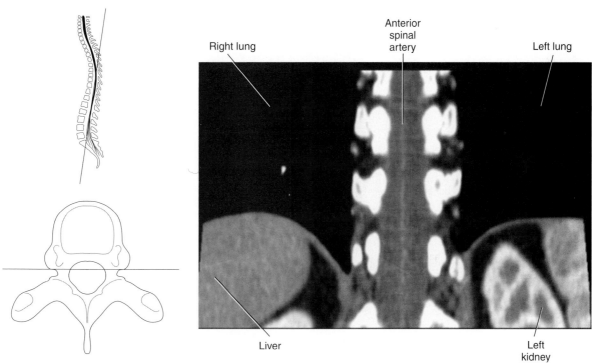

Figure 4.115
Coronal CT reformat with anterior spinal artery.

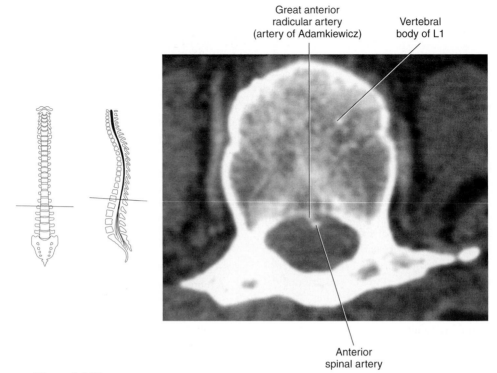

Figure 4.116
Axial CT scan with anterior spinal artery and great anterior radicular artery (artery of Adamkiewicz).

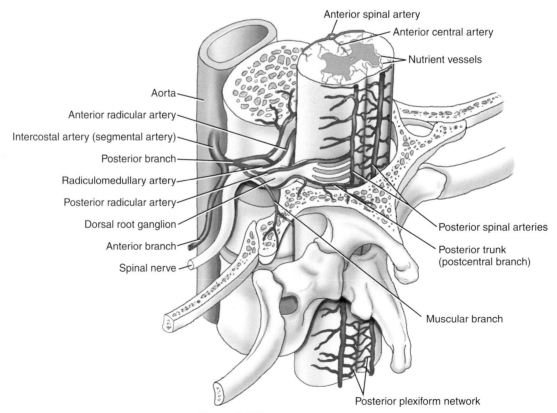

Figure 4.117
Oblique view of radicular arteries.

Intercostal artery
(spinal branch)

Spinal
muscles

Rib

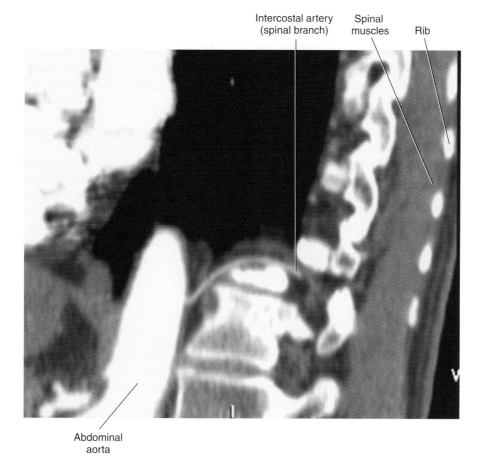

Abdominal
aorta

Figure 4.118
Coronal oblique CT curved-reformat with arteries of the spinal cord.

Spinal Veins

VEINS OF THE SPINAL CORD   The veins that drain the spinal cord follow the same segmental organization as their arterial counterparts. The central gray matter of the cord is drained by the **anterior** and **posterior central veins** located in the anterior median fissure and posterior sulcus, respectively. The outer white matter is drained by small **radial veins** that encircle the spinal cord within the pia mater. The venous blood collected by these tiny veins drains into the **anterior** and **posterior median (spinal) veins** created by the longitudinal venous channels within the pia mater on the anterior and posterior surfaces of the spinal cord (Figure 4.119). The anterior median vein parallels the anterior spinal artery, and the posterior median vein typically presents as the largest vascular structure on the posterior surface of the spinal cord. The anterior and posterior median veins drain into the **anterior** and **posterior radicular veins** that parallel the ventral and dorsal nerve roots and eventually empty into the **intervertebral veins** that accompany the spinal nerves through the intervertebral foramina.

VEINS OF THE VERTEBRAL COLUMN   The veins of the vertebral column form an extensive network of **internal** and **external venous plexuses,** named according to their corresponding location to the vertebral column (Figures 4.119 and 4.120). The **internal venous plexuses** lie within the vertebral canal in the epidural space and are divided into **anterior** and **posterior internal plexuses.** The anterior internal venous plexuses are found on either side of the anterior longitudinal ligament, and the single posterior internal venous plexus lies anterior to the ligamentum flavum.

The valveless **external venous plexuses** communicate freely with the vertebral veins and intracranial venous sinuses and are located at the outer surfaces of the vertebral column. They can be divided into the anterior and posterior external plexuses. The **anterior external plexuses** run directly in front of the vertebral bodies and the **posterior external plexuses** run along the posterior aspect of the vertebral arches (Figure 4.121). The anterior sections of the internal and external plexuses communicate via a network of veins that drain the vertebral bodies called the **basivertebral veins.** The basivertebral veins emerge from the posterior surfaces of the vertebral bodies, creating large channels that join with the anterior internal venous plexuses (Figure 4.122). The internal and external venous plexuses, along with the radicular veins, drain into the intervertebral veins, ending in the vertebral, intercostal, lumbar, and sacral veins.

> Because the vertebral venous plexuses are valveless, an increase in intraabdominal pressure (e.g., coughing, straining) may cause backflow of blood into the basivertebral veins of the spine or dural sinuses of the brain. This creates a potential pathway for metastatic disease or other pathology to spread to the central nervous system.

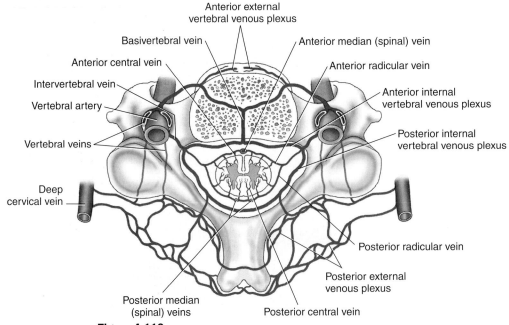

Figure 4.119

Axial view of venous drainage of vertebral column and spinal cord.

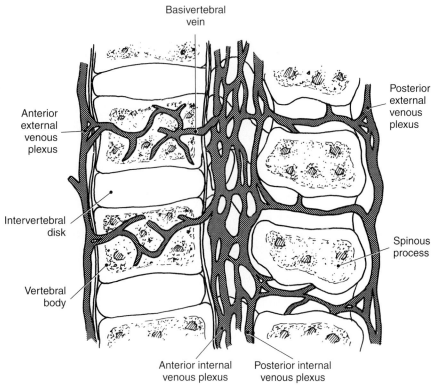

Basivertebral
vein

Anterior
external
venous
plexus

Posterior
external
venous
plexus

Intervertebral
disk

Spinous
process

Vertebral
body

Anterior internal
venous plexus

Posterior internal
venous plexus

Figure 4.120
Sagittal view of venous plexuses of the spine.

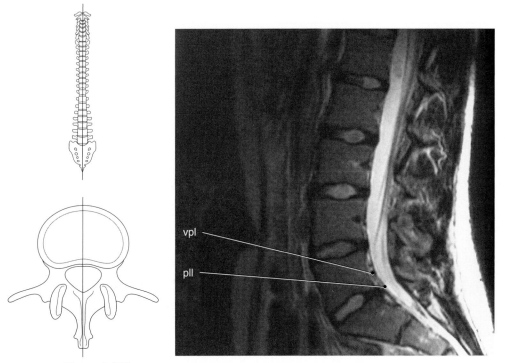

vpl

pll

Figure 4.121
Sagittal, T2-weighted MR scan of lumbar spine showing internal venous plexus.

KEY: **vpl,** Venous plexus; **pll,** posterior longitudinal ligament.

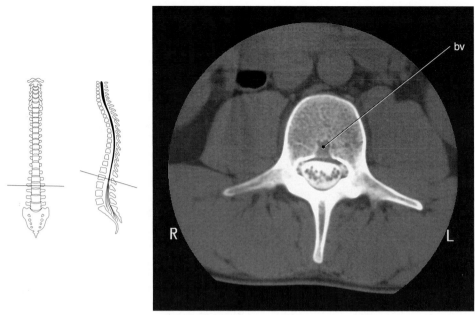

Figure 4.122
Axial CT scan of lumbar vertebra demonstrating basivertebral vein.

KEY: bv, Basivertebral vein.

REFERENCES

Agur AM: *Grant's atlas of anatomy,* Baltimore, 1996, Williams & Wilkins.

Ballinger PW: *Merrill's atlas of radiographic positions and radiologic procedures,* ed 10, St. Louis, 2003, Mosby.

English AW: *Wolf-Heidegger's atlas of human anatomy,* ed 5, Basel, Switzerland, 2000, S. Karger.

Frick H, Leonhardt H, Starck D, et al: *Human anatomy 1,* New York, 1991, Thieme Medical Publishers.

Frick H, Leonhardt H, Starck D, et al: *Human anatomy 2,* New York, 1991, Thieme Medical Publishers.

Gray H: *Gray's anatomy,* ed 15, New York, 1995, Barnes & Noble.

Harnsberger HR: *Handbook of head and neck imaging,* ed 2, St. Louis, 1995, Mosby.

Hayman LA: *Clinical brain imaging: Normal structure and functional anatomy,* St. Louis, 1992, Mosby.

Hendelman WJ: *Student's atlas of neuroanatomy,* Philadelphia, 1994, Saunders.

Jacob S: *Atlas of human anatomy,* Philadelphia, 2002, Churchill Livingstone.

Larsen WJ: *Anatomy: development function clinical correlations,* Philadelphia, 2002, Saunders.

Leblanc A: *Atlas of hearing and balance organs,* New York, 1999, Springer-Verlag.

Mancuso AA: *Workbook for MRI and CT of the head and neck,* ed 2, Baltimore, 1989, Williams & Wilkins.

Martini FH: *Fundamentals of anatomy and physiology,* ed 3, Englewood Cliffs, NJ, 1995, Prentice-Hall.

Mosby's medical, nursing, and allied health dictionary, ed 6, St. Louis, 2002, Mosby.

Netter FH: *The Ciba collection: nervous system,* Summitt, NJ, 1957, Ciba Pharmaceutical Products.

Orrison WW, Lewine JD, Sanders JA, et al: *Functional brain imaging,* St. Louis, 1995, Mosby.

Osborn AG: *Diagnostic neuroradiology,* St. Louis, 1994, Mosby.

Osborn AG, Tong KA: *Handbook of neuroradiology: brain and skull,* ed 2, St. Louis, 1996, Mosby.

Palastanga N, Field D, Soames R, et al: *Anatomy and human movement,* ed 4, Philadelphia, 2002, Butterworth-Heinemann.

Standring S: *Gray's anatomy,* ed 39, Philadelphia, 2005, Churchill Livingstone.

Som PM, Curtin HD: *Head and neck imaging,* ed 3, St. Louis, 1996, Mosby Year Book.

Stark DD, Bradley WG: *Magnetic resonance imaging,* ed 3, St. Louis, 1999, Mosby.

Taveras JM: *Neuroradiology,* ed 3, Baltimore, 1996, Williams & Wilkins.

Valvassori GE, Mahmood FM, Carter BL: *Imaging of the head and neck,* New York, 1995, Thieme Medical Publishers.

Warner JJ: *Atlas of neuroanatomy: with systems organization and case correlations,* Philadelphia, 2001, Butterworth-Heinemann.

NECK

A sharp tongue and a dull mind are usually found in the same head.

PROVERB

The neck has a large amount of complex anatomy situated in a relatively small area. Recent advances in medical imaging have enhanced the ability to differentiate among the structures of the neck (Figure 5.1). This chapter demonstrates sectional anatomy of the following structures:

ORGANS
>   Pharynx
>   Larynx
>   Esophagus and Trachea
>   Salivary Glands
>   Thyroid Gland
>   Cervical Lymph Nodes

MUSCLES
>   Pharyngeal Muscles
>   Laryngeal Muscles
>   Muscles within the Anterior
>   Triangle
>   Muscles within the Posterior
>   Triangle
>   Fascial Planes and Spaces

VASCULAR STRUCTURES
>   Carotid Arteries
>   Vertebral Arteries
>   Jugular Veins
>   Carotid Sheath

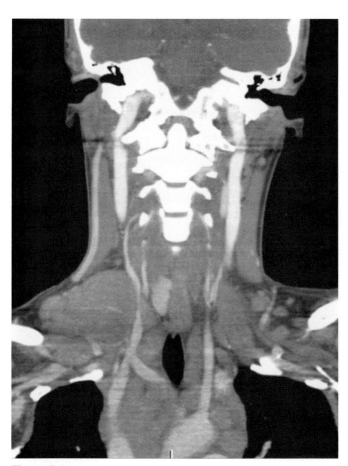

Figure 5.1
Coronal CT reformat demonstrating massive cervical lymphadenopathy.

ORGANS

The organs of the neck are attached to one another by connective tissue. They are located primarily in the anterior and middle portions of the neck and include the pharynx, larynx, esophagus, trachea, salivary glands, thyroid gland, and cervical lymph nodes.

Pharynx

The **pharynx** is a funnel-shaped fibromuscular tube approximately 12 cm long that acts as an opening for both the respiratory and digestive systems. The pharynx extends from the base of the skull and ends inferiorly as the continuation of the esophagus. The pharynx is divided into three sections: nasopharynx, oropharynx, and laryngopharynx (Figures 5.2 and 5.3).

The **nasopharynx** is the most superior portion of the pharynx. It is an extension of the nasal cavities with which it shares the nasal mucosa. The nasopharynx has a respiratory function to allow for the passage of air from the nasal cavity to the larynx. Posteriorly, the boundaries of the nasopharynx are the clivus and upper cervical spine. It is bordered inferiorly by the **soft palate** and extends down to the level of the **uvula,** which is a process on the posterior edge of the soft palate. In the roof and posterior wall of the nasopharynx is a collection of lymphoid tissue known as **pharyngeal tonsils.** The pharyngeal tonsils have a protective immune function of initiating early activation of specific defense mechanisms (Figures 5.2 and 5.4 through 5.7). Within the lateral wall of the nasopharynx, posterior to the inferior nasal conchae, is the opening of the **auditory tube (eustachian tube),** which connects the middle ear to the nasopharynx.

The **oropharynx** is a posterior extension of the oral cavity and extends from the soft palate to the level of the hyoid bone (Figures 5.8 and 5.9). It is separated from the larynx by the epiglottis. Two additional pairs of lymphoid tissue are found within the oropharynx: the **palatine tonsils,** which are located on the lateral walls and the smaller **lingual tonsils,** which are situated on the base of the tongue. On each side of the union of the base of the tongue and the epiglottis are two pouchlike openings called **valleculae.** The valleculae are common sites for foreign objects to become lodged within the neck (Figures 5.2 through 5.5, 5.10, and 5.11).

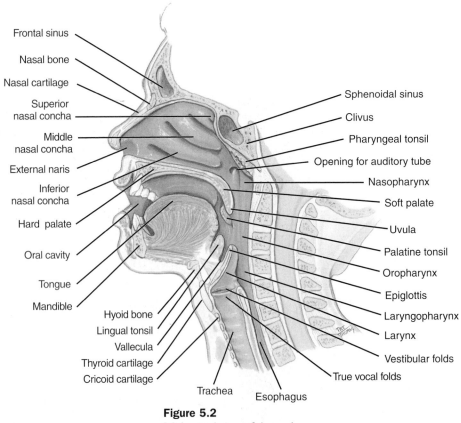

Figure 5.2
Midsagittal view of the neck.

KEY: **na,** Nasopharynx; **or,** oropharynx; **la,** laryngopharynx.

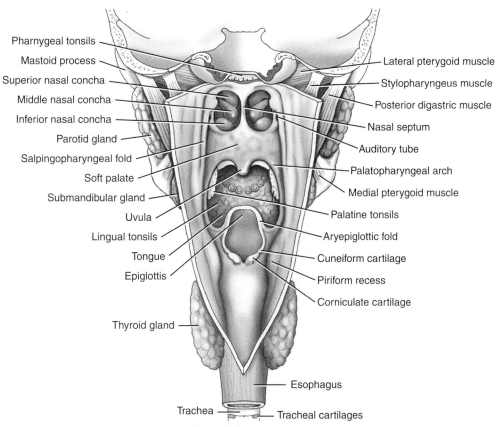

Pharyngeal tonsils
Mastoid process
Superior nasal concha
Middle nasal concha
Inferior nasal concha
Parotid gland
Salpingopharyngeal fold
Soft palate
Submandibular gland
Uvula
Lingual tonsils
Tongue
Epiglottis
Thyroid gland

Lateral pterygoid muscle
Stylopharyngeus muscle
Posterior digastric muscle
Nasal septum
Auditory tube
Palatopharyngeal arch
Medial pterygoid muscle
Palatine tonsils
Aryepiglottic fold
Cuneiform cartilage
Piriform recess
Corniculate cartilage
Esophagus
Trachea
Tracheal cartilages

Figure 5.3
Posterior view of pharynx.

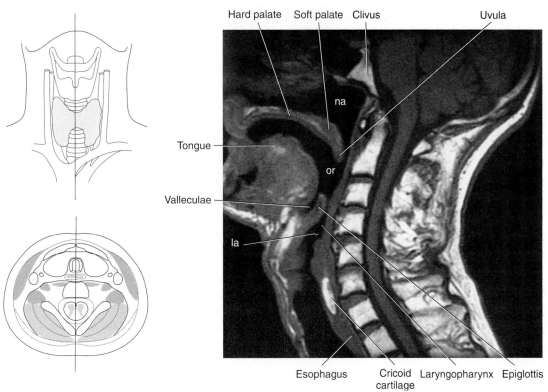

Hard palate   Soft palate   Clivus   Uvula
na
Tongue
or
Valleculae
la
Esophagus   Cricoid   Laryngopharynx   Epiglottis
cartilage

Figure 5.4
Midsagittal, T1-weighted MR scan of pharyngeal divisions.

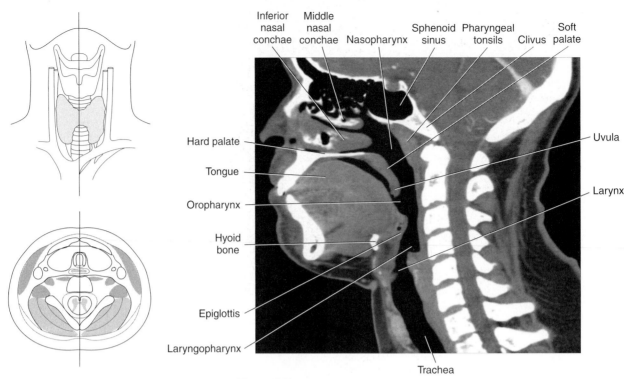

Inferior nasal conchae   Middle nasal conchae   Nasopharynx   Sphenoid sinus   Pharyngeal tonsils   Clivus   Soft palate

Hard palate

Tongue

Oropharynx

Hyoid bone

Epiglottis

Laryngopharynx

Uvula

Larynx

Trachea

Figure 5.5
Sagittal CT reformat of pharynx.

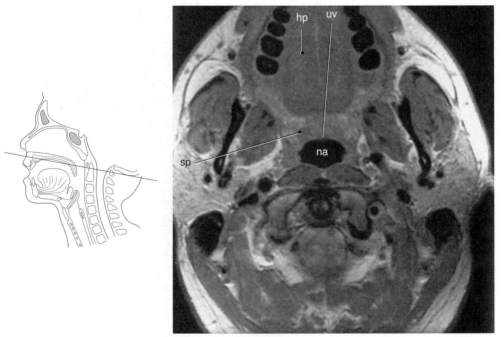

Figure 5.6
Axial, T1-weighted MR scan of nasopharynx.

KEY: hp, Hard palate; **uv,** uvula; **sp,** soft palate; **na,** nasopharynx.

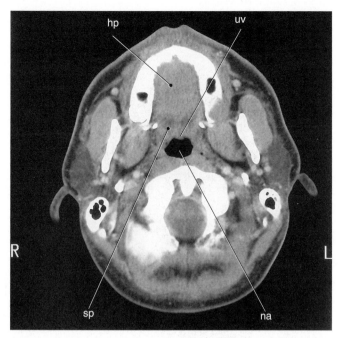

Figure 5.7
Axial CT scan of nasopharynx.

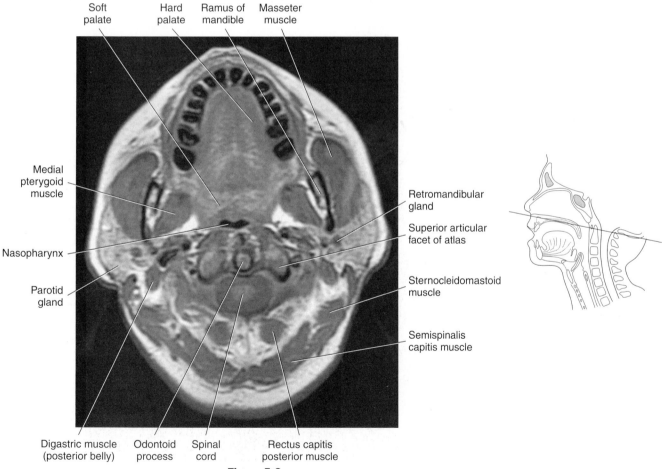

Figure 5.8
Axial, T1-weighted MR scan of nasopharynx.

KEY: hp, Hard palate; **uv,** uvula; **sp,** soft palate; **na,** nasopharynx.

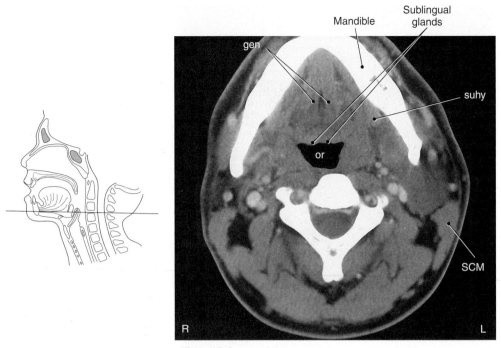

Figure 5.9
Axial CT scan of oropharynx.

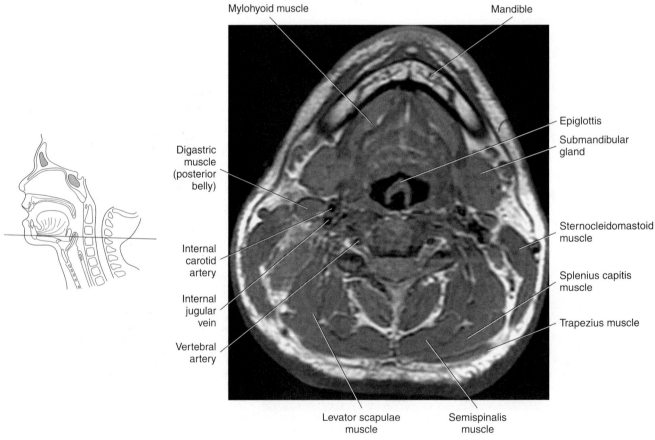

Figure 5.10
Axial, T1-weighted MR scan of valleculae.

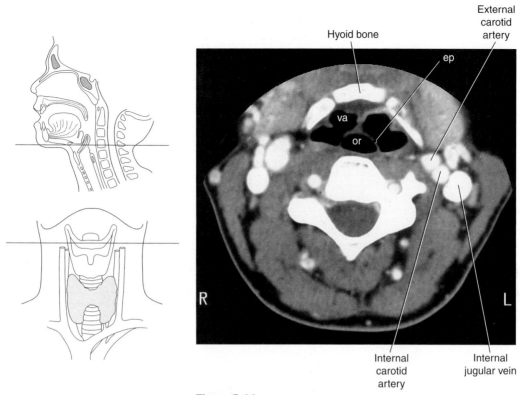

Figure 5.11
Axial CT scan of valleculae.

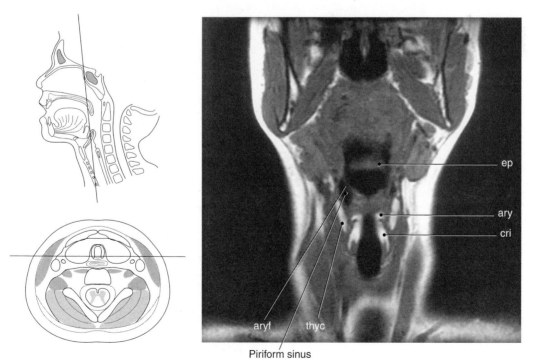

Figure 5.12
Coronal, T1-weighted MR scan of larynx.

KEY: ep, Epiglottis; **va,** vallecula; **or,** oropharynx; **ary,** arytenoids cartilage; **cri,** cricoid cartilage; **thyc,** thyroid cartilage; **aryf,** arytenoids fold.

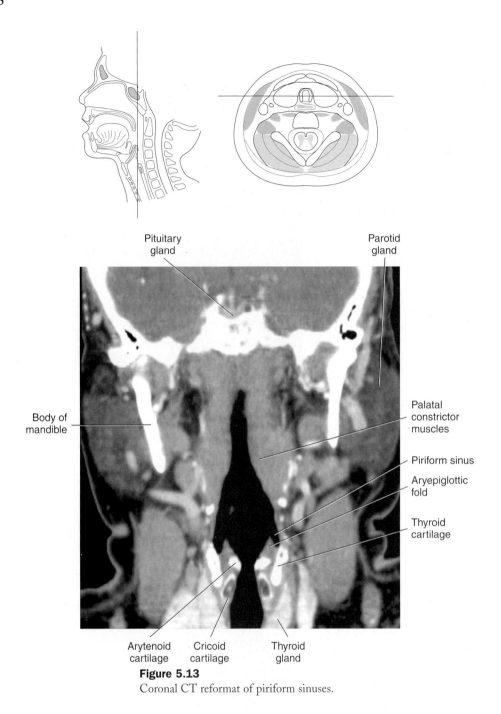

Pituitary gland

Parotid gland

Body of mandible

Palatal constrictor muscles

Piriform sinus

Aryepiglottic fold

Thyroid cartilage

Arytenoid cartilage   Cricoid cartilage   Thyroid gland

Figure 5.13
Coronal CT reformat of piriform sinuses.

The narrow **laryngopharynx** continues from the oropharynx and lies between the hyoid bone and the entrance to the larynx and esophagus. It continues as the esophagus at the level of the cricoid cartilage of the larynx. Within the anterior walls of the laryngopharynx, along either side of the larynx are two depressions or cavities termed the **piriform sinuses (recesses).** These sinuses divert food away from the entrance of the larynx so that it can continue into the esophagus (Figures 5.2 through 5.5 and 5.12 through 5.15).

> **The pharyngeal tonsils, when enlarged, are frequently referred to as the *adenoids.***

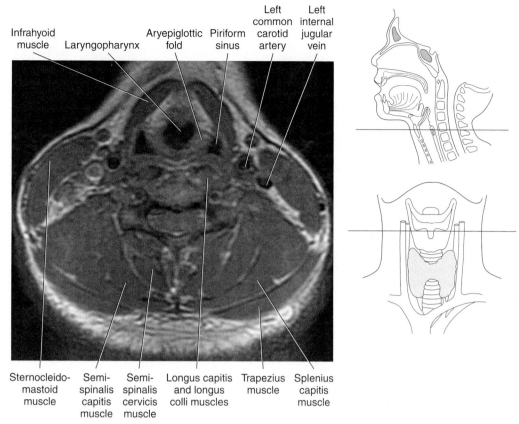

Infrahyoid muscle
Laryngopharynx
Aryepiglottic fold
Piriform sinus
Left common carotid artery
Left internal jugular vein

Sternocleido-mastoid muscle
Semi-spinalis capitis muscle
Semi-spinalis cervicis muscle
Longus capitis and longus colli muscles
Trapezius muscle
Splenius capitis muscle

Figure 5.14
Axial, T1-weighted MR scan of laryngopharynx.

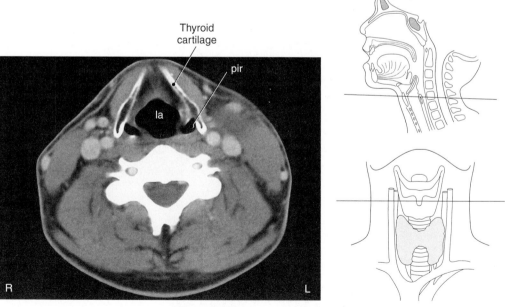

Thyroid cartilage
pir
la

R   L

Figure 5.15
Axial CT scan of laryngopharynx.

KEY: **pir,** Piriform sinus; **la,** larynx.

Larynx

The **larynx** is the bony skeleton that surrounds and protects the vocal cords and is commonly called the *voice box*. It begins at the laryngopharynx and continues to the trachea and marks the beginning of the respiratory pathway by allowing for the passage of air into the trachea. The larynx consists of an outer skeleton made up of nine cartilages that extend from approximately the third to the sixth cervical vertebrae. These cartilages are connected to one another by ligaments and are moved by numerous muscles. Three of the cartilages are unpaired and include the thyroid, epiglottis, and cricoid. The three paired cartilages are the arytenoid, corniculate, and cuneiform (Figures 5.16 through 5.19). The largest and most superior is the **thyroid cartilage.** It consists of a right and a left lamina that unite anteriorly to form a shield to protect the vocal cords (Figures 5.20 and 5.21). The anterior union of the lamina forms a vertical projection commonly referred to as the *Adam's apple.* On the posterior aspect of this projection is the attachment for the epiglottis. The **epiglottis** differs from the other cartilages in that it is elastic and allows for movement. During swallowing, the epiglottis folds back over the larynx, preventing the entry of liquids or solid food into the respiratory

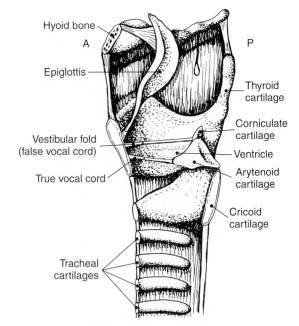

Figure 5.16
Midsagittal view of larynx.

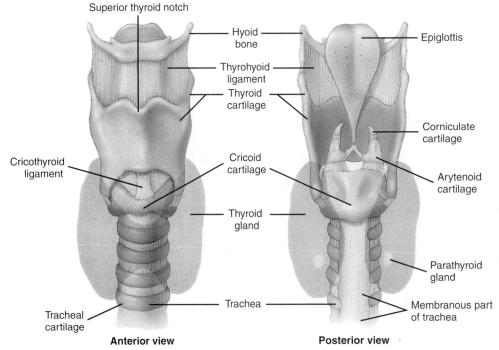

Figure 5.17
Anterior and posterior views of larynx.

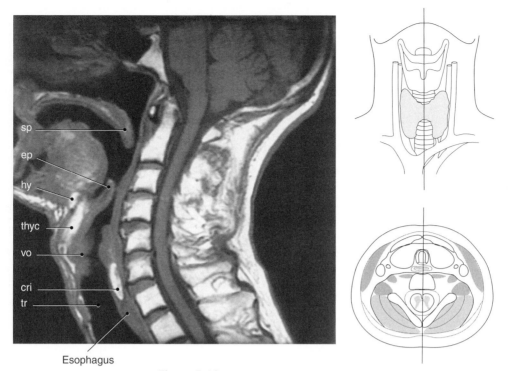

sp

ep

hy

thyc

vo

cri

tr

Esophagus

Figure 5.18
Sagittal, T1-weighted MR scan of larynx.

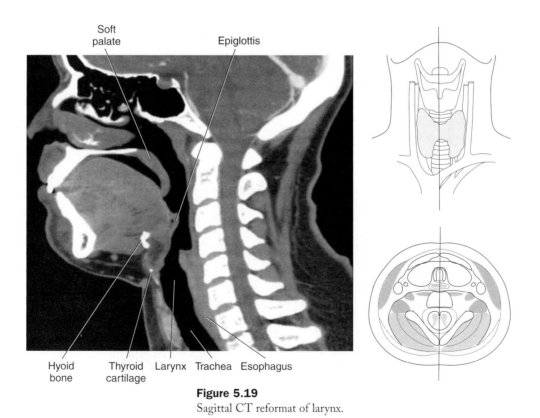

Soft
palate

Epiglottis

Hyoid   Thyroid   Larynx   Trachea Esophagus
bone   cartilage

Figure 5.19
Sagittal CT reformat of larynx.

KEY: **sp,** Soft palate; **ep,** epiglottis; **hy,** hyoid bone; **thyc,** thyroid cartilage; **vo,** vocal cords; **cri,** cricoid cartilage; **tr,** trachea.

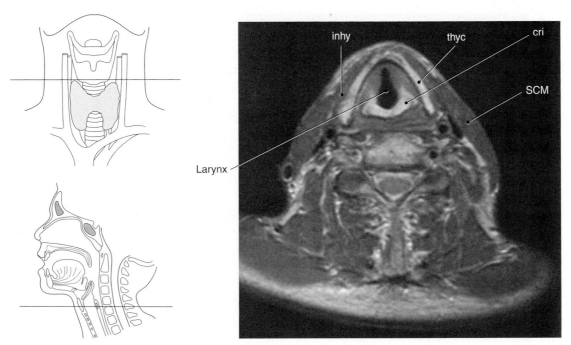

Figure 5.20
Axial, T1-weighted MR scan of neck with thyroid cartilage.

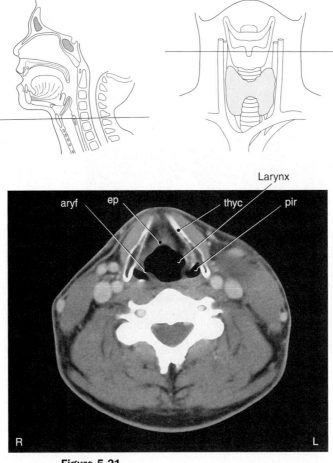

Figure 5.21
Axial CT scan of neck with thyroid cartilage.

passageways (Figures 5.18, 5.19, 5.22, and 5.23). The paired **arytenoid cartilages** are shaped like pyramids and are situated at the posterior aspect of the larynx just on top of the cricoid cartilage (Figures 5.17, 5.24, and 5.25). Articulating with the superior surface of the arytenoid cartilages are the small, horn-shaped **corniculate cartilages.** These cartilages are involved in the opening and closing of the glottis for the production of sound. The small, curved **cuneiform cartilages** lie within the folds of tissue termed the *aryepiglottic folds* that extend between the lateral aspect of the arytenoid cartilage and epiglottis. The **cricoid cartilage** is a complete ring that forms the base of the larynx on which the other laryngeal cartilages rest. The cricoid cartilage marks the junction between the larynx and the trachea and the beginning of the esophagus (Figures 5.26 and 5.27).

> Resultant swelling of the epiglottis because of bacterial or viral infection can be very dangerous (acute epiglottitis). This condition can result in closure of the glottis and suffocation.

The inner structures of the larynx include the false and true vocal cords and the aryepiglottic folds. The false and true vocal cords consist of two pair of ligaments that extend from the arytenoid cartilages to the posterior laminal surface of the thyroid cartilage and are separated by a space termed the *ventricle* (Figure 5.16). The superior pair of ligaments are called the **vestibular folds or false vocal cords** because they are not directly concerned in the production of voice. The inferior pair are the **true vocal cords** named accordingly for their involvement in the production of sound. The true vocal cords extend toward the midline in a closed position during phonation. With quiet respiration the true vocal cords are in a relaxed position, creating an opening between them called the **glottis (rima glottidis)** (Figures 5.24, 5.25, 5.28, and 5.29). The glottis is the part of the larynx most directly involved with voice production. The **aryepiglottic folds** consist of tissue projecting off the arytenoid cartilages to the inferior margin of the epiglottis. These folds form the lateral margins of the entrance to the larynx. Located lateral to these folds, between the larynx and thyroid cartilage, are two mucosal pouches called the **piriform sinuses** whose medial borders form the lateral walls of the larynx (Figures 5.12 through 5.15).

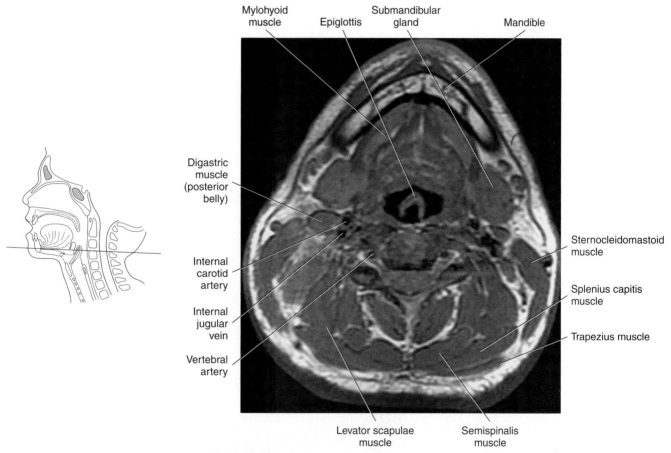

Figure 5.22
Axial, T1-weighted, MR scan of neck with epiglottis.

KEY: inhy, Infrahyoid muscle; **thyc,** thyroid cartilage; **vo,** vocal cords; **cri,** cricoid cartilage; **SCM,** sternocleidomastoid muscle; **aryf,** arytenoids fold; **ep,** epiglottis; **pir,** piriform sinus; **man,** mandible; **va,** vallecula.

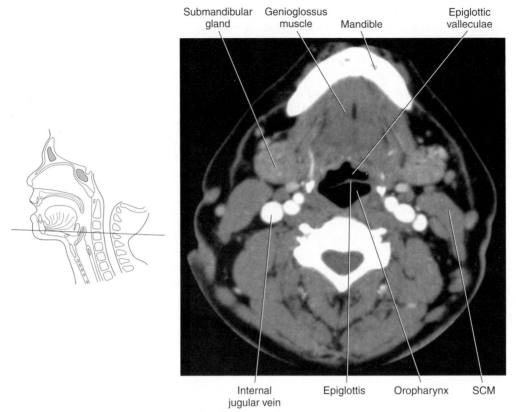

Submandibular gland   Genioglossus muscle   Mandible   Epiglottic valleculae

Internal jugular vein   Epiglottis   Oropharynx   SCM

Figure 5.23
Axial CT scan of neck with epiglottis.

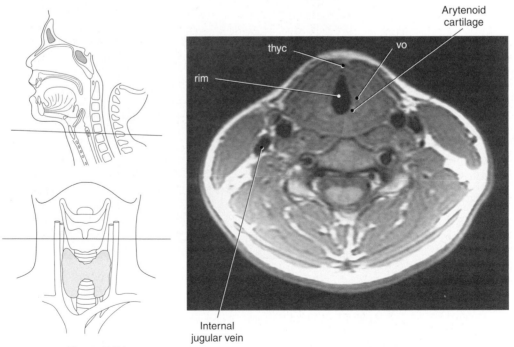

Arytenoid cartilage

thyc   vo

rim

Internal jugular vein

Figure 5.24
Axial, T1-weighted MR scan of larynx with vocal cords and arytenoid cartilages.

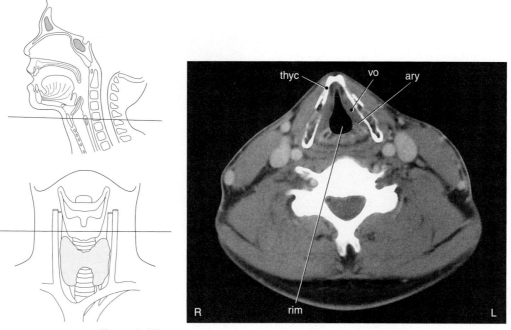

Figure 5.25
Axial CT scan of larynx with vocal cords and arytenoid cartilages.

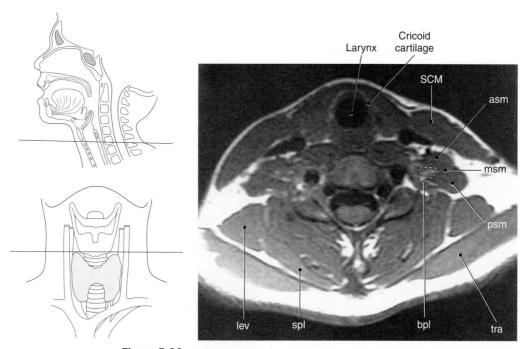

Figure 5.26
Axial, T1-weighted MR scan of larynx with cricoid cartilage.

KEY: **rim,** Rima glottis; **thyc,** thyroid cartilage; **vo,** vocal cords; **ary,** arytenoids cartilage;
SCM, sternocleidomastoid muscle; **asm,** anterior scalene muscle; **msm,** middle scalene muscle;
psm, posterior scalene muscle; **tra,** trapezius muscle; **bpl,** brachial plexus; **spl,** splenius capitus;
lev, levator scapula.

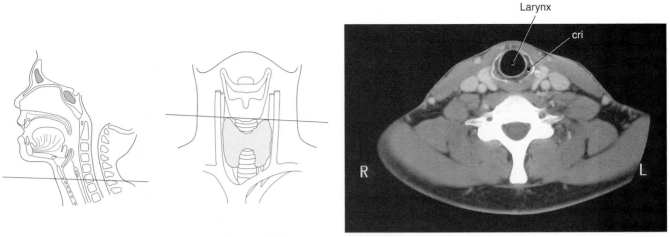

Figure 5.27
Axial CT scan of larynx with cricoid cartilage.

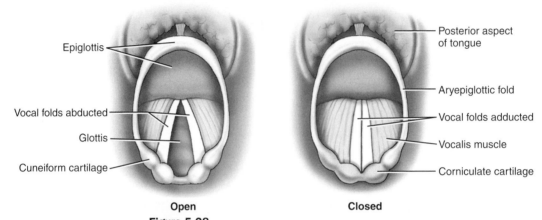

Open   **Closed**
Figure 5.28
Superior view of glottis in open and closed positions.

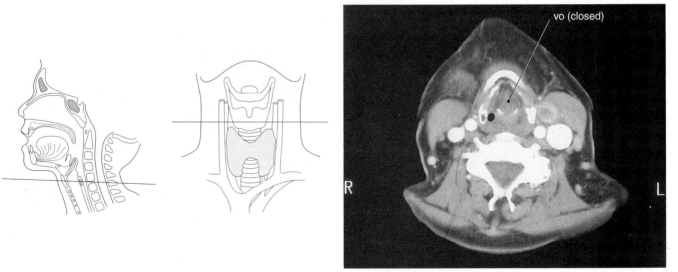

Figure 5.29
Axial CT scan of larynx with closed vocal cords.

KEY: cri, Cricoid cartilage; **vo (closed),** vocal cords (closed).

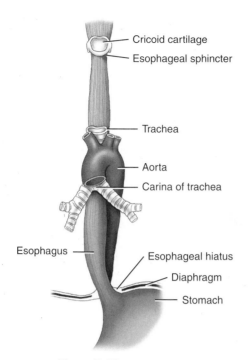

Figure 5.30
Anterior view of esophagus.

Esophagus and Trachea

The esophagus and trachea allow for the transmission of food to the stomach and air to the lungs. The **esophagus** is a muscular tube that extends down from the laryngopharynx to the cardiac orifice of the stomach (Figures 5.30 through 5.32). It begins posterior to the cricoid cartilage, then descends through the thoracic cavity between the trachea and anterior longitudinal ligament of the vertebrae. The esophagus then enters the abdominal cavity through an opening in the diaphragm termed the *esophageal hiatus* to meet the stomach (Figure 5.30). There are two narrowed areas, or sphincters, of the esophagus: esophageal and cardiac. The esophageal sphincter is situated at the entrance of the esophagus and functions to prevent air from entering the esophagus. The inferior or cardiac sphincter prevents reflux from the stomach into the esophagus. The **trachea,** considered the airway, extends from the larynx to the lungs and lies immediately anterior to the esophagus (Figures 5.30 through 5.32). Considered an elastic tube, the trachea is reinforced by many C-shaped pieces of cartilage that maintain an open passageway for air. The cartilages are closed posteriorly by elastic connective tissue that allows for the passage of food through the esophagus. At approximately the level of T5, the trachea bifurcates at a level termed the *carina* into the right and left mainstem bronchi.

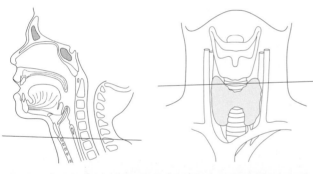

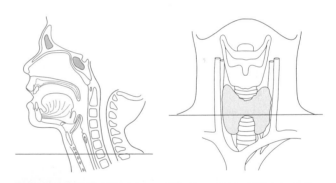

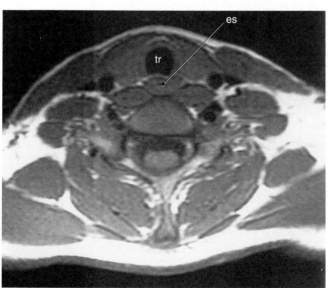

Figure 5.31
Axial, T1-weighted MR scan of esophagus and trachea.

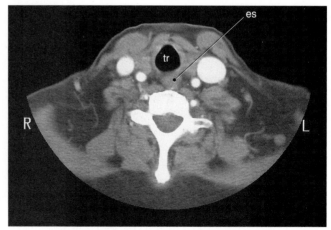

Figure 5.32
Axial CT scan of esophagus and trachea.

KEY: tr, Trachea; **es,** esophagus.

Salivary Glands

The **salivary glands** collectively produce and empty saliva into the oral cavity by way of ducts to begin the process of digestion. Each pair of salivary glands has a distinctive cellular organization and produces saliva with slightly different properties. There are three large paired salivary glands: parotid, submandibular, and sublingual (Figure 5.33). The largest of the pairs are the **parotid glands,** which are situated in front of the auricle, wedged between the ramus of the mandible and the sternocleidomastoid muscle (Figures 5.34 through 5.37). The parotid glands extend inferiorly from the level of the external auditory meatus to the angle of the mandible. Their appearance differs from that of the other salivary glands because of the amount of fat they contain. The **parotid duct (Stensen's duct)** emerges from the anterior edge of the gland. It passes under the zygomatic arch to enter the oral cavity opposite the second upper molar. The **submandibular glands** border the posterior half of the mandible, extending from the angle of the mandible to the level of the hyoid bone (Figures 5.38 through 5.40). The **submandibular duct (Wharton's duct)** opens into the oral cavity on either side of the lingual frenulum immediately posterior to the teeth. The **sublingual glands** are

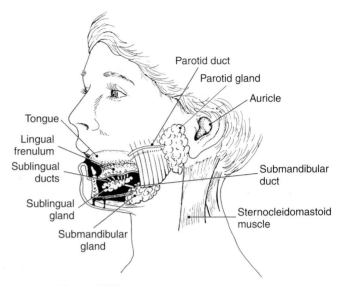

Figure 5.33
Lateral view of salivary glands and lymph nodes.

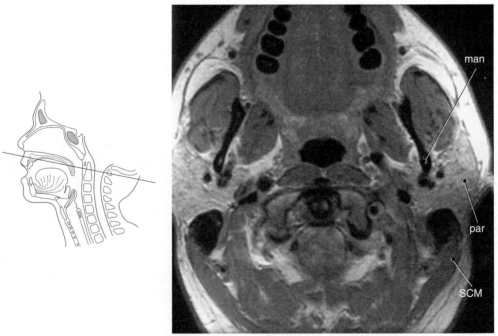

Figure 5.34
Axial, T1-weighted MR scan of neck with parotid gland.

KEY: man, Mandible; **par,** parotid gland; **SCM,** sternocleidomastoid muscle.

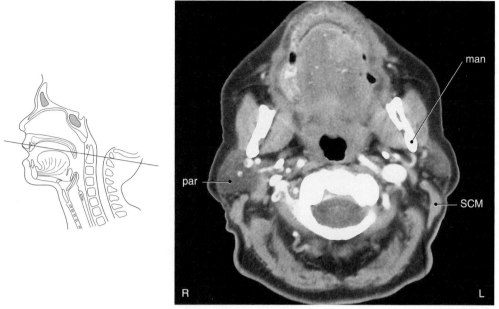

Figure 5.35
Axial CT scan of neck with parotid gland.

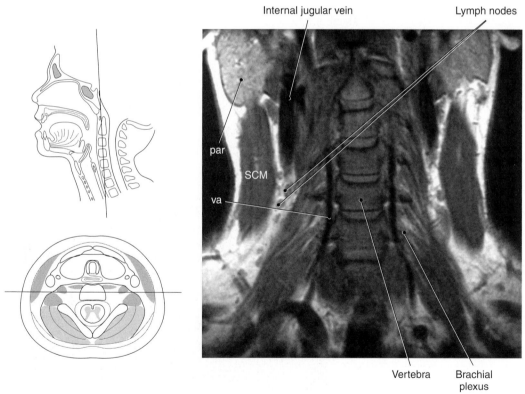

Figure 5.36
Coronal, T1-weighted MR scan of parotid glands.

KEY: man, Mandible; **SCM,** sternocleidomastoid muscle; **par,** parotid gland; **va,** vallecula.

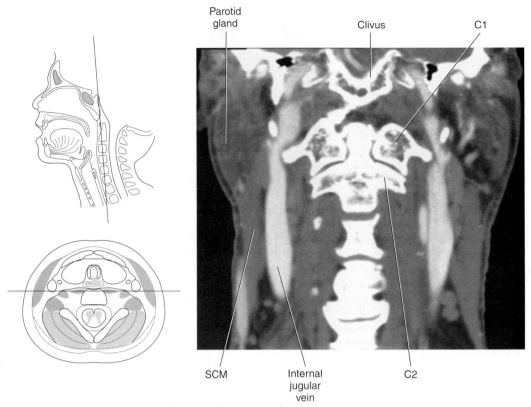

Figure 5.37
Coronal CT reformat of parotid glands.

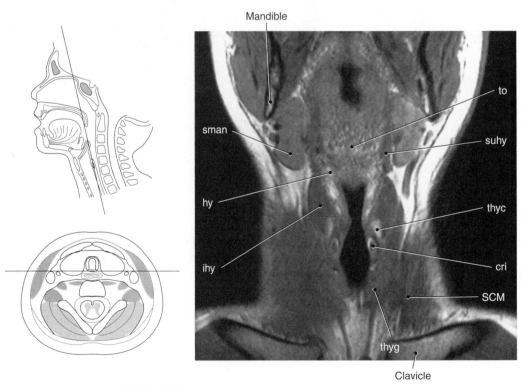

Figure 5.38
Coronal, T1-weighted MR scan of submandibular glands.

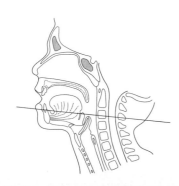

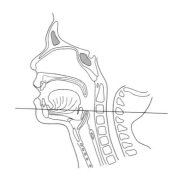

Genioglossus muscle   Tongue   Submandibular gland   Sternocleidomastoid muscle

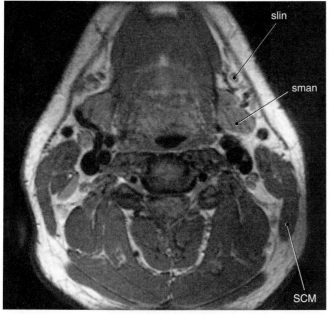

slin

sman

SCM

Figure 5.39
Axial, T1-weighted MR scan of neck with submandibular and sublingual glands.

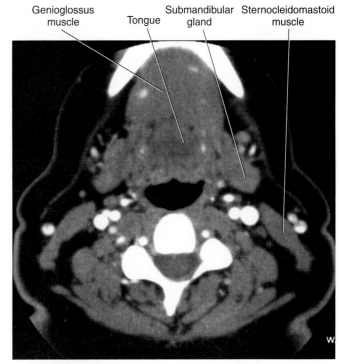

Figure 5.40
Axial CT scan of neck with submandibular glands.

KEY: sman, Submandibular gland; **hy,** hyoid bone; **ihy,** infrahyoid muscle; **to,** tongue; **suhy,** suprahyoid muscle; **thyc,** thyroid cartilage; **cri,** cricoid cartilage; **SCM,** sternocleidomastoid muscle; **thyg,** thyroid gland; **slin,** sublingual gland.

---

the smallest of the salivary glands and lie under the tongue on the floor of the mouth (Figure 5.39). Numerous (10-20) **sublingual ducts (Rivinus's ducts)** open in a line along the floor of the mouth. Some of these ducts may fuse and form the Bartholin's duct, which opens into or adjacent to the submandibular duct (Figure 5.33).

> **The mumps virus often targets the salivary glands, most commonly the parotid gland. Infection usually occurs between 5 and 9 years of age. Because of an effective mumps vaccine, the incidence of this disease has been reduced dramatically.**

Thyroid Gland

The **thyroid gland** is an endocrine gland located at the level of the cricoid cartilage. It consists of two lobes that are joined together anteriorly by the **isthmus** (Figures 5.41 and 5.42). In the axial plane, the thyroid gland appears as a wedge-shaped structure, hugging both sides of the trachea (Figures 5.43 and 5.44). The thyroid gland excretes the hormones, thyroxine (T_4), triiodothyronine (T_3), and calcitonin, which affect almost every cell in the body. Thyroxine and triiodothyronine stimulate cell metabolism and are essential for normal body growth. Calcitonin lowers the blood calcium level and promotes bone formation. Also involved with metabolism of calcium as well as phosphorus are the parathyroid hormones (PTH), which are produced by the **parathyroid glands.** The parathyroid glands are located on the posterior surface of the thyroid lobes and are usually four in number.

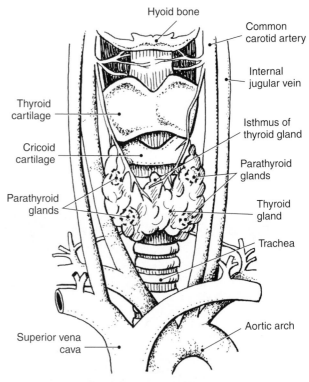

Figure 5.41
Anterior view of thyroid gland.

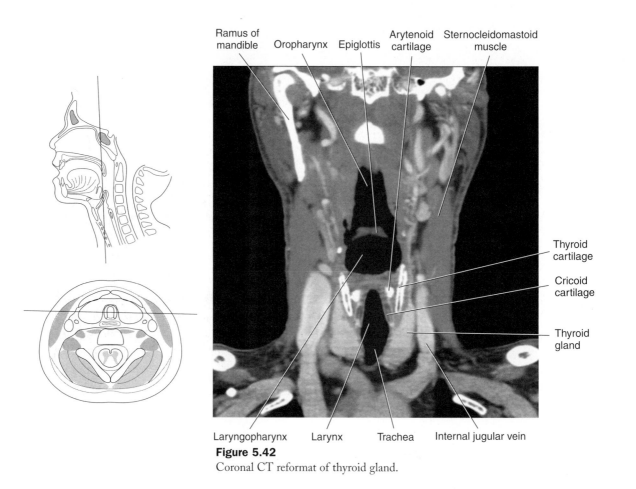

Figure 5.42
Coronal CT reformat of thyroid gland.

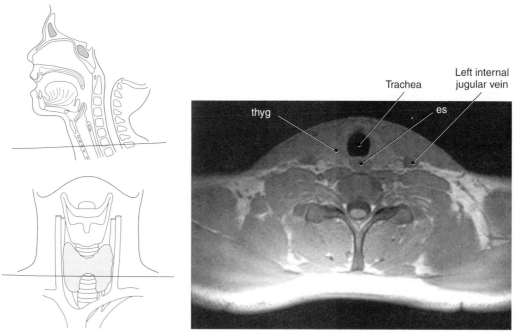

Figure 5.43
Axial, T1-weighted MR scan of thyroid gland.

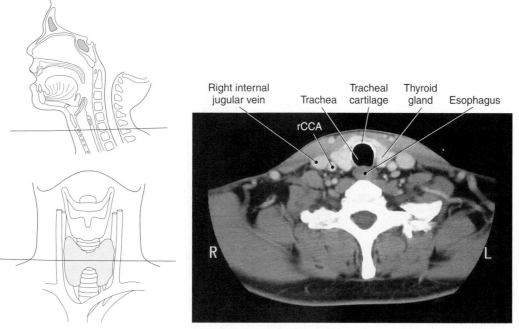

Figure 5.44
Axial CT scan of thyroid gland.

KEY: thyg, Thyroid gland; **es,** esophagus; **rJV,** right jugular vein; **rCCA,** right common carotid artery.

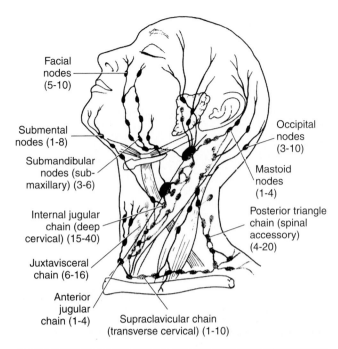

Facial nodes (5-10)

Submental nodes (1-8)

Submandibular nodes (sub-maxillary) (3-6)

Internal jugular chain (deep cervical) (15-40)

Juxtavisceral chain (6-16)

Anterior jugular chain (1-4)

Supraclavicular chain (transverse cervical) (1-10)

Occipital nodes (3-10)

Mastoid nodes (1-4)

Posterior triangle chain (spinal accessory) (4-20)

Cervical Lymph Nodes

The neck has an extensive lymphatic network containing more than one third of the body's total number of lymph nodes. Typically, as many as 75 lymph nodes are located on each side of the neck (Figures 5.45 and 5.46). **Lymph nodes** are clustered in regions throughout the vessels of the lymphatic system. The lymph vessels carry fluid from the interstitial spaces to the regional lymph nodes that filter the lymphatic fluid of harmful foreign particles before being emptied into the venous blood supply. In the cervical region, nodes are grouped along the

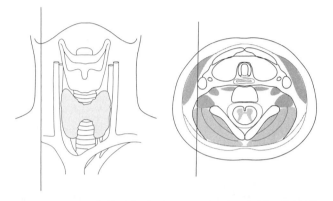

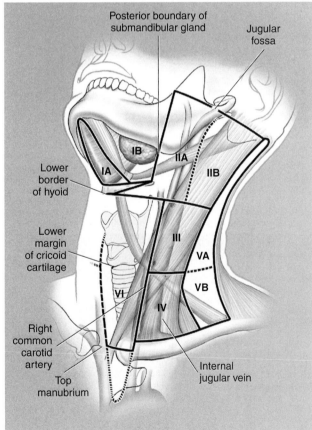

Posterior boundary of submandibular gland

Jugular fossa

IB

IA

IIA

IIB

Lower border of hyoid

III

VA

Lower margin of cricoid cartilage

VI

VB

IV

Right common carotid artery

Top manubrium

Internal jugular vein

Figure 5.45
Top, Oblique view of cervical lymph nodes. *Bottom,* Regional classification of cervical lymph nodes.

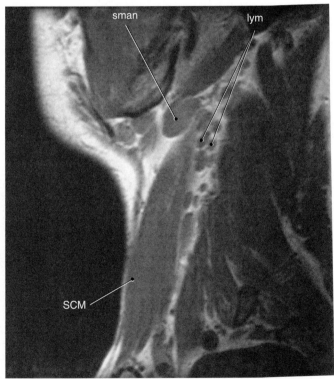

sman

lym

SCM

Figure 5.46
Sagittal, T1-weighted MR scan of lymph nodes.

lower border of the jaw, in front of and behind the ears, and deep in the neck along the larger blood vessels. They drain the skin of the scalp and face, tissues of the nasal cavity, oral cavity, pharynx, trachea, upper esophagus, thyroid gland, and salivary glands. The lymph nodes of the neck can be classified or divided into six levels or regions for ease of identification, both clinically and surgically (Table 5.1 and Figure 5.45). The lymph nodes as well as the muscles, fascial spaces, and vascular structures can be identified on sequential images found in Figures 5.47 through 5.64.

KEY: sman, Submandibular gland; **lym,** lymph nodes; **SCM,** sternocleidomastoid muscle.

TABLE 5-1 Neck Lymph Nodes*

NODE	LOCATION	PRIMARY AREAS OF DRAINAGE
Level I		
Submental	• Midline behind the tip of the mandible	• Anterior mouth, lower lip, and chin
Submandibular	• Midpoint between the tip of the mandible and the mandibular angle	• Floor of the mouth cheek, nose, and submandibular gland, and anterior oral cavity
Level II		
Upper internal jugular vein	• Upper third of the internal jugular vein. Extends from the skull base to the level of the carotid bifurcation or hyoid bone. Bounded posteriorly by the sternocleidomastoid (SCM) muscle	• Soft palate, tonsils, posterior tongue, piriform sinus, and larynx above the vocal folds, parotid gland, superficial cervical, and submandibular nodes
Level III		
Middle internal jugular vein	• Extends from carotid bifurcation or hyoid bone down to the cricoid cartilage	• Supraglottic larynx, lower piriform sinus and posterior cricoid, deep nasopharynx and oropharynx, oral cavity and laryngopharynx
Level IV		
Lower internal jugular vein	• Extends superiorly from the omohyoid muscle to the clavicle inferiorly and bordered laterally by the SCM muscle	• Thyroid, trachea, subglottic larynx, and upper esophagus
Level V (Posterior Triangle Nodes)		
Spinal accessory	• Bordered anterior by the SCM muscle, posterior by the trapezius muscle, and inferiorly by the clavicle	• Occipital, postauricular, suprascapular, posterior aspect of the scalp, lateral aspect of the neck, and the shoulder
Transverse cervical		
Supraclavicular		
Level VI (Anterior Triangle Nodes)		
Paratracheal	• Frontal compartment. Extend from hyoid bone to the suprasternal notch. Defined laterally by carotid artery on both sides.	• Thyroid lobes, parathyroid glands, subglottic larynx, trachea, and upper esophagus
Pretracheal		
Surrounding the midline visceral structures	• Located between pharynx and prevertebral fascia	• Posterior region of the nasal cavity, sphenoid and ethmoid sinuses, hard and soft palate, and nasopharynx

*The retropharyngeal nodes are not included in this classification scheme.

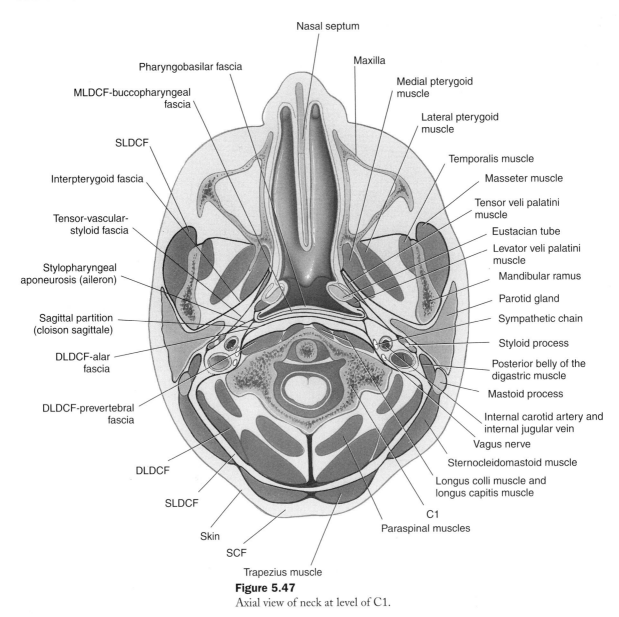

Figure 5.47
Axial view of neck at level of C1.

KEY: **DLDCF,** Deep layer, deep cervical fascia; **MLDCF,** middle layer, deep cervical fascia; **SCF,** superficial cervical fascia; **SLDCF,** superficial layer, deep cervical fascia.

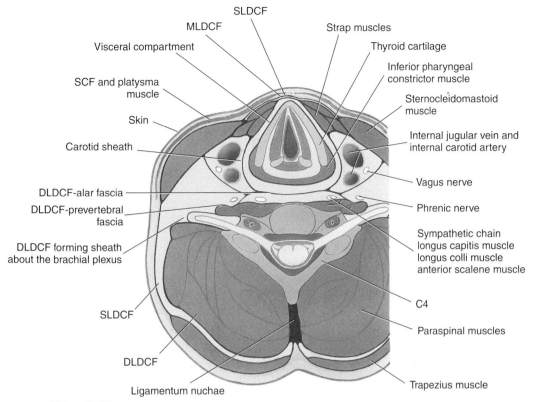

Figure 5.48
Axial view of neck at level of C4. *DLDCF,* Deep layer, deep cervical fascia; *MLDCF,* middle layer, deep cervical fascia; *SCF,* superficial caervical fascia; *SLDCF,* superficial layer, deep cervical fascia.

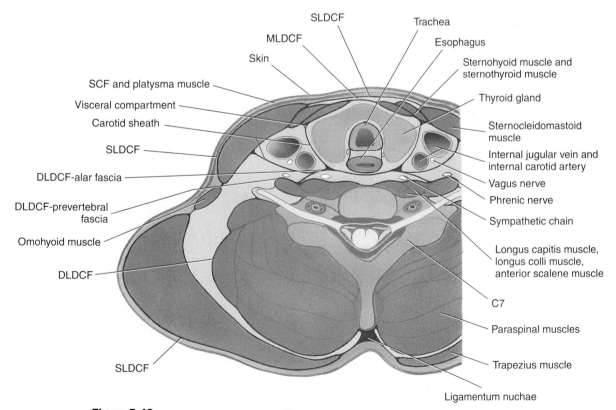

Figure 5.49
Axial view of neck at level of C7. *DLDCF,* Deep layer, deep cervical fascia; *MLDCF,* middle layer, deep cervical fascia; *SCF,* superficial caervical fascia; *SLDCF,* superficial layer, deep cervical fascia.

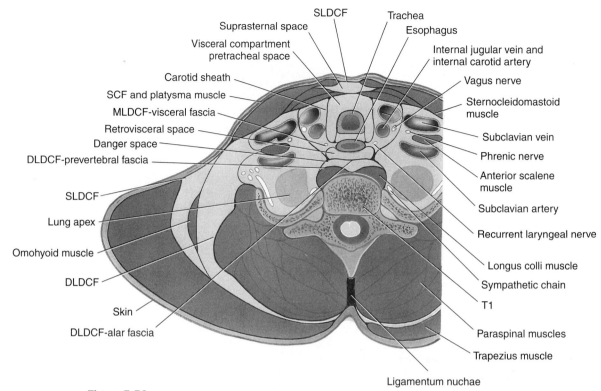

Figure 5.50
Axial view of neck at level of T1. *DLDCF,* Deep layer, deep cervical fascia; *MLDCF,* middle layer, deep cervical fascia; *SCF,* superficial caervical fascia; *SLDCF,* superficial layer, deep cervical fascia.

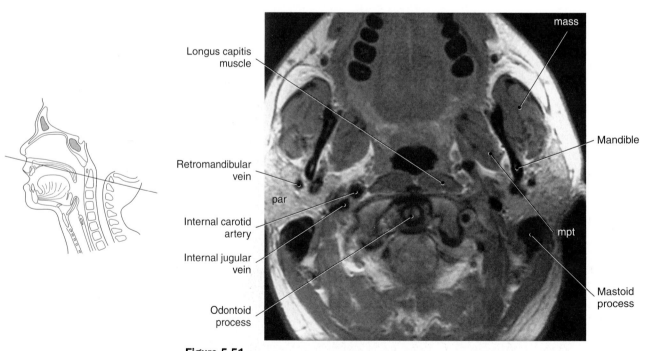

Figure 5.51
Axial, T1-weighted MR scan of neck with parotid gland.

KEY: mass, Masseter muscle; **mpt,** medial pterygoid muscle; **par,** parotid gland; **ECA,** external carotid artery; **ICA,** internal carotid artery; **VA,** vertebral artery.

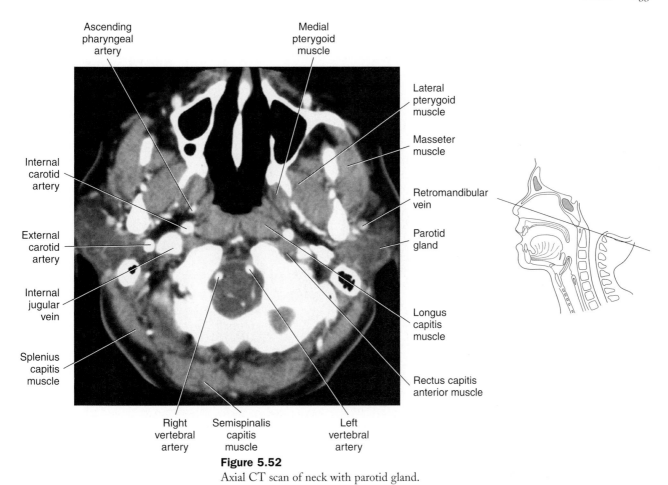

Ascending pharyngeal artery

Medial pterygoid muscle

Lateral pterygoid muscle

Masseter muscle

Retromandibular vein

Parotid gland

Internal carotid artery

External carotid artery

Internal jugular vein

Splenius capitis muscle

Longus capitis muscle

Rectus capitis anterior muscle

Right vertebral artery

Semispinalis capitis muscle

Left vertebral artery

Figure 5.52
Axial CT scan of neck with parotid gland.

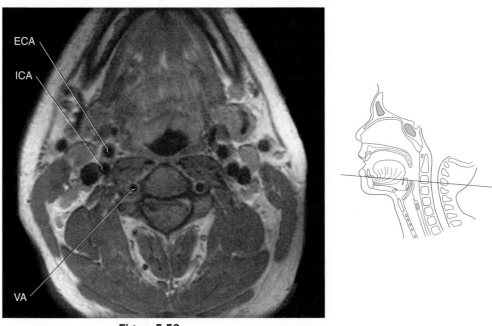

ECA

ICA

VA

Figure 5.53
Axial, T1-weighted MR scan of neck with oropharynx.

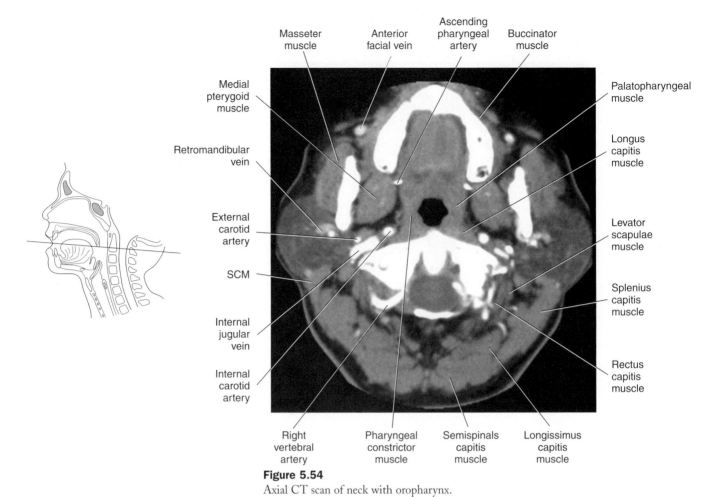

Masseter muscle

Anterior facial vein

Ascending pharyngeal artery

Buccinator muscle

Medial pterygoid muscle

Retromandibular vein

External carotid artery

SCM

Internal jugular vein

Internal carotid artery

Palatopharyngeal muscle

Longus capitis muscle

Levator scapulae muscle

Splenius capitis muscle

Rectus capitis muscle

Right vertebral artery

Pharyngeal constrictor muscle

Semispinals capitis muscle

Longissimus capitis muscle

Figure 5.54
Axial CT scan of neck with oropharynx.

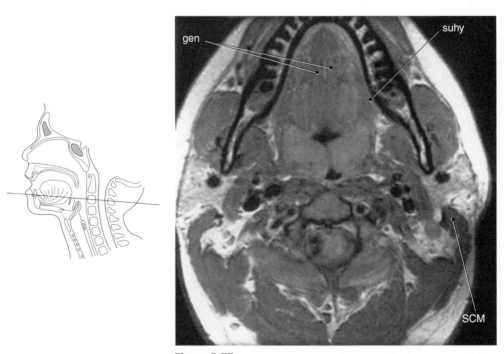

gen

suhy

SCM

Figure 5.55
Axial, T1-weighted MR scan of neck.

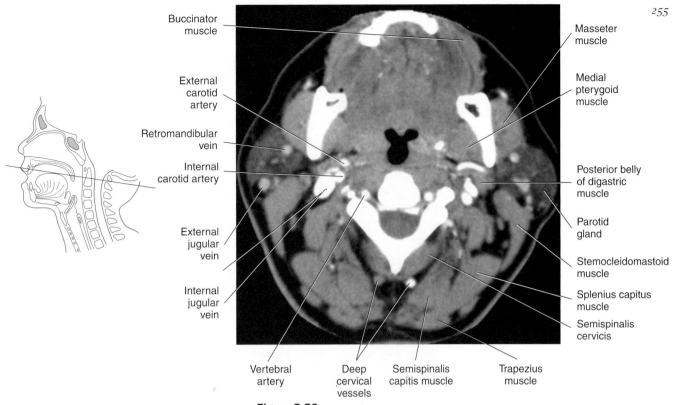

Buccinator muscle

External carotid artery

Retromandibular vein

Internal carotid artery

External jugular vein

Internal jugular vein

Masseter muscle

Medial pterygoid muscle

Posterior belly of digastric muscle

Parotid gland

Stemocleidomastoid muscle

Splenius capitus muscle

Semispinalis cervicis

Vertebral artery

Deep cervical vessels

Semispinalis capitis muscle

Trapezius muscle

Figure 5.56

Axial CT scan of neck with uvula.

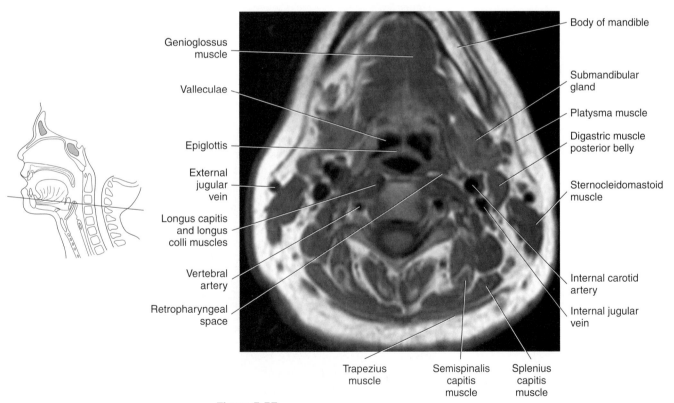

Genioglossus muscle

Valleculae

Epiglottis

External jugular vein

Longus capitis and longus colli muscles

Vertebral artery

Retropharyngeal space

Body of mandible

Submandibular gland

Platysma muscle

Digastric muscle posterior belly

Sternocleidomastoid muscle

Internal carotid artery

Internal jugular vein

Trapezius muscle

Semispinalis capitis muscle

Splenius capitis muscle

Figure 5.57

Axial, T1-weighted MR scan of neck with epiglottis.

KEY: gen, Genioglossus muscle; **suhy,** suprahyoid muscle; **SCM,** sternocleidomastoid muscle.

256

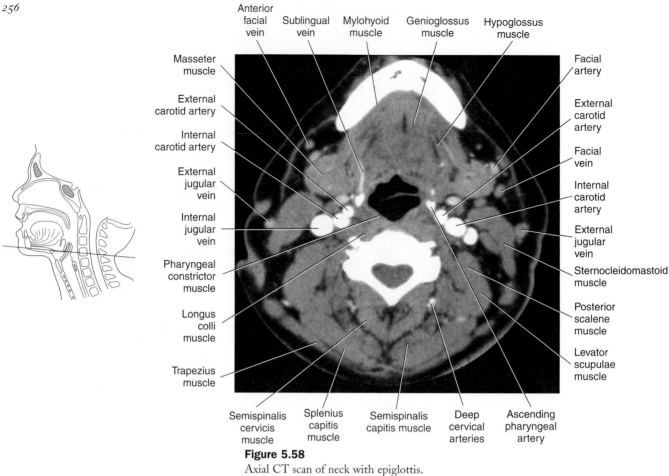

Anterior facial vein
Sublingual vein
Mylohyoid muscle
Genioglossus muscle
Hypoglossus muscle

Masseter muscle
External carotid artery
Internal carotid artery
External jugular vein
Internal jugular vein
Pharyngeal constrictor muscle
Longus colli muscle
Trapezius muscle

Facial artery
External carotid artery
Facial vein
Internal carotid artery
External jugular vein
Sternocleidomastoid muscle
Posterior scalene muscle
Levator scupulae muscle

Semispinalis cervicis muscle
Splenius capitis muscle
Semispinalis capitis muscle
Deep cervical arteries
Ascending pharyngeal artery

Figure 5.58
Axial CT scan of neck with epiglottis.

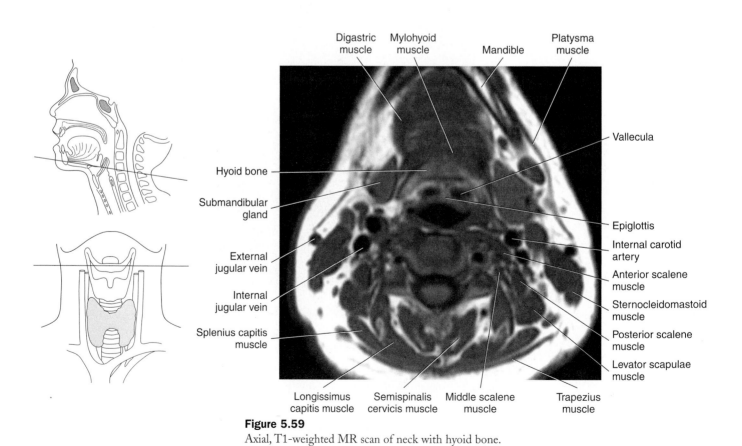

Digastric muscle
Mylohyoid muscle
Mandible
Platysma muscle

Hyoid bone
Submandibular gland
External jugular vein
Internal jugular vein
Splenius capitis muscle

Vallecula
Epiglottis
Internal carotid artery
Anterior scalene muscle
Sternocleidomastoid muscle
Posterior scalene muscle
Levator scapulae muscle

Longissimus capitis muscle
Semispinalis cervicis muscle
Middle scalene muscle
Trapezius muscle

Figure 5.59
Axial, T1-weighted MR scan of neck with hyoid bone.

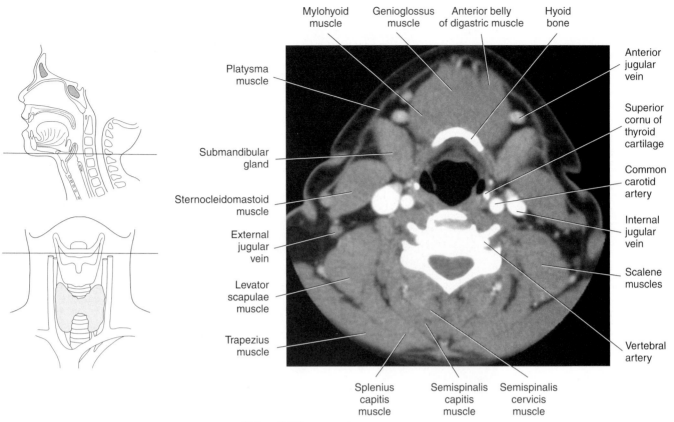

Figure 5.60
Axial CT scan of neck with hyoid bone.

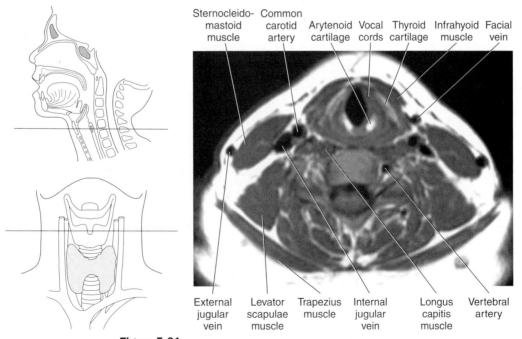

Figure 5.61
Axial, T1-weighted MR scan of neck with thyroid cartilage.

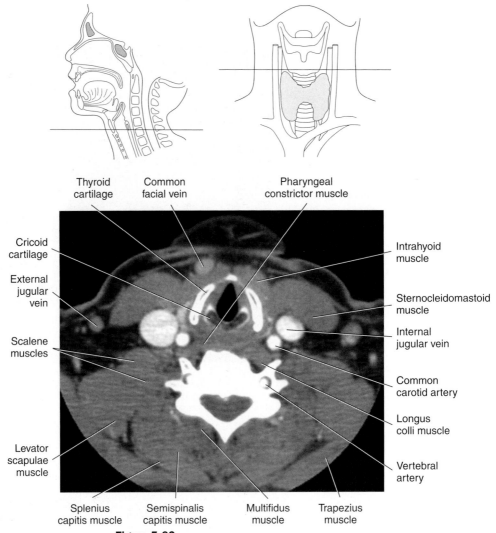

Figure 5.62

Axial CT scan of neck with thyroid cartilage.

Thyroid cartilage

Common facial vein

Pharyngeal constrictor muscle

Cricoid cartilage

External jugular vein

Scalene muscles

Levator scapulae muscle

Intrahyoid muscle

Sternocleidomastoid muscle

Internal jugular vein

Common carotid artery

Longus colli muscle

Vertebral artery

Splenius capitis muscle

Semispinalis capitis muscle

Multifidus muscle

Trapezius muscle

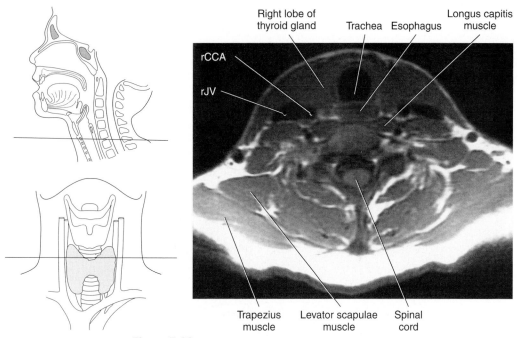

Figure 5.63
Axial, T1-weighted MR scan of neck with thyroid gland.

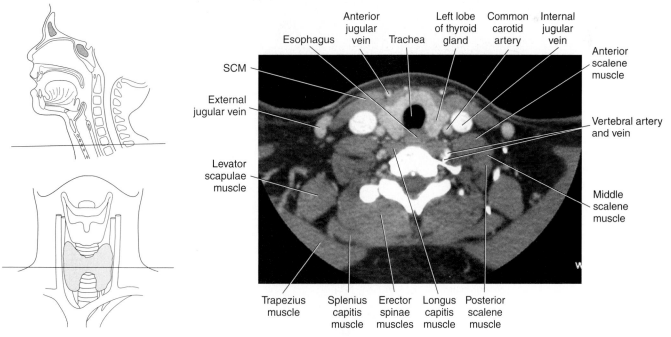

Figure 5.64
Axial CT scan of neck with thyroid gland.

MUSCLES

Numerous muscles are located within the neck. Each muscle can be difficult to identify individually because the margins seem to blend together in cross-section images. This section of text addresses only the largest and most significant muscles of the neck region.

Pharyngeal Muscles

The pharyngeal muscles include the circular layer of constrictors and the inner longitudinal layers (Table 5.2). There are three overlapping **constrictor muscles (superior, middle, inferior)** that are responsible for constricting the pharynx and inducing peristaltic waves during swallowing (Figure 5.65). The three inner longitudinal muscles include the **stylopharyngeus, palotopharyngeus,** and **salpingopharyngeus** muscles, all involved with elevating the pharynx and larynx during swallowing and speaking. The extrinsic muscles of the tongue are responsible for changing the position of the tongue and include the **genioglossus, hyoglossus, styloglossus,** and **palatoglossus** muscles (Figure 5.66).

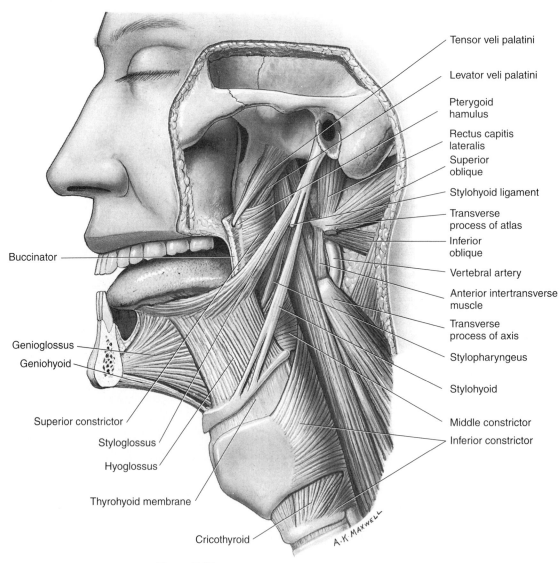

Figure 5.65
Sagittal view of pharyngeal and tongue muscles.

TABLE 5-2   Pharyngeal Muscles

PHARYNGEAL MUSCLES	ORIGIN	INSERTION	ACTION
External (Circular) Muscles			
Superior constrictors Middle constrictors Inferior constrictors	• Pterygoid hamulus, posterior end of mandible, and side of tongue • Stylohyoid ligament, greater and lesser horns of hyoid bone • Sides of thyroid and cricoid cartilages	• Pharyngeal tubercle and median raphe of pharynx • Median raphe of pharynx • Median raphe of pharynx	All constrict pharynx, induce peristaltic waves during swallowing
Longitudinal (Internal) Muscles			
Stylopharyngeus Palatopharyngeus Salpingopharyngeus	• Styloid process of temporal bone • Hard palate and palatine aponeurosis • Cartilaginous part of auditory tube	• Posterior/superior borders of thyroid cartilage • Side of pharynx and esophagus, posterior border of lamina of thyroid cartilage • Blends with palatopharyngeus muscle	All elevate pharynx and larynx during swallowing and speaking
Tongue Muscles			
Genioglossus Hyoglossus Styloglossus Palatoglossus	• Mental spine of mandible • Greater horn and body of hyoid bone • Styloid process, temporal bone • Oral surface of palatine aponeurosis	• Ventral surface tongue; anterior hyoid bone • Base of tongue • Lateral margin of tongue • Side and dorsum of tongue	• Moves tongue forward • Moves tongue backward • Moves tongue upward and backward • Elevates posterior tongue

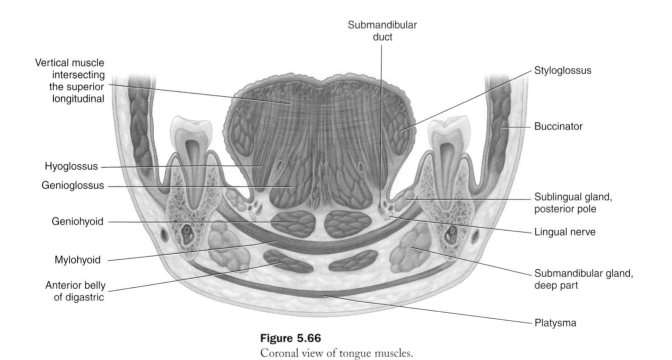

Figure 5.66
Coronal view of tongue muscles.

Laryngeal Muscles

The laryngeal muscles control the position and tension of the vocal folds. They can be divided into two groups: muscles acting on the false vocal cords **(aryepiglottic, arytenoid, and thyroarytenoid)** and muscles acting on the true vocal cords **(arytenoids, posterior and lateral cricoarytenoids, and vocalis)** (Table 5.3 and Figures 5.67 and 5.68). The **aryepiglotticus** is a continuation of the oblique arytenoid muscles and functions as a sphincter to close the laryngeal inlet during swallowing.

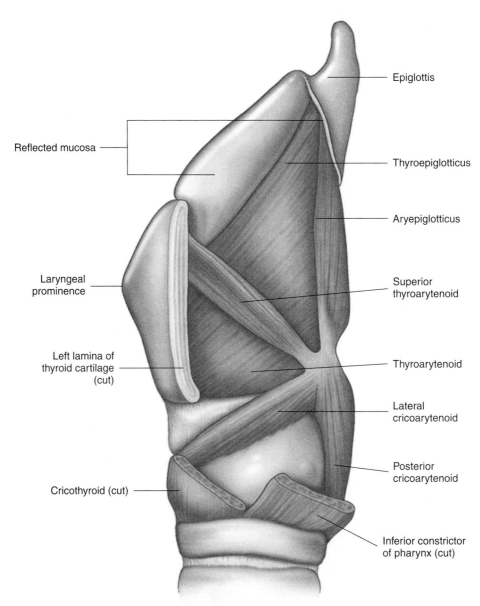

Epiglottis

Reflected mucosa

Thyroepiglotticus

Aryepiglotticus

Laryngeal prominence

Superior thyroarytenoid

Left lamina of thyroid cartilage (cut)

Thyroarytenoid

Lateral cricoarytenoid

Posterior cricoarytenoid

Cricothyroid (cut)

Inferior constrictor of pharynx (cut)

Figure 5.67
Sagittal view of laryngeal muscles.

TABLE 5-3 Laryngeal Muscles

LARYNGEAL MUSCLES	ORIGIN	INSERTION	ACTION
Lateral cricoarytenoid	Superolateral rim of cricoid cartilage	Muscular process of arytenoid cartilage	Adduction, lengthens vocal cords
Posterior cricoarytenoid	Lateral half cricoid cartilage	Posterior surface of arytenoid cartilage	Abducts the vocal cords
Arytenoid transverse oblique	• Dorsolateral arytenoid cartilage	• Dorsolateral arytenoid cartilage, opposite side	• Powerful vocal fold adductor
	• Posterior base arytenoid cartilage	• Fibers course diagonally to apex opposite arytenoid cartilage	• Adducts vocal fold
Aryepiglotticus	Apex of arytenoid cartilage	Epiglottic cartilage, aryepiglottic fold	Draws the epiglottis downward
Cricothyroid	Arch of cricoid cartilage	Thyroid cartilage	Changes the length/tension of vocal cords
Thyroarytenoid	Inner surface of thyroid cartilage	Anterolateral surface of arytenoid cartilage	Shortens vocal folds
Vocalis	Posterior surface of thyroid cartilage	Vocal process of arytenoid cartilage	Adjusts the tension of the vocal cords

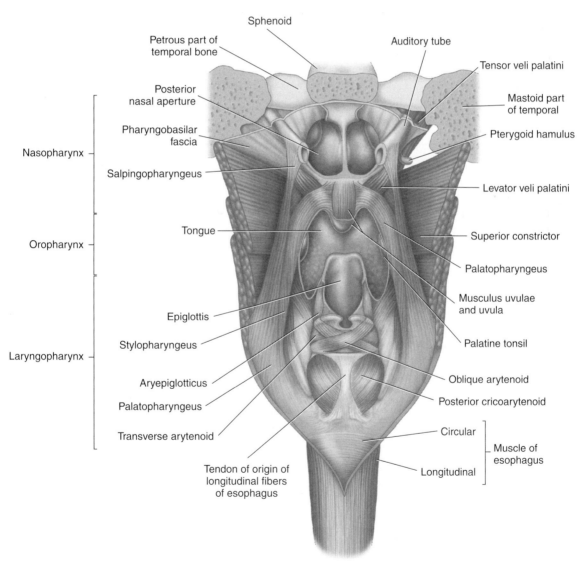

Figure 5.68
Posterior view of laryngeal muscles.

Muscles within the Anterior Triangle

The neck is frequently divided by the **sternocleidomastoid muscle (SCM)** into two areas called the *anterior* and *posterior triangles*. Everything anteromedial to the SCM is considered part of the anterior triangle, and everything posterior to the SCM is considered part of the posterior triangle. The SCM is a broad straplike muscle that originates on the sternum and clavicle and inserts on the mastoid tip of the temporal bone. It functions to turn the head from side to side and to flex the neck (Figure 5.69).

The muscles of the anterior triangle are referred to as the *muscles of the throat* and can be divided into the suprahyoid and infrahyoid muscle groups (Figures 5.69 and 5.70). These muscle groups are named according to their location in relation to the horseshoe-shaped hyoid bone. The hyoid bone lies in the anterior surface of the neck superior to the thyroid cartilage and below the mandible; it forms a base for the tongue. The suprahyoid and infrahyoid muscles aid in the movement of the hyoid bone and larynx. The **suprahyoid muscles (digastric, mylohyoid, stylohyoid, geniohyoid)** connect the hyoid bone to the temporal bone and mandible and elevate the hyoid and floor of the mouth and tongue during swallowing and speaking. **The infrahyoid muscles (thyrohyoid, sternohyoid, sternothyroid, omohyoid)** are often called *strap muscles* because of their ribbonlike appearance. They act primarily to depress the hyoid bone and extend inferiorly to insert on the sternum, thyroid cartilage, and scapula (Table 5.4 and sequential images in Figures 5.47 through 5.64).

TABLE 5-4   Neck Muscles

	ORIGIN	INSERTION	ACTION
Front of Neck—Anterior Triangle			
Platysma	• Base of mandible and skin of lower face	• Fascia and skin over pectoralis major and deltoid muscles	• Changes facial expression
Sternocleidomastoid (SCM)		• Mastoid process, lateral half of superior nuchal line	• Flexes head and neck
Sternal head	• Upper manubrium		
Clavicular head	• Sternal end of clavicle		
Scalene Muscles			
Anterior	• Anterior tubercle of transverse processes of C3-C6	• Scalene tubercle of 1st rib	• Elevates 1st rib, flexes cervical vertebrae
Medius	• Transverse processes of C3-C7	• 1st rib, occasionally 2nd rib	• Same as anterior
Posterior	• Posterior tubercle of transverse processes of C5-C6	• 2nd rib, sometimes 3rd rib	• Laterally flexes head; rotates head and neck
Infrahyoid Muscles			
Thyrohyoid	• Hyoid cartilage	• Inferolateral border hyoid bone	• Lower hyoid bone, raise larynx
Sternohyoid	• Superior border of manubrium	• Passes over thyroid cartilage, inserts on hyoid bone	• Lower hyoid bone
Sternothyroid	• Manubrium and medial end	• Thyroid cartilage	• Lower larynx
Omohyoid	• 1st costal cartilage superior border of scapula	• Inferolateral border hyoid bone	• Lower hyoid bone and larynx
Suprahyoid Muscles			
Digastric	• Posterior belly—mastoid notch of temporal bone; anterior belly—lower border of mandible	• Ends as intermediate tendon between the two bellies that attaches to hyoid bone	• Jaw opener (speech muscle) • Elevate floor of the mouth • Move hyoid bone posterior/superior
Mylohyoid	• Body of mandible	• Mandibular symphysis and midpoint of hyoid bone	• Jaw opener
Stylohyoid	• Styloid process	• Superior surface of hyoid bone near minor horn	
Geniohyoid	• Mandibular symphysis	• Body of hyoid bone	
Prevertebral Muscles			
Longus capitis	• Anterior tubercles of transverse processes of C3-C6	• Basilar part of occipital bone	• Flex head
Longus colli	• Bodies of C5-T3; anterior tubercles of transverse processes C2-C5	• Anterior arch C1, anterior tubercles of the transverse processes of C5-C6, anterior bodies of C2-C4	• Flex neck, rotates and bends neck laterally
Back of Neck—Posterior Triangle			
Trapezius	• Occipital bone and spinous processes of C7-T12	• Clavicle, acromion, scapular spine	• Elevates the scapula
Levator scapulae	• Transverse processes of upper four cervical vertebrae	• Vertebral border of the scapula	• Raises the scapula
Splenius capitis	• Lower cervical and upper thoracic vertebrae	• Occipital bone	• Extends head
Splenius cervicis	• Spinous processes of T1-T6 and ligamentum nuchae	• Posterior tubercles of transverse processes of C1-C4	• Extends head

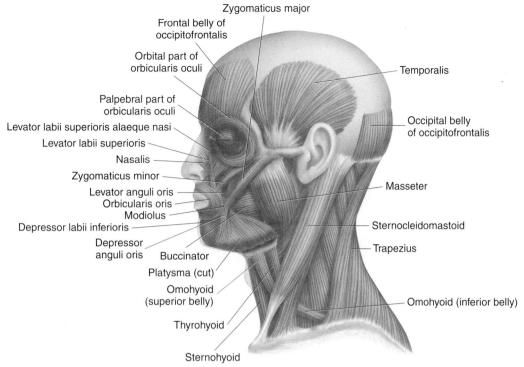

Figure 5.69
Sagittal view of sternocleidomastoid muscle and neck muscles within the anterior and posterior triangles.

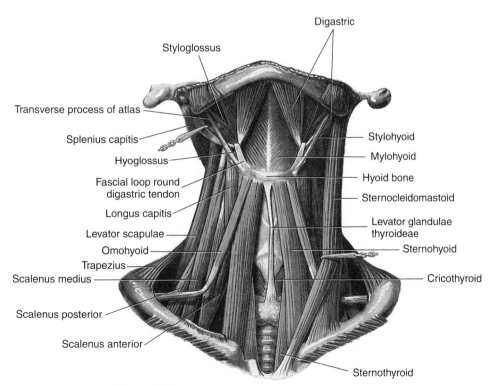

Figure 5.70
Anterior view of suprahyoid and infrahyoid neck muscles.

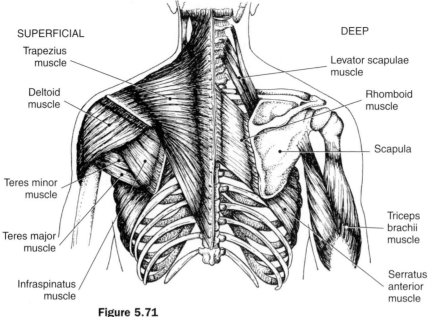

SUPERFICIAL

Trapezius
muscle

Deltoid
muscle

Teres minor
muscle

Teres major
muscle

Infraspinatus
muscle

DEEP

Levator scapulae
muscle

Rhomboid
muscle

Scapula

Triceps
brachii
muscle

Serratus
anterior
muscle

Figure 5.71
Posterior view of trapezius and levator scapulae muscles.

Muscles within the Posterior Triangle

The muscles of the posterior triangle include the trapezius, splenius capitis, levator scapulae, and anterior, middle, and posterior scalene muscles. The **trapezius muscle,** a superficial muscle located on the posterior portion of the neck, acts to elevate the scapula. It originates from the occipital bone and spinous processes of C7-T12 to insert on the clavicle, acromion, and spine of the scapula (Figures 5.71 and 5.72). Located just anterior to the trapezius muscle, the **splenius capitis muscle** arises from the lower cervical and upper thoracic vertebrae to insert on the occipital bone and acts to extend the head. The **levator scapulae muscle** is located in the posterolateral portion of the neck. It arises from the transverse processes of the upper four cervical vertebrae to insert on the vertebral border of the scapula and acts to raise the scapula. The scalene muscle group **(anterior, middle, and posterior scalene muscles)** is located in the anterolateral portion of the neck. The muscles originate from the transverse processes of the cervical vertebrae to insert on the first two ribs. Together, the scalene muscles act to elevate the upper two ribs and flex the neck. The anterior and middle scalene muscles can serve as a landmark for the brachial plexus because it courses between them. (These muscles are listed in Table 5.4 and identified on Figures 5.47 through 5.64.) Two other prominent muscle groups found in the neck are the erector spinae and transversospinal, which are discussed in Chapter 4.

Fascial Planes and Spaces

The suprahyoid and infrahyoid regions of the neck can be further divided by **fascial planes** that separate the anatomy of each region into compartments or spaces that contain distinct anatomic structures (Figure 5.73). Each compartment or space is associated with pathology specific to the anatomic structures contained within it. Knowledge of the anatomy in these compartments improves the ability to predict the spread of infection throughout the soft tissue structures in the neck (Table 5.5).

The **suprahyoid region** can be divided into eight main spaces: parapharyngeal, masticator, parotid, carotid, pharyngeal mucosa, retropharyngeal, prevertebral, and danger spaces. The **infrahyoid region** contains six main spaces: Four continuous with the suprahyoid spaces (carotid, retropharyngeal, prevertebral, and danger spaces), and two new spaces (posterior cervical and visceral spaces) (Figures 5.50 and 5.73).

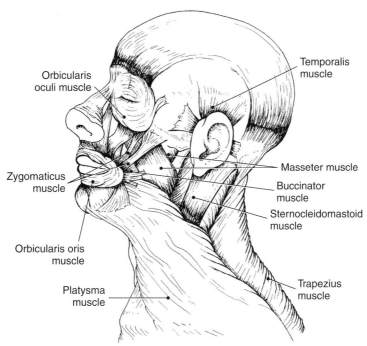

Figure 5.72
Sagittal view of superficial neck muscles.

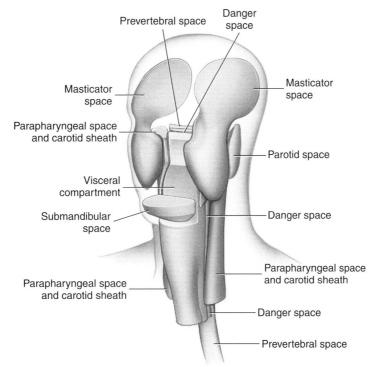

Figure 5.73
Oblique view of fascial planes and spaces of the neck.

TABLE 5-5   Fascial Planes and Spaces of the Neck

	LOCATION	ANATOMY	PATHOLOGY
Suprahyoid Neck			
Parapharyngeal space (PPS)	Extends from skull base to hyoid bone, lying medial to foramen ovale and posterior to pharyngeal mucosa. Communicates with RPS, PS, MS	Fat, vasculature, branches of trigeminal nerve	Abscess from adjacent space
Pharyngeal mucosal space (PMS)	Extends from the skull base to the cricoid cartilage. Consists of the muscosal surface of the naso-, oro-, and hypopharynx.	Mucosal surface, lymph tissue of Waldeyer's ring, tonsils, minor salivary glands, eustachian tube, levator and constrictor muscles	Squamous cell carcinoma (SCCA), lymphoma, salivary gland tumors, Thornwaldt's cyst
Masticator space (MS)	Extends from the inferior mandible to the skull base, anterolateral to the PPS. The space extends from the inferior edge of the mandible to the skull base medially and lies along the skull laterally.	Mandible, masticator, temporalis, and pterygoid muscles attached to mandible, branch of trigeminal nerve	Odontogenic abscess, sarcoma, invasive carcinoma, rhabdomyosarcoma, hemangioma
Parotid space (PS)	Space posterior to MS and lateral to the CS and PPS. Extends from the external auditory meatus to the inferior edge of the mandible	Parotid gland and duct, facial nerve, intraparotid lymph nodes, retromandibular vein and branches of external carotid artery	Warthin's tumor, pleomorphic adenoma, hemangioma, SCCA, metastatic disease to lymph nodes
Carotid space (CS)	Potential cavity within the carotid sheath, which extends into the mediastinum	Carotid and jugular vessels, lymph nodes, cranial and sympathetic nerves	Paraganglioma, schwannoma, metastatic disease to lymph nodes, blood clots
Retropharyngeal space (RPS)	Area of loose connective tissue posterior to the pharynx and esophagus and anterior to prevertebral fascia, ending at about the level of the carina Communicates with the pretracheal space	Fat, lymph nodes draining the adenoids, nasal cavities, nasopharynx, and posterior ethmoid sinuses	Adenopathy, metastatic SCCA, lymphoma
Danger space (DS)	Lies posterior to RPS and anterior to prevertebral fascia Runs from the skull base to the diaphragm	Fat	Infection, tumor spread from RPS
Perivertebral space (PVS)	Located midline behind the RPS. Extends from skull base to the coccyx. Divided into prevertebral portion anteriorly and paraspinal portion posteriorly.	Vertebral column, longus colli muscles, scalene muscles, brachial plexus, phrenic nerve, vertebral artery and vein, spinal cord, paraspinal muscles	Vertebral body mass, infection, degenerative osteophyte, chordoma
Infrahyoid Neck			
Carotid space (CS)	As above	As above	As above
Retropharyngeal space (RPS)	As above	As above	As above
Danger space (DS)	As above	As above	As above
Prevertebral space (PVS)	As above	As above	As above
Visceral space (VS)	Extends from the thyroid cartilage into the anterior superior mediastinum to aortic arch	Thyroid gland, parathyroid glands, larynx, trachea, esophagus, lymph nodes, recurrent laryngeal nerves	Thyroid tumors, nodal disease, esophageal tumors, laryngeal SCCA
Posterior cervical space (PCS)	Posterior to VS and posterolateral to CS lying between the sternocleidomastoid and trapezius muscles	Fat, spinal accessory nerve, lymph nodes, preaxillary brachial plexus	Adenopathy, nerve sheath tumors, congenital cystic lesions

VASCULATURE STRUCTURES

The extracranial or main vessels of the neck include the carotid and vertebral arteries and the jugular veins (Table 5.6). These vessels are located primarily in the lateral portions of the neck (Figures 5.74 through 5.77).

Carotid Arteries

The **right common carotid artery** arises from the brachiocephalic artery posterior to the sternoclavicular joint. The **left common carotid artery** arises directly from the aortic arch. The common carotid arteries lie medial to the internal jugular vein and bifurcate into the internal and external carotid arteries at approximately the level of the thyroid cartilage (C3-C4) (Figure 5.75). The **internal carotid artery** ascends the neck,

almost in a vertical plane, to enter the base of the skull through the carotid canal of the temporal bone. The internal carotid artery has no branches in the neck, but branches in the head to supply blood to the orbit and brain. As the **external carotid artery** ascends the neck, it passes through the parotid gland to the level of the temporomandibular joint, where it bifurcates into its terminal branches to supply blood to the face and neck. These branches include the superior thyroid, lingual, facial, occipital, posterior auricular, and ascending pharyngeal arteries (Table 5.6 and Figures 5.74 and 5.75). The external carotid artery changes position in relation to the internal carotid artery as it ascends the neck. At its lower level, the external carotid artery is anterior and medial to the internal carotid artery then becomes anterior and lateral to the internal carotid artery at its higher level (Figures 5.51 through 5.64).

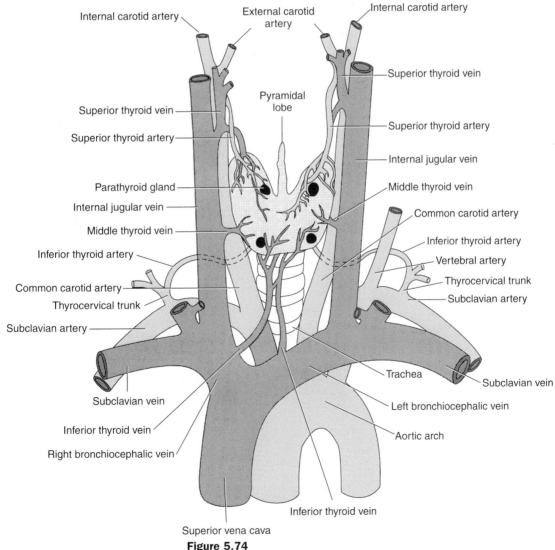

Figure 5.74

Coronal view of extracranial vasculature.

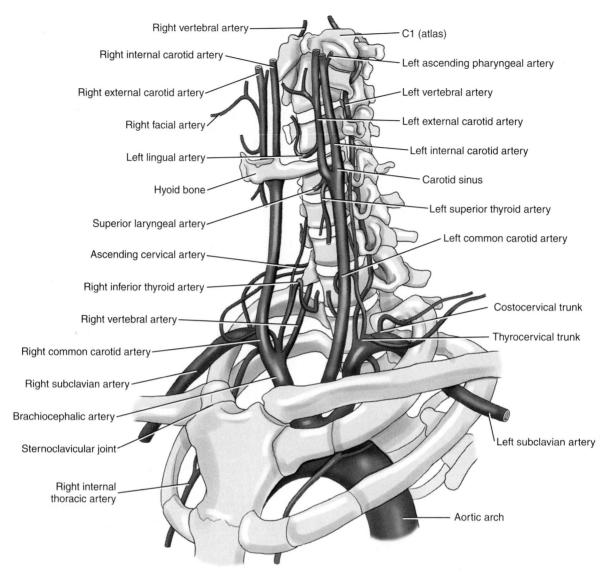

Figure 5.75
Sagittal oblique view of extracranial arteries.

ARTERIES OF THE NECK	ORIGIN	BRANCHES
Common carotid artery		Internal and external carotid arteries
Left common carotid	Aortic arch	
Right common carotid	Right brachiocephalic artery	
Internal carotid artery	Common carotid artery	Ophthalmic, anterior and middle cerebral arteries
External carotid artery	Common carotid artery	Superior thyroid, lingual, facial, occipital, posterior auricular, and ascending pharyngeal arteries
Vertebral arteries	Subclavian artery	Posterior inferior cerebellar artery
Unite to form basilar artery		

TABLE 5-6 Arteries of the Neck

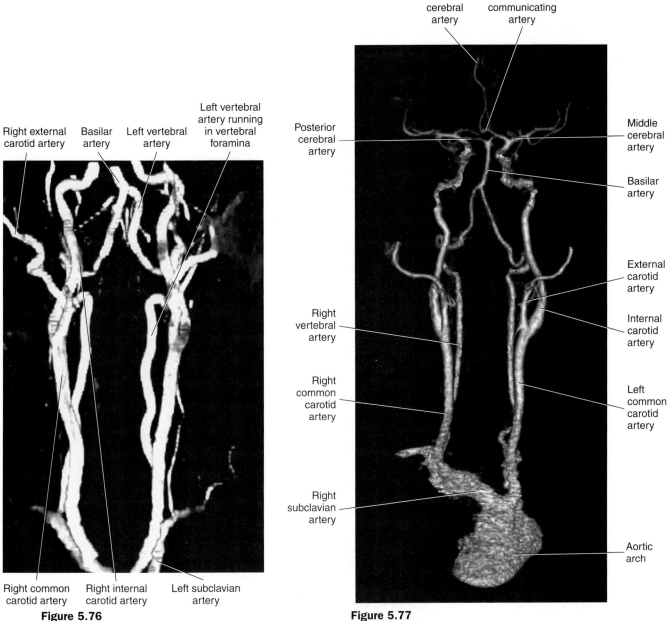

Figure 5.76
MR angiogram of extracranial arteries.

Right external carotid artery
Basilar artery
Left vertebral artery
Left vertebral artery running in vertebral foramina
Right common carotid artery
Right internal carotid artery
Left subclavian artery

Figure 5.77
CT angiogram of intracranial and extracranial arteries.

Anterior cerebral artery
Anterior communicating artery
Posterior cerebral artery
Middle cerebral artery
Basilar artery
Right vertebral artery
External carotid artery
Internal carotid artery
Right common carotid artery
Left common carotid artery
Right subclavian artery
Aortic arch

Vertebral Arteries

The **vertebral arteries** begin as a branch of the subclavian artery and ascend the neck through the transverse foramina of C6-C1, where the arteries enter the foramen magnum and join to form the basilar artery. The vertebral and basilar arteries supply blood to the posterior aspect of the brain (Figures 5.51 through 5.64 and 5.75 through 5.77).

Jugular Veins

The **internal jugular veins** drain blood from the brain and superficial parts of the face and neck and are typically the largest of the vascular structures of the neck (Table 5.7). The internal jugular veins commence at the jugular foramen in the posterior cranial fossa and descend the lateral portion of the neck to unite with the **subclavian vein** to form the **brachio-cephalic vein** (Figures 5.74 and 5.78). Commonly, the right internal jugular vein is larger than the left because it is the continuation of the sigmoid sinus from the head. The internal jugular veins typically run lateral to the common carotid artery and posterior to the internal carotid artery at the upper levels of the neck. Tributaries of the internal jugular vein include the inferior petrosal sinus, facial, lingual, pharyngeal, superior and middle thyroid veins, and often the occipital vein (Figure 5.78).

Blood from the lateral region of the face is drained by the **retromandibular vein** that courses inferiorly through the parotid gland, to continue as the external jugular vein. The **external jugular veins** begin near the angle of the mandible and cross the SCM just beneath the skin to empty into the subclavian vein. Tributaries of the external jugular veins include the retromandibular and anterior jugular veins and occasionally the occipital veins. The **anterior jugular vein** begins at approximately the level of the hyoid bone and drains blood from the lower lip. This vessel passes beneath the SCM to open into the termination of the external jugular vein. Jugular veins are identified on Figures 5.51 through 5.64.

The **vertebral veins** descend within the transverse foramina of the cervical vertebrae along with the vertebral arteries to drain the cervical spinal cord and the posterior surface of the skull.

Carotid Sheath

The **carotid sheath** is a compartment composed of cervical fascia that encloses the common and internal carotid arteries, the internal jugular vein and associated lymph nodes, and the vagus nerve (Figure 5.79).

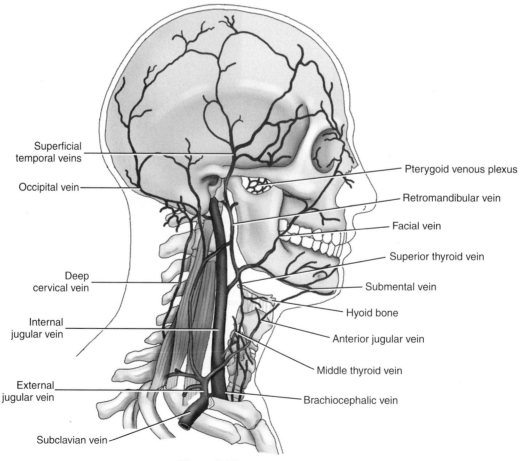

Figure 5.78
Sagittal view of extracranial veins.

TABLE 5-7   Veins of the Neck

VEINS OF THE NECK	TERMINATION	TRIBUTARIES
Internal jugular vein	Subclavian vein	Inferior petrosal sinus, facial, lingual, pharyngeal, superior and middle thyroid, and occasionally the occipital veins
External jugular vein	Subclavian vein	Retromandibular, anterior jugular, temporal, and maxillary veins and occasionally the occipital vein
Vertebral veins	Brachiocephalic vein	Internal and external vertebral venous plexuses and deep cervical veins

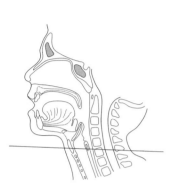 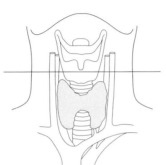 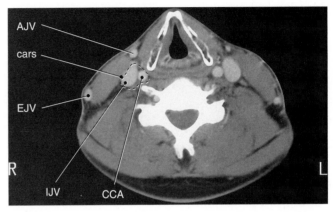

Figure 5.79
Axial CT scan of neck with carotid sheath.

KEY: **AJV,** Anterior jugular vein; **cars,** carotid artery sheath; **EJV,** external jugular vein; **IJV,** internal jugular vein; **CCA,** common carotid artery.

REFERENCES

Agur AM: *Grant's atlas of anatomy,* Baltimore, 1996, Williams & Wilkins.

Applegate E: *The anatomy and physiology learning system,* ed 2, Philadelphia, 2000, Saunders.

Applegate E: *The sectional anatomy learning system,* ed 2, Philadelphia, 2002, Saunders.

Ballinger PW: *Merrill's atlas of radiographic positions and radiologic procedures,* St. Louis, ed 10, 2003, Mosby.

Curry RA, Tempkin BB: *Ultrasonography: an introduction to normal structure and functional anatomy,* Philadelphia, 1995, Saunders.

English AW: *Wolf-Heidegger's atlas of human anatomy,* ed 5 Basel, Switzerland, 2000, Karger.

Gray H: *Gray's anatomy,* ed 15, New York, 1995, Barnes & Noble.

Haaga JR, Lanzieri CF, Gilkeson RC, et al: *CT and MR imaging of the whole body,* ed 4, Philadelphia, 2003, Mosby.

Harnsberger HR: *Handbook of head and neck imaging,* ed 2, St. Louis, 1995, Mosby.

Jacob S: *Atlas of human anatomy,* Philadelphia, 2002, Churchill Livingstone.

Larsen WJ: *Anatomy: Development function clinical correlations,* Philadelphia, 2002, Saunders.

Mancuso AA: *Workbook for MRI and CT of the head and neck,* ed 2, Baltimore, 1989, Williams & Wilkins.

Martini FH: *Fundamentals of anatomy and physiology,* ed 3, Englewood Cliffs, NJ, 1995, Prentice-Hall.

Mosby's medical, nursing, and allied health dictionary, ed 6, St. Louis, 2002, Mosby.

Palastanga N, Field D, Soames R, et al: *Anatomy and human movement,* ed 4, Philadelphia, 2002, Butterworth-Heinemann.

Ryan S, McNicholas M: *Anatomy for diagnostic imaging,* Philadelphia, 1994, Saunders.

Sandring S: *Gray's anatomy,* ed 39, Philadelphia, 2005, Churchill Livingstone.

Seidel HM, Ball JW, Dains JE, et al: *Mosby's guide to physical examination,* ed 4, St. Louis, 1999, Mosby.

Som PM, Curtin HD: *Head and neck imaging,* ed 3, St. Louis, 1996, Mosby.

Stark DD, Bradley WG: *Magnetic resonance imaging,* ed 3, St. Louis, 1999, Mosby.

Valvassori GE, Mahmood FM, Carter BL: *Imaging of the head and neck,* Basel, Switzerland, 1995, Thieme Medical Publishers.

CHAPTER 6

THORAX

Anyone who would attempt to operate on the heart should lose the respect of his colleagues.

CHRISTIAN ALBERT THEODOR BILLROTH, 1881

Many structures of the chest are in constant motion. Although physiologic motion can make imaging difficult, a thorough knowledge of chest anatomy and physiology can improve diagnostic imaging of this area. (Figure 6.1) This chapter demonstrates sectional anatomy of the following structures:

BONY THORAX
    Thoracic Apertures

LUNGS

PLEURAL CAVITIES

BRONCHI

MEDIASTINUM
    Thymus Gland
    Trachea and Esophagus

LYMPHATIC SYSTEM
    Lymph Nodes
    Lymph Vessels

HEART AND VASCULATURE
    Superficial Landmarks
    Pericardium
    Heart Wall
    Chambers
    Cardiac Valves
    Semilunar Valves

GREAT VESSELS
    Circulation of Blood through the Heart
    Off-Axis Cardiac Imaging
    Branches of the Aortic Arch
    Tributaries of the Superior Vena Cava

CORONARY CIRCULATION
    Coronary Arteries
    Cardiac Veins

AZYGOS VENOUS SYSTEM

MUSCLES

BREAST

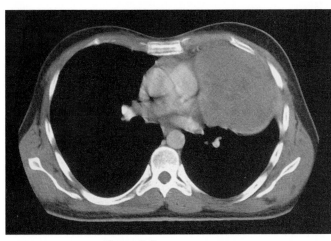

Figure 6.1
Axial CT with chest mass.

BONY THORAX

The bony thorax functions to protect the organs of the thorax and to aid in respiration. It consists of the **thoracic vertebrae, sternum, ribs, and costal cartilages** (Figure 6.2). The 12 thoracic vertebrae make up the posterior boundary of the thoracic cage. The anterior boundary is created by the sternum, located midline. The sternum has three components: manubrium, body, and xiphoid process (Figures 6.3 and 6.4). The triangular-shaped **manubrium** is the most superior portion and articulates with the first two pairs of ribs and the clavicles. It articulates with the clavicle at the clavicular notch to form the **sternoclavicular joints** (Figure 6.5). A common landmark, the **jugular notch,** is located on the superior border of the manubrium at approximately the level of T2-T3. The manubrium and body of the sternum come together at an angle to form a ridge known as the **sternal angle,** which is located at approximately the level of T4-T5. The slender **body** of the sternum has several indentations along its sides where it articulates with the cartilage of the third through seventh ribs (Figures 6.6 and 6.7). The small **xiphoid** process is located on the inferior border of the sternum and is a site for muscle attachments (Figure 6.8).

Forming the lateral borders of the thoracic cage are the 12 pairs of **ribs.** The spaces between adjacent ribs are referred to as the **intercostal spaces.** All 12 pairs of ribs articulate posteriorly with the thoracic spine. The ribs consist of a **head, neck, tubercle,** and **body** (Figures 6.7 and 6.8). The facets of the head of the rib articulate with the vertebral bodies at the **costovertebral joints,** whereas the facets of the tubercles articulate with the transverse processes of the vertebrae to form the **costotransverse joints.** The first 7 pairs of ribs (true ribs) articulate anteriorly with the sternum by costal cartilage. The lower 5 pairs of ribs are considered false ribs because they do not attach directly to the sternum. The costal cartilage of the eighth, ninth, and tenth ribs attach to the costal cartilage of the seventh rib. The eleventh and twelfth ribs are considered floating because they attach only to the thoracic vertebrae and contain no neck or tubercle, just vertebral and sternal ends (Figure 6.2).

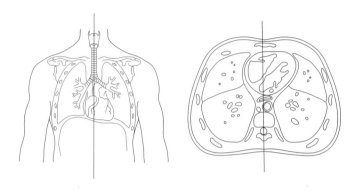

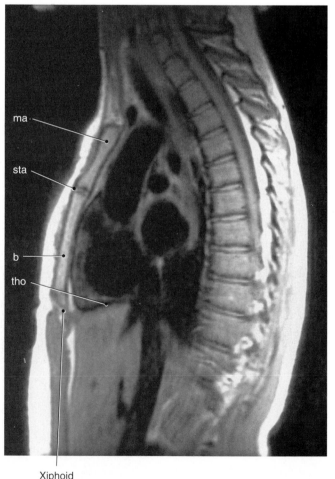

Figure 6.3
Sagittal, T1-weighted MR scan of thoracic cage.

Figure 6.2
Anterior view of thoracic cage. *SC joint,* Sternoclavicular joint.

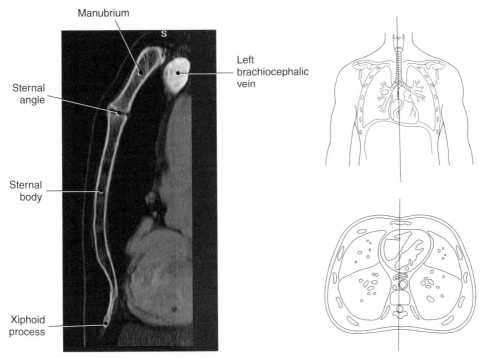

Figure 6.4
Sagittal CT reformat of sternum.

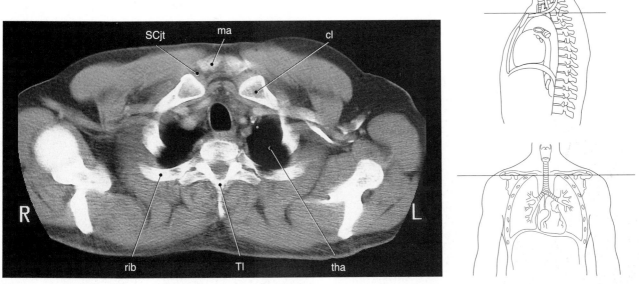

Figure 6.5
Axial CT scan of thoracic inlet.

KEY: **ma,** Manubrium; **sta,** sternal angle; **b,** body; **tho,** thoracic outlet; **SCjt,** sternoclavicular joint; **cl,** clavicle; **tha,** thoracic aperture; **T1,** first thoracic vertebra; **rib,** first rib.

Thoracic Apertures

There are two openings, or apertures, associated with the bony thorax. The superior aperture is formed by the first thoracic vertebra, first pair of ribs and their costal cartilages, and manubrium. This aperture, known as the **thoracic inlet,** allows for the passage of nerves, vessels, and viscera from the neck into the thoracic cavity. The inferior aperture is much larger and is made up of the twelfth thoracic vertebra, twelfth pair of ribs and costal margins, and xiphoid sternal junction. This aperture is known as the **thoracic outlet** (Figures 6.2, 6.5, and 6.8).

KEY: **ra,** Right atrium; **a,** aorta; **rv,** right ventricle; **la,** left atrium; **xi,** xiphoid process.

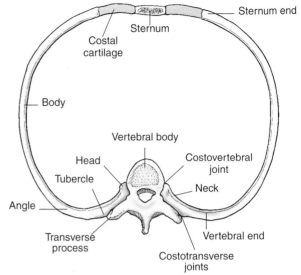

Figure 6.7
Axial view of costovertebral and costotransverse joints.

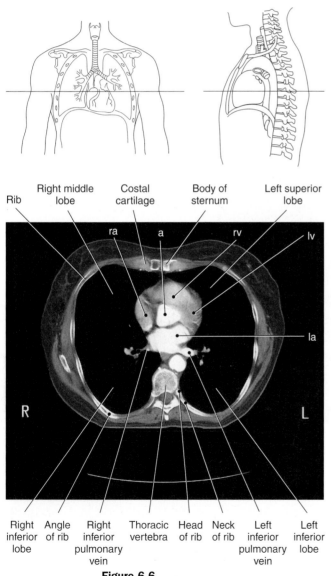

Figure 6.6
Axial CT scan of sternum.

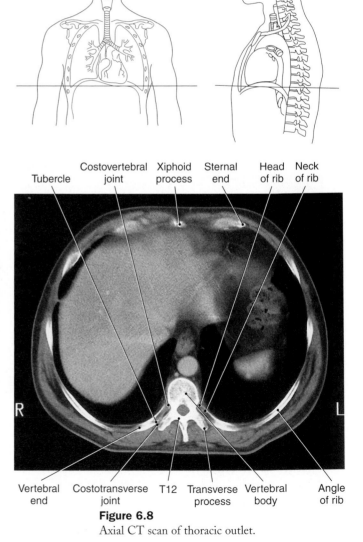

Figure 6.8
Axial CT scan of thoracic outlet.

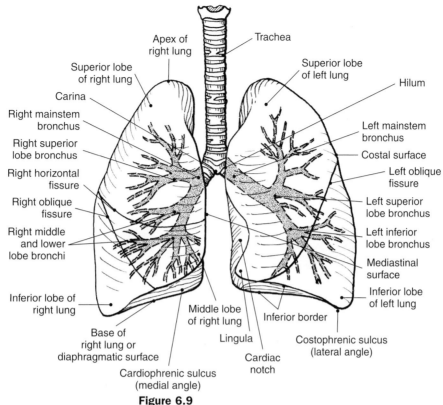

Apex of
right lung

Trachea

Superior lobe
of right lung

Superior lobe
of left lung

Carina

Hilum

Right mainstem
bronchus

Left mainstem
bronchus

Right superior
lobe bronchus

Costal surface

Right horizontal
fissure

Left oblique
fissure

Right oblique
fissure

Left superior
lobe bronchus

Right middle
and lower
lobe bronchi

Left inferior
lobe bronchus

Mediastinal
surface

Inferior lobe of
right lung

Inferior lobe
of left lung

Base of
right lung or
diaphragmatic surface

Middle lobe
of right lung

Inferior border

Costophrenic sulcus
(lateral angle)

Lingula

Cardiophrenic sulcus
(medial angle)

Cardiac
notch

Figure 6.9
Anterior view of bronchial tree.

LUNGS

The **lungs** are the organs of respiration, where gaseous exchange occurs between the respiratory air and blood. They are composed of a spongelike material, the parenchyma, and surrounded by a layer of serous membrane. The large conical-shaped lungs extend up to or slightly above the level of the first rib at their **apex** and down to the dome of the diaphragm at their wide concave-shaped **bases or diaphragmatic surfaces** (Figure 6.9). Each lung has a **mediastinal or medial surface** that is apposed to the mediastinum, and a **costal surface** that is apposed to the inner surface of the rib cage. Each lung also has an inferior, anterior, and posterior border. The **inferior border** extends into the costodiaphragmatic recess of the pleural cavity, and the **anterior border** of each lung extends into the costomediastinal recess of the pleural cavity (Figure 6.10). Two prominent angles can be identified at the medial and lateral edges of the lung bases. The **medial angle** is termed the **cardiophrenic sulcus,** and the **lateral angle** is termed the **costophrenic sulcus** (Figures 6.11 and 6.12). The lungs are divided into **lobes** by **fissures** that are lined by pleura and may extend as far as the hilum (Figure 6.13). The right lung has three lobes (superior [upper], middle, and inferior [lower]), whereas the left lung has just superior (upper) and inferior (lower) lobes (Figures 6.6 and 6.11 through 6.13). The inferior lobe of the right lung is separated from the middle and superior lobes by the **oblique fissure,** termed *oblique* because

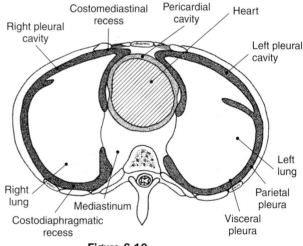

Costomediastinal
recess

Pericardial
cavity

Heart

Right pleural
cavity

Left pleural
cavity

Right
lung

Mediastinum

Left
lung

Costodiaphragmatic
recess

Parietal
pleura

Visceral
pleura

Figure 6.10
Axial cross section of pleura.

of its posterosuperior to anteroinferior course. Separating the middle lobe from the superior lobe is the **horizontal fissure** (Figures 6.9 and 6.14, *A*). An oblique fissure also separates the superior and inferior lobes of the left lung (Figure 6.11). The left lung has a large notch on the medial surface of its superior lobe called the **cardiac notch** and a tonguelike projection off its inferoanterior surface termed the **lingula.** Each lung has an

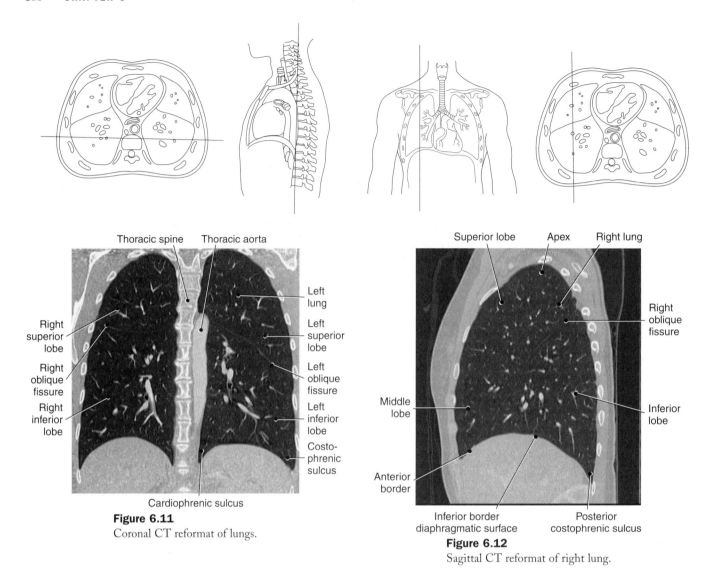

Figure 6.11
Coronal CT reformat of lungs.

Figure 6.12
Sagittal CT reformat of right lung.

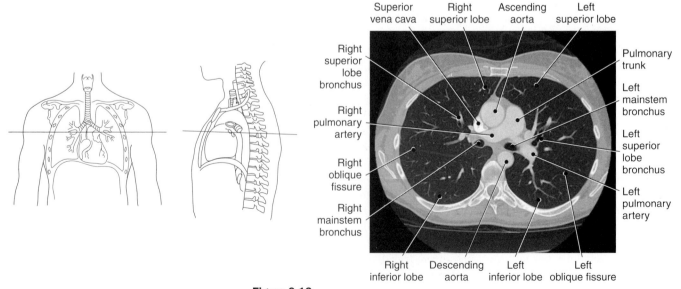

Figure 6.13
Axial CT scan of lungs with fissures.

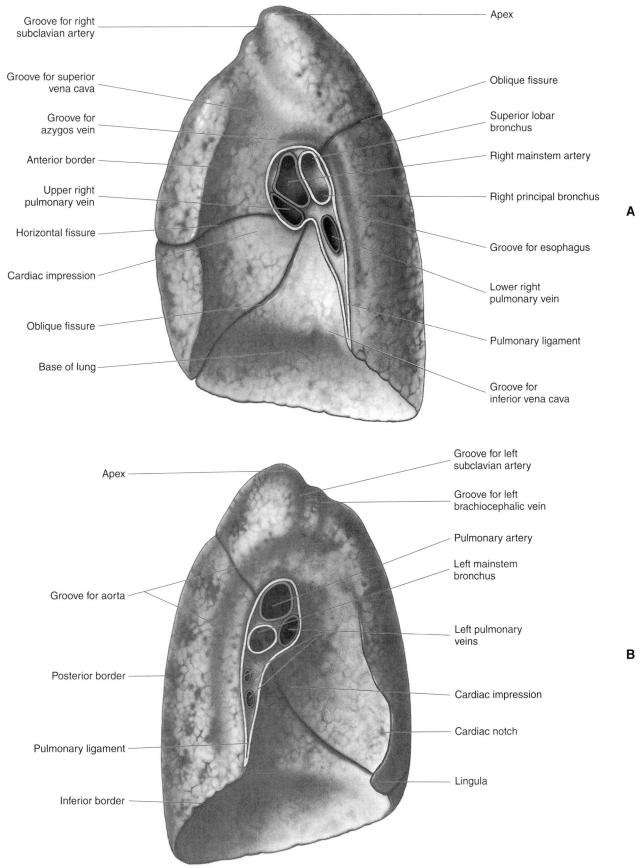

Groove for right subclavian artery

Groove for superior vena cava

Groove for azygos vein

Anterior border

Upper right pulmonary vein

Horizontal fissure

Cardiac impression

Oblique fissure

Base of lung

Apex

Oblique fissure

Superior lobar bronchus

Right mainstem artery

Right principal bronchus

Groove for esophagus

Lower right pulmonary vein

Pulmonary ligament

Groove for inferior vena cava

A

Groove for left subclavian artery

Groove for left brachiocephalic vein

Pulmonary artery

Left mainstem bronchus

Left pulmonary veins

Cardiac impression

Cardiac notch

Lingula

Apex

Groove for aorta

Posterior border

Pulmonary ligament

Inferior border

B

Figure 6.14
Medial view of lungs. **A,** Right lung. **B,** Left lung.

opening on the medial surface termed the **hilum** (Figures 6.14 through 6.16). This opening acts as a passage for mainstem bronchi, blood vessels, lymph vessels, and nerves to enter or leave the lung and is commonly referred to as the *root of the lung.*

> **Cystic disease of the lung encompasses a wide variety of pathologic processes that are characterized by "holes" or abnormal air-containing spaces within the lung parenchyma.**

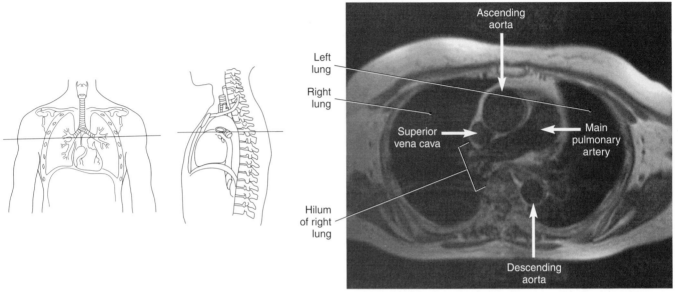

Figure 6.15
Axial, T1-weighted MR scan of lungs at hilum.

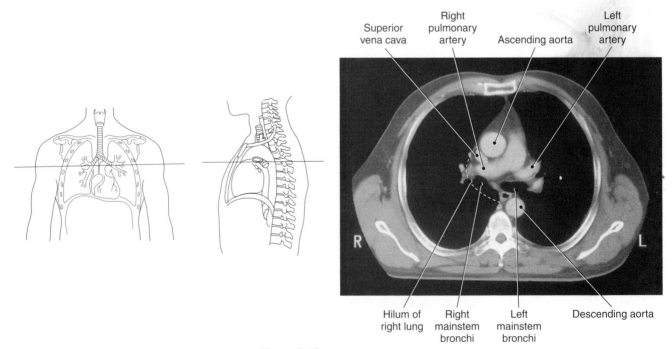

Figure 6.16
Axial CT scan of lungs at hilum.

PLEURAL CAVITIES

Each lung lies within a single pleural cavity that is lined by a serous membrane, or **pleura.** The pleura can be divided into two layers. The **parietal pleura,** the outer layer, is continuous with the thoracic wall and diaphragm and moves with these structures during respiration. The **visceral pleura** is the inner layer that closely covers the outer surface of the lung and continues into the fissures to cover the individual lobes as well. Both membranes secrete a small amount of pleural fluid that provides lubrication between the surfaces during breathing. Deep pockets or recesses of the pleural cavities are the **costomediastinal** and **costodiaphragmatic** recesses. The costomediastinal recesses are located at the point where the mediastinum and costal cartilages meet anteriorly, and the costodiaphragmatic recesses are located where the diaphragm and ribs connect inferiorly. These recesses serve as expansions to provide additional pleural space where parts of the lung can glide during inspiration (Figures 6.10 and 6.17).

BRONCHI

The **trachea** bifurcates into the left and right **mainstem (primary) bronchi** at approximately the level of T5. This location is commonly referred to as the **carina** (Figure 6.9). The right main bronchus is wider, shorter, and more vertical in orientation then the left. At the hilum the mainstem bronchi enter the lung and divide into **secondary or lobar bronchi.** Secondary bronchi correspond to the lobes of the lungs, thus with three divisions on the right (superior, middle, inferior) and two divisions on the left (superior and inferior) (Figures 6.9, and 6.18 through 6.20). There is further division of the secondary bronchi into **tertiary or segmental bronchi** that extend into each segment of the lobes **(bronchopulmonary segments)** (Figure 6.21 and Table 6.1). There are typically 10 segments within each lung. Each bronchopulmonary segment is functionally independent and can be individually removed surgically. The bronchial tree continues to divide many times into smaller **bronchi,** then into **bronchioles** (Figure 6.22). Each bronchiole continues to divide until it reaches the terminal end as **alveoli,** which are the functional units of the respiratory system. Gaseous exchange between alveolar air and capillary blood occurs through the wall of the alveoli.

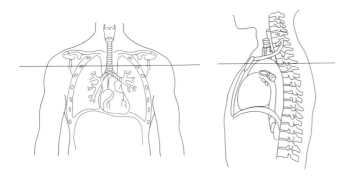

> **Lung cancer remains the leading cause of cancer-related deaths in both men and women in the United States.**

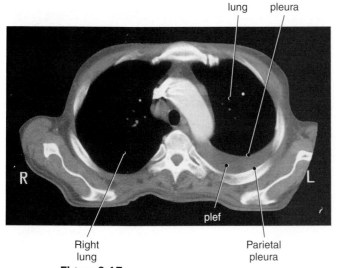

Figure 6.17
Axial CT scan of lungs with pleural effusion.

TABLE 6-1   Bronchopulmonary Segments

LOBE	RIGHT LUNG	LEFT LUNG
Superior lobe	Apical segment	Apical segment
	Posterior segment	Posterior segment
	Anterior segment	Anterior segment
		Superior lingular segment
		Inferior lingular segment
Middle lobe	Lateral segment	
	Medial segment	
Inferior lobe	Superior segment	Superior (apical) segment
	Medial basal segment	Medial basal segment
	Anterior basal segment	Anterior basal segment
	Lateral basal segment	Lateral basal segment
	Posterior basal segment	Posterior basal segment

KEY: plef, Pleural effusion.

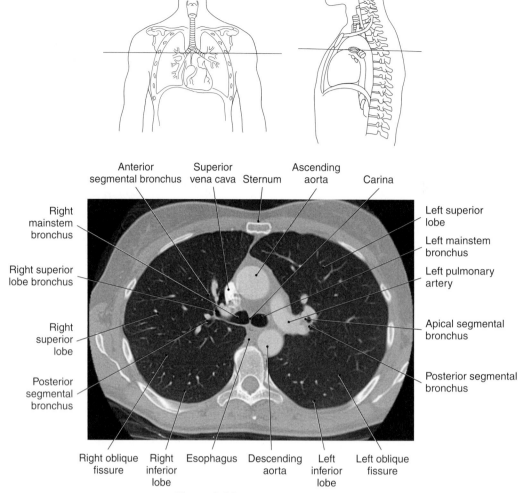

Figure 6.18
Axial CT scan of mainstem bronchi.

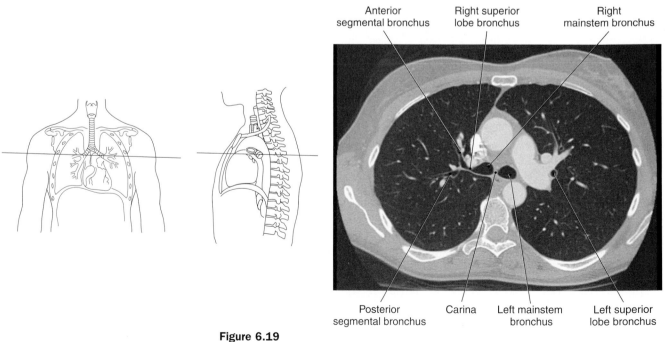

Figure 6.19
Axial CT scan of left superior lobe bronchus.

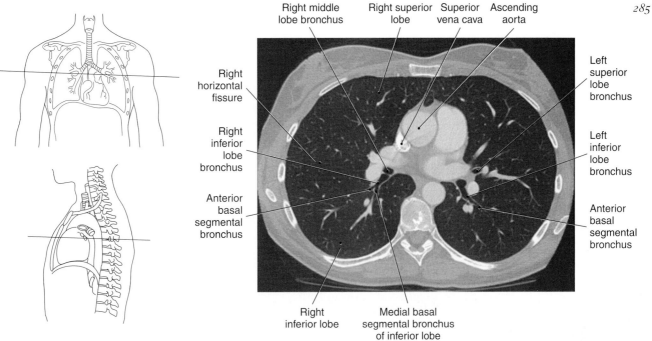

Figure 6.20

Axial CT scan of right inferior lobe bronchus.

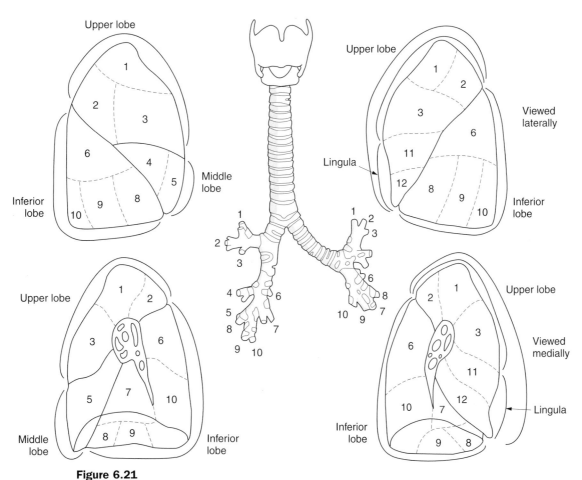

Figure 6.21

Trachea and bronchopulmonary segments. Bronchopulmonary segments: *1*, apical;
2, posterior; *3*, anterior; *4*, lateral; *5*, medial; *6*, apical basal; *7*, medial basal; *8*, anterior basal;
9, lateral basal; *10*, posterior basal; *11*, superior; *12*, inferior.

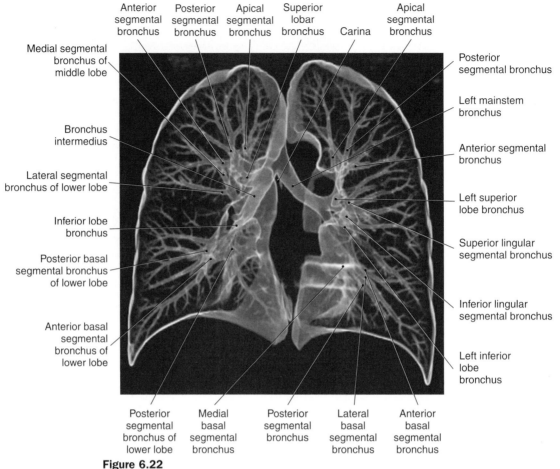

Anterior segmental bronchus
Posterior segmental bronchus
Apical segmental bronchus
Superior lobar bronchus
Carina
Apical segmental bronchus
Medial segmental bronchus of middle lobe
Posterior segmental bronchus
Left mainstem bronchus
Bronchus intermedius
Anterior segmental bronchus
Lateral segmental bronchus of lower lobe
Left superior lobe bronchus
Inferior lobe bronchus
Superior lingular segmental bronchus
Posterior basal segmental bronchus of lower lobe
Inferior lingular segmental bronchus
Anterior basal segmental bronchus of lower lobe
Left inferior lobe bronchus
Posterior segmental bronchus of lower lobe
Medial basal segmental bronchus
Posterior segmental bronchus
Lateral basal segmental bronchus
Anterior basal segmental bronchus

Figure 6.22
Coronal, CT 3D volume-rendered image of central and peripheral airways.

MEDIASTINUM

The **mediastinum** is the midline region of the thoracic cavity located between the two pleural cavities of the lungs. It extends from the superior thoracic aperture to the diaphragm and is bordered anteriorly by the sternum and posteriorly by thoracic vertebrae. The mediastinum can be subdivided into compartments for descriptive purposes. The superior and inferior compartments are made by drawing an imaginary line between the sternal angle and the intervertebral disk of T4-T5. The **superior compartment** constitutes the upper portion of the mediastinum. It contains the thymus gland and acts as a conduit for structures as they enter and leave the thoracic cavity. The **inferior compartment** can be further divided into anterior, middle, and posterior compartments (Figure 6.23). The **anterior compartment** is located anterior to the pericardial sac and posterior to the sternum. The **middle compartment** is the area that contains the pericardial sac, heart, and roots of the great vessels. The **posterior compartment** is the area lying posterior to the pericardium and anterior to the inferior eight thoracic vertebrae. Structures located within the mediastinum include the thymus gland, trachea, esophagus, lymph nodes, thoracic duct, heart and great vessels, and various nerves.

Thymus Gland

The **thymus gland** is a triangular-shaped bilobed gland of lymph tissue, located in the superior portion of the mediastinum just behind the manubrium (Figures 6.24 through 6.26). It is considered the primary lymphatic organ responsible for the development of cellular immunity. T-lymphocytes within the blood reach the thymus as stem cells, where they are stored while they undergo T-cell differentiation and maturation. The thymus gland produces a hormone, **thymosin,** that is responsible for the development and maturation of lymphocytes. The thymus gland reaches its maximum size during puberty and gradually diminishes in size in the adult.

> The thymus gland is large in children. In the newborn, it is often larger than the heart. It gradually decreases in size with increasing age and is replaced by mediastinal fat.

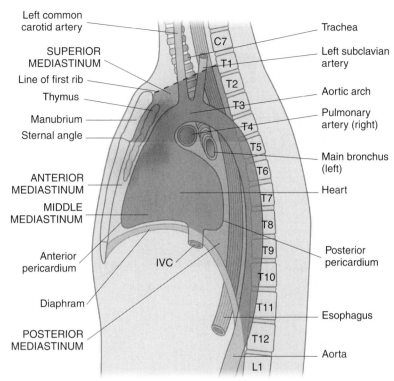

Figure 6.23
Sagittal view of mediastinal compartments. *IVC*, Inferior vena cava.

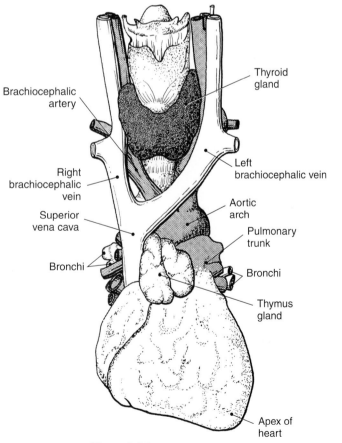

Figure 6.24
Anterior view of thymus gland.

288

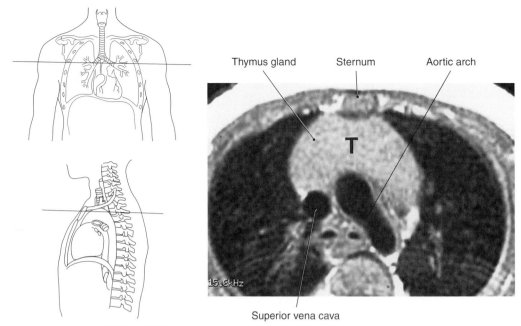

Figure 6.25
Axial, T1-weighted MR scan of pediatric chest with thymus gland.

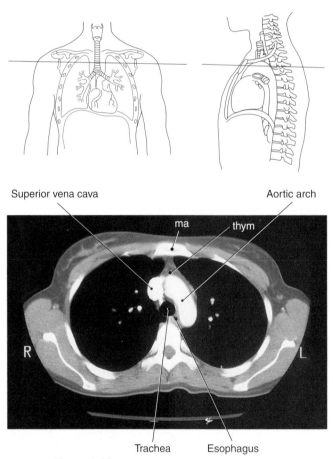

Figure 6.26
Axial CT scan of adult chest with thymus gland.

KEY: **ma,** Manubrium; **thym,** thymus gland.

Trachea and Esophagus

Throughout its course in the mediastinum, the trachea runs anterior to the esophagus. In cross section, the trachea appears as a round air-filled structure to the point at which it bifurcates at the carina (Figures 6.9 and 6.18). The esophagus appears as an oval-shaped structure that descends through the diaphragm to enter the stomach at the gastroesophageal junction (Figures 6.27 and 6.28).

KEY: rbV, Right brachiocephalic vein; **brA,** brachiocephalic artery; **lbV,** left brachiocephalic vein; **lCCA,** left common carotic artery; **lSA,** left subclavian vein; **tr,** trachea; **es,** esophagus.

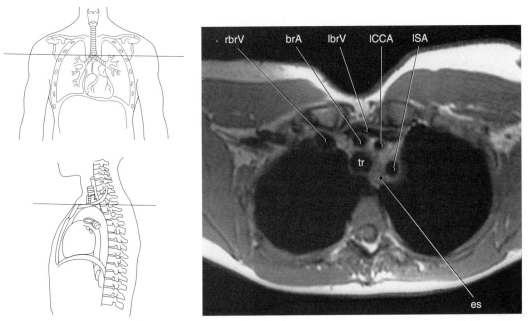

Figure 6.27
Axial, T1-weighted MR scan of trachea and esophagus.

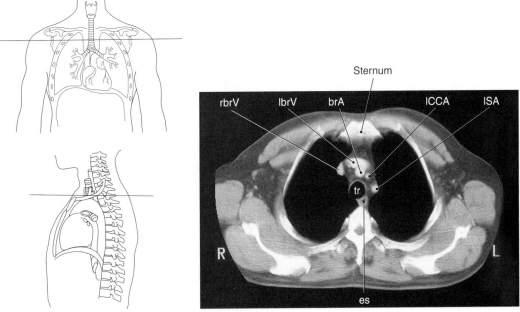

Figure 6.28
Axial CT scan of trachea and esophagus.

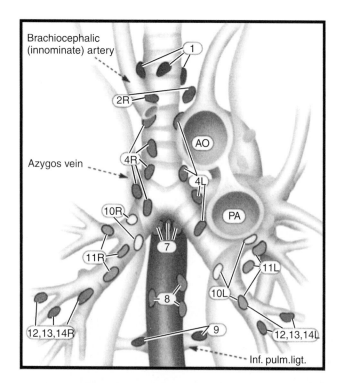

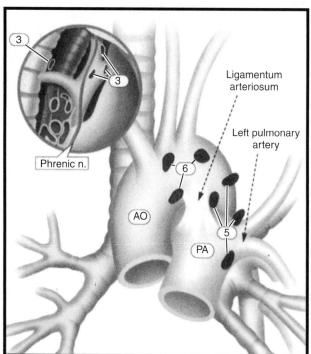

Figure 6.29
Coronal view with distribution of mediastinal lymph nodes. *L*, Left; *R*, right; *1*, highest mediastinal nodes; *2*, upper paratracheal nodes; *3*, prevascular and retrotracheal nodes; *4*, lower paratracheal (including azygos) nodes; *5*, subaortic nodes; *6*, paraaortic nodes; *7*, subcarinal; *8*, paraesophageal nodes; *9*, pulmonary ligament; *10*, hilar nodes; *11*, interlobar nodes; *12*, lobar nodes; *13*, segmental nodes; *14*, segmental nodes.

KEY: AO, aorta; **PA**, pulmonary artery; **Inf. pulm. ligt.**, inferior pulmonary ligament; **Phrenic n.**, phrenic nerve; **S**, superior vena cava; **A**, aorta.

LYMPHATIC SYSTEM

Lymph Nodes

Lymph nodes in the mediastinum are generally clustered around the great vessels, esophagus, bronchi, and carina. Mediastinal lymph nodes are classified according to their location and are grouped into 14 regional nodal stations for use in lung cancer staging (Figure 6.29 and Table 6.2). Lymph vessels and nodes can be difficult to visualize in cross section unless they are enlarged as a result of an abnormality (Figures 6.30 and 6.31).

> The supraclavicular lymph nodes are commonly referred to as the *sentinel lymph nodes* because their enlargement alerts the medical professional to the possibility of malignant disease in the thoracic and/or abdominal cavities.

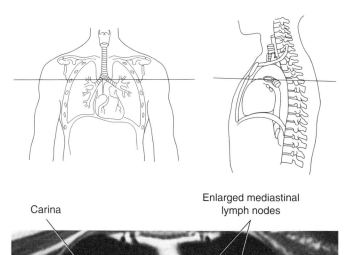

Figure 6.30
Axial, T1-weighted MR scan of chest with enlarged lymph nodes in the precarinal and aortopulmonary window regions.

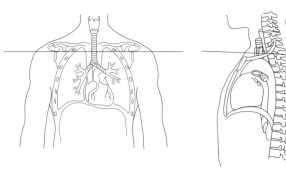

TABLE 6-2 Regional Nodal Stations for Staging Lung Cancer

NODES	LOCATION
N_2 Nodes	
Superior Mediastinal Nodes	
2R Right upper paratracheal nodes	Between intersection of caudal margin of innominate artery with trachea and the apex of the lung (suprainnominate nodes)
2L Upper left paratracheal nodes	Between top of aortic arch and apex of the lung (supraaortic nodes)
4R Right lower paratracheal nodes	Between intersection of caudal margin of innominate artery with trachea and cephalic border of azygos vein
4L Left lower paratracheal nodes	Between top of aortic arch and carina—medial to ligamentum arteriosum
10R Right tracheobronchial angle nodes	From cephalic border of azygos vein to origin of right upper lobe bronchus
10L Left tracheobronchial angle nodes	Between carina and left upper lobe—medial to ligamentum arteriosum
Aortic Nodes	
5 Aortopulmonary nodes	Subaortic and paraaortic nodes lateral to the ligamentum arteriosum—proximal to first branch of left pulmonary artery
6 Anterior mediastinal nodes	Anterior to ligamentum arteriosum
Inferior Mediastinal Nodes	
7 Subcarinal nodes	Caudal to the carina
8 Paraesophageal nodes	Dorsal to the posterior wall of the trachea and to the right or left of the midline of the esophagus
9 Pulmonary ligament nodes	Nodes within the pulmonary ligament
N_3 Nodes	
13 Interlobar nodes	
12 Lobar nodes	
13 Segmental nodes	
14 Subsegmental nodes	

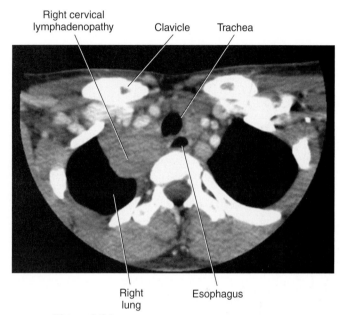

Figure 6.31
Axial CT scan of chest with enlarged lymph nodes.

Lymph Vessels

The lymphatic system consists of a network of lymphatic vessels that carry lymph fluid (excess interstitial fluid) away from the tissue and into the venous circulation. Small lymph vessels (capillaries) can be found accompanying the arteries and veins throughout the body. The tiny lymph vessels increase in size until they reach their terminal collecting vessels; the thoracic duct and the right lymphatic duct. The **thoracic duct** is the main vessel of the lymph system, draining all of the lymph fluid from tissues below the diaphragm and from the left side of the body above the diaphragm. It begins inferior to the diaphragm at the level of L2 and passes from the abdominal cavity into the thorax through the aortic hiatus of the diaphragm. It ascends the thorax, between the azygos vein and the descending aorta, and empties into the left subclavian vein at the level of the clavicle. The smaller **right lymphatic duct** collects lymph from the right upper side of the body and is formed by the merging of various lymphatic trunks near the right clavicle. This duct empties into the right subclavian vein (Figure 6.32).

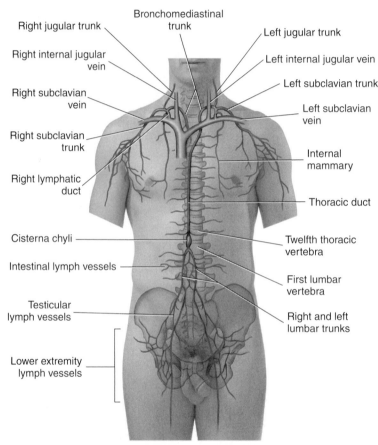

Figure 6.32
Thoracic and right lymphatic ducts.

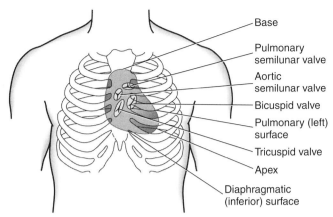

Figure 6.33
Superficial landmarks of the heart with borders, surfaces, apex, and base.

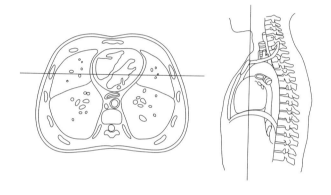

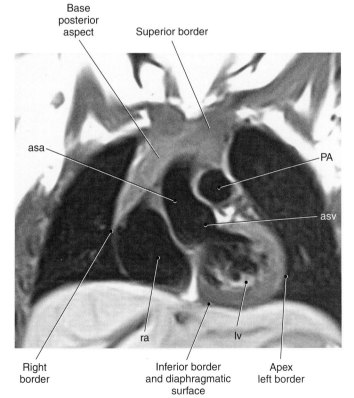

Figure 6.34
Coronal, T1-weighted MR scan of surfaces and borders of heart.

HEART AND VASCULATURE

Superficial Landmarks

The **heart** is a hollow, four-chambered muscular organ located within the middle mediastinum. It is approximately the size of a large clenched fist and is situated obliquely in the chest with one third of its mass lying to the right of the median plane and two thirds to the left. The heart can be described as being roughly trapezoid shaped (Figure 6.33). The superficial relationships of the heart include the base, apex, three surfaces (sternocostal, diaphragmatic, pulmonary), and four borders (right, inferior, left, and superior). The broad **base (posterior aspect)** is the most superior and posterior portion of the heart. It is formed by both atria, primarily the left atrium, and gives rise to the great vessels. The **apex** is formed by the left ventricle and points inferiorly, anteriorly, and to the left. It is located at the level of the fifth intercostal space, just medial to the mid-clavicular line. The **sternocostal (anterior surface)** is formed primarily by the right atrium and right ventricle with a small contribution from the left ventricle. The **diaphragmatic (inferior surface)** rests on the central tendon of the diaphragm and is formed by both ventricles and a small portion of the right atrium. The **pulmonary (left surface)** is formed mainly by the left ventricle and fills the cardiac notch of the left lung. The borders of the heart represent the external surfaces of the cardiovascular silhouette in radiographic profile. The borders include the **right border,** formed by the right atrium and located between the superior and inferior venae cavae; the **left border,** formed by the apex of the heart or the left ventricle; the **superior border,** formed by the right and left atria; and the **inferior border,** which is formed primarily by the right ventricle with a small contribution from the left ventricle (Figures 6.33 through 6.35).

> Carditis, an inflammation of the heart, can often lead to valvular heart disease. When infection damages or destroys the heart valves, valve leakage, heart failure, and death can ensue.

KEY: asa, Ascending aorta; **PA,** pulmonary arteries; **asv,** aortic similar valve; **lv,** left ventricle; **ra,** right atrium.

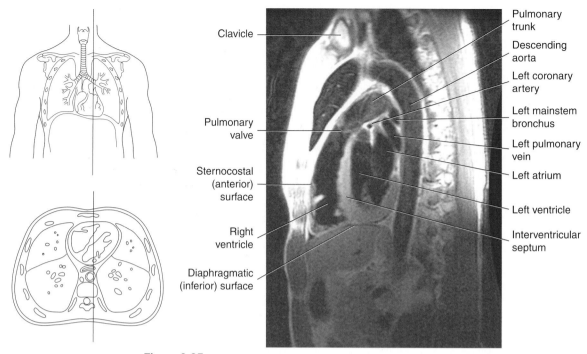

Figure 6.35
Sagittal, T1-weighted MR scan of surfaces and borders of heart.

Pericardium

The heart is enclosed in a pericardial sac that surrounds the heart and the proximal portions of the great vessels entering and leaving the heart. The **fibrous pericardium** is attached to the central tendon of the diaphragm and is pierced by the inferior vena cava. The inner surface of the fibrous pericardium consists of a double-layered serous membrane termed the **serous pericardium.** The serous pericardial layers are the **parietal layer** that lines the inner surface of the fibrous pericardium and the **visceral layer (epicardium)** that covers the outer surface of the heart and the roots of the great vessels. Located between the two layers is a potential space **(pericardial cavity)** containing a thin film of serous fluid that acts as a lubricant to reduce friction to the tissues caused by heart movement. Located between the pericardium and the heart wall is a layer of epicardial fat that is typically more prominent near the venous inflow and arterial outflow of the heart (Figures 6.36 through 6.38).

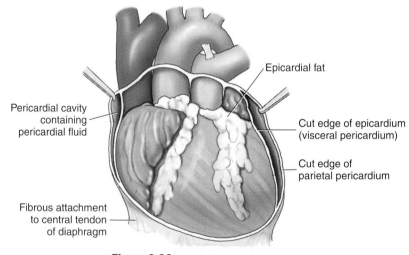

Figure 6.36
Anterior view of heart with pericardium.

Ten percent of the total cardiac volume of each heartbeat is required solely for supply to the heart muscle.

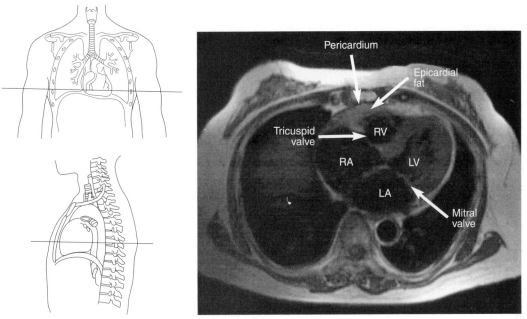

Figure 6.37
Axial, T1-weighted MR scan of heart with pericardium.

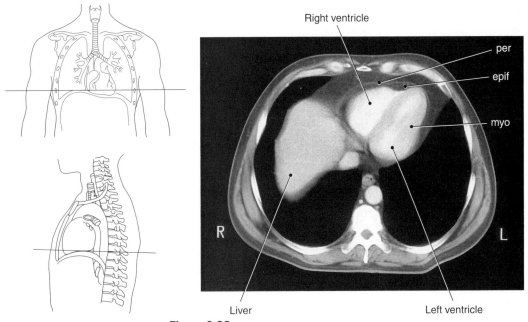

Figure 6.38
Axial CT scan of heart with pericardium.

KEY: RV, Right ventricle; **LV,** left ventricle; **LA,** left atrium; **RA,** right atrium; **per,** pericardium; **epif,** epicardial fat; **myo,** myocardium.

Heart Wall

The walls of the heart consist of three layers: (1) **epicardium,** the thin outer layer that is in contact with the pericardium; (2) **myocardium,** the thick middle layer consisting of strong cardiac muscle; and (3) **endocardium,** the thin, endothelial layer lining the inner surface. The endothelial layer also lines the valves of the heart and is continuous with the inner lining of the blood vessels. The heart is divided into four chambers: the right and left atria and the right and left ventricles. The two superior collecting chambers called *atria* are divided by the **interatrial septum.** During embryonic development an oval opening exists within the interatrial septum called the **foramen ovale.** This opening allows blood flow between the right and left atria during fetal lung development. At birth, the foramen ovale closes, leaving a small depression in the septal wall called the **fossa ovalis** in the adult heart. The two inferior pumping chambers called *ventricles* are divided by the **interventricular septum** (Figure 6.39).

Chambers

The **right atrium** forms the right border of the heart and receives deoxygenated blood from the body via the superior and inferior venae cavae and from the coronary sinus and cardiac veins that drain the myocardium. A small muscular embryonic appendage, the **right auricle,** projects upward and toward the left from the right atrium, covering the root of the aorta (Figure 6.40). The **right ventricle** lies on the diaphragm and comprises the largest portion of the anterior surface of the heart. It receives deoxygenated blood from the right atrium and forces it into the pulmonary trunk for conveyance to the lungs. Projecting off the inferior surface of the ventricular walls are conical-shaped projections of cardiac muscle called **papillary muscles** that anchor the cusps of the tricuspid valve to the right ventricle (Figure 6.39). The **left atrium** lies posterior to the right atrium and is the most posterior surface of the heart. It also has an embryonic appendage, the **left auricle,** that projects to the left of the pulmonary trunk over the superior surface of the heart. The left atrium receives oxygenated blood directly from the lungs via the four pulmonary veins (two on each side). The **left ventricle** forms the apex, left border, and most of the inferior surface of the heart. It receives oxygenated blood from the left atrium and pumps it into the aorta for distribution throughout the systemic circuit. The myocardium of the left ventricle is normally three times thicker than that of the right ventricle, reflecting the force necessary to pump blood to the distant sites of the systemic circulation (Figures 6.41 through 6.52). Two **papillary muscles** project from the ventricular walls to anchor the bicuspid valve to the ventricle (Figures 6.39 and 6.47).

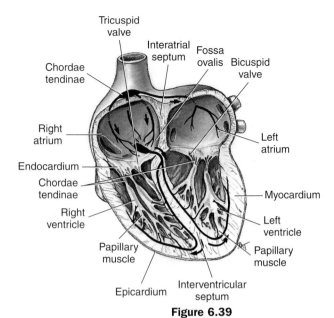

Figure 6.39
Coronal view of heart wall and chambers.

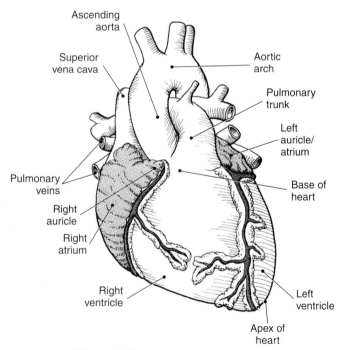

Figure 6.40
Coronal view of anterior surface of heart.

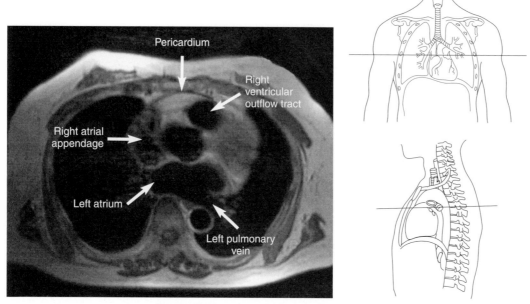

Figure 6.41
Axial, T1-weighted MR scan of right ventricle.

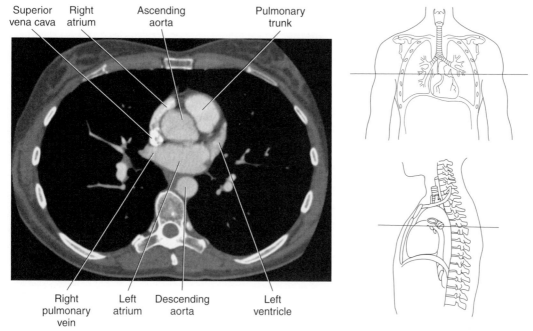

Figure 6.42
Axial CT scan of right ventricle.

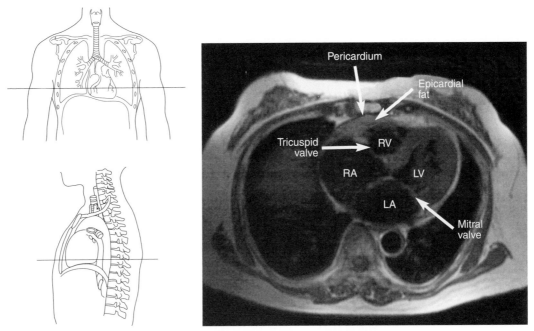

Figure 6.43
Axial, T1-weighted MR scan of left atrium.

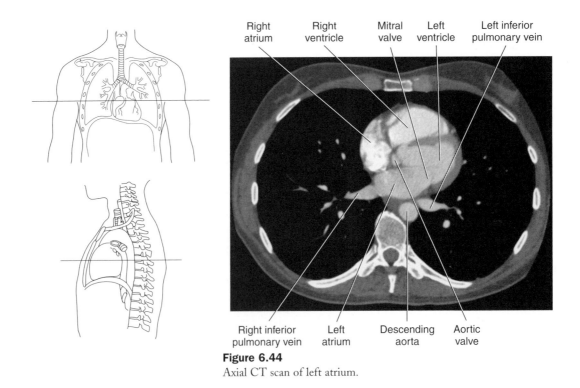

Figure 6.44
Axial CT scan of left atrium.

KEY: RV, Right ventricle; **LV,** left ventricle; **LA,** left atrium; **RA,** right atrium.

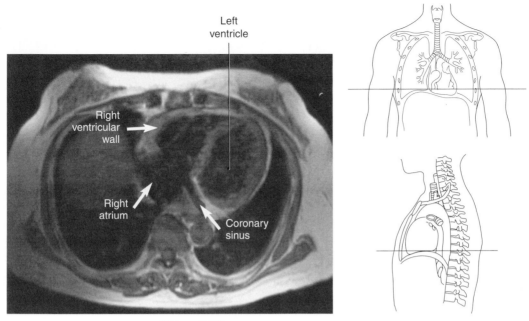

Figure 6.45
Axial, T1-weighted MR scan of right atrium.

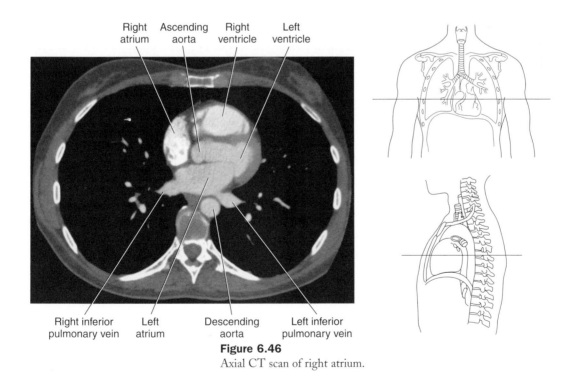

Figure 6.46
Axial CT scan of right atrium.

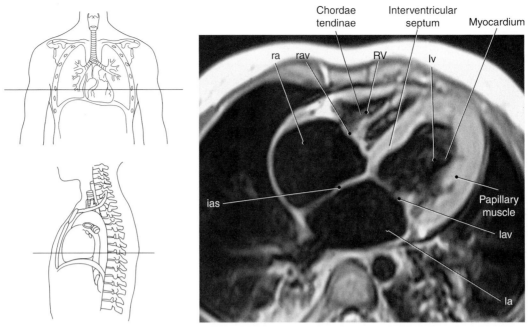

Figure 6.47
Axial, T1-weighted MR scan with four-chamber view of heart.

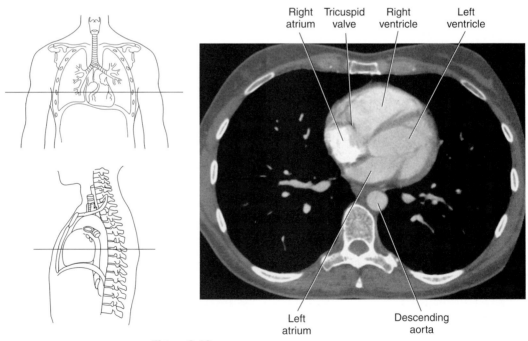

Figure 6.48
Axial CT scan with four-chamber view of heart.

KEY: ra, Right atrium; **rav,** right atrioventricular valve; **RV,** right ventricle; **lv,** left ventricle; **lav,** left atrioventricular valve; **la,** left atrium; **ias,** intraatrial septum.

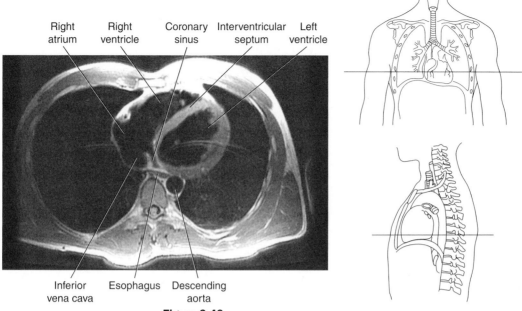

Right atrium Right ventricle Coronary sinus Interventricular septum Left ventricle

Inferior vena cava Esophagus Descending aorta

Figure 6.49
Axial, T1-weighted MR scan of ventricles.

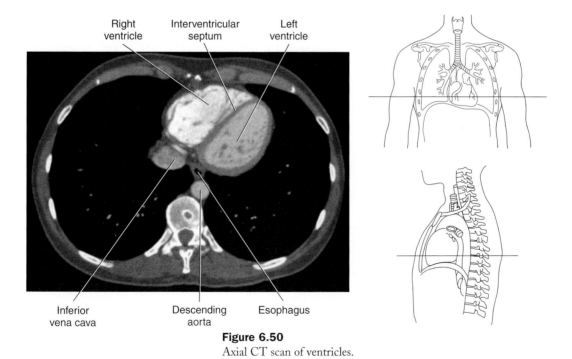

Right ventricle Interventricular septum Left ventricle

Inferior vena cava Descending aorta Esophagus

Figure 6.50
Axial CT scan of ventricles.

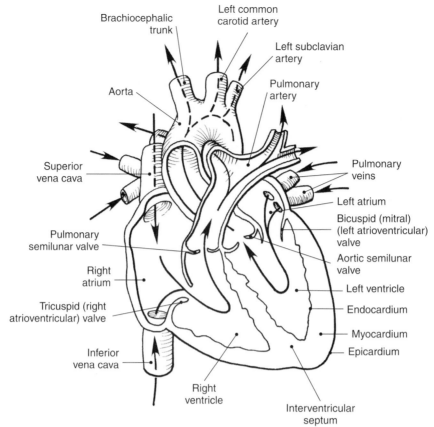

Brachiocephalic trunk

Left common carotid artery

Left subclavian artery

Pulmonary artery

Aorta

Superior vena cava

Pulmonary veins

Left atrium

Bicuspid (mitral) (left atrioventricular) valve

Aortic semilunar valve

Left ventricle

Endocardium

Myocardium

Epicardium

Pulmonary semilunar valve

Right atrium

Tricuspid (right atrioventricular) valve

Inferior vena cava

Right ventricle

Interventricular septum

Figure 6.51
Coronal view of heart with four chambers and cardiac valves.

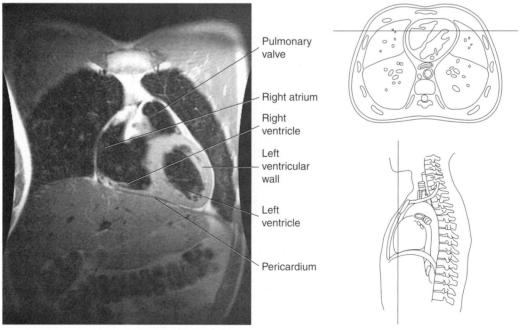

Pulmonary valve

Right atrium

Right ventricle

Left ventricular wall

Left ventricle

Pericardium

Figure 6.52
Coronal, T1-weighted MR scan of pulmonary valve.

Cardiac Valves

Four valves are located in the heart that function to maintain one-way directional blood flow throughout the heart. The valves can be divided into two groups: atrioventricular and semilunar (Figure 6.51).

ATRIOVENTRICULAR VALVES The two **atrioventricular valves** are found at the entrances to both ventricles and function to prevent backflow of blood between the atria and ventricles during ventricular contraction. These valves have leaflets that are attached to the papillary muscles by thin cords of fibrous tissue called **chordae tendineae.** The **right atrioventricular valve,** with three leaflets, is called the **tricuspid valve,** and the **left atrioventricular valve,** with two leaflets, is called the **bicuspid (mitral) valve** (Figures 6.39, 6.43, 6.44, 6.47, and 6.48).

Semilunar Valves

The **semilunar valves** are located at the junction where the ventricles meet the great vessels, separating the ventricles from the circulatory system. These valves are called semilunar because of their three crescent-shaped cusps and function to prevent the flow of blood back into the ventricles during ventricular relaxation. The **pulmonary semilunar valve** is located at the juncture of the right ventricle and pulmonary artery, and the **aortic semilunar valve** lies between the left ventricle and ascending aorta (Figures 6.51 through 6.53).

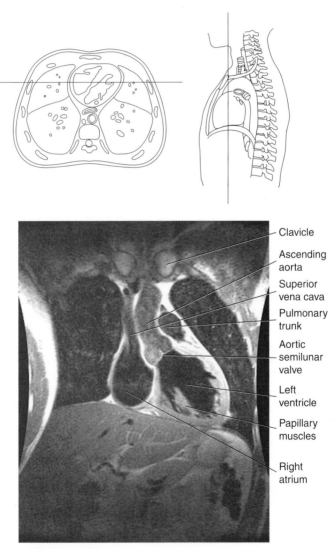

Clavicle

Ascending aorta

Superior vena cava

Pulmonary trunk

Aortic semilunar valve

Left ventricle

Papillary muscles

Right atrium

Figure 6.53
Coronal, T1-weighted MR scan of aortic valve.

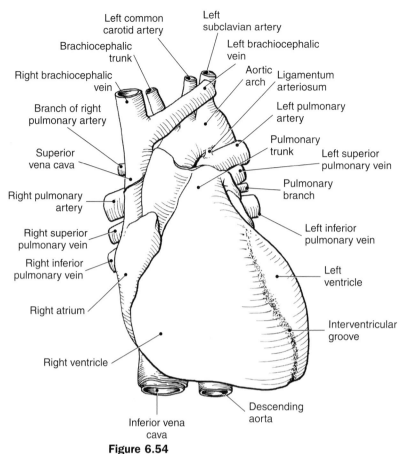

Left common
carotid artery

Left
subclavian artery

Brachiocephalic
trunk

Left brachiocephalic
vein

Right brachiocephalic
vein

Aortic
arch

Ligamentum
arteriosum

Branch of right
pulmonary artery

Left pulmonary
artery

Superior
vena cava

Pulmonary
trunk

Left superior
pulmonary vein

Right pulmonary
artery

Pulmonary
branch

Right superior
pulmonary vein

Left inferior
pulmonary vein

Right inferior
pulmonary vein

Left
ventricle

Right atrium

Interventricular
groove

Right ventricle

Descending
aorta

Inferior vena
cava

Figure 6.54

Anterior view of heart and great vessels.

GREAT VESSELS

Blood travels to and from the heart through the **great vessels,** which include the aorta, pulmonary arteries and veins, and superior and inferior venae cavae (Figures 6.54 and 6.55). The **aorta** is the largest artery of the body and can be divided into the ascending aorta, aortic arch, and descending aorta. The **ascending aorta** begins at the base of the left ventricle at the level of the sternal angle, then curves superiorly and posteriorly as the **aortic arch** over the root of the left lung. The top of the aortic arch is approximately at T3 (Figures 6.56 and 6.57). The arch continues as the **descending aorta** posterior to the left bronchus and pulmonary trunk, on the left side of the vertebral body of T4 (Figures 6.58 and 6.59). The descending aorta passes slightly anterior and to the left of the vertebral column as it descends through the thoracic and abdominal cavities (Figure 6.60). While in the thoracic cavity, the descending aorta is commonly called the **thoracic aorta,** and while in the abdominal cavity, it is called the **abdominal aorta.** The **pulmonary trunk** is the origin of the right and left pulmonary arteries and lies entirely within the pericardial sac. It arises from the right ventricle and ascends in front of the ascending aorta, courses posteriorly and to the left, where it bifurcates at the level of the sternal angle (T4) into the right and left pulmonary arteries (Figures 6.61 through 6.63). The pulmonary

trunk is attached to the aortic arch by a fibrous cord called the **ligamentum arteriosum,** the remnant of an important fetal blood vessel (ductus arteriosus) that links the pulmonary and systemic circuits during fetal development (Figures 6.54 and 6.61). The **right pulmonary artery** courses laterally, posterior to the ascending aorta and superior vena cava, and anterior to the esophagus and right mainstem bronchus, to the hilum of the right lung. At the root of the right lung, the right pulmonary artery divides into two branches, with the lower branch supplying the middle and inferior lobes and the upper branch supplying the superior lobe (Figures 6.61 through 6.64). The **left pulmonary artery,** shorter and smaller than the right, is also the most superior of the pulmonary vessels. It travels horizontally, arching over the left mainstem bronchus, and enters the hilum of the left lung just superior to the left mainstem bronchus (Figures 6.61 through 6.64). Within the lungs, each pulmonary artery descends posterolateral to the main bronchus and divides into lobar and segmental arteries, continuing to branch out and to follow along with the smallest divisions of the bronchial tree (Figures 6.61 and 6.64). Located inferior to the pulmonary arteries are the four **pulmonary veins,** two each (superior and inferior) extending from each lung to enter the left atrium (Figures 6.54, 6.55, 6.61, and 6.64 through 6.68). They commence in a capillary network along the walls of the alveoli, where they are continuous with the

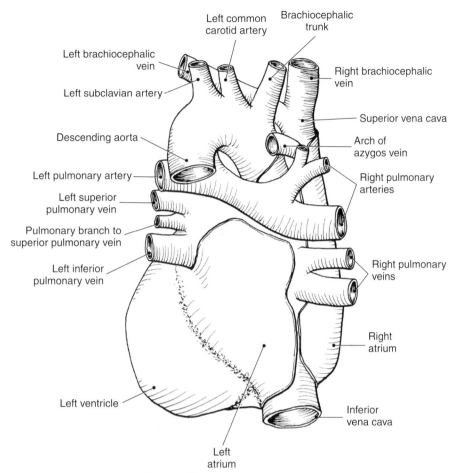

Figure 6.55
Posterior view of heart and great vessels.

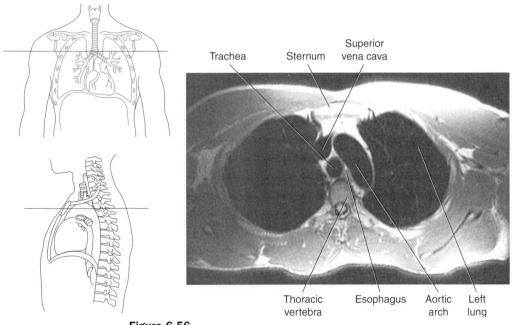

Figure 6.56
Axial, T1-weighted MR scan of chest with aortic arch.

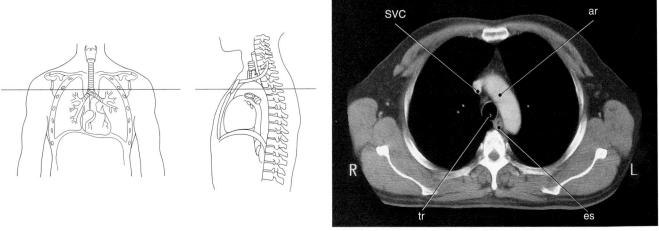

Figure 6.57
Axial CT scan of chest with aortic arch.

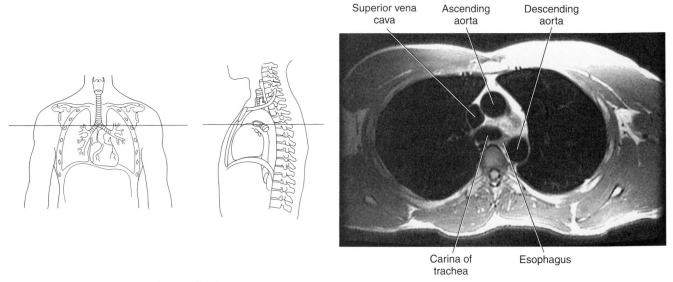

Figure 6.58
Axial, T1-weighted MR scan of chest with ascending and descending aorta.

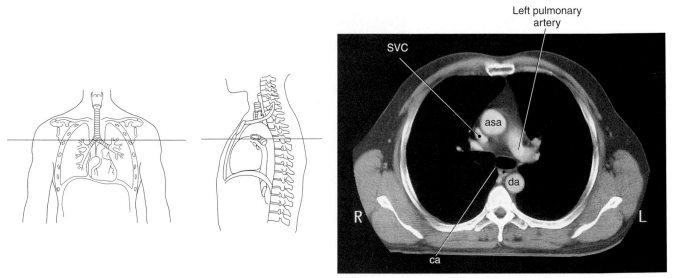

Figure 6.59
Axial CT scan of chest with ascending and descending aorta.

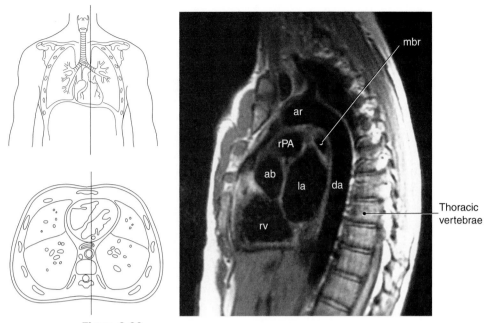

Figure 6.60
Sagittal, T1-weighted MR scan with aortic arch and descending aorta.

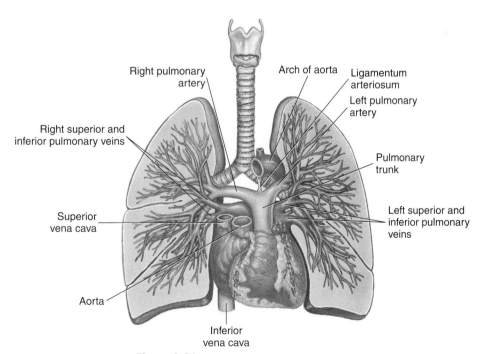

Figure 6.61
Anterior view of pulmonary arteries and veins.

KEY: SVC, Superior vena cava; **ar,** aortic arch; **es,** esophagus; **tr,** trachea; **asa,** ascending aorta; **da,** descending aorta; **ca,** carina; **mbr,** mainstem bronchi; **rPA,** right pulmonary artery; **ab,** aortic bulb; **la,** left atrium; **rv,** right ventricle.

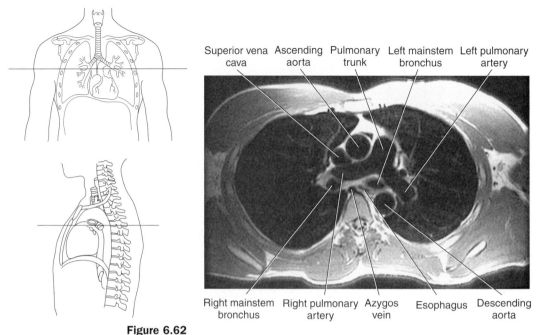

Figure 6.62
Axial, T1-weighted MR scan of chest with pulmonary trunk.

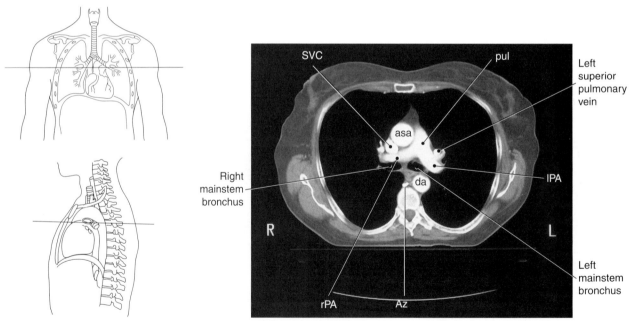

Figure 6.63
Axial CT scan of chest with pulmonary trunk.

KEY: **SVC,** Superior vena cava; **pul,** pulmonary trunk; **asa,** ascending aorta; **da,** descending aorta; **rPA,** right pulmonary artery; **Az,** azygous vein; **IPA,** left pulmonary artery.

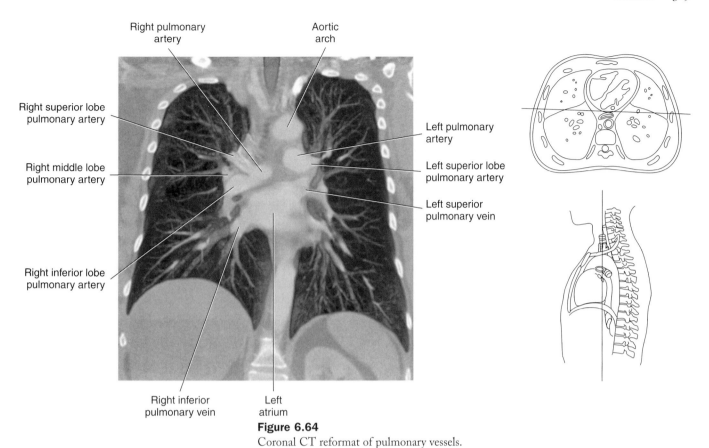

Right pulmonary artery

Aortic arch

Right superior lobe pulmonary artery

Right middle lobe pulmonary artery

Right inferior lobe pulmonary artery

Left pulmonary artery

Left superior lobe pulmonary artery

Left superior pulmonary vein

Right inferior pulmonary vein

Left atrium

Figure 6.64
Coronal CT reformat of pulmonary vessels.

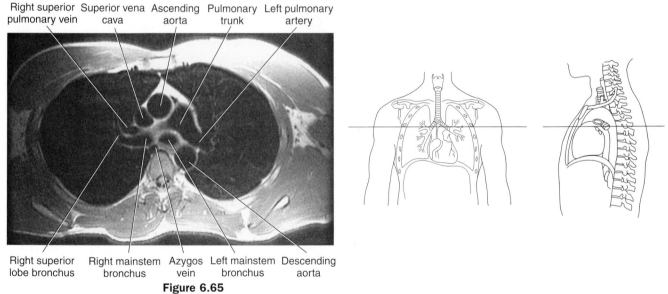

Right superior pulmonary vein

Superior vena cava

Ascending aorta

Pulmonary trunk

Left pulmonary artery

Right superior lobe bronchus

Right mainstem bronchus

Azygos vein

Left mainstem bronchus

Descending aorta

Figure 6.65
Axial, T1-weighted MR scan of chest with right superior pulmonary vein.

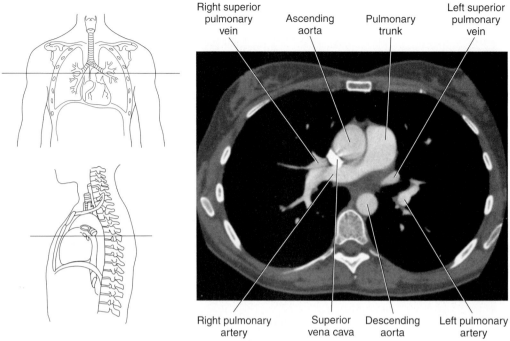

Figure 6.66
Axial CT scan of chest with superior pulmonary veins.

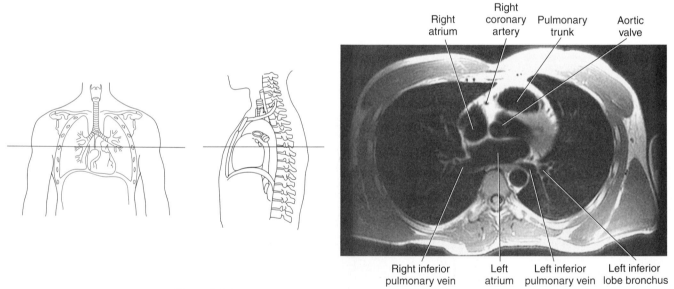

Figure 6.67
Axial, T1-weighted MR scan of chest with inferior pulmonary veins.

capillaries of the pulmonary arteries. The venous capillaries merge to form small vessels that unite successively to eventually form a single trunk for each lobe: three for the right and two for the left lung. Frequently the trunk from the middle lobe of the right lung unites with the trunk from the upper lobe, forming just two trunks on the right side prior to entering the left atrium. The **right superior pulmonary vein** collects blood from the upper lobe segments of the right lung and passes anterior and inferior to the right pulmonary artery, behind the superior vena cava. The **right inferior pulmonary vein** receives blood from the right lower lobes of the lung and crosses behind the right atrium to the left atrium (Figures 6.61 and 6.69 through 6.71). The **left superior pulmonary vein** receives blood from the left upper lobe of the left lung and courses anterior and inferior to the left main bronchus as it enters the left atrium. The **left inferior pulmonary vein** drains the inferior lobe of the left lung and passes toward the left atrium anterior to the bronchi (Figures 6.61 and 6.72 through 6.74). The pulmonary veins course more horizontally than the pulmonary arteries and are ultimately oriented toward the left

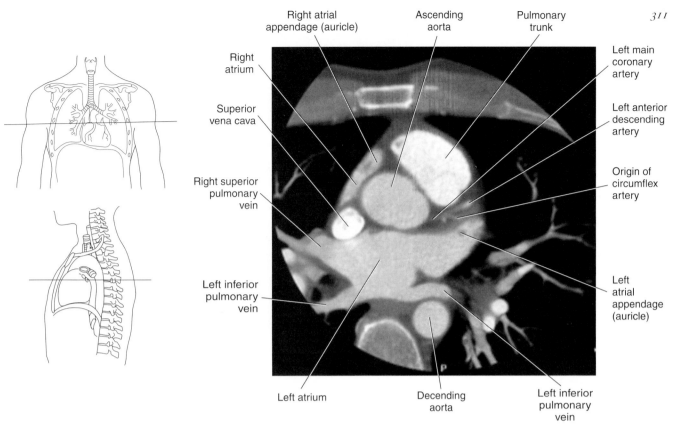

Right atrial appendage (auricle)

Ascending aorta

Pulmonary trunk

Right atrium

Left main coronary artery

Superior vena cava

Left anterior descending artery

Right superior pulmonary vein

Origin of circumflex artery

Left atrial appendage (auricle)

Left inferior pulmonary vein

Left atrium

Decending aorta

Left inferior pulmonary vein

Figure 6.68
Axial CT scan of chest with inferior pulmonary veins.

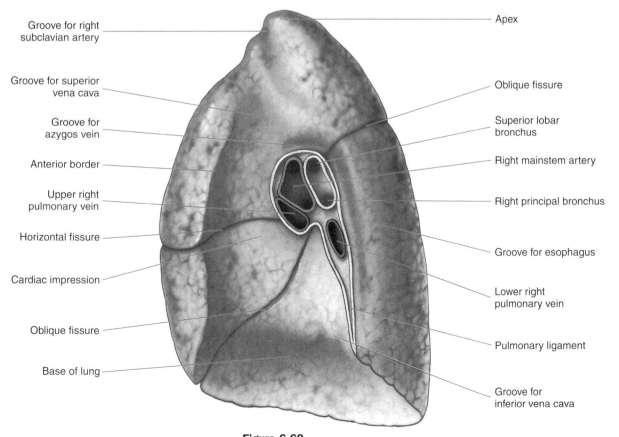

Groove for right subclavian artery

Apex

Groove for superior vena cava

Oblique fissure

Groove for azygos vein

Superior lobar bronchus

Anterior border

Right mainstem artery

Upper right pulmonary vein

Right principal bronchus

Horizontal fissure

Groove for esophagus

Cardiac impression

Lower right pulmonary vein

Oblique fissure

Pulmonary ligament

Base of lung

Groove for inferior vena cava

Figure 6.69
Medial surface of right lung.

312

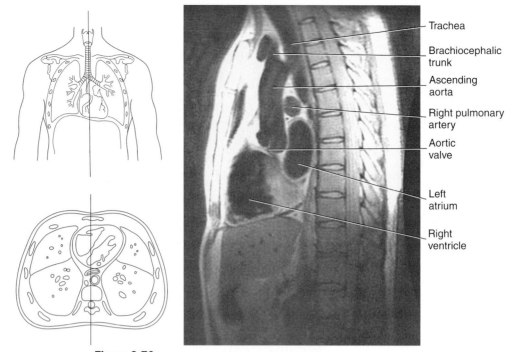

Figure 6.70
Sagittal, T1-weighted MR scan of right mediastinum and diaphragm.

- Trachea
- Brachiocephalic trunk
- Ascending aorta
- Right pulmonary artery
- Aortic valve
- Left atrium
- Right ventricle

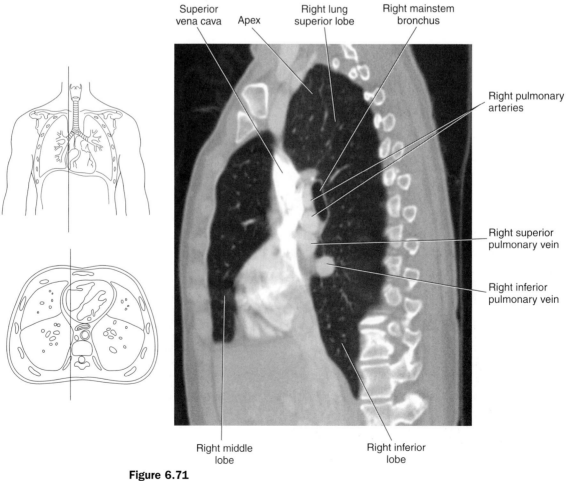

Superior vena cava

Apex

Right lung superior lobe

Right mainstem bronchus

Right pulmonary arteries

Right superior pulmonary vein

Right inferior pulmonary vein

Right middle lobe

Right inferior lobe

Figure 6.71
Sagittal CT reformat of right mediastinum and pulmonary vessels.

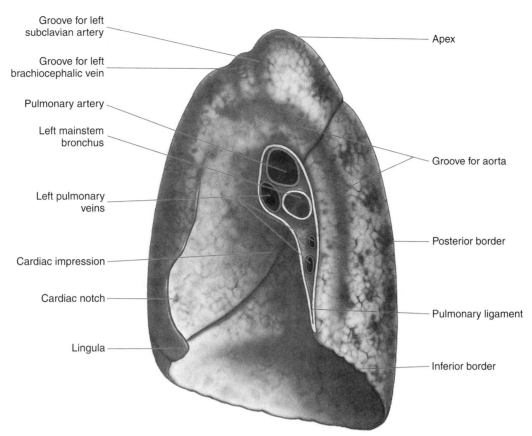

Figure 6.72
Medial surface of left lung.

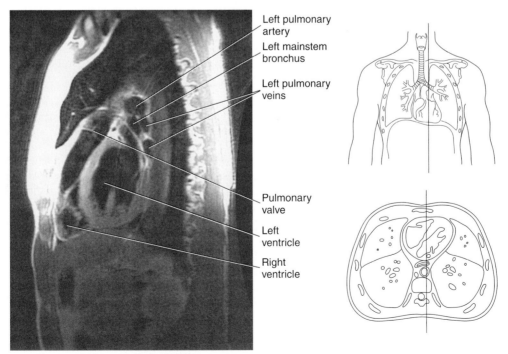

Figure 6.73
Sagittal, T1-weighted MR scan of left mediastinum.

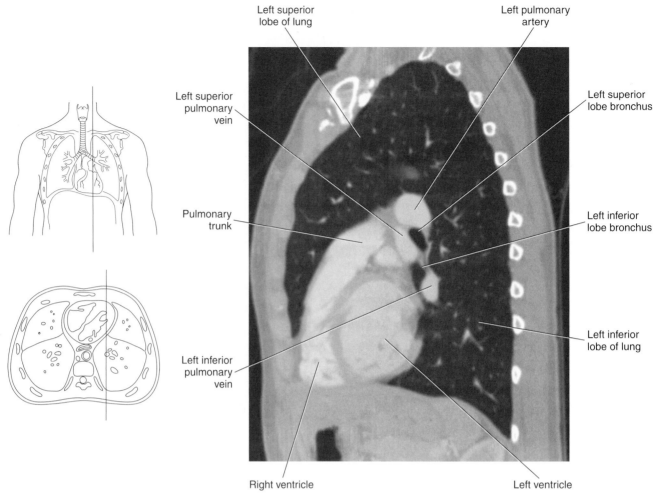

Figure 6.74
Sagittal CT reformat of left mediastinum and pulmonary vessels.

atrium. At the root of the lungs, the pulmonary veins are anterior to the pulmonary arteries, which are anterior to the bronchus. While within the lungs, the branches of the pulmonary arteries are anterior to the bronchi, which are anterior to the pulmonary veins. The superior and inferior venae cavae are the largest veins of the body. The **superior vena cava** is formed by the junction of the brachiocephalic veins, posterior to the right first costal cartilage, and carries blood from the thorax, upper limbs, head, and neck (Figure 6.24). As it travels inferiorly, it is located posterior and lateral to the ascending aorta before entering the upper portion of the right atrium (Figures 6.54 through 6.59). The **inferior vena cava** is formed by the junction of the common iliac veins in the pelvis and ascends the abdomen to the right of the abdominal aorta and anterior to the vertebral column. It passes through the caval hiatus of the diaphragm and almost immediately enters the inferior portion of the right atrium (Figures 6.75 and 6.76).

> **Obstruction of a pulmonary artery or one of its branches is known as a *pulmonary embolism*. This condition prevents blood flow to the alveoli and, if left in place for several hours, will result in permanent collapse of the alveoli. It is commonly caused by thrombosis from the lower extremities.**

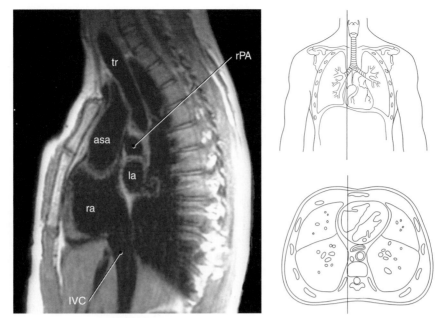

Figure 6.75
Sagittal, T1-weighted MR scan of inferior vena cava.

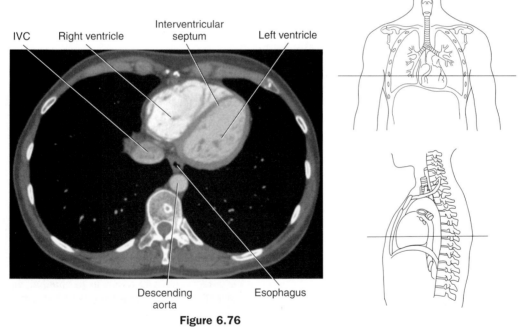

Figure 6.76
Axial CT scan of inferior vena cava.

KEY: tr, Trachea; **rPA,** right pulmonary artery; **asa,** ascending aorta; **la,** left atrium; **ra,** right atrium; **IVC,** inferior vena cava.

Circulation of Blood through the Heart

Deoxygenated blood is brought to the right atrium from the peripheral tissues by the inferior and superior venae cavae. The right atrium contracts, forcing blood through the tricuspid (right atrioventricular) valve into the right ventricle. The right ventricle pumps blood through the pulmonary semilunar valve to the pulmonary arteries, which enter into the lungs. Oxygenated blood returns to the heart via the pulmonary veins, which enter the left atrium. The left atrium forces blood through the bicuspid (mitral) valve into the left ventricle, where it is then pumped through the aortic semilunar valve to the aorta (Figure 6.51).

Off-Axis Cardiac Imaging

In an effort to standardize nomenclature for tomographic imaging of the heart, the Cardiac Imaging Committee of the Council on Clinical Cardiology of the American Heart Association published a statement recommending that all cardiac imaging modalities use the same nomenclature for defining tomographic imaging planes. Their recommendation stated that "all cardiac imaging modalities should define, orient, and display the heart using the long axis of the left ventricle and selected planes oriented at 90-degree angles relative to the long axis." Their second recommendation stated, "The names for the 90-degree–oriented cardiac planes used in all imaging modalities should be short axis, vertical long axis, and horizontal long axis. These correspond to the short-axis, apical two-chamber, and apical four-chamber planes traditionally used in 2D echocardiography" (Figure 6.77). We will follow these recommendations for labeling cardiac images throughout this text. In magnetic resonance (MR) imaging, each successive

acquisition provides the landmarks for planning the next acquisition (view) and provides a logical method to obtain 90-degree viewing of the heart according to its intrinsic short and long axes. Several different methods can be used to obtain views of the cardiac planes during an examination, of which we provide an example of one method. To obtain the **vertical long axis** (VLA) view, an oblique coronal image can be positioned parallel to the interventricular septum, directly through the left atrium and ventricle (Figures 6.78 and 6.79). This plane closely approximates the right anterior oblique projection used in

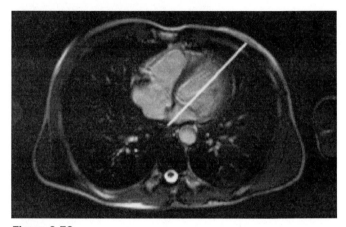

Figure 6.78
Axial, T1-weighted MR scout for planning vertical long axis images.

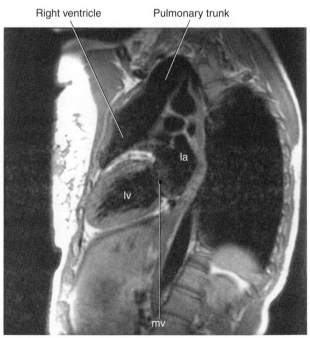

Figure 6.79
Resulting, T1-weighted vertical long axis MR image.

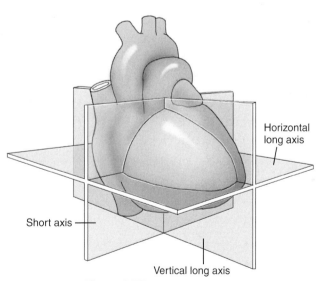

Figure 6.77
Off-axis planes (views) of heart.

cineangiography and the two-chamber view used in echo-cardiography. The **horizontal long axis** (HLA) view can be obtained by angling an oblique coronal image to bisect the left ventricle, mitral valve, and left atrium (Figures 6.80 and 6.81). The HLA view demonstrates the four cardiac chambers and is comparable with the four-chamber plane used in echo-cardiography. The **short axis** (SA) view can be obtained by using the HLA image to prescribe an oblique plane through the right and left ventricles, oriented perpendicular to the interventricular septum (Figures 6.82 and 6.83).

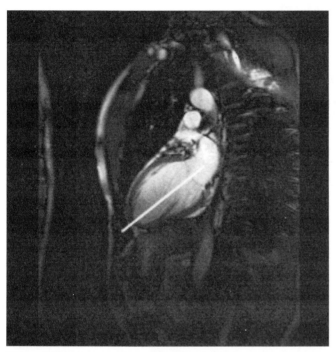

Figure 6.80
T1-weighted vertical long axis MR image for planning HLA images.

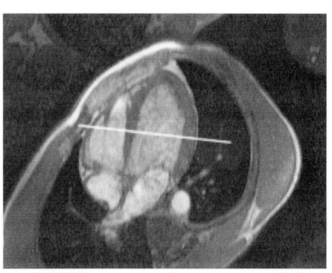

Figure 6.81
Resulting, T1-weighted horizontal long axis MR image.

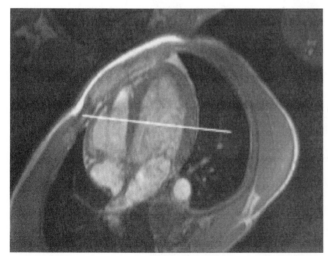

Figure 6.82
T1-weighted horizontal long axis MR image for planning SA images.

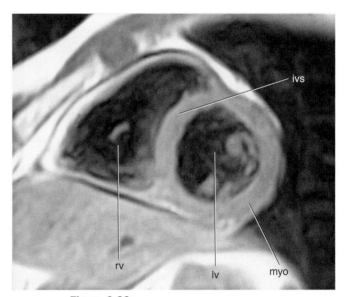

Figure 6.83
Short axis, T1-weighted MR image or heart.

KEY: ivs, Interventricular septum; **myo,** myocardium; **lv,** left ventricle; **rv,** right ventricle.

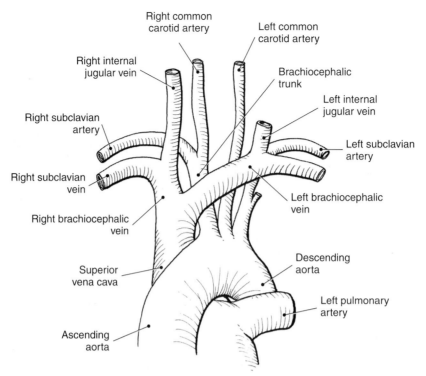

Figure 6.84
Great vessels in the superior mediastinum.

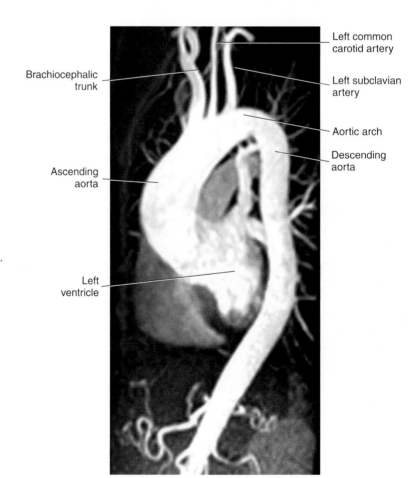

Figure 6.85
MR angiogram of aortic arch.

Branches of the Aortic Arch

The three main branches of the aortic arch are the brachiocephalic trunk, left common carotid artery, and left subclavian artery (Figure 6.84). The **brachiocephalic (innominate) trunk** is the first major vessel and the largest branch arising from the aortic arch. It ascends obliquely to the upper border of the right sternoclavicular joint, where it divides into the right common carotid and right subclavian arteries (Figures 6.85 and 6.86). The **right common carotid artery** ascends the neck lateral to the trachea to the level of C4, where it divides into the right external and internal carotid arteries. The **right subclavian artery** curves posterior to the clavicle into the axillary region, where it becomes the right **axillary artery**. The **left common carotid artery** is the second vessel to branch from the aortic arch. It arises just behind the left sternoclavicular joint and ascends into the neck along the left side of the trachea to the level of C4, where it bifurcates into the left external and internal carotid arteries. The **left subclavian artery** arises from the aortic arch posterior to the left common carotid artery and arches laterally toward the axilla in a manner similar to that of the right subclavian artery, where it continues as the left axillary artery (Figures 6.85 through 6.88). The right and left **internal thoracic arteries** arise from the respective subclavian artery at the base of the neck. They run deep to the ribs, just lateral to the sternum, to supply blood to the anterior portion of the thorax (Figure 6.89). The common carotid arteries supply blood to the head and neck, whereas the subclavian arteries supply blood to the upper extremities.

The internal thoracic arteries create an important anastomotic pathway between the subclavian artery and external iliac vessels in the event that the descending aorta is blocked.

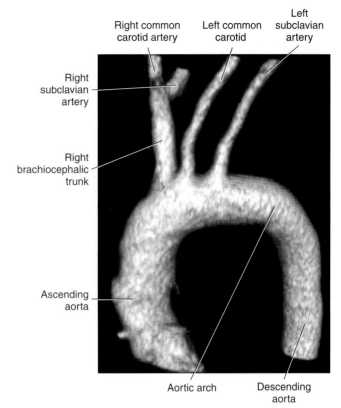

Figure 6.86
3D CT angiogram of aortic arch.

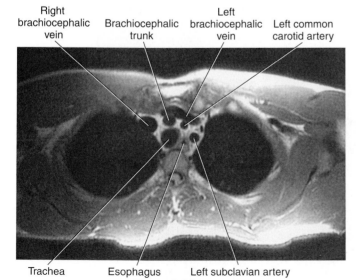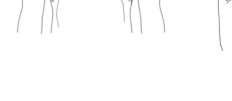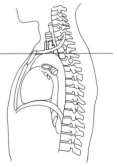

Figure 6.87
Axial, T1-weighted MR scan of chest with branches of aortic arch and brachiocephalic veins.

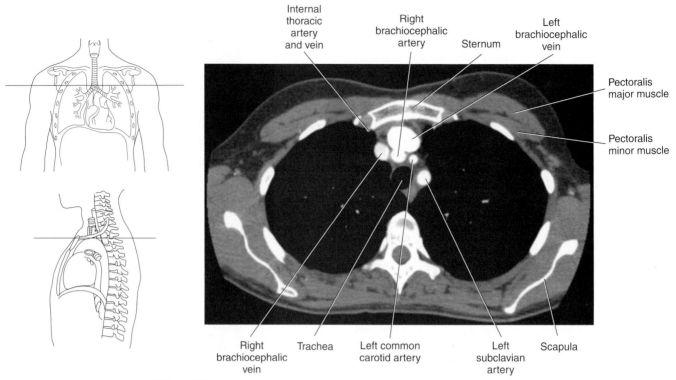

Figure 6.88
Axial CT scan of chest with branches of aortic arch and brachiocephalic veins.

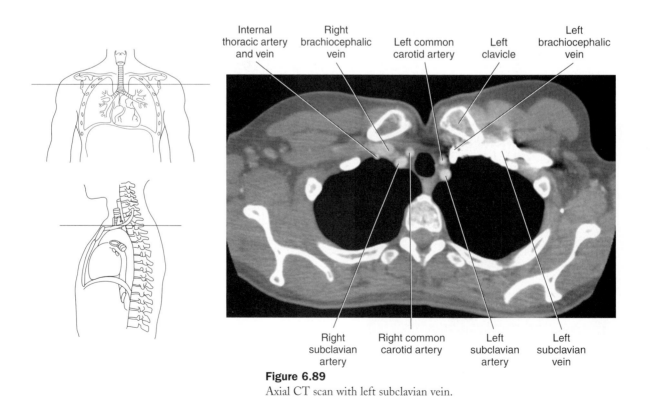

Figure 6.89
Axial CT scan with left subclavian vein.

Tributaries of the Superior Vena Cava

The superior vena cava receives blood from the head and neck via the **internal** and **external jugular veins** and from the upper extremities via the subclavian veins (Figures 6.84 and 6.90). The **subclavian veins** arise from the axillary veins and course posterior to the clavicles. They receive blood from the external jugular veins before uniting with the internal jugular veins behind the sternoclavicular joints, where they continue as the **brachiocephalic veins.** The left brachiocephalic vein courses across the midline, anterior to the branches of the aorta, to unite with the right brachiocephalic vein just posterior to the costal cartilage of the right first rib. The union of the two brachiocephalic veins forms the superior vena cava, which empties into the right atrium of the heart (Figures 6.75 and 6.76).

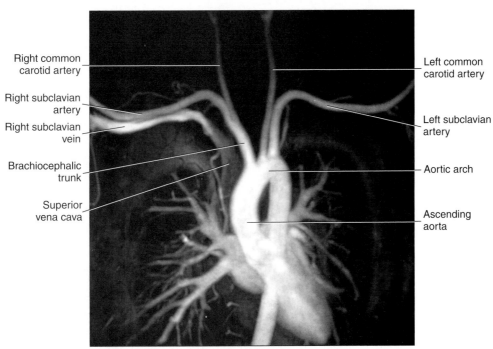

Figure 6.90
MR angiogram with right brachiocephalic vein

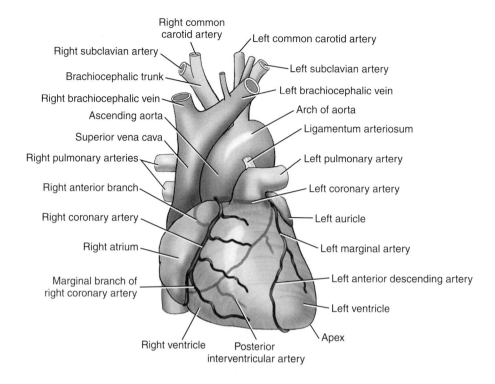

A

Right common
carotid artery

Right subclavian artery

Brachiocephalic trunk

Right brachiocephalic vein

Ascending aorta

Superior vena cava

Right pulmonary arteries

Right anterior branch

Right coronary artery

Right atrium

Marginal branch of
right coronary artery

Right ventricle

Left common carotid artery

Left subclavian artery

Left brachiocephalic vein

Arch of aorta

Ligamentum arteriosum

Left pulmonary artery

Left coronary artery

Left auricle

Left marginal artery

Left anterior descending artery

Left ventricle

Apex

Posterior
interventricular artery

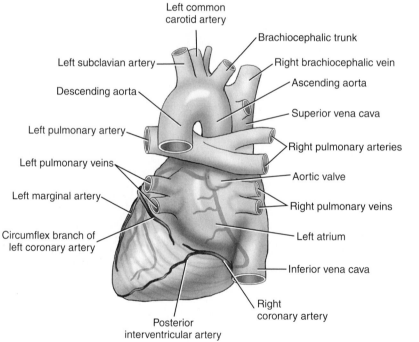

B

Left common
carotid artery

Left subclavian artery

Descending aorta

Left pulmonary artery

Left pulmonary veins

Left marginal artery

Circumflex branch of
left coronary artery

Brachiocephalic trunk

Right brachiocephalic vein

Ascending aorta

Superior vena cava

Right pulmonary arteries

Aortic valve

Right pulmonary veins

Left atrium

Inferior vena cava

Right
coronary artery

Posterior
interventricular artery

Figure 6.91
Heart with coronary vessels. **A,** Anterior view. **B,** Posterior view.

CORONARY CIRCULATION

The cardiac muscle requires a continuous supply of oxygen and nutrients, which is supplied by the **coronary circulation.** The coronary circulation consists of arteries that supply blood to the heart and the cardiac veins that provide venous drainage. The vessels of the coronary circulation frequently vary in their development and distribution of blood to the heart.

Coronary Arteries

The two main coronary arteries are the first vessels to branch off the ascending aorta (Figures 6.91 and 6.92). The **right coronary artery** arises from the base or root of the aorta **(right aortic sinus)** and passes anteriorly between the pulmonary trunk and right atrium to descend in the **coronary (atrioventricular) groove.** As it reaches the diaphragmatic surface, it gives off a **right marginal branch** that runs toward the apex of the heart. The right coronary artery then turns to the left and enters the **posterior interventricular groove,** where it gives off the **posterior interventricular branch (posterior descending artery).** The posterior interventricular branch continues to descend along the interventricular groove toward the apex, where it anastomoses with the left anterior descending artery of the left coronary artery. The right coronary artery and

its branches supply the right atrium, right ventricle, interventricular septum, and the sinoatrial (SA) and atrioventricular (AV) nodes. It also supplies a portion of the left atrium and ventricle (Figures 6.92 through 6.96). The **left coronary artery** arises from the **left aortic sinus** and passes to the left between the pulmonary trunk and left atrium to reach the coronary groove (Figures 6.91 and 6.92). Soon after reaching the coronary groove, the left coronary artery divides into the circumflex and left anterior descending (interventricular) arteries. The **circumflex artery** winds around the left border of the heart to the posterior surface, where it gives off the **left marginal artery.** The **left anterior descending artery** (LAD) descends in the **anterior interventricular groove** toward the apex of the heart, where it reaches the diaphragmatic surface to anastomose with the posterior descending artery. The left coronary artery and its branches supply the interventricular septum, including the AV bundles, and most of the left ventricle and atrium (Figures 6.97 through 6.99).

> The left anterior descending artery (LAD) is also known as the "widow maker" because many men die of blockage to this artery.

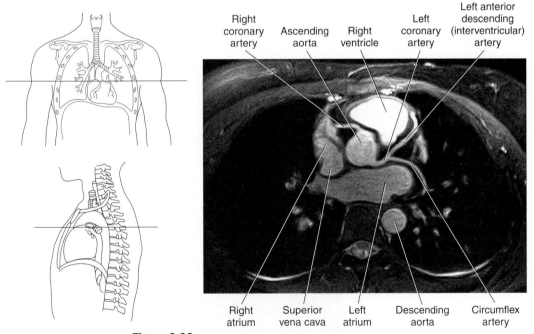

Figure 6.92
Axial, MRA of heart with right proximal coronary artery.

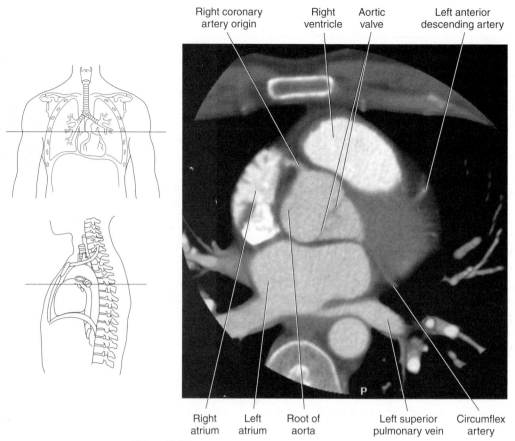

Right coronary artery origin   Right ventricle   Aortic valve   Left anterior descending artery

Right atrium   Left atrium   Root of aorta   Left superior pulmonary vein   Circumflex artery

Figure 6.93
CT scan of heart with right proximal coronary artery.

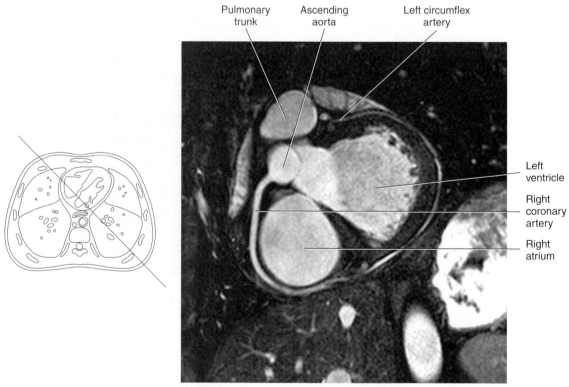

Pulmonary trunk   Ascending aorta   Left circumflex artery

Left ventricle

Right coronary artery

Right atrium

Figure 6.94
MRA of heart with right coronary artery.

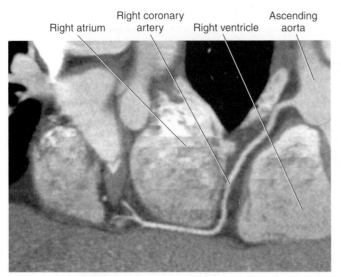

Right atrium | Right coronary artery | Right ventricle | Ascending aorta

Figure 6.95
CT curved reformat of heart with right coronary artery.

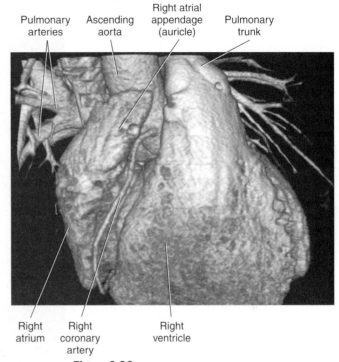

Pulmonary arteries | Ascending aorta | Right atrial appendage (auricle) | Pulmonary trunk

Right atrium | Right coronary artery | Right ventricle

Figure 6.96
3D CT angiogram of right coronary artery.

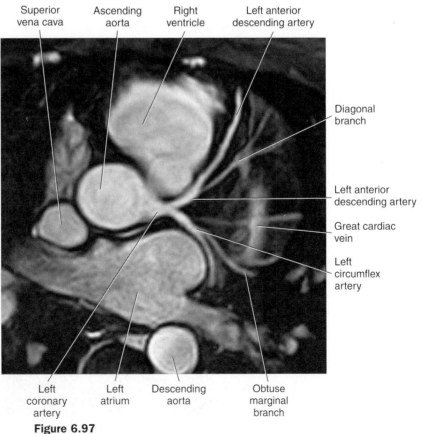

Superior vena cava | Ascending aorta | Right ventricle | Left anterior descending artery

Diagonal branch

Left anterior descending artery

Great cardiac vein

Left circumflex artery

Left coronary artery | Left atrium | Descending aorta | Obtuse marginal branch

Figure 6.97
Axial MR angiogram of heart with left coronary artery.

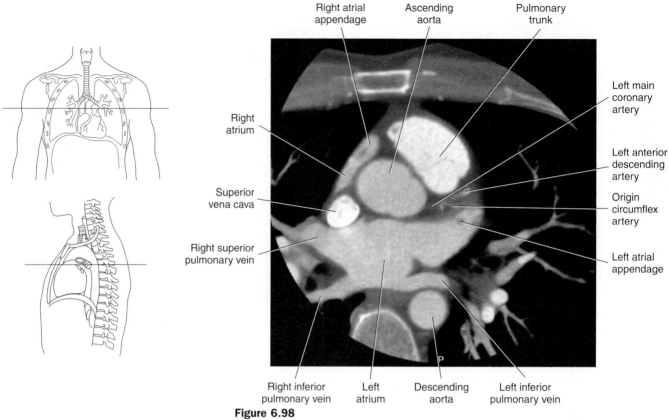

Figure 6.98
CT scan of heart with left coronary artery.

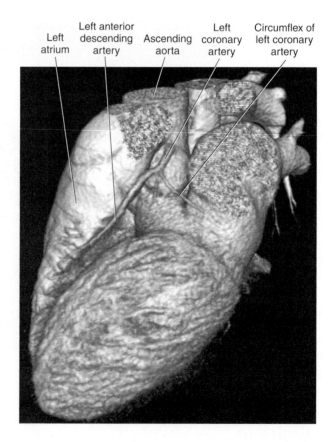

Figure 6.99
3D CT angiogram of left coronary arteries.

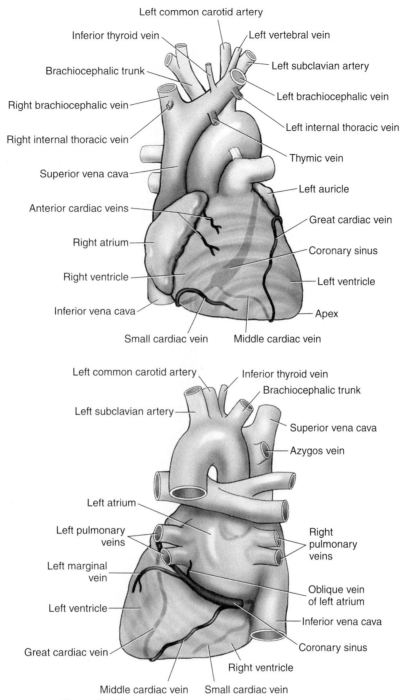

Figure 6.100
Heart with cardiac veins. **A,** Anterior view. **B,** Posterior view.

Cardiac Veins

Most of the venous return from the heart is carried by the **coronary sinus** as it runs along the posterior section of the coronary sulcus and terminates in the right atrium immediately to the left of the inferior vena cava. The **coronary sinus** is a wide venous channel situated in the posterior part of the coronary sulcus and is the main vein of the heart (Figures 6.100 through 6.102). Its tributaries include the great, small, and middle cardiac veins; the left posterior ventricular vein; and the oblique vein of the left atrium. The **great cardiac vein,** the main tributary of the coronary sinus, arises near the apex of the heart and ascends in the anterior interventricular groove along with the anterior interventricular artery to the base of the ventricles. It receives blood from the left posterior ventricular

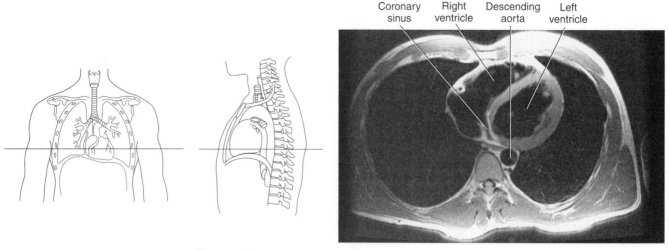

Figure 6.101
Axial, T1-weighted MR scan of heart with coronary sinus.

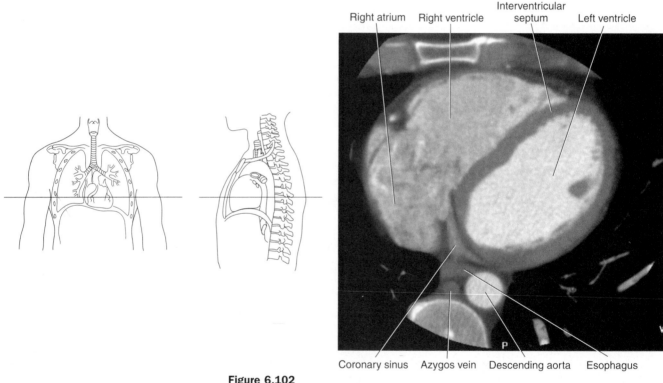

Figure 6.102
Axial CT scan of heart with coronary sinus.

vein and the left marginal vein before emptying into the coronary sinus. **The small (right) cardiac vein** runs in the coronary sulcus between the right atrium and ventricle and joins the coronary sinus from the right side. It receives blood from the right atrium and ventricle. The **middle (posterior) cardiac vein** commences at the apex of the heart and ascends along the posterior interventricular groove to the base of the heart, where it drains into the coronary sinus near the drainage site of the small cardiac vein. It receives blood from the pos-

terior surface of both ventricles. The **left posterior ventricular vein** carries blood from the posterior wall of the left ventricle as it runs along the diaphragmatic surface of the left ventricle to drain into either the great cardiac vein or the coronary sinus. The **oblique vein of the left atrium,** a small vessel, descends obliquely over the posterior wall of the left atrium and enters the left end of the coronary sinus. Two small **anterior cardiac veins** drain directly into the right atrium (Figure 6.100).

Superior vena cava

Left superior intercostal vein

Azygos vein

Posterior intercostal veins

Accessory hemiazygos vein

Posterior intercostal veins

Posterior intercostal veins

Hemiazygos vein

Left renal vein

Inferior vena cava

Ascending lumbar vein

Lumbar veins

Figure 6.103
Anterior view of azygos venous system.

AZYGOS VENOUS SYSTEM

The azygos venous system, which provides collateral circulation between the inferior and superior venae cavae, can be divided into the **azygos** and **hemiazygos veins** (Figure 6.103). Together, they drain blood from most of the posterior thoracic wall and from the bronchi, pericardium, and esophagus. The azygos vein ascends along the right side of the vertebral column, whereas the hemiazygos vein ascends along the left side. The hemiazygos vein crosses to the right behind the aorta to join the azygos vein at approximately T7-T9. The azygos vein then arches over the hilum of the right lung to empty into the posterior superior vena cava (Figures 6.104 and 6.105).

KEY: **da,** Descending aorta; **hemi,** hemiazygos vein; **Az,** azygous vein; **es,** esophagus.

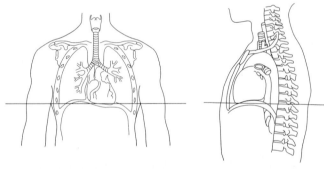

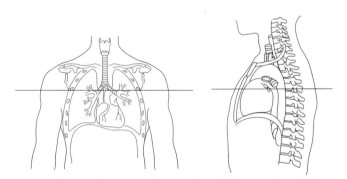

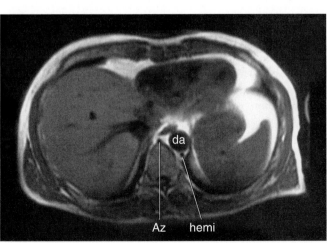

Figure 6.104
Axial, T1-weighted MR scan of abdomen with azygos and hemiazygos veins.

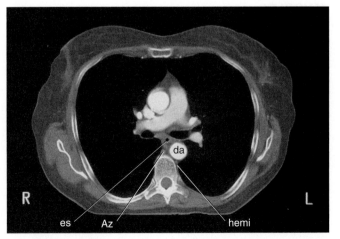

Figure 6.105
Axial CT scan of chest with azygos and hemiazygos veins.

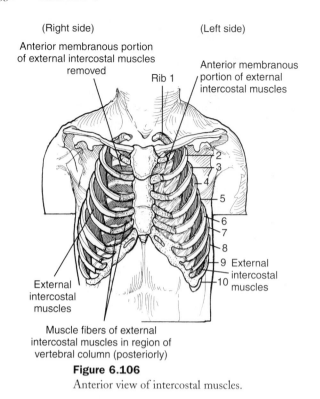

(Right side)   (Left side)

Anterior membranous portion
of external intercostal muscles
removed

Rib 1

Anterior membranous
portion of external
intercostal muscles

2
3
4
5
6
7
8
9 External
10 intercostal
muscles

External
intercostal
muscles

Muscle fibers of external
intercostal muscles in region of
vertebral column (posteriorly)

Figure 6.106
Anterior view of intercostal muscles.

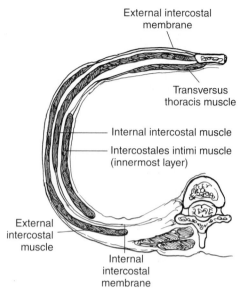

External intercostal
membrane

Transversus
thoracis muscle

Internal intercostal muscle

Intercostales intimi muscle
(innermost layer)

External
intercostal
muscle

Internal
intercostal
membrane

Figure 6.107
Axial view of intercostal muscles.

TABLE 6-3   Muscles of the Thorax

MUSCLE	ORIGIN	INSERTION	ACTION
Intercostal	Inferior border of ribs	Superior border of ribs below	Fixes intercostal spaces during respiration and aids forced inspiration by elevating ribs.
Serratus posterior superior	Spinous processes and supraspinous ligaments of C7-T2	Posterior aspect of 2nd-5th ribs	Assists forced inspiration
Serratus posterior inferior	Spinous processes and supraspinous ligaments of T11-L2	Posterior aspect of 9th-12th ribs	Assists in forced expiration
Diaphragm	Xiphoid process, costal margin, fascia over the quadratus lumborum, and psoas major muscles. Vertebral bodies L1-L3	Central tendon of the diaphragm	Pushes the abdominal viscera inferiorly, increasing the volume of the thoracic cavity for inspiration

MUSCLES

Muscles associated with respiration are the intercostal, serratus posterior superior, serratus posterior inferior, and the diaphragm (Table 6.3). The spaces between the ribs, or the intercostal spaces, are filled with three layers of **intercostal muscles (external, internal, and innermost layer)** (Figures 6.106 through 6.108). These muscles act together to elevate the ribs and expand the thoracic cavity, as well as keep the intercostal spaces somewhat rigid. The **serratus posterior superior muscle** spans from C7-T2 to ribs 2 to 5 and acts to assist forced inspiration, whereas the **serratus posterior inferior muscle** spans from T11-L2 to ribs 9 to 12 and acts to assist forced expiration (Figures 6.109 through 6.110). The **diaphragm** is a large dome-shaped muscle that spans the entire thoracic outlet and separates the thoracic cavity from the abdominal cavity (Figure 6.111). It is the chief muscle of inspiration because it enlarges the thoracic cavity vertically as the domes move

inferiorly and flatten. The muscle fibers of the diaphragm converge to be inserted into a **central tendon,** which is situated near the center of the diaphragm immediately below the pericardium, with which it is partially blended. The diaphragm is attached to the lumbar spine via two tendinous structures termed **crura** (Figures 6.111 through 6.113). The right crus arises from the anterior surfaces of L1-L3, whereas the left crus arises from the corresponding parts of L1-L2 only. The left and right crura join together across the ventral aspect of the abdominal aorta to form the medial arcuate ligament. Three major openings, or hiatuses, of the diaphragm allow for the passage of vessels and organs from the thorax to the abdomen. The **aortic hiatus** allows for the passage of the descending aorta, azygos vein, and thoracic duct. The **caval hiatus** allows for the passage of the inferior vena cava and the right phrenic nerve. The **esophageal hiatus** allows for the passage of the esophagus and the vagus nerve.

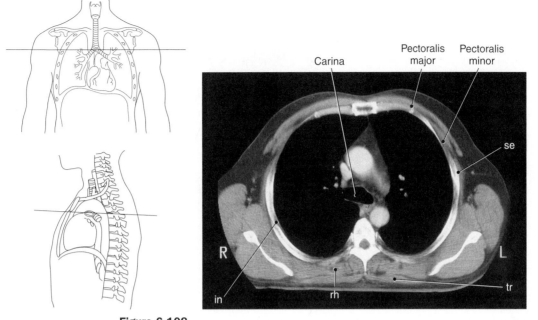

Carina   Pectoralis major   Pectoralis minor

se

R   L

in   rh   tr

Figure 6.108
Axial CT scan of chest at level of carina with thoracic muscles.

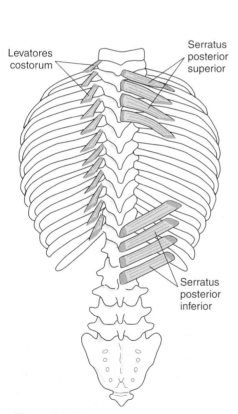

Levatores costorum   Serratus posterior superior

Serratus posterior inferior

Figure 6.109
Posterior view of posterior serratus muscles.

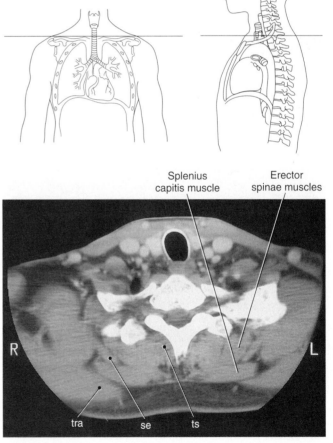

Splenius capitis muscle   Erector spinae muscles

R   L

tra   se   ts

Figure 6.110
Axial CT scan of chest with serratus posterior superior muscle.

KEY: se, Serratus posterior superior; **tr,** trachea; **rh,** rhomboid muscle; **in,** intercostals; **ts,** transversospinal muscles; **tra,** trapezius muscle.

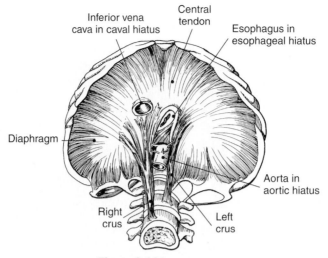

Figure 6.111
Inferior view of diaphragm.

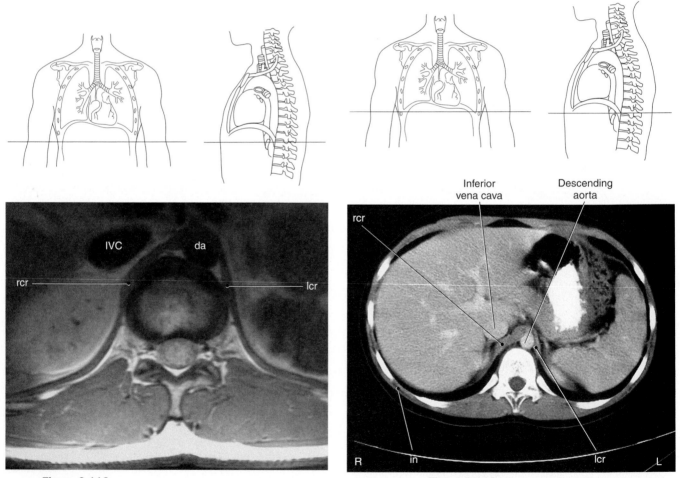

Figure 6.112
Axial, T1-weighted MR scan of abdomen with crura.

Figure 6.113
Axial CT scan of chest with crura.

KEY: **rcr,** Right crus; **IVC,** inferior vena cava; **da,** descending aorta; **lcr,** left crus; **in,** intercostals.

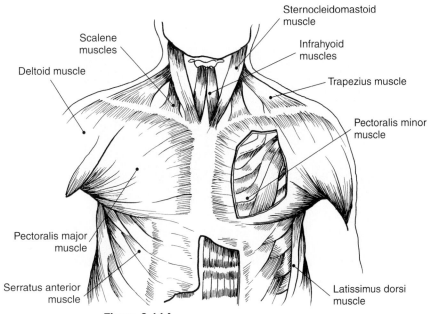

Figure 6.114
Anterior view of muscles associated with thorax.

TABLE 6-4   Muscles of the Anterior and Lateral Wall of the Thorax

MUSCLE	ORIGIN	INSERTION	ACTION
Pectoralis major	Clavicular head—medial half of clavicle. Sternal head—lateral manubrium and sternum, six upper costal cartilages	Bicipital groove of humerus and deltoid tuberosity	Flexes and adducts and medially rotates arm and accessory for inspiration
Pectoralis minor	Anterior surface of 3rd-5th ribs	Coracoid process of the scapula	Elevates ribs of scapula, protracts scapula, and assists serratus anterior
Subclavius	First rib and cartilage	Inferior surface of the clavicle	Depresses the shoulder and assists pectoralis in inspiration
Serratus anterior	Angles of superior 8th or 9th ribs	Medial border of scapula	Laterally rotates and protracts scapula

Muscles Connecting the Upper Extremity to the Anterior and Lateral Thoracic Walls

Muscles of the anterior and lateral thoracic region are pectoralis major, subclavius, pectoralis minor, and serratus anterior. Muscles associated with the movement of the upper extremity such as the pectoralis, subclavius, and serratus anterior can also function as accessory muscles for respiration (Figure 6.114 and Table 6.4). For example, the **pectoralis muscles (major and minor),** located on the anterior surface of the chest, primarily aid in the movement of the upper limb, but the pectoralis major muscle can also act to expand the thoracic cavity on deep inspiration (Figures 6.115 and 6.116). The **subclavius,** a small triangular-shaped muscle located between the clavicle and first rib acts alone to stabilize the clavicle and depress the shoulder. However, conjointly with the pectoralis muscles, the subclavius muscles act to raise the ribs, drawing them upward and expanding the chest, thus becoming important agents in forced inspiration. Additionally, the **serratus anterior muscles** aid in respiration. The serratus (sawlike) anterior muscle is visualized on the lateral border of the thorax. It extends from the medial border of the scapula to the lateral surface of the first rib through eighth ribs. The primary action of the serratus anterior muscle is to laterally rotate and protract the scapula. It can, however assist in raising the ribs for inspiration (Figure 6.114; see also Chapter 9).

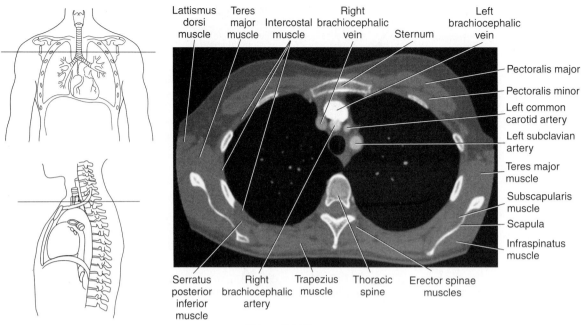

Figure 6.115

Axial CT scan with pectoralis muscle.

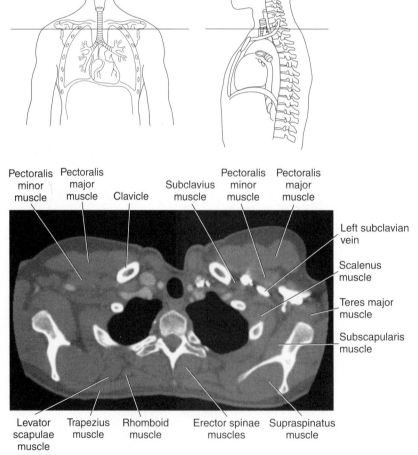

Figure 6.116

Axial CT scan with subclavius muscle.

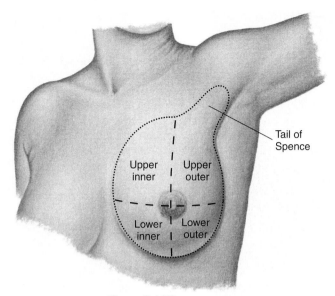

Figure 6.117
Anterior view of left breast.

BREAST

The female **breast,** or **mammary gland,** lies within the sub-cutaneous tissue overlying the pectoralis major muscle. Typically the breast extends laterally from the sternum to the axilla and inferiorly from the second to the seventh ribs. For examination purposes, the breast can be divided into **four quadrants** (upper inner, upper outer, lower outer, lower inner) and the **tail of Spence** (Figure 6.117). The breast consists of three layers of tissue: subcutaneous layer, mammary layer, and retromammary layer (Figure 6.118). The **subcutaneous layer** contains the skin and all of the subcutaneous fat. The **mammary layer** consists of glandular tissue, excretory (lactiferous) ducts, and connective tissues. The **glandular tissue** consists of 15 to 20 lobes arranged radially around a centrally located nipple. The glandular lobes are embedded in connective tissue and fat, which give the breast its size and shape. **Excretory (lactiferous) ducts** extend from each lobe to the nipple, where they terminate as small openings. Cords of connective tissue coursing throughout the mammary layer, from the dermis to the thoracic fascia, are known as the **suspensory ligaments** of the breast or **Cooper's ligaments.** These ligaments provide support for the breasts. The **retromammary layer** contains muscle, deep connective tissue, and retromammary fat (Figures 6.119 and 6.120).

Axillary lymph nodes drain the lymphatics from the breast, arm, and integument of the back. They are frequently clustered around the axillary vessels, the lower border of the pectoralis major muscle, and the lower margin of the posterior wall.

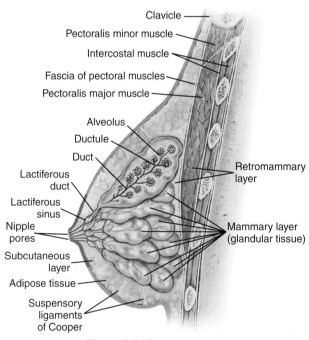

Figure 6.118
Sagittal view of female breast.

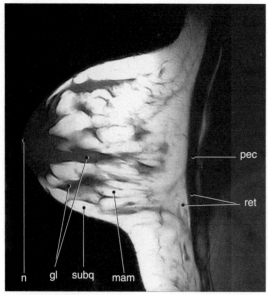

Figure 6.119
Sagittal, T1-weighted MR scan of female breast.

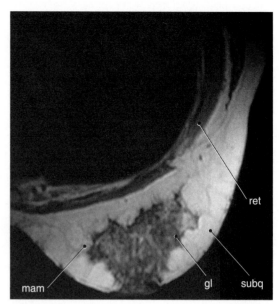

Figure 6.120
Axial, T1-weighted MR scan of female breast.

KEY: pec, Pectoralis major muscle; **ret,** retromammary layer; **mam,** mammary layer; **subq,** subcutaneous layer; **gl,** glandular; **n,** nipple.

REFERENCES

Agur AM: *Grant's atlas of anatomy,* Baltimore, 1996, Williams & Wilkins.

Applegate E: *The anatomy and physiology learning system,* ed 2, Philadelphia, 2000, Saunders.

Applegate E: *The sectional anatomy learning system,* ed 2, Philadelphia, 2002, Saunders.

Ballinger PW: *Merrill's atlas of radiographic positions and radiologic procedures,* ed 10, St. Louis, 2003, Mosby.

Blackwell, GG, Cranney GB, Pohost GM, et al: *MRI: cardiovascular system,* New York, 1992, Gower Medical Publishing.

Cerqueira MD, Weissman NJ, Dilsizian V, et al: Standardized myocardial segmentation and nomenclature for tomographic imaging of the heart: a statement for healthcare professionals from the Cardiac Imaging Committee of the Council on Clinical Cardiology of the American Heart Association, *Circulation* 105:539, 2002.

English AW: *Wolf-Heidegger's atlas of human anatomy,* ed 5, Basel, Switzerland, 2000, Karger.

Gray H: *Gray's anatomy,* ed 38, Philadelphia, 1995, Churchill Livingstone.

Sandring S: *Gray's anatomy,* ed 39, Philadelphia, 2005, Churchill Livingstone.

Haaga JR, Lanzieri CF, Gilkeson RC, et al: *CT and MR imaging of the whole body,* ed 4, Philadelphia, 2003, Mosby.

Harnsberger HR: *Handbook of head and neck imaging,* ed 2, St. Louis, 1995, Mosby.

Jacob S: *Atlas of human anatomy,* Philadelphia, 2002, Churchill Livingstone.

Larsen WJ: *Anatomy: development function clinical correlations,* Philadelphia, 2002, Saunders.

Manning WJ, Pennel DJ: *Cardiovascular magnetic resonance,* Philadelphia, 2002, Churchill Livingstone.

Martini FH: *Fundamentals of anatomy and physiology,* ed 3, Englewood Cliffs, NJ, 1995, Prentice-Hall.

Miller SW: *Cardiac radiology: the requisites,* St. Louis, 1996, Mosby.

Mosby's medical, nursing, and allied health dictionary, ed 6, St. Louis, 2002, Mosby.

Palastanga N, Field D, Soames R, et al: *Anatomy and human movement,* ed 4, Philadelphia, 2002, Butterworth-Heinemann.

Seidel HM, Ball JW, Dains JE, et al: *Mosby's guide to physical examination,* ed 4, St. Louis, 1999, Mosby.

Som PM, Curtin HD: *Head and neck imaging,* ed 3, St. Louis, 1996, Mosby.

Stark DD, Bradley WG: *Magnetic resonance imaging,* ed 3, St. Louis, 1999, Mosby.

ABDOMEN

A man's liver is his carburetor.

ANONYMOUS

The abdominal cavity houses many critical structures that have a large array of functions. It is for this reason that cross-section imaging of the abdomen is so essential in visualizing these various organs and body systems (Figure 7.1). This chapter demonstrates cross-section anatomy of the following structures:

ABDOMINAL CAVITY
    Peritoneum
    Peritoneal Spaces
    Retroperitoneum
    Retroperitoneal Spaces

LIVER
    Surface Anatomy
    Segmental Anatomy
    Portal Hepatic System
    Vasculature

GALLBLADDER AND BILIARY SYSTEM

PANCREAS

SPLEEN

ADRENAL GLANDS

URINARY SYSTEM

STOMACH

INTESTINES

ABDOMINAL AORTA AND BRANCHES
    Paired Parietal (Dorsal) Branches
    Paired Visceral Branches
    Unpaired Visceral Branches

INFERIOR VENA CAVA AND TRIBUTARIES
    Inferior Phrenic Veins
    Lumbar Veins
    Gonadal Veins
    Renal Veins
    Suprarenal Veins
    Hepatic Veins

LYMPH NODES

MUSCLES OF THE ABDOMINAL WALL

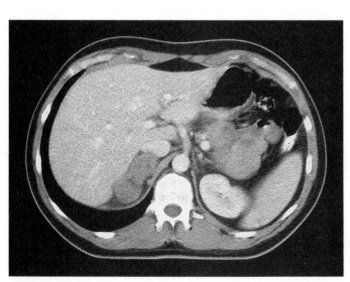

Figure 7.1
Axial CT scan of abdomen with right adrenal mass associated with an abnormal retrocaval lymph node.

ABDOMINAL CAVITY

The abdominal cavity is the region located between the diaphragm and sacral promontory (Figure 7.2). The abdominal and pelvic cavities are commonly divided into four quadrants or nine distinct regions (see Chapter 1). Contents of the abdominal cavity include the liver, gallbladder and biliary system, pancreas, spleen, adrenal glands, kidneys, ureters, stomach, intestines, and vascular structures.

Peritoneum

The walls of the abdominal cavity are lined by a thin serous membrane called the **peritoneum.** This membrane is divided into two layers: the **parietal peritoneum,** which lines the abdominal walls, and the **visceral peritoneum,** which covers the organs (Figures 7.3). The two layers of peritoneum are separated by a film of serous fluid for lubrication to allow organs to move against each other without friction. The peritoneum forms a cavity that encloses the following organs of the abdomen: liver (except for the bare area), gallbladder, spleen, stomach, ovaries, and majority of intestines (Figures 7.4 and 7.5). In males, the **peritoneal cavity** is a closed cavity, but in females it communicates with the exterior through the uterine tubes, uterus, and vagina (Figure 7.6, *A* and *B*). The peritoneal cavity consists of the **greater sac** and **lesser sac (omental bursae).** The greater sac is located between the inner surface of the anterior abdominal wall and the outer surface of the abdominal viscera. It is bounded between the parietal and visceral peritoneum. The greater sac communicates with the lesser sac through the **epiploic foramen (of Winslow).** The lesser sac is located primarily between the posterior surface of

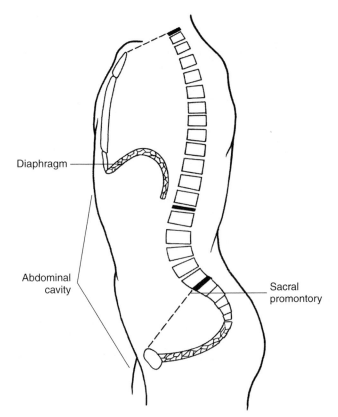

Figure 7.2
Sagittal view of the abdominal cavity.

KEY: **li,** Liver; **p,** peritoneum; **pa,** pancreas; **st,** stomach; **sp,** spleen.

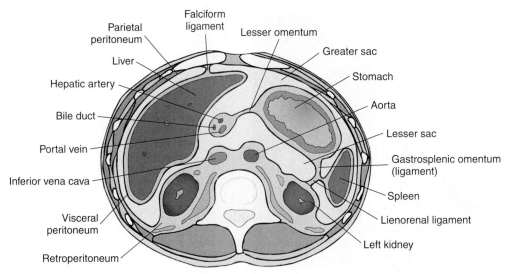

Figure 7.3
Axial view of abdomen with greater and lesser sac, falciform, gastrosplenic, and lienorenal ligaments.

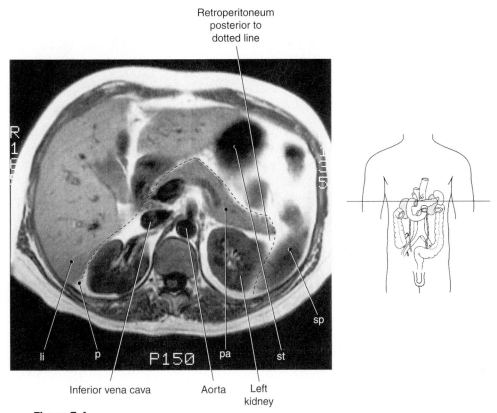

Figure 7.4
Axial, T1-weighted MR scan of peritoneal and retroperitoneal structures (separated by *dotted line*).

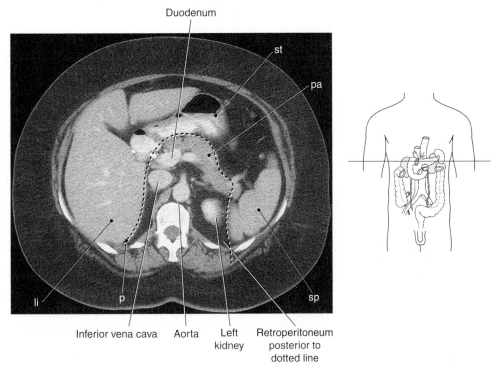

Figure 7.5
Axial CT scan of peritoneal and retroperitoneal structures (separated by *dotted line*).

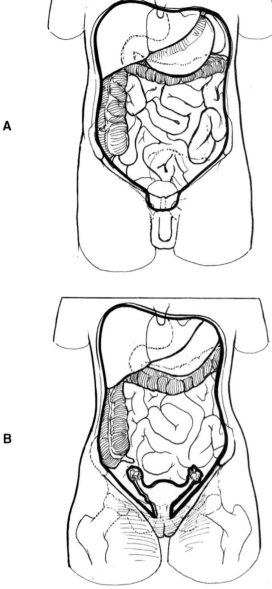

A

B

Figure 7.6
Coronal view of peritoneum. **A,** Male peritoneum. **B,** Female peritoneum.

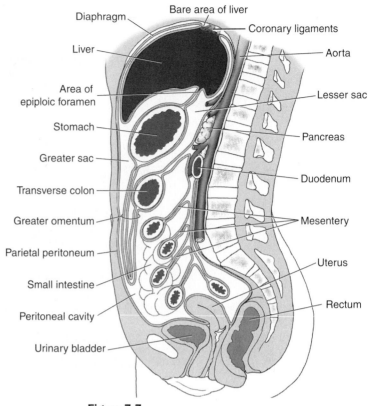

Figure 7.7
Sagittal view of peritoneum and peritoneal cavity.

TABLE 7-1   Peritoneal Ligaments

LIGAMENTS	LOCATION
Gastrocolic ligaments	Apron portion of the greater omentum attached to the transverse colon
Gastrosplenic ligaments (gastrolienal ligament)	The left portion of the greater omentum that connects the hilum of the spleen to the greater curvature and fundus of the stomach
Splenorenal (lienorenal) ligament	Connecting the spleen and kidney
Gastrophrenic ligament	Superior portion of greater omentum attached to the diaphragm and posterior aspect of the fundus and esophagus
Hepatorenal ligament	Connects the liver with the kidney
Hepatoesophageal ligament	Connects the liver with the esophagus
Hepatogastric ligament	Connects the liver with the lesser curvature of the stomach
Hepatoduodenal ligament	Connects the superior region of the duodenum to the liver
Falciform ligament	Extends from the liver to the anterior abdominal wall and diaphragm
Round ligament (ligamentum teres)	Remnant of the left umbilical vein, lying in the free edge of the falciform ligament
Coronary ligaments (superior and inferior)	Reflections of the peritoneum that surround the bare area of the liver
Triangular (left and right)	Where the layers of the coronary ligament meet to the left and right, respectively
Phrenocolic ligament	Attaches the left flexure of the colon and the diaphragm.

the stomach and the posterior abdominal wall (Figures 7.3 and 7.7 through 7.9)

Numerous folds of peritoneum extend between organs, serving to hold them in position and at the same time enclose the vessels and nerves proceeding to each part. These folds or double layers of peritoneum are termed *mesentery, omenta,* and *peritoneal ligaments.* The **mesentery** is a double layer of peritoneum, which encloses the intestine and attaches it to the abdominal wall. An **omentum** is a mesentery or double layer of peritoneum that is attached to the stomach. The normal omentum is usually imperceptible on routine scans, visible only when fluid is present. The **greater omentum** is a fat-laden fold of peritoneum that drapes down from the greater curvature of the stomach and connects the stomach with the spleen, and transverse colon, whereas the **lesser omentum** attaches the duodenum and lesser curvature of the stomach to the liver (Figures 7.10 through 7.13). Numerous **peritoneal ligaments** serve to connect an organ with another organ or abdominal wall. These peritoneal ligaments are not ligaments in the classic sense but are distinct regions of mesentery connecting the structures for which they are named. Three regions of the greater omentum that are characterized as peritoneal ligaments include **gastrocolic, gastrosplenic,** and **gastrophrenic.** These ligaments attach the greater omentum

to the transverse colon, hilum of the spleen and greater curvature and fundus of the stomach, diaphragm, and esophagus (Figures 7.3, 7.11, and 7.12). Ligaments of the lesser omentum include the **hepatogastric** and **hepatoduodenal,** which serve to connect the stomach and duodenum to the liver. Ligaments associated specifically with the liver are the **round ligament (ligamentum teres),** which represents the obliterated umbilical vein and attaches the internal surface of the umbilicus within the free inferior margin of the falciform ligament. The **falciform ligament** extends from the liver to the anterior abdominal wall and diaphragm and forms a plane that divides the liver anatomically into right and left lobes (Figures 7.14 and 7.15). The **coronary ligaments** surround the superior pole of the liver and attach the liver to the diaphragm, forming the margins of the bare area (Figures 7.7, 7.8, and 7.16). Additional peritoneal ligaments are described in Table 7.1.

> Inflammation of the peritoneal cavity is termed *peritonitis.* Acute peritonitis is most commonly caused by the leaking of infection through a perforation in the bowel.

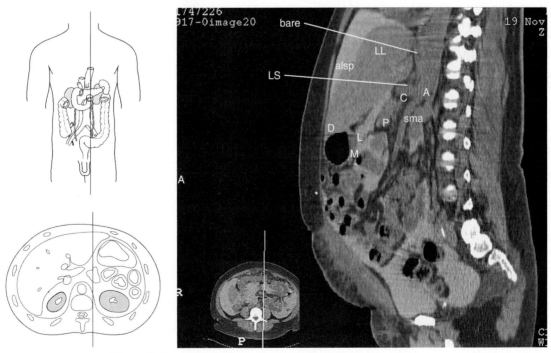

Figure 7.8
Sagittal CT reformat of abdomen with lesser sac and peritoneal spaces.

KEY: **bare,** Bare area of liver; **LS,** lesser sac; **alsp,** anterior left subphrenic space; **LL,** liver; **D,** duodenum; **L,** lesser sac; **M,** mesocolon; **P,** pancreas; **sma,** superior mesenteric artery; **C,** celiac artery; **A,** aorta.

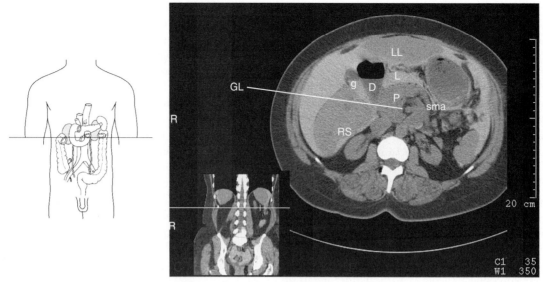

Figure 7.9
Axial CT scan of abdomen and peritoneal spaces.

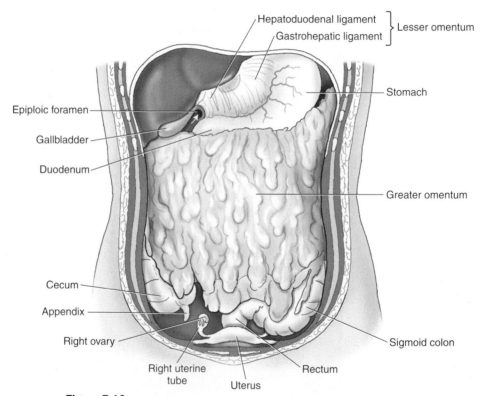

Figure 7.10
Anterior view of abdomen with mesentery and lesser and greater omentum.

KEY: **GL**, gastrohepatic ligament; **LL**, liver; **L**, lesser sac; **g**, gallbladder; **D**, duodenum; **P**, pancreas; **sma**, superior mesenteric artery; **RS**, right subhepatic space; **IVC**, inferior vena cava; **SpV**, splenic vein; **st**, stomach; **sp**, spleen; **hi**, hilum; **GO**, greater omentum; **TL**, triangular ligaments; **alsp**, anterior left subphrenic space; **SP**, splenic recess; **av**, splenic artery and vein; **MC**, mesocolon.

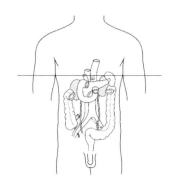

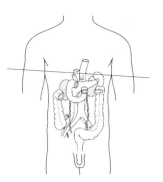

Greater omentum   Gastrosplenic ligament

Pancreas   Gastrosplenic ligament   Greater omentum   Spleen

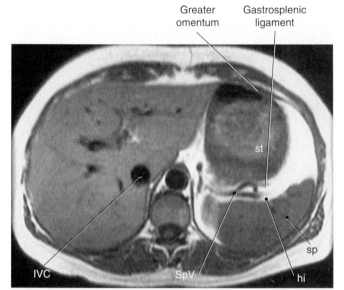

st

IVC   SpV   hi   sp

Figure 7.11
Axial, T1-weighted MR scan of abdomen with greater omentum and gastrosplenic ligament.

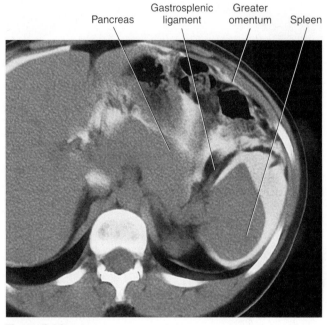

Figure 7.12
Axial CT scan of abdomen with greater omentum and gastrosplenic ligament.

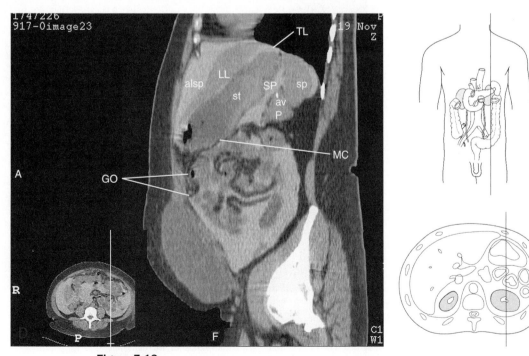

Figure 7.13
Sagittal CT reformat of abdomen with greater omentum and peritoneal spaces.

344

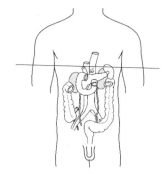

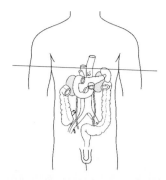

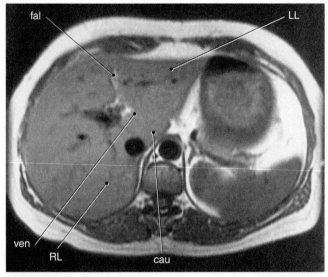

Figure 7.14
Axial, T1-weighted MR scan of abdomen with falciform ligament.

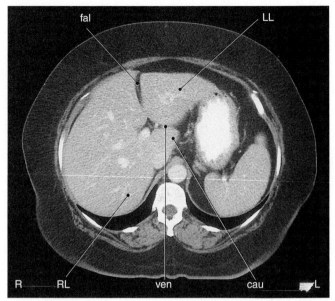

Figure 7.15
Axial CT scan of abdomen with falciform ligament.

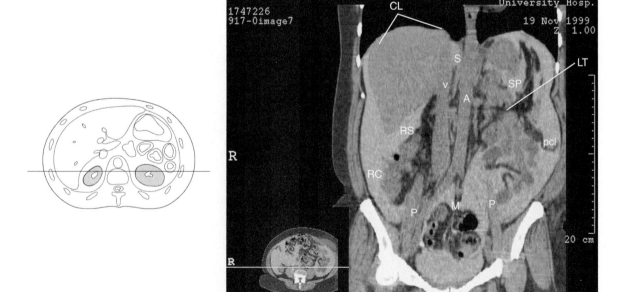

Figure 7.16
Coronal CT reformat of liver and coronary ligaments.

KEY: fal, Falciform ligament; **LL,** left lobe of liver; **ven,** ligamentum venosum; **RL,** right lobe of liver; **cau,** caudate lobe of liver; **CL,** coronary ligaments; **S,** superior recess of the lesser sac; **v,** vena cava; **A,** aorta; **SP,** splenic recess; **RS,** right subhepatic space; **LT,** ligament of Treitz; **pcl,** phrenicocolic ligament; **RC,** paracolic space; **P,** psoas muscles; **M,** mesentery of small bowel.

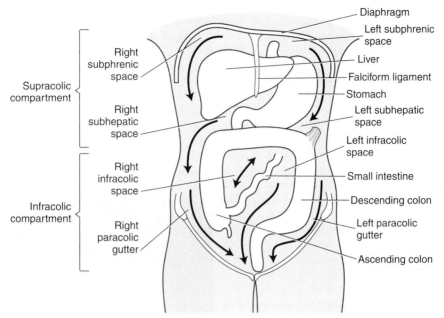

Figure 7.17
Anterior view of peritoneal spaces.

Peritoneal Spaces

The peritoneal cavity contains potential spaces resulting from folds of peritoneum that extend from the viscera to the abdominal wall. These spaces can be divided into the **supra-colic** and **infracolic compartments** (Figure 7.17). The supra-colic compartment is located above the transverse colon and contains the right and left **subphrenic spaces** and right and left **subhepatic spaces.** The subphrenic spaces are located between the diaphragm and the anterior portion of the liver. They are divided into right and left compartments by the falciform ligament (Figures 7.18 and 7.19). The subhepatic spaces are located posterior and inferior between the liver and the abdominal viscera. The right subhepatic space, located between the liver and kidney, contains **Morison's pouch,** which is the deepest point of the abdominal cavity in a supine patient and a common site for collection of fluid (Figures 7.20 and 7.21).

Below the transverse colon is the **infracolic compartment,** which consists of the right and left **infracolic spaces** and the **paracolic gutters.** The right and left infracolic spaces are divided by the mesentery of the small intestine. The right and left paracolic gutters are troughlike spaces located lateral to the ascending and descending colon (Figures 7.17 and 7.22 and Table 7.2). The deeper right gutter is a common site for free fluid collections.

TABLE 7-2   Peritoneal and Retroperitoneal Spaces

SPACE	LOCATION
Peritoneal Spaces	
Supracolic Compartment	*Above Transverse Colon*
Subphrenic space	Between diaphragm and anterior liver
Right	Right and left spaces divided by falciform
Left	ligament
Subhepatic space	Posterior and inferior to liver
Right	Between right lobe of liver and kidney;
	contains Morison's pouch
Left	Between left lobe of liver and kidney;
	includes lesser omentum
Infracolic Compartment	*Below Transverse Colon*
Infracolic spaces	
Right and left	Divided by mesentery of small intestine
Paracolic gutters	
Right	Between ascending colon and right
	abdominal wall
Left	Between descending colon and left
	abdominal wall
Retroperitoneal Spaces	
Pararenal Spaces	
Anterior	Between renal (Gerota's) fascia and
	posterior surface of peritoneum
Posterior	Between renal (Gerota's) fascia and muscles
	of posterior abdominal wall
Perirenal Space	
Right	Around kidney and adrenal glands;
Left	completely enclosed by renal (Gerota's)
	fascia

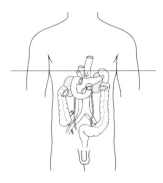

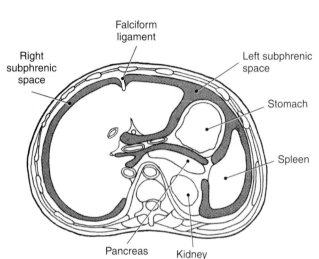

Figure 7.18
Axial view of subphrenic spaces.

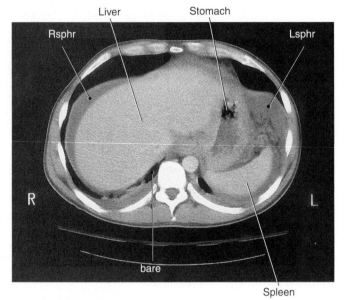

Figure 7.19
Axial CT scan of abdomen with subphrenic spaces.

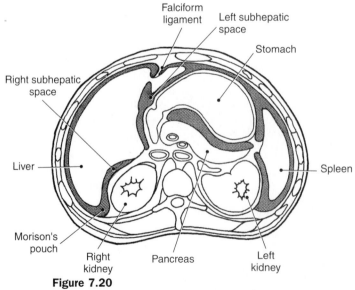

Figure 7.20
Axial view of subhepatic spaces and Morison's pouch.

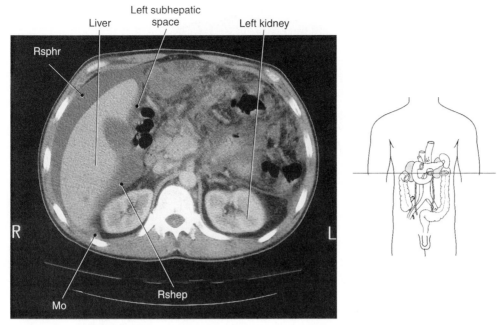

Figure 7.21
Axial CT scan of abdomen with subhepatic spaces and Morison's pouch.

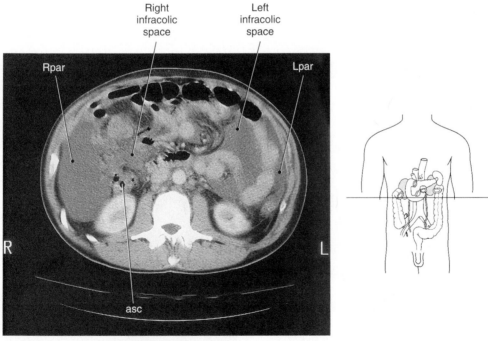

Figure 7.22
Axial CT scan of abdomen with paracolic gutters.

KEY: Rsphr, Right subphrenic compartment; **Lsphr,** left subphrenic compartment; **bare,** bare area of liver; **Mo,** Morison's pouch; **Rshep,** right subhepatic space; **Rpar,** right paracolic gutter; **Lpar,** left paracolic gutter; **asc,** ascending colon.

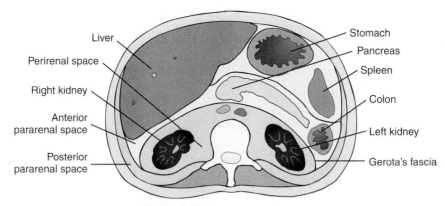

Figure 7.23
Axial view of retroperitoneal space.

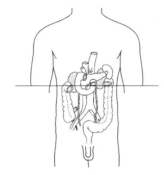

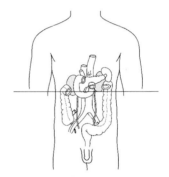

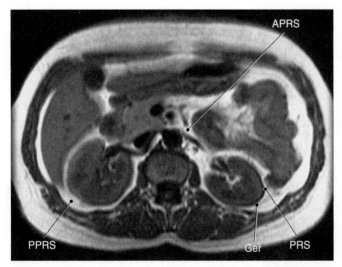

Figure 7.24
Axial, T1-weighted MR scan of abdomen with kidneys and pararenal spaces.

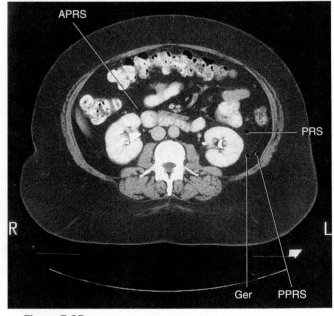

Figure 7.25
Axial CT scan of abdomen with kidneys and pararenal spaces.

KEY: APRS, Anterior pararenal space; **PPRS,** posterior pararenal space; **Ger,** Gerota's fascia; **PRS,** perirenal space.

Retroperitoneum

Structures located posterior to the peritoneum, yet lined by it anteriorly, are considered to be in the **retroperitoneum** and include the kidneys, ureters, adrenal glands, pancreas, duodenum, aorta, inferior vena cava, bladder, uterus, and prostate gland. In addition, the ascending and descending colon and most of the duodenum are situated in the retroperitoneum (Figures 7.3 through 7.5)

Retroperitoneal Spaces

The retroperitoneum can be divided into compartments or spaces that include the anterior and posterior pararenal spaces and left and right perirenal spaces (Figure 7.23). The **anterior pararenal space** is located between the anterior surface of the **renal fascia (Gerota's fascia)** and the posterior position of the peritoneum. It contains the retroperitoneal portions of the ascending and descending colon, the pancreas, and the duodenum. The **posterior pararenal space** is located between the posterior renal fascia and the muscles of the posterior abdominal wall. There are no solid organs located in this space, just fat and vessels (Figures 7.24 and 7.25). The left and right **perirenal spaces** are the areas located directly around the kidneys and are completely enclosed by renal fascia. The perirenal spaces contain the kidneys, adrenal glands, lymph nodes, blood vessels, and perirenal fat. The perirenal fat separates the adrenal glands from the kidneys and provides cushioning for the kidney (Figure 7.26 and Table 7.2).

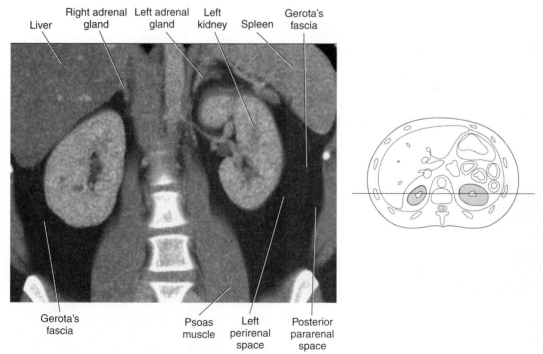

Figure 7.26
Coronal CT reformat of kidneys and perirenal spaces.

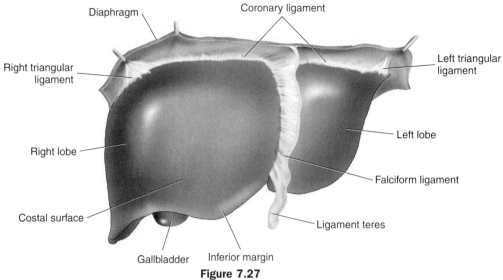

Figure 7.27
Anterior view of liver.

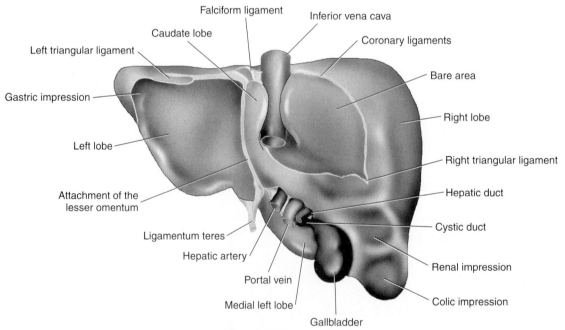

Figure 7.28
Posterior view of liver.

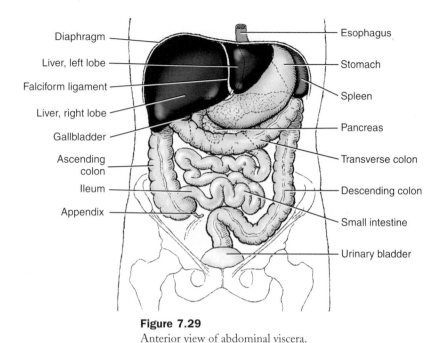

Figure 7.29
Anterior view of abdominal viscera.

LIVER

The **liver** is a large, complex organ with numerous functions that include metabolic regulation, hematologic regulation, and bile production. It is the largest organ of the abdomen, occupying a major portion of the right hypochondriac and epigastric regions, sometimes extending into the left hypochondriac and umbilical regions. The liver is bordered superiorly, laterally, and anteriorly by the right hemidiaphragm (Figures 7.27 and 7.28). The medial surface is bordered by the stomach, duodenum, and transverse colon; the inferior surface is bordered by the hepatic flexure of the colon; and the posterior surface is bordered by the right kidney (Figure 7.29). The liver is surrounded by a strong connective tissue capsule **(Glisson's capsule)** that gives shape and stability to the soft hepatic tissue. It is also entirely covered by peritoneum except for the **gallbladder fossa,** the surface apposed to the inferior vena cava (IVC), and the **bare area** (liver surface between the superior and inferior coronary ligaments) (Figures 7.7, 7.8, 7.19, and 7.28).

Within the liver there are several main grooves or fissures that are useful in defining the lobes and boundaries of the hepatic segments. The **umbilical fissure (fissure for ligamentum teres)** divides the left hepatic lobe into medial and lateral segments. The **fissure for the ligamentum venosum** separates the caudate lobe from the left lobe, and the **trans-**

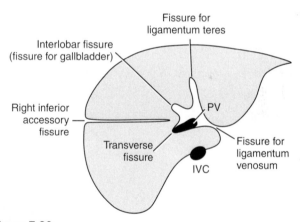

Figure 7.30
Axial view of liver with fissures. *PV,* Portal vein; *IVC,* inferior vena cava.

verse fissure (portal) contains the horizontal portions of the right and left portal veins. The **interlobar fissure (main lobar fissure),** also called the *fissure for the gallbladder,* divides the right from left lobes of the liver (Figure 7.30). The hilum of the liver, the **porta hepatis,** is located on the inferomedial border of the liver. It is the central location for vessels to enter and exit the liver (Figure 7.28).

Surface Anatomy

The liver can be divided into lobes according to surface anatomy or into segments according to vascular supply. The four lobes commonly used for reference based on surface anatomy are the left, right, caudate, and quadrate. The **left lobe** is the most anterior of the liver lobes, extending across the midline. It is separated from the **right lobe** by the **interlobar fissure,** an imaginary line drawn through the gallbladder fossa and the middle hepatic vein to the inferior vena cava. The smallest lobe is the **caudate lobe,** which is located on the inferior and posterior liver surface, sandwiched between the IVC and the **ligamentum venosum.** The **quadrate lobe** is located on the anteroinferior surface of the left lobe between the gallbladder and the ligamentum teres. The round, cordlike, **ligamentum teres** is a remnant of the fetal umbilical vein and runs along the free edge of the falciform ligament. The **falciform ligament** provides the structural support that attaches the upper surfaces of the liver to the diaphragm and upper abdominal wall (Figures 7.27, 7.28, 7.29, and 7.31 through 7.34).

KEY: fal, Falciform ligament; **LL,** left lobe of liver; **ven,** ligamentum venosum; **RL,** right lobe of liver; **cau,** caudate lobe of liver.

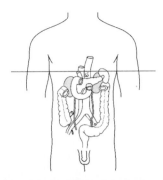

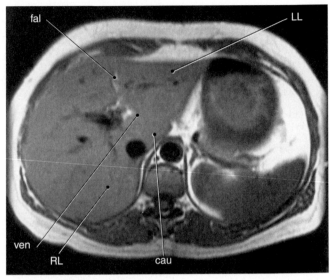

Figure 7.31
Axial, T1-weighted MR scan of abdomen with lobes of liver.

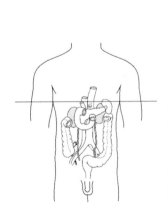

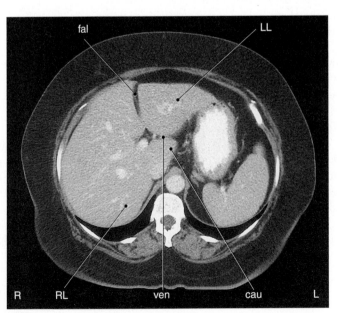

Figure 7.32
Axial CT scan of abdomen with lobes of liver.

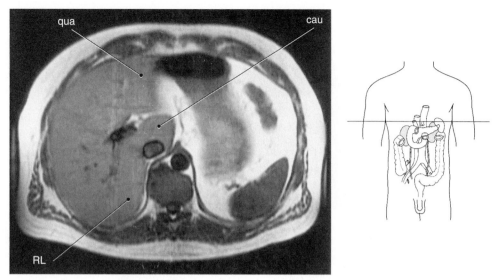

Figure 7.33
Axial, T1-weighted MR scan of liver with quadrate lobe.

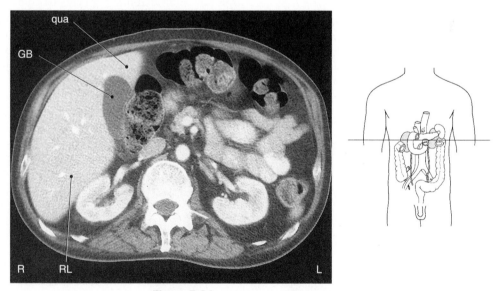

Figure 7.34
Axial CT scan of liver with quadrate lobe.

KEY: **qua,** Quadrate lobe of liver; **cau,** caudate lobe of liver; **RL,** right lobe of liver; **GB,** gallbladder.

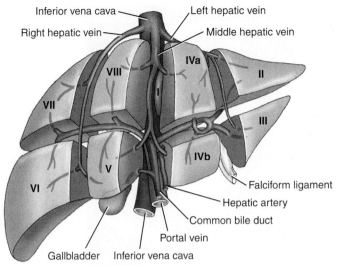

Figure 7.35
Anterior view of segmentation of liver.

Segmental Anatomy

Current practice favors dividing the liver into eight segments, according to its vascular supply, which can aid in surgical resection. According to the French anatomist Couinaud, the liver can be divided into segments based on the branching of the portal and hepatic veins. The three main hepatic veins divide the liver longitudinally into four sections (Figure 7.35). The middle hepatic vein divides the liver into right and left lobes. The right lobe is divided into medial and lateral sectors by the right hepatic vein, and the left lobe is divided into medial and lateral sectors by the left hepatic vein. Each section is then subdivided transversely by the right and left portal veins, creating nine segments numbered counterclockwise from the IVC. Each segment can be considered functionally independent with its own hepatic artery, portal vein, and bile duct and drained by a branch of the hepatic vein (Figures 7.36 through 7.47).

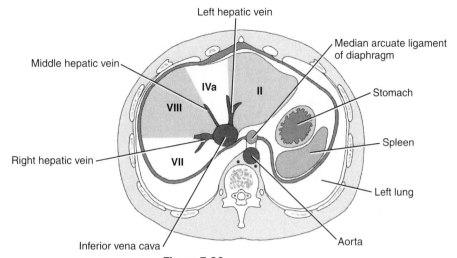

Figure 7.36
Axial view of liver segments.

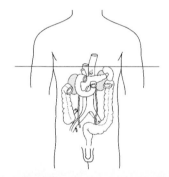

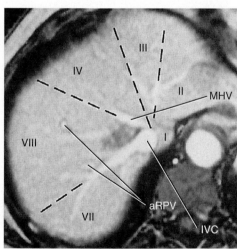

Figure 7.37
Axial, T1-weighted MR scan of liver segments.

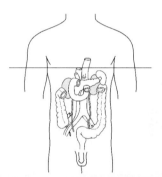

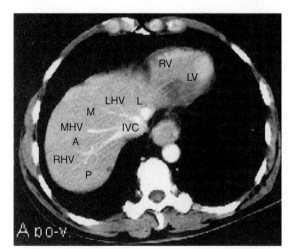

Figure 7.38
Axial CT scan of liver segments.

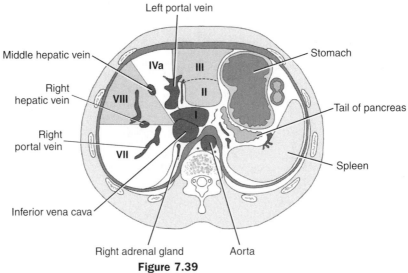

Figure 7.39
Axial view of liver segments.

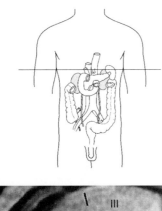

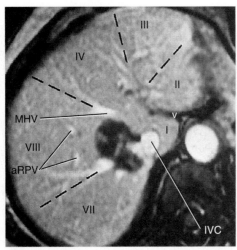

Figure 7.40
Axial, T1-weighted MR scan of liver segments.

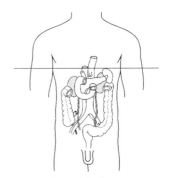

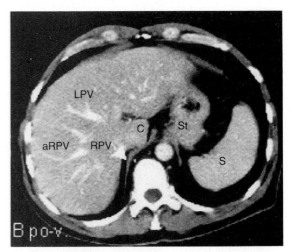

Figure 7.41
Axial CT scan of liver segments.

KEY: **v,** Ligamentum venosum; **MHV,** middle hepatic vein; **IVC,** inferior vena cava; **aRPV,** anterior branches of right portal vein; **LPV,** left portal vein; **aRPV,** anterior branches of right portal vein; **RPV,** right portal vein; **C,** caudate lobe; **St,** stomach; **S,** spleen.

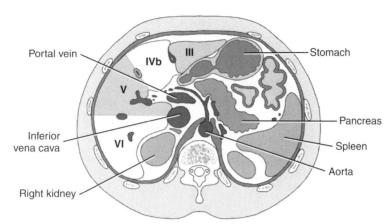

Figure 7.42
Axial view of liver segments.

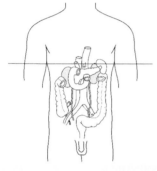

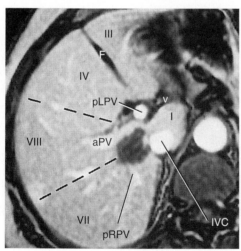

Figure 7.43
Axial, T1-weighted MR scan of liver segments.

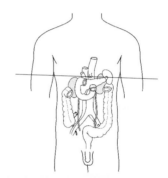

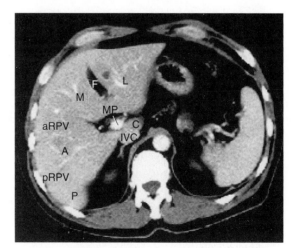

Figure 7.44
Axial CT scan of liver segments.

KEY: **F,** Falciform ligament; **A,** anterior segment of right lobe; **pLPV,** proximal left portal vein; **IVC,** inferior vena cava; **pRPV,** posterior branch of right portal vein; **v,** ligamentum venosum; **M,** medial segment of left lobe; **L,** lateral segment of left lobe; **MP,** main portal vein; **C,** caudate lobe; **aRPV,** anterior branches of right portal vein; **A,** anterior segment of right lobe; **pRPV,** posterior branches of right portal vein; **P,** posterior segment of right lobe.

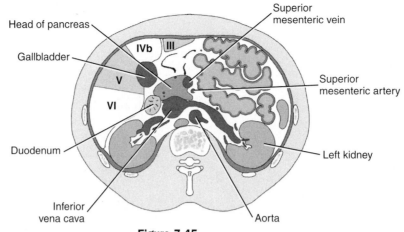

Figure 7.45
Axial view of liver segments.

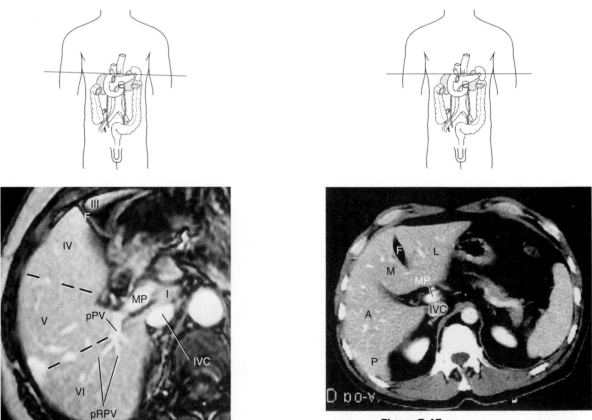

Figure 7.46
Axial, T1-weighted MR scan of liver segments.

Figure 7.47
Axial CT scan of liver segments.

KEY: **F,** Falciform ligament; **pPV,** posterior branch of portal vein; **MP,** main portal vein; **IVC,** inferior vena cava; **pRPV,** posterior branch of right portal vein; **M,** medial segment of left lobe; **L,** lateral segment of left lobe; **A,** anterior segment of right lobe; **P,** posterior segment of right lobe.

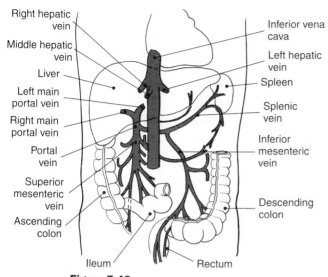

Figure 7.48
Anterior view of portal hepatic system.

Portal Hepatic System

The liver receives nutrient-rich blood from the gastrointestinal tract via the **portal hepatic system** (Figures 7.35 and 7.48). The major vessel of this system is the **portal vein,** which is formed in the retroperitoneum by the union of the superior mesenteric and splenic veins, posterior to the neck of the pancreas (Figures 7.49 through 7.52). It passes obliquely to the right, posterior to the hepatic artery within the lesser omentum, and enters the liver at the porta hepatis. At the **porta hepatis,** the portal vein branches into **right** and **left main portal veins** that then follow the course of the right and left hepatic arteries (Figures 7.53 and 7.54). The right portal vein first sends branches to the caudate lobe, then divides into anterior and posterior branches that subdivide into superior and inferior branches to supply the right lobe of the liver. The left portal vein initially courses to the left, then turns medially toward the ligamentum teres. It branches to supply the lateral segments (segments II and III) of the left lobe and the superior and inferior segmental branches of segment IV.

KEY: li, Liver; **p,** peritoneum; **pa,** pancreas; **st,** stomach; **sp,** spleen.

Portal hypertension is caused by obstruction of blood flow in the portal hepatic system. This condition can lead to splenomegaly and ascites.

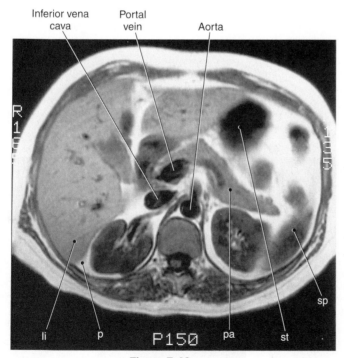

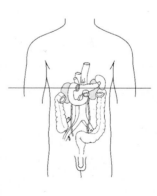

Figure 7.49
Axial, T1-weighted MR scan of liver and portal vein.

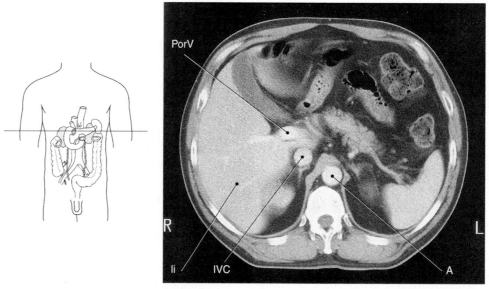

Figure 7.50
Axial CT scan of liver and portal vein.

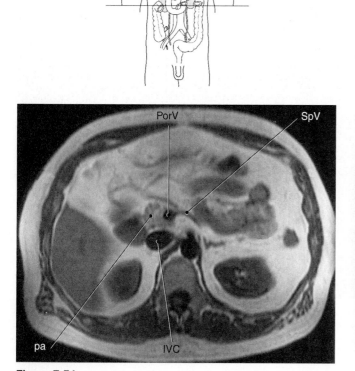

Figure 7.51
Axial, T1-weighted MR scan of abdomen with portal and splenic veins.

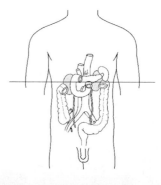

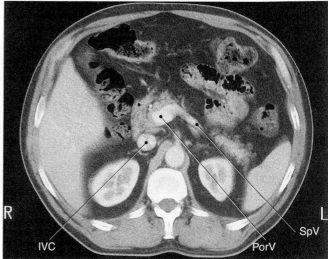

Figure 7.52
Axial CT scan of abdomen with portal and splenic veins.

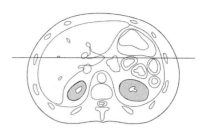

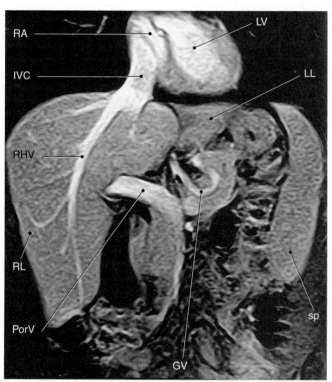

Figure 7.53
Coronal MRV of portal system.

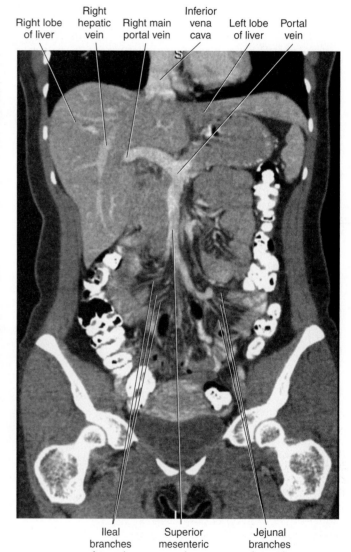

Figure 7.54
Coronal CT reformat of portal system.

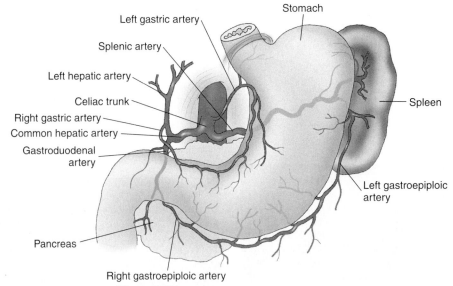

Figure 7.55
Anterior view of celiac trunk and hepatic artery.

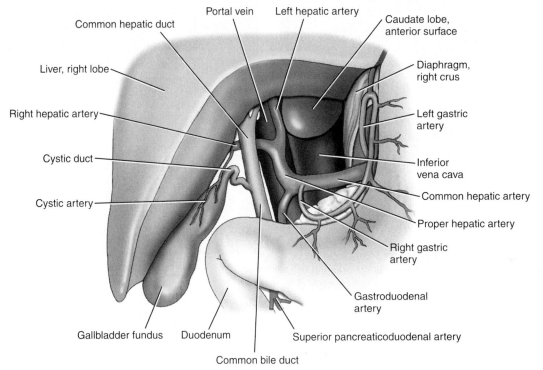

Figure 7.56
Anterior view of hepatic artery, common bile duct, and portal vein.

KEY: CHA, Common hepatic artery; **Ce,** celiac axis; **SpA,** splenic artery.

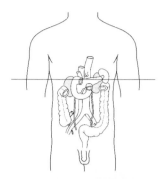

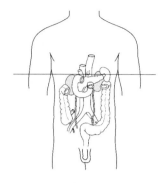

Right hepatic
artery

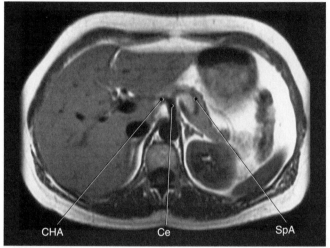

CHA   Ce   SpA

Figure 7.57
Axial, T1-weighted MR scan of abdomen with celiac trunk and
hepatic artery.

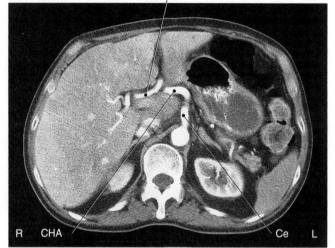

R   CHA   Ce   L

Figure 7.58
Axial CT scan of abdomen with celiac trunk and hepatic artery.

Vasculature

The liver is unusual in that it has a dual blood supply, receiving
arterial blood (20%-25%) from the common hepatic artery and
nutrient-rich venous blood (75%-80%) from the portal vein.
The **common hepatic artery** usually arises as one of the three
branches off the celiac artery, coursing to the right to enter
the lesser omentum anterior to the portal vein (Figures 7.55
through 7.58). It branches into the right gastric and gastroduodenal arteries just above the duodenum and continues in
the hepatoduodenal ligament as the **proper hepatic artery.**
While within or just before entering the porta hepatis, the
proper hepatic artery divides into left and right hepatic arteries
that continue to branch and supply the lobes of the liver.
The **right hepatic artery** is larger than the left and supplies the
majority of the right lobe of the liver. It passes posterior to the
uncinate process of the pancreas and runs along the posterior
wall of the bile duct into the right hepatic lobe. The **left
hepatic artery** is located between the lesser curvature of the
stomach and approaches the liver in the lesser omentum and
branches to supply the caudate, quadrate, and medial and

lateral segments of the left lobe of the liver (Figure 7.59). The
venous drainage of the liver occurs via the small interlobar and
intersegmental hepatic vessels that merge into the three major
hepatic veins, emptying directly into the IVC, just below the
diaphragm (Figure 7.60). The **right hepatic vein,** the largest,
lies between the right anterior and posterior hepatic segments,
drains segments V, VI, and VII, and enters the IVC at the
right lateral aspect. The **middle hepatic vein** lies in the interlobar fissure, drains segments IV, V, and VIII, then enters the
IVC at the anterior or right anterior surface. The smallest
hepatic vein, the **left hepatic vein,** courses between the medial
and lateral segments of the left lobe, drains segments II
and III, then enters the left anterior surface of the IVC
(Figures 7.61 and 7.62). Frequently, the middle and left hepatic
veins converge to form a common trunk before emptying into
the IVC just below the diaphragm. The **IVC** lies in a groove
along the posterior wall of the liver and ascends into the
thoracic cavity through the **caval hiatus** of the diaphragm
and enters the right atrium of the heart (Figures 7.61
through 7.64).

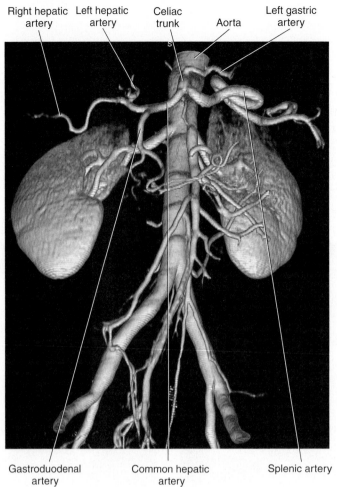

Right hepatic artery • Left hepatic artery • Celiac trunk • Aorta • Left gastric artery

Gastroduodenal artery • Common hepatic artery • Splenic artery

Figure 7.59

CTA of celiac trunk and hepatic artery.

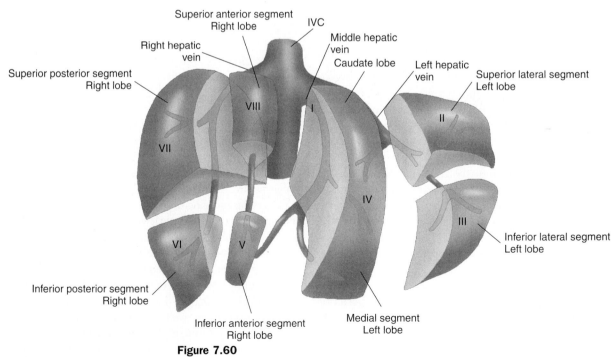

Superior anterior segment Right lobe • IVC

Right hepatic vein • Middle hepatic vein

Superior posterior segment Right lobe • Caudate lobe • Left hepatic vein • Superior lateral segment Left lobe

VIII • I • II

VII

IV • III • Inferior lateral segment Left lobe

VI • V

Inferior posterior segment Right lobe

Inferior anterior segment Right lobe • Medial segment Left lobe

Figure 7.60

Couinaud's segmentation of the liver with hepatic veins.

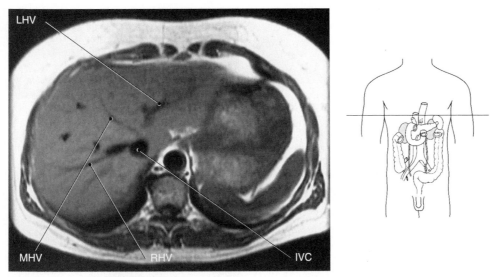

Figure 7.61
Axial, T1-weighted MR scan of abdomen with hepatic veins.

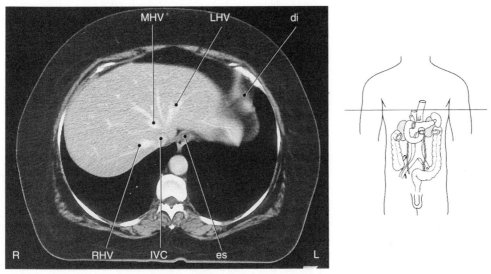

Figure 7.62
Axial CT scan of liver with hepatic veins.

KEY: LHV, Left hepatic vein; **MHV,** middle hepatic vein; **RHV,** right hepatic vein; **IVC,** inferior vena cava; **di,** diaphragm; **es,** esophagus.

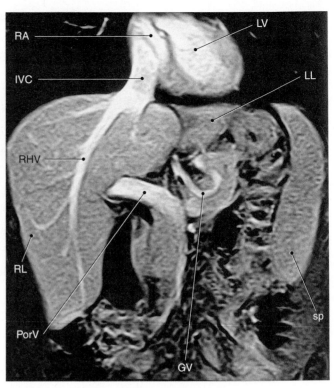

Figure 7.63
MRV with hepatic and portal veins.

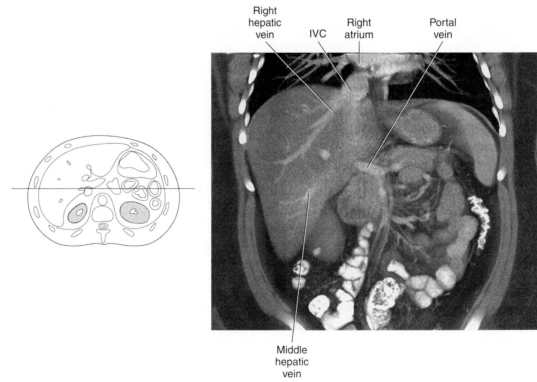

Figure 7.64
Coronal CT reformat of hepatic and portal veins.

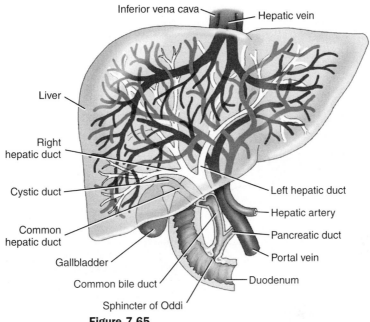

Figure 7.65
Anterior view of intrahepatic biliary system.

GALLBLADDER AND BILIARY SYSTEM

The **biliary system** is composed of the gallbladder and bile ducts (both intrahepatic and extrahepatic) that serve to drain the liver of bile and then store it until it is transported to the duodenum to aid in digestion (Figure 7.65). The hollow pear-shaped **gallbladder** is located in the **gallbladder fossa** on the anteroinferior portion of the right lobe of the liver, closely associated with the **main lobar fissure.** It functions as the reservoir for storing and concentrating bile before being transported to the duodenum. The gallbladder can be divided into a fundus, body, and neck (Figures 7.66 to 7.71). The **fundus** is the rounded distal portion of the gallbladder sac that is frequently in contact with the anterior abdominal wall. The widest portion, the **body,** gently tapers superiorly into the neck. The narrow **neck** lies to the right of the porta hepatis and continues as the **cystic duct.** The neck contains circular muscles that create spiral folds within the mucosa that are called the **spiral valves of Heister** (Figure 7.67). These valves are especially prominent at the bend formed by the neck and cystic duct, a common area for gallbladder impaction during acute or chronic cholecystitis. The gallbladder has a muscular wall that contracts when stimulated by cholecystokinin, forcing bile through the extrahepatic biliary system into the duodenum. Bile, formed within the liver, is collected for transport to the gallbladder by the intrahepatic bile ducts. The **intrahepatic bile ducts** run beside the hepatic arteries and portal veins throughout the liver parenchyma. The intrahepatic ducts merge into successively larger ducts as they follow a course from the periphery to the central portion of the liver, eventually forming the **right** and **left hepatic ducts** (Figures 7.65 to 7.68). The right and left hepatic ducts unite at the porta hepatis to form the proximal portion of the **common hepatic duct** (CHD), which marks the beginning of the **extrahepatic biliary system** (Figure 7.66). The CHD is located anterior to the portal vein and lateral to the hepatic artery in its caudal descent from the porta hepatis. As the CHD descends in the free border of the lesser omentum, it is joined from the right by the cystic duct to form the **common bile duct** (CBD). The CBD continues a caudal descent along with the hepatic artery and portal vein within the hepatoduodenal ligament (Figure 7.65). It curves slightly to the right, away from the portal vein, then courses posterior and medial to the first part of the duodenum behind the head of the pancreas (Figures 7.69 through 7.76). The CBD follows a groove on the posterior surface of the pancreatic head, then pierces the medial wall of the second part of the duodenum along with the **main pancreatic duct (duct of Wirsung)** through the **ampulla of Vater** (Figure 7.66). The ends of both ducts are surrounded by the circular muscle fibers of the **sphincter of Oddi** (Figure 7.67).

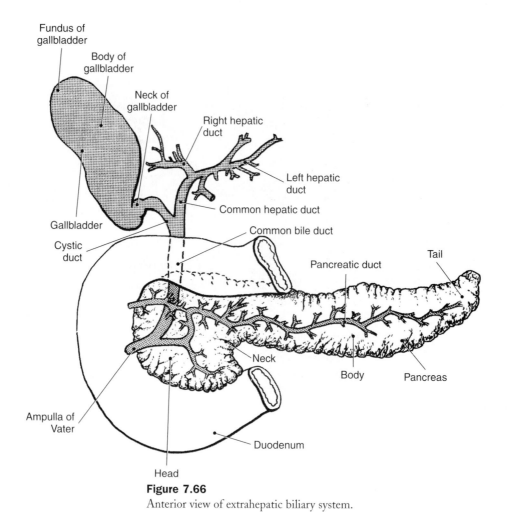

Figure 7.66
Anterior view of extrahepatic biliary system.

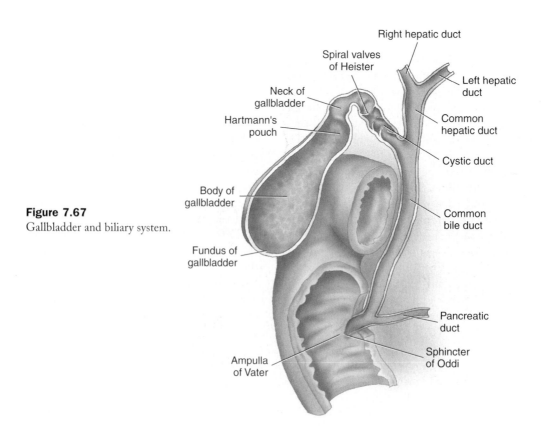

Figure 7.67
Gallbladder and biliary system.

Intrahepatic
ducts

Stomach

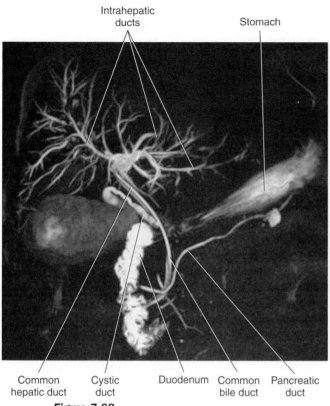

Common   Cystic   Duodenum   Common   Pancreatic
hepatic duct duct   bile duct   duct

Figure 7.68
MR cholongiopancreatogram of biliary system.

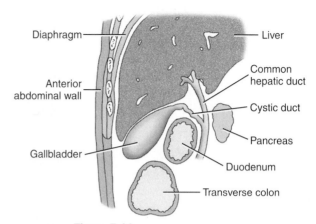

Diaphragm

Anterior
abdominal wall

Gallbladder

Liver

Common
hepatic duct

Cystic duct

Pancreas

Duodenum

Transverse colon

Figure 7.69
Sagittal view of liver and gallbladder.

KEY: **PorV,** Portal vein; **li,** liver; **k,** kidney; **GB,** gallbladder.

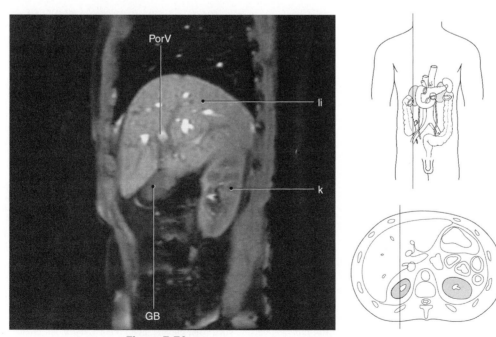

PorV

li

k

GB

Figure 7.70
Sagittal, T2-weighted MR scan of liver and gallbladder.

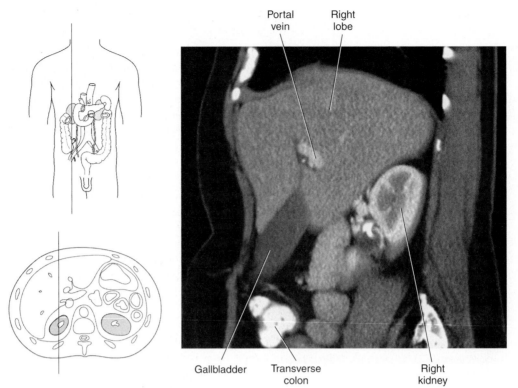

Figure 7.71
Sagittal CT reformat of liver and gallbladder.

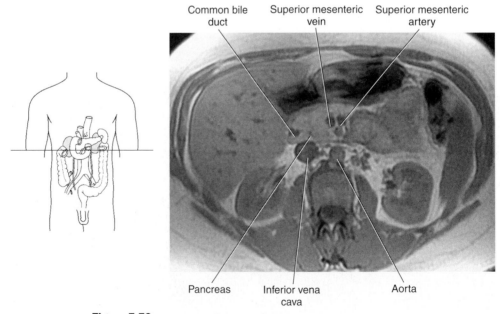

Figure 7.72
Axial, T1-weighted MR scan of abdomen and common bile duct.

KEY: **CHD,** Common hepatic duct; **HAb,** hepatic artery branch; **IPorV,** left branch of portal vein; **rPorV,** right branch of portal vein.

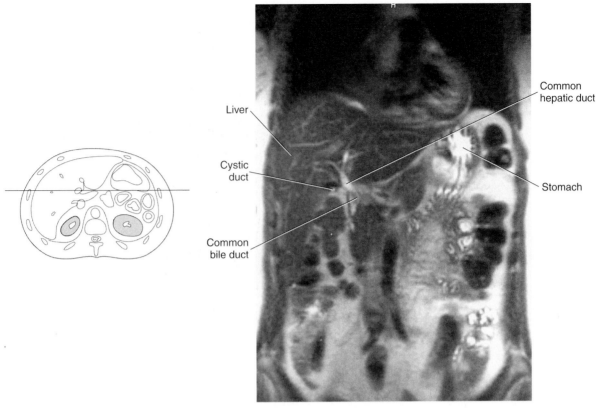

Figure 7.73
Coronal, T1-weighted MR scan of abdomen and common bile duct.

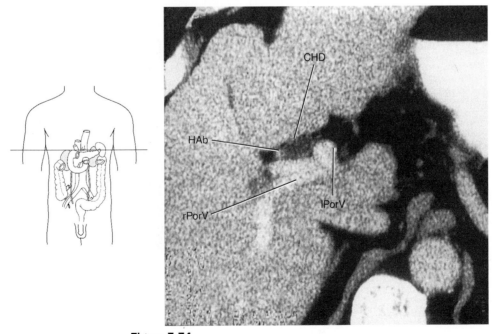

Figure 7.74
Axial CT scan of abdomen and common bile duct.

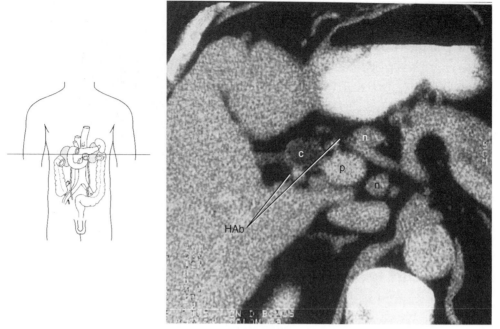

Figure 7.75
Axial CT scan of abdomen and common bile duct.

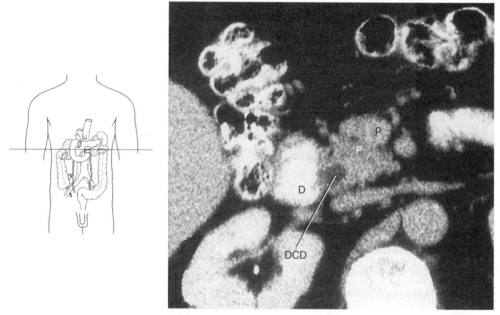

Figure 7.76
Axial CT scan of abdomen and common bile duct.

KEY: **c,** Common duct; **HAb,** hepatic artery branches; **p,** main portal vein; **n,** lymph nodes; **D,** duodenum; **DCD,** distal common duct; **P,** pancreatic head.

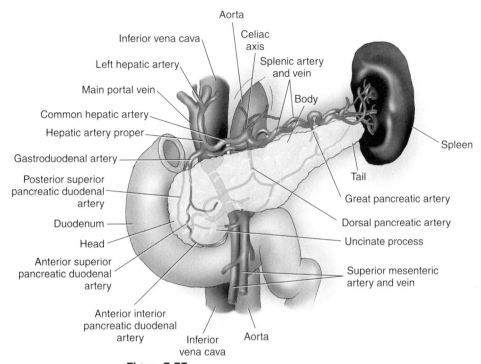

Aorta

Inferior vena cava

Celiac axis

Left hepatic artery

Splenic artery and vein

Main portal vein

Body

Common hepatic artery

Hepatic artery proper

Gastroduodenal artery

Spleen

Posterior superior pancreatic duodenal artery

Tail

Duodenum

Great pancreatic artery

Head

Dorsal pancreatic artery

Anterior superior pancreatic duodenal artery

Uncinate process

Anterior interior pancreatic duodenal artery

Superior mesenteric artery and vein

Inferior vena cava

Aorta

Figure 7.77
Anterior view of pancreas and adjacent structures.

PANCREAS

The **pancreas** is a long, narrow retroperitoneal organ that lies posterior to the stomach and extends transversely at an oblique angle between the duodenum and splenic hilum. The pancreas can be divided into the head, uncinate process, neck, body, and tail (Figure 7.77). The broad, flat **head** of the pancreas lies inferior and to the right of the body and tail, nestled in the curve of the second portion of the duodenum at approximately the level of L2-L3. The head is anterior to the IVC and renal veins. Two vessels can be commonly seen running through the head: the common bile duct in the right posterior aspect and the gastroduodenal artery in the anterior aspect (Figures 7.78 and 7.79). The **uncinate process** is a medial and posterior extension of the head, lying between the superior mesenteric vein and inferior vena cava (Figure 7.77). The **neck,** the constricted portion of the gland, is located between the pancreatic head and body. Located just posterior to the neck is the **portal splenic confluence,** where the portal vein is formed by the merging of the superior mesenteric and splenic veins (Figure 7.77). The **body** is the largest and most anterior portion of the pancreas, extending transversely to the left, anterior to the aorta and superior mesenteric artery (Figures 7.80 and 7.81). The splenic vein runs along the posterior surface of the body on its route to the portal splenic confluence. The body tapers superiorly and posteriorly into the **pancreatic tail.** The tail extends into to the left anterior pararenal space, anterior to the left kidney, to end at the splenic hilum (Figures 7.77 and 7.80 through 7.82). The pancreas has both an **endocrine**

(insulin, glucagon) and **exocrine** (digestive enzymes) function. It delivers its endocrine hormones into the draining venous system and its enzymes into the small intestines. The endocrine hormones help control plasma glucose concentration. **Insulin's** chief role is to regulate cellular absorption and utilization of glucose, thereby affecting carbohydrate, protein and lipid metabolism in body tissues. **Glucagon,** acting in opposition to insulin, tends to raise plasma sugar levels by increasing the rate of glycogen breakdown and glucose synthesis in the liver. Pancreatic enzymes include **amylase** for the digestion of starch, **lipase** for the digestion of lipids, **peptidases** for protein digestion, and **sodium bicarbonate** to neutralize gastric acid. The pancreatic enzymes are carried to the duodenum via a system of ducts. The main pancreatic duct **(duct of Wirsung)** begins in the tail and runs the length of the gland to the **ampulla of Vater,** where it empties, together with the common bile duct, into the duodenum through the sphincter of Oddi (Figures 7.66 and 7.82). The arterial supply of the pancreas comes from branches of the celiac and superior mesenteric arteries. Venous blood drains from the pancreas into the portal vein via the superior mesenteric or splenic vein. The pancreas is unencapsulated and has a distinct lobulated appearance, making identification easy in cross section.

> **Acute pancreatitis can lead to the leakage of powerful digestive enzymes. As the enzymes "digest" the surrounding tissue, pancreatic necrosis results.**

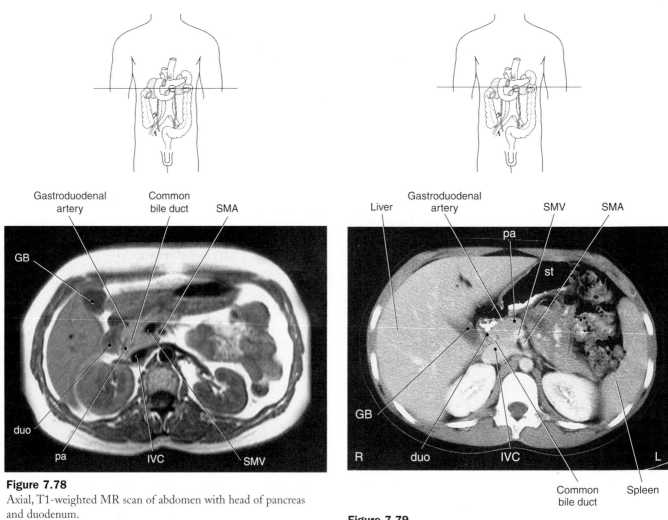

Figure 7.78
Axial, T1-weighted MR scan of abdomen with head of pancreas and duodenum.

Figure 7.79
Axial CT scan of abdomen with head of pancreas and duodenum.

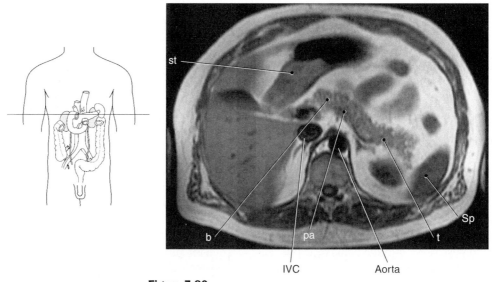

Figure 7.80
Axial, T1-weighted MR scan of pancreas.

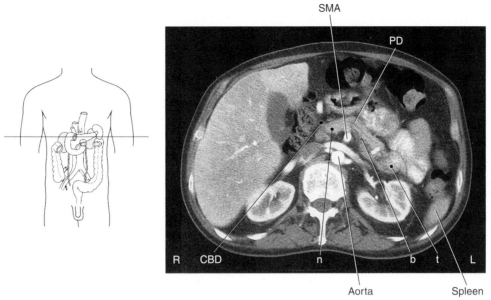

Figure 7.81
Axial CT scan of pancreas and pancreatic duct.

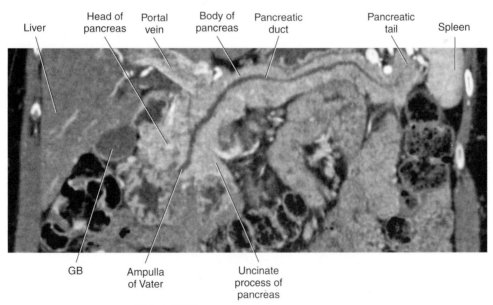

Figure 7.82
Coronal CT curved-reformat of pancreatic duct.

KEY: GB, Gallbladder; **duo,** duodenum; **pa,** pancreas; **IVC,** inferior vena cava; **SMV,** superior mesenteric vein; **st,** stomach; **b,** body of pancreas; **t,** tail of pancreas; **Sp,** spleen; **SMA,** superior mesenteric artery; **PD,** pancreatic duct; **CBD,** common bile duct; **n,** neck of pancreas.

SPLEEN

The **spleen** is the largest lymph organ in the body composed of lymphoid tissue. The cellular components of the spleen create a highly vascular, spongy parenchyma called **red** and **white pulp.** The red pulp contains large quantities of blood, and the white pulp contains lymphoid tissue and white blood cells. The spleen is an intraperitoneal organ that is covered entirely with peritoneum except at its small bare area at the splenic hilum. It is located posterior to the stomach in the left upper quadrant of the abdomen, protected by the ninth through eleventh ribs. The spleen is bordered on its medial side by the left kidney, splenic flexure of the colon, and pancreatic tail. The posterior border of the spleen is in contact with the diaphragm, pleura, left lung, and ribs. The spleen is attached to the greater curvature of the stomach and the left kidney by the **gastrosplenic** and **lienorenal ligaments,** respectively (Figure 7.83). The spleen receives its arterial blood from the splenic artery and is drained via the splenic vein. The splenic artery and vein enter and exit the spleen at the splenic hilum between the gastric and renal depressions (Figures 7.84 and 7.85). The spleen is a highly vascular organ that functions to produce white blood cells, filter abnormal blood cells from the blood, store iron from red blood cells, and initiate the immune response. Normal splenic parenchyma is homogeneous; however, immediately after intravenous contrast injection, the spleen can have a heterogeneous appearance on early arterial phase images (Figure 7.85).

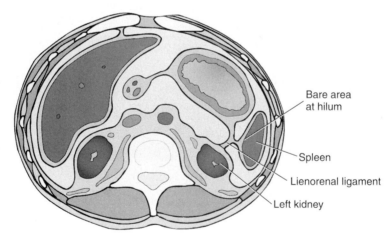

Bare area at hilum

Spleen

Lienorenal ligament

Left kidney

Figure 7.83
Axial view of the abdomen with greater and lesser sac, falciform and gastrosplenic and lienorenal ligaments.

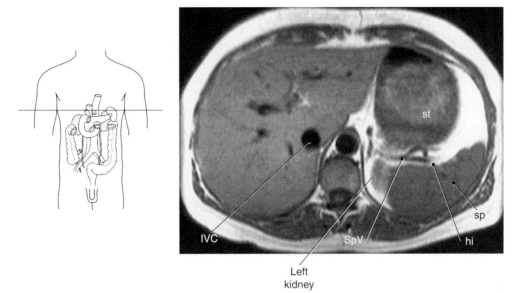

Figure 7.84
Axial, T1-weighted MR scan of spleen.

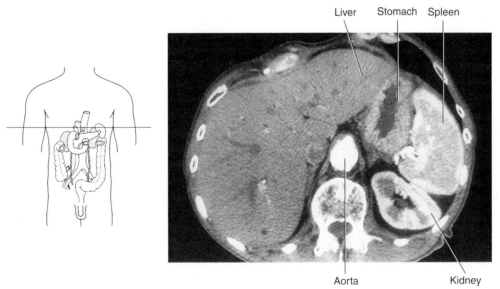

Figure 7.85
Axial CT scan of spleen.

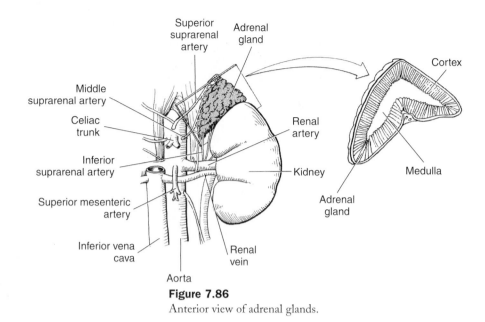

Figure 7.86

Anterior view of adrenal glands.

ADRENAL GLANDS

The paired **adrenal (suprarenal) glands** are retroperitoneal organs located superior to each kidney (Figures 7.86 and 7.87). They are separated from the superior surface of the kidneys by **perirenal fat** and are enclosed, along with the kidneys, by **Gerota's fascia** (Figure 7.88). The **right adrenal gland** is located just posterior to the IVC, medial to the posterior segment of the right hepatic lobe, and lateral to the right crus of the diaphragm. It is generally lower and more medial than the left adrenal gland and commonly appears as an inverted V on cross section (Figures 7.89 through 7.91). The **left adrenal gland** lies anteromedial to the upper pole of the left kidney. It is located in a triangle formed by the aorta, pancreatic tail, and left kidney (Figure 7.92). It commonly appears as a triangular or Y-shaped configuration (Figures 7.93 and 7.94). The posterior surfaces of both the right and left glands border the **crus** of the diaphragm. Each adrenal gland has an outer cortex and an inner medulla that function independently (Figure 7.86). The **adrenal cortex** produces more than two dozen steroids, collectively called **adrenocortical steroids** or just **corticosteroids.** The corticosteroids are broken into three main categories: **glucocorticoids,** which affect glucose metabolism; **mineralocorticoids,** which regulate sodium and potassium levels; and **androgens** and **estrogens,** which are responsible for promoting normal development of bone and reproductive organs. The **adrenal medulla** produces the hormones **epinephrine** and **norepinephrine,** which accelerate metabolism and energy and are responsible for the body's "fight or flight" response. The adrenal glands receive arterial blood from the superior, middle, and inferior adrenal arteries. The drainage of the right gland is via a short suprarenal vein that empties directly into the IVC. The left gland is drained by the left suprarenal vein, which empties into the left renal vein.

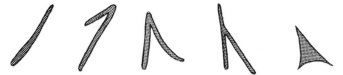

Figure 7.87
Axial view with common configurations of adrenal glands.

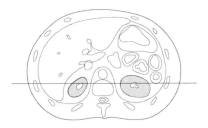

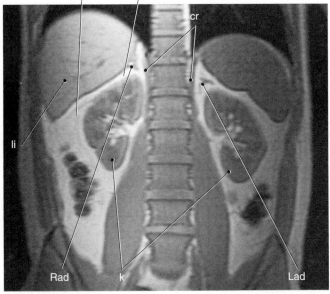

Figure 7.88
Coronal, T1-weighted MR scan with adrenal glands.

KEY: cr, Crus; **li,** liver; **Rad,** right adrenal gland; **k,** kidney; **Lad,** left adrenal gland.

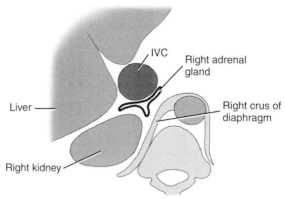

Figure 7.89
Axial view of right adrenal gland.

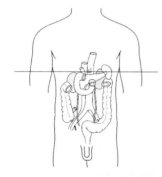

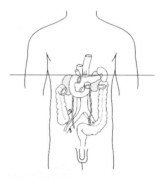

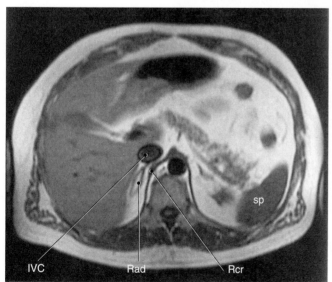

Figure 7.90
Axial, T1-weighted MR scan of right adrenal gland.

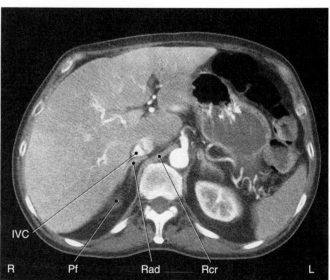

Figure 7.91
Axial CT scan of right adrenal gland.

KEY: **IVC,** Inferior vena cava; **Rad,** right adrenal gland; **Rcr,** right crus; **sp,** spleen; **Pf,** perirenal fat.

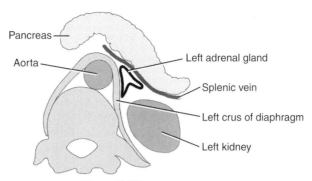

Figure 7.92
Axial view of left adrenal gland.

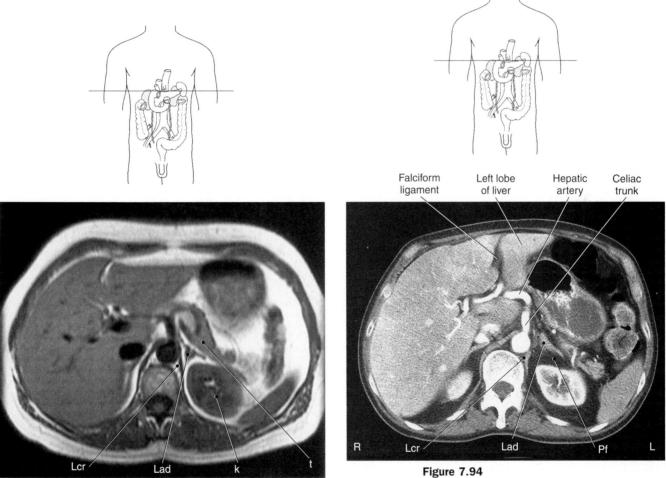

Figure 7.93
Axial, T1-weighted MR scan of left adrenal gland.

Figure 7.94
Axial CT scan of left adrenal gland.

KEY: Lcr, Left crus; **Lad,** left adrenal gland; **k,** kidney; **t,** tail of pancreas; **Pf,** perirenal fat.

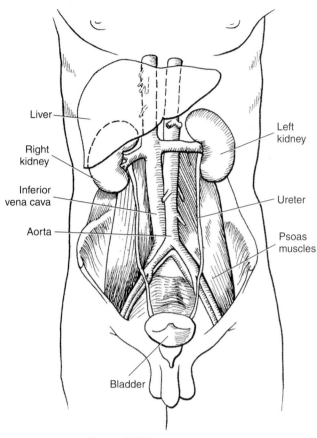

Figure 7.95
Anterior view of urinary system.

URINARY SYSTEM

The structures of the urinary system include the kidneys, ureters, bladder, and urethra. Those that are located within the abdomen are the kidneys and ureters (Figure 7.95). The bladder and urethra are located in the pelvis and are discussed in Chapter 8. The **kidneys** are retroperitoneal bean-shaped organs that lie in the **paravertebral gutters** against the posterior abdominal wall (Figure 7.96). They lie at an oblique orientation, with the upper poles more medial and posterior than the lower poles. They are located on each side of the spine between T12 and L4 and are embedded in **perirenal fat** (Figure 7.97). The right kidney is usually slightly lower due to displacement by the liver (Figures 7.98 and 7.99). Each kidney is composed of an outer cortex and an inner medulla. The **renal cortex** comprises the outer one third of the renal tissue and has extensions between the renal pyramids of the medulla. The cortex contains the functional subunit of the kidney, the **nephron,** which consists of the **glomerulus** and **convoluted tubules** and is responsible for filtration of urine (Figure 7.100). The **renal medulla** consists of segments called **renal pyramids** that radiate from the **renal sinus** to the outer surface of the kidney. The striated-appearing pyramids contain the **loops of Henle** and collecting tubules and function as the beginning of the collecting system. Arising from the apices of the pyramids are the cup-shaped minor calyces. Each kidney has 7 to 14 **minor calyces** that merge into 2 or 3 **major calyces.** The major calyces join to form the **renal pelvis,** which is the largest dilated portion of the collecting system and is continuous with the ureters (Figure 7.100). The fat-filled cavity surrounding the renal pelvis is called the *renal sinus.*

Surrounding the kidneys and perirenal fat is another protective layer called the **renal fascia (Gerota's fascia).** The renal fascia functions to anchor the kidneys to surrounding structures in an attempt to prevent bumps and jolts to the body from injuring the kidneys. In addition, the renal fascia acts as a barrier, limiting the spread of infection that may arise from the kidneys. The medial indentation in the kidney is called the **hilum;** it allows the renal artery and vein and ureters to enter and exit the kidney (Figures 7.97 and 7.101 through 7.104). The kidneys can be divided into five segments according to their vascular supply: **apical, anterosuperior (upper anterior), anteroinferior (middle inferior), inferior,** and **posterior** (Figure 7.105). The segmental classification helps with surgical planning for partial nephrectomies. The **ureters** are paired muscular tubes that transport urine to the urinary bladder. Each ureter originates at the renal pelvis and descends anteriorly and medially to the psoas muscles, just anterior to the transverse processes of the lumbar spine (Figures 7.104 through 7.106). The ureters then enter the posterior wall of the bladder at an oblique angle (Figure 7.107). The primary function of the urinary system is to filter blood, produce and excrete urine, and help maintain normal body physiology.

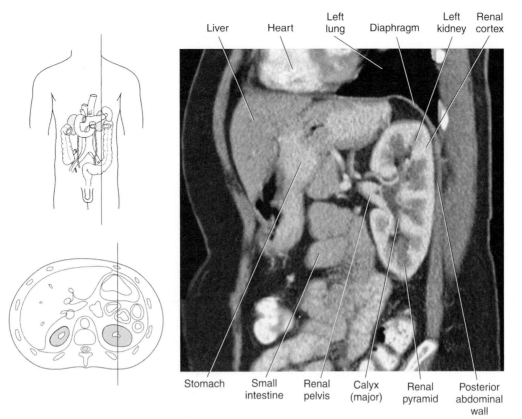

Figure 7.96
Sagittal CT reformat of left kidney.

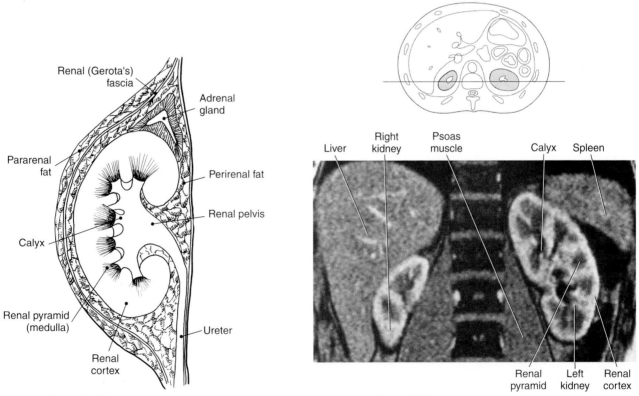

Figure 7.97
Coronal midsection view of kidney.

Figure 7.98
Coronal, T1-weighted MR scan of kidneys.

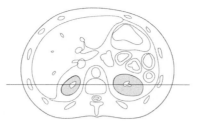

Liver   T12   Renal
pelvis   Calyx   Renal pyramid
(medulla)   Spleen

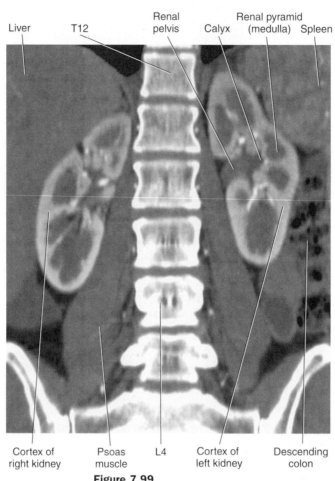

Cortex of
right kidney   Psoas
muscle   L4   Cortex of
left kidney   Descending
colon

Figure 7.99
Coronal CT reformat of kidneys.

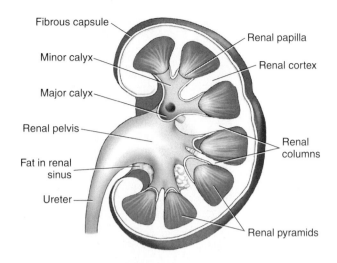

Fibrous capsule

Minor calyx

Major calyx

Renal pelvis

Fat in renal sinus

Ureter

Renal papilla

Renal cortex

Renal columns

Renal pyramids

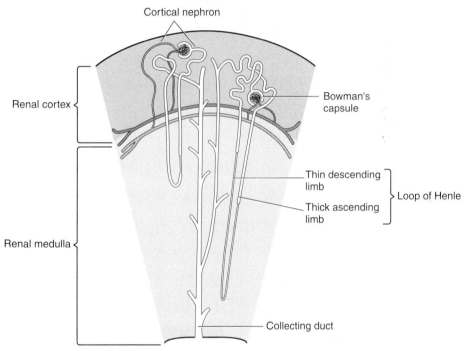

Cortical nephron

Renal cortex

Renal medulla

Bowman's capsule

Thin descending limb

Thick ascending limb

Loop of Henle

Collecting duct

Figure 7.100

Coronal midsection view of internal structures of kidney.

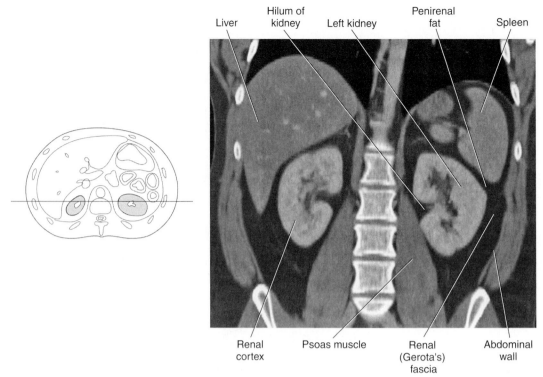

Figure 7.101
Coronal CT reformat of kidneys in nephrogram phase.

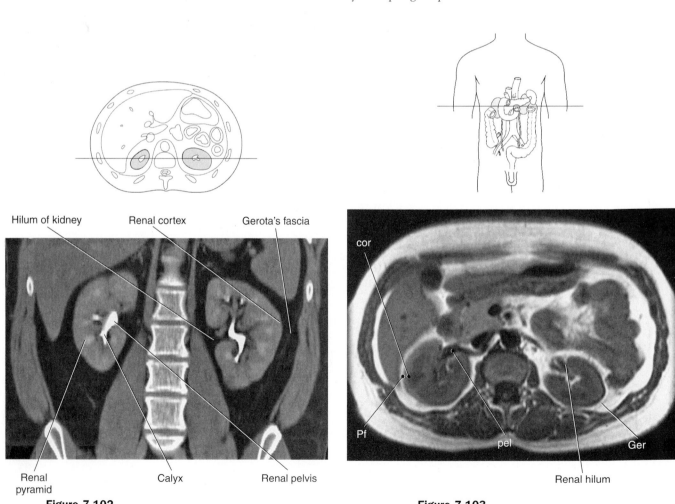

Figure 7.102
Coronal CT reformat of kidneys in excretory phase.

Figure 7.103
Axial, T1-weighted MR scan of kidney.

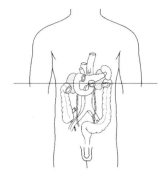

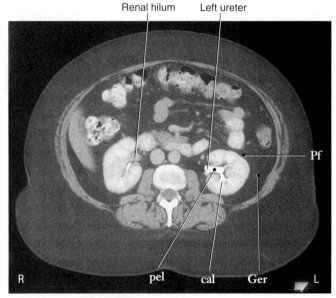

Renal hilum   Left ureter

Pf

pel   cal   Ger

R   L

Figure 7.104
Axial CT scan of kidney.

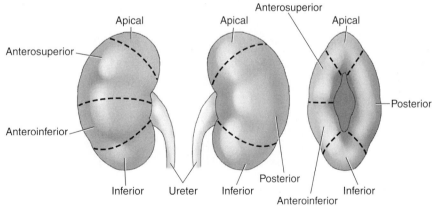

Apical   Anterosuperior

Apical   Apical

Anterosuperior   Posterior

Anteroinferior

Inferior   Ureter   Inferior   Posterior   Anteroinferior   Inferior

Figure 7.105
Segments of kidney.

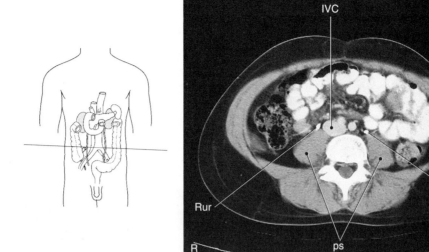

Figure 7.106
Axial CT with ureters.

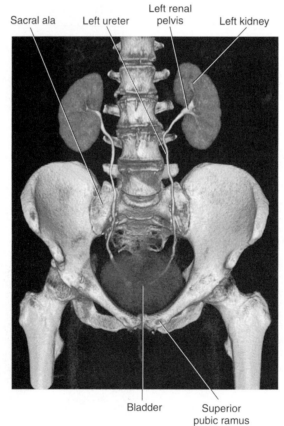

Figure 7.107
CT urogram.

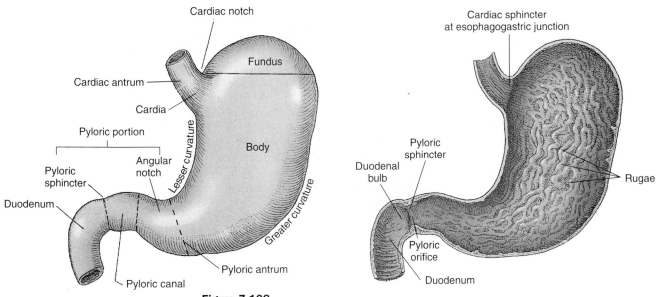

Figure 7.108
Stomach. *Left,* Anterior surface. *Right,* Internal surface.

STOMACH

The **stomach** is the dilated portion of the digestive system that acts as a food reservoir and is responsible for the early stages of digestion. It has four major functions: (1) storage of food, (2) mechanical breakdown of food, (3) dissolution of chemical bonds via acids and enzymes, and (4) production of intrinsic factor. The stomach is located under the left dome of the diaphragm, with the superior portion joining the esophagus at the **cardiac orifice** (cardiac sphincter), creating the **esophagogastric junction** (Figures 7.108 through 7.110). The stomach has two borders called the **lesser** and **greater curvatures.** Between the two curvatures is the largest portion of the stomach, termed the **body** (Figures 7.111 to 7.113). On the superior surface of the body is a rounded surface called the **fundus** (Figure 7.110). The inferior portion **(pyloric antrum)** empties into the duodenum through the **pyloric sphincter** (Figure 7.114). The anterior surface is in contact with the diaphragm, anterior abdominal wall, and left lobe of the liver. Located posterior to the stomach is the gastric portion of the spleen, the left adrenal gland and kidney, and the body and tail of the pancreas. When empty, the inner surface of the stomach creates prominent folds called **rugae** that allow the stomach to expand with the ingestion of food (Figures 7.108 and 7.110). The average adult produces 2 to 3 L per day of gastric juices that contain mucus, hydrochloric acid, intrinsic factor, and the digestive enzymes of pepsinogen and lipase. The stomach can hold up to 3 L of food, which it mixes with digestive juices to form chyme. The stomach is one of the most vascular organs within the body. The arterial blood is supplied by branches of the gastric, splenic, and gastroduodenal arteries (Figure 7.55). Venous drainage corresponds to the arterial supply. The gastric veins usually drain directly into the portal vein or into the superior mesenteric vein.

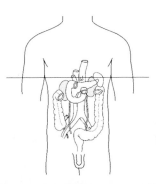

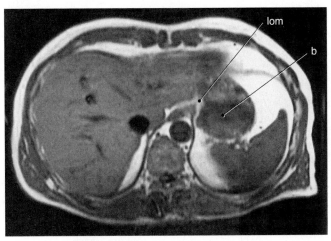

Figure 7.109
Axial, T1-weighted MR scan of stomach.

KEY: lom, Lesser omentum; **b,** body of pancreas.

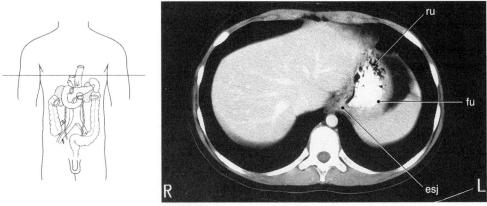

Figure 7.110
Axial CT scan of esophagogastric junction.

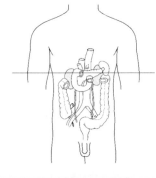

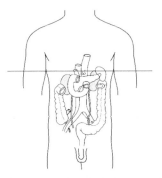

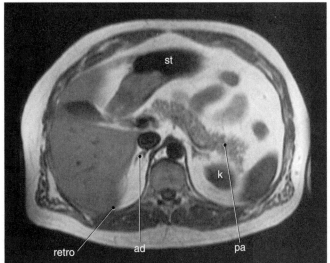

Figure 7.111
Axial, T1-weighted MR scan of stomach.

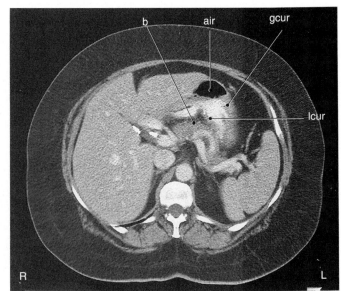

Figure 7.112
Axial CT scan of stomach.

KEY: **ru,** Rugae; **fu,** fundus of stomach; **esj,** esophagogastric junction; **st,** stomach; **k,** kidney; **retro,** retroperitoneum; **ad,** adrenal gland; **pa,** pancreas; **b,** body of pancreas; **air,** air; **gcur,** greater curvature; **lcur,** lesser curvature.

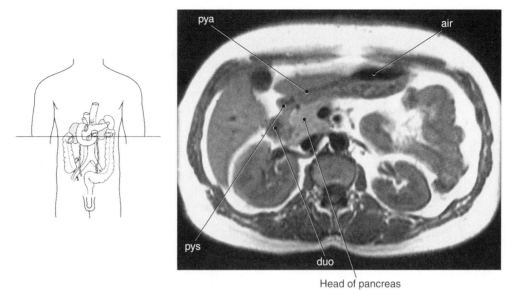

Figure 7.113
Axial, T1-weighted MR scan of pyloric antrum and pyloric sphincter.

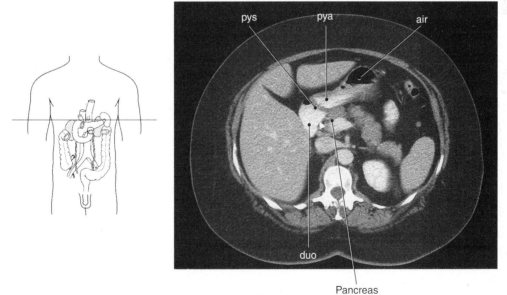

Figure 7.114
Axial CT scan of stomach with pyloric antrum and pyloric sphincter.

KEY: **pya,** Pyloric antrum; **air,** air in stomach; **pys,** pyloric sphincter; **duo,** duodenum.

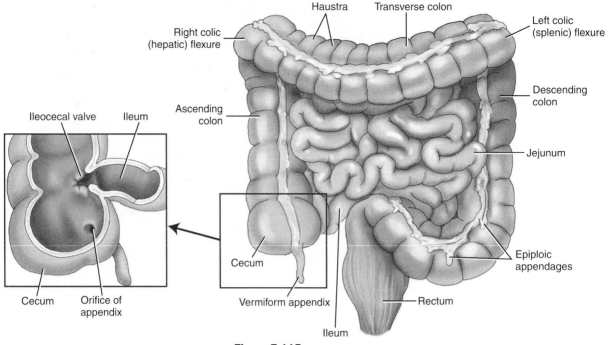

Figure 7.115
Anterior view of small bowel.

INTESTINES

The **small intestine (small bowel)** is located between the pylorus and ileocecal valve and consists of loops of bowel averaging 6 to 7 meters in length. It can be subdivided into the duodenum, jejunum, and the ileum (Figures 7.115 and 7.116). The proximal portion of the small intestine is the **duodenum,** which begins at the gastric pylorus and curves around the head of the pancreas, forming the letter C (Figures 7.113 through 7.117). The duodenum is mostly retroperitoneal, making it less mobile than the rest of the small intestine. Although quite short, the duodenum is divided into four portions. The **first (superior) portion** is formed by the first 2 inches of the duodenum, the conical-shaped **duodenal bulb.** It is the most common site for peptic ulcer formation. The **second (descending) portion** is formed by the next 4 inches of duodenum that descends along the right side of the vertebral column; it contains the ampulla of Vater and receives pancreatic and biliary drainage. The **third (horizontal) portion** is about 10 cm long and runs horizontally in front of the third lumbar vertebra. In its horizontal course from right to left, the third portion of the duodenum runs anterior to the superior vena cava (SVC), aorta, and inferior mesenteric artery and posterior to the superior mesenteric artery. The **fourth (ascending) portion** is about 2.5 cm in length and ascends on the left side of the aorta to the level of the L2 vertebra, where it meets up with the jejunum at the **duodenojejunal flexure.** The duodenojejunal flexure is fixed in place by the **ligament of Treitz,** a suspensory ligament created from the connective tissue around the celiac axis and left crus of the diaphragm (Figure 7.117). This location marks the entry of the small bowel into the peritoneal cavity. The remainder of the small intestine, the jejunum and ileum, is suspended from the posterior abdominal wall by a fan-shaped mesentery. The **jejunum** is approximately 2.5 meters long and occupies the left upper abdomen or umbilical region of the abdomen (Figures 7.115 through 7.119). This section of small bowel is where the bulk of chemical digestion and nutrient absorption occurs. The jejunum contains numerous circular folds that give it a feathery appearance on barium or computed tomography (CT) examinations. The lower three fifths of the small intestine, the **ileum,** is the longest portion of the small intestine, averaging 3.5 meters long and located in the right lower abdomen (Figures 7.115, 7.116, and 7.119 through 7.121). It is in the ileum that intrinsic factor from the stomach combines with vitamin B_{12} for absorption in the terminal ileum. Vitamin B_{12} is essential for normal red blood cell (RBC) formation and nervous system function. The loops of ileum terminate at the **ileocecal valve,** a sphincter that controls the flow of material from the ileum into the cecum of the large intestine (Figures 7.118, 7.122, and 7.123). The mesentery serves as a route for blood vessels, lymphatics, and nerves to reach the small intestine. The segments of the small intestine receive blood from branches of the superior mesenteric artery and are drained by branches of the superior mesenteric vein.

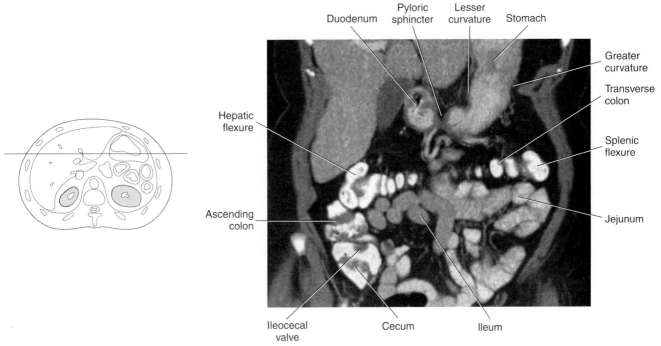

Figure 7.116
Coronal CT reformat of small bowel.

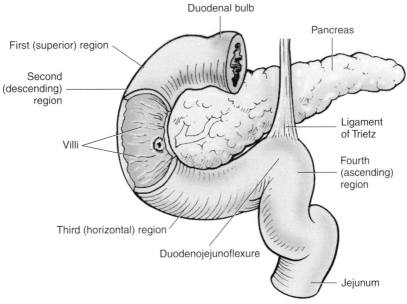

Figure 7.117
Anterior view of duodenum and ligament of Treitz.

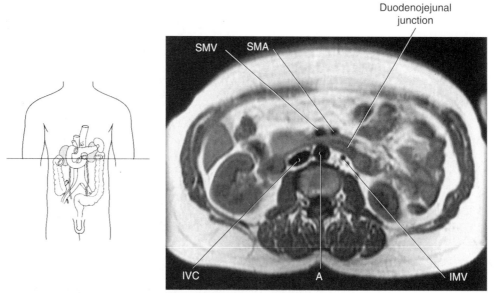

Figure 7.118
Axial, T1-weighted MR scan at duodenojejunal junction.

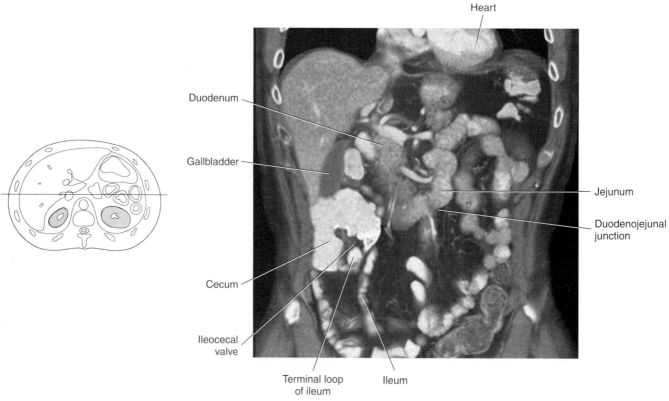

Figure 7.119
Coronal CT reformat of small bowel with duodenojejunal junction.

KEY: **SMV,** superior mesenteric vein; **SMA,** superior mesenteric artery; **IVC,** inferior vena cava; **A,** aorta; **IMV,** inferior mesenteric vein; **reab,** rectus abdominis; **la,** linea alba; **trab,** transverse abdominis; **iob,** internal oblique; **eob,** external oblique; **quad,** quadratus lumborum.

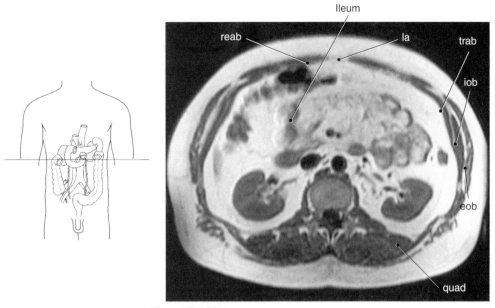

Figure 7.120
Axial, T1-weighted MR scan with ileum.

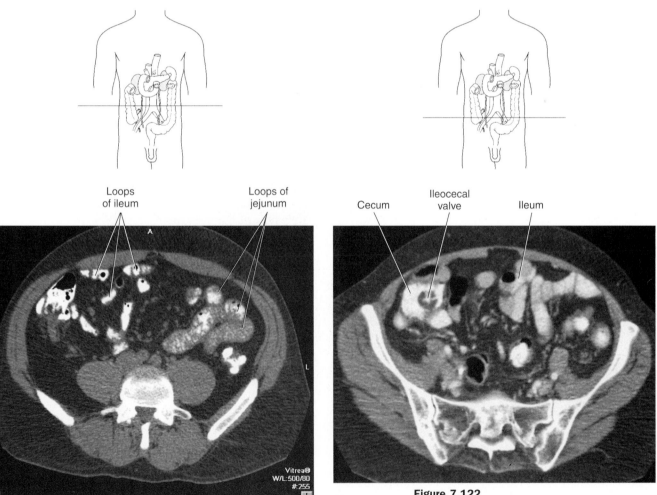

Figure 7.121
Axial CT scan with ileum.

Figure 7.122
Axial CT scan with ileocecal valve.

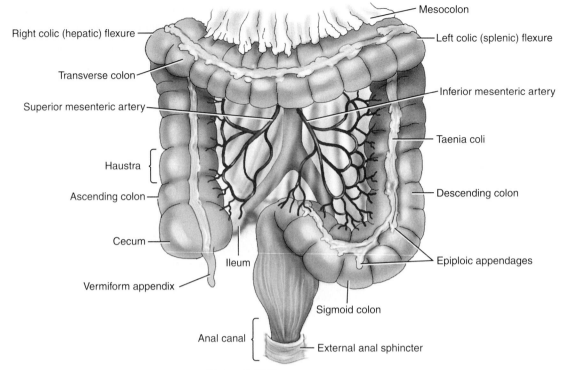

Figure 7.123
Anterior view of large intestine.

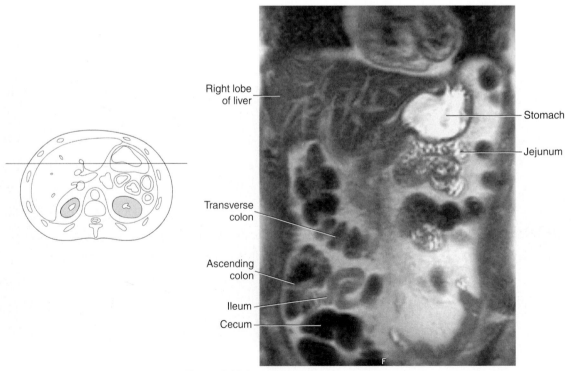

Figure 7.124
Coronal, T1-weighted, MR scan of cecum.

The **large intestine (large bowel)** lies inferior to the stomach and liver and almost completely frames the small intestine (Figures 7.115 and 7.123). The large intestine has a larger diameter and thinner walls than the small intestine and is approximately 1.5 meters long, starting at the ileocecal junction and ending at the anus. The outer, longitudinal muscle of the large intestine forms three thickened bands called **taenia coli** that gather the cecum and colon into a series of pouchlike folds called **haustra.** On the outer surface of the large intestine are small fat-filled sacs of omentum called the **epiploic appendages.** The three main divisions of the large intestine are the cecum, colon, and rectum (Figure 7.123). The **cecum** is a pouchlike section of the proximal portion of the large intestine located at the ileocecal valve. The slender **vermiform appendix** attaches to the posteromedial surface of the cecum (Figures 7.123 through 7.125). The **colon** is the longest portion of the large intestine and can be subdivided into four distinct portions: ascending, transverse, descending, and sigmoid (Figures 7.126 and 7.127). The **ascending colon** is retroperitoneal and commences at the cecum, ascending the right lateral wall of the abdomen to the level of the liver. It

then curves sharply to the left, creating the hepatic flexure (Figures 7.123, 7.128, and 7.129). The **hepatic flexure** marks the beginning of the transverse colon. The **transverse colon** travels horizontally across the anterior abdomen toward the spleen, where it bends sharply downward, creating the **splenic flexure** and the beginning of the descending colon (Figures 7.130 and 7.131). The transverse colon is located within the peritoneal cavity and is the largest and most mobile portion of the large intestine, making its position quite variable in the patient. The **descending colon** is retroperitoneal and continues inferiorly along the left lateral abdominal wall to the iliac fossa, where it curves to become the S-shaped sigmoid colon posterior to the bladder (Figure 7.123). The **sigmoid colon** joins the rectum, which is the terminal portion of the colon (Figures 7.132 and 7.133). The rectum is considered a pelvic organ and is covered in greater detail in Chapter 8. The superior and inferior mesenteric arteries and veins supply and drain blood from the large intestine. The major functions of the large intestine include the reabsorption of water and the storage and elimination of fecal material.

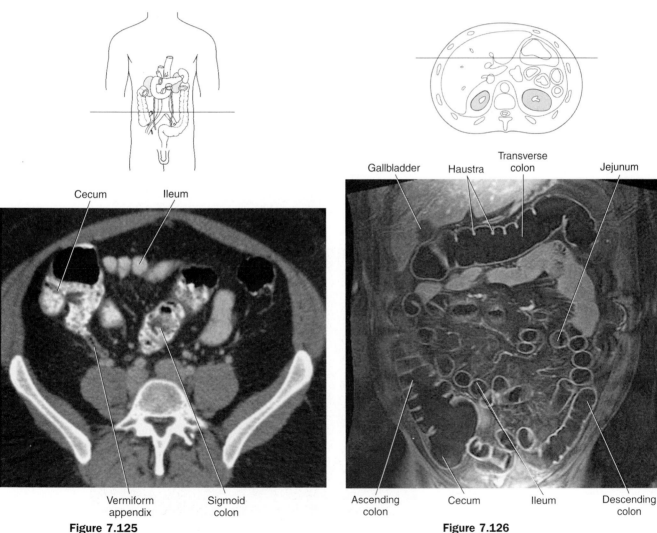

Figure 7.125
Axial CT scan of cecum and appendix.

Figure 7.126
Coronal MR colonography.

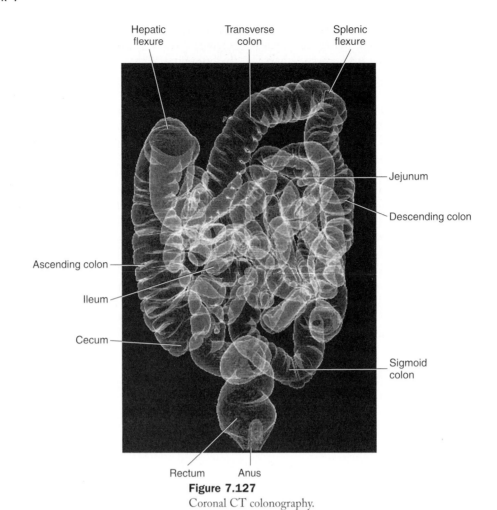

Figure 7.127
Coronal CT colonography.

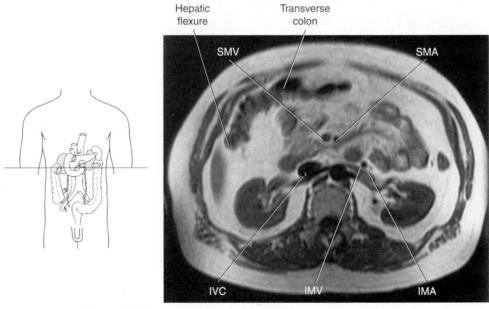

Figure 7.128
Axial, T1-weighted MR scan of hepatic flexure and transverse colon.

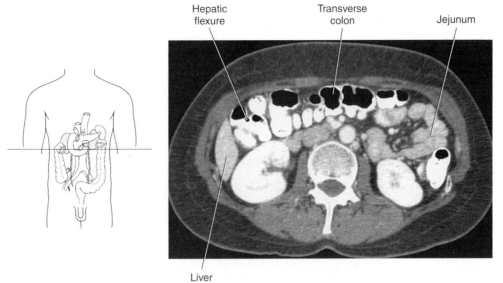

Figure 7.129
Axial CT scan of hepatic flexure and transverse colon.

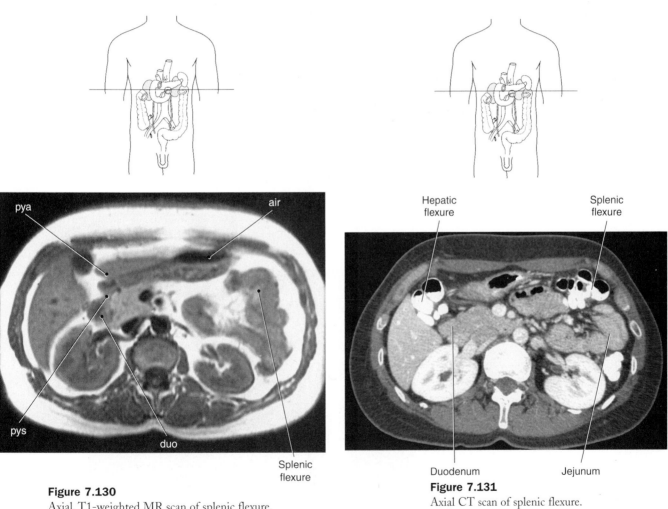

Figure 7.130
Axial, T1-weighted MR scan of splenic flexure.

Figure 7.131
Axial CT scan of splenic flexure.

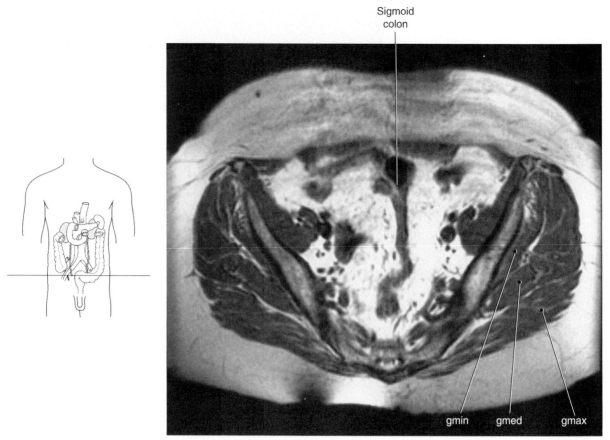

Sigmoid
colon

gmin   gmed   gmax

Figure 7.132
Axial, T1-weighted MR scan of sigmoid colon.

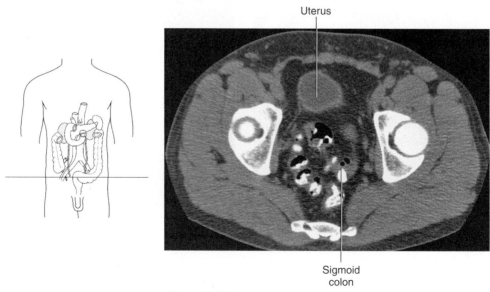

Uterus

Sigmoid
colon

Figure 7.133
Axial CT scan of sigmoid colon.

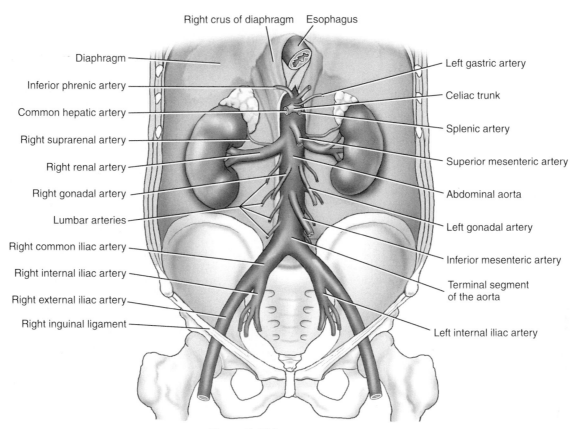

Right crus of diaphragm   Esophagus

Diaphragm

Inferior phrenic artery

Common hepatic artery

Right suprarenal artery

Right renal artery

Right gonadal artery

Lumbar arteries

Right common iliac artery

Right internal iliac artery

Right external iliac artery

Right inguinal ligament

Left gastric artery

Celiac trunk

Splenic artery

Superior mesenteric artery

Abdominal aorta

Left gonadal artery

Inferior mesenteric artery

Terminal segment
of the aorta

Left internal iliac artery

Figure 7.134
Anterior view of abdominal aorta.

KEY: **gmin,** gluteus minimus; **gmed,** gluteus medius; **gmax,** gluteus maximus.

ABDOMINAL AORTA AND BRANCHES

The **abdominal aorta** is a retroperitoneal structure beginning, as an extension of the thoracic aorta, at the aortic hiatus of the diaphragm. The abdominal aorta has a gradual diminishment of its diameter as it descends the abdomen just left of the midline next to the vertebral bodies. It delivers blood to all the abdominopelvic organs and structures. At approximately the level of L4, the abdominal aorta bifurcates into the right and left **common iliac** arteries. The branches of the abdominal aorta can be divided into the paired **(dorsal) parietal branches,** including the inferior phrenic and lumbar arteries; paired **visceral branches,** including the suprarenal, renal, and gonadal arteries; and unpaired **(ventral) visceral branches** that include the celiac trunk, splenic, superior mesenteric, and inferior mesenteric arteries (Figures 7.134 through 7.136). Each of these branches has a typical configuration that is described within this text; however, many normal variations of these vessels may occur.

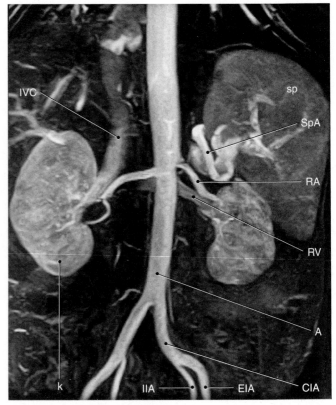

Figure 7.135
MR angiogram of abdominal aorta.

Figure 7.136
CT angiogram of abdominal aorta.

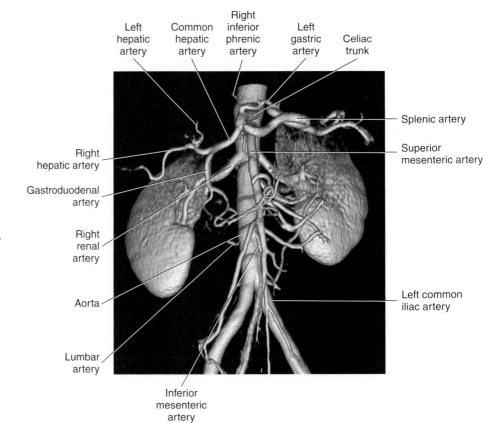

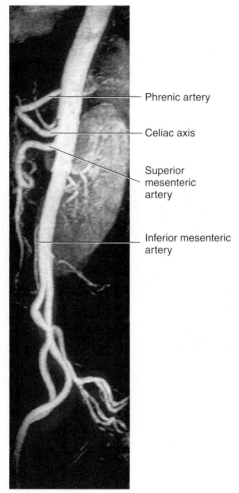

Figure 7.137
Sagittal MR angiogram of abdominal aorta.

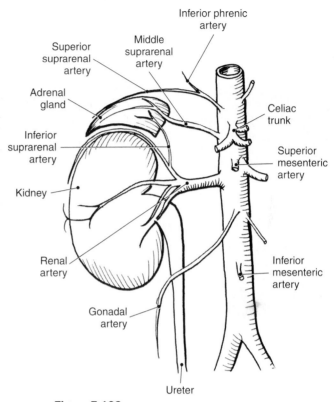

Figure 7.138
Anterior view of paired branches of the abdominal aorta.

Paired Parietal (Dorsal) Branches

The parietal (dorsal) branches supply the diaphragm and trunk wall and include the inferior phrenic and lumbar arteries. The paired **inferior phrenic arteries** are first to branch from the lateral surface of the abdominal aorta just as it descends through the aortic hiatus. The **right inferior phrenic artery** passes upward on the right side behind the IVC, and the **left inferior phrenic artery** passes behind the stomach and the abdominal part of the esophagus (Figures 7.134 and 7.137). The phrenic arteries extend to supply the inferior surface of the diaphragm and dispatch the **superior suprarenal arteries** to the upper pole of the suprarenal glands (Figure 7.138).

Four pair of **lumbar arteries** arise from the posterior wall of the abdominal aorta at the level of L1-L4 (Figures 7.134 and 7.136). The lumbar arteries supply the posterior abdominal wall, lumbar vertebrae, and the inferior end of the spinal cord (see Chapter 4 for branches of the lumbar arteries). Extending from the dorsal wall of the aorta, somewhat above the aortic bifurcation, is the **median sacral artery,** which continues caudally in front of the sacrum. It gives off the fifth pair of lumbar arteries as lateral branches and terminates anterior to the apex of the coccyx.

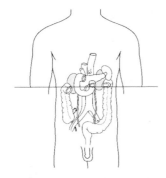

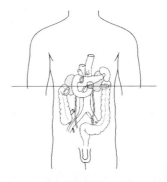

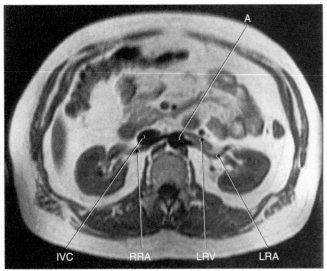

Figure 7.139
MRA of abdomen with renal arteries and veins.

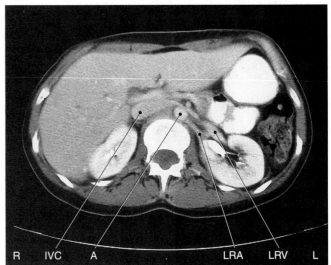

Figure 7.140
Axial CT scan of abdomen with renal arteries and veins.

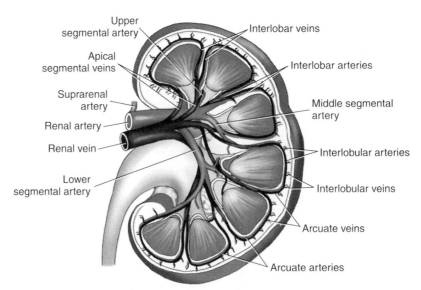

Figure 7.141
Anterior view of renal vasculature.

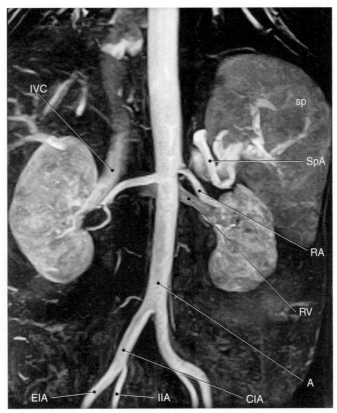

Figure 7.142
MRA of renal arteries.

Paired Visceral Branches

SUPRARENAL ARTERIES   The **middle suprarenal arteries** exit the lateral walls of the aorta near the base of the superior mesenteric artery. These arteries course laterally and slightly superiorly to supply the adrenal glands. The **superior suprarenal** arteries are branches of the inferior phrenic arteries, and the **inferior suprarenal arteries** extend from the renal arteries (Figures 7.134 and 7.138).

RENAL ARTERIES   The two large **renal arteries** arise from the lateral walls of the aorta just below the superior mesenteric artery. Each vessel travels horizontally to the hilum of the corresponding kidney (Figures 7.134 through 7.136). Because of the position of the aorta on the left side of the vertebral column, the right renal artery is slightly longer than the left renal artery. The right renal artery passes posterior to the inferior vena cava and right renal vein on its course to the right kidney (Figure 7.139). Typically, the left kidney is higher than the right kidney, which means the left renal artery is generally slightly superior to the right (Figure 7.140). As each

renal artery reaches the renal hilum, it typically divides into anterior and posterior branches from which five segmental arteries—**apical, upper, middle, lower, and posterior**—arise (Figures 7.141 through 7.143). Each segmental artery further divides into lobar arteries, one for each pyramid and adjoining cortex.

> **Renal artery stenosis causes renal ischemia and can result in secondary hypertension.**

GONADAL ARTERIES   The **gonadal arteries** originate from the anterior wall of the aorta just inferior to the renal arteries. They descend along the psoas muscles to reach their respective organs (Figures 7.134, 7.144, and 7.145). In the male, the gonadal arteries are termed the **testicular arteries,** which supply the testes and scrotum, whereas the gonadal arteries in the female are termed the **ovarian arteries** and supply the ovaries, uterine tubes, and uterus.

KEY: **A,** Aorta; **IVC,** inferior vena cava; **RRA,** right renal artery; **LRV,** left renal vein; **LRA,** left renal artery; **EIA,** external iliac artery; **IIA,** internal iliac artery; **CIA,** common iliac artery; **RV,** renal vein; **RA,** renal artery; **SpA,** splenic artery; **sp,** spleen.

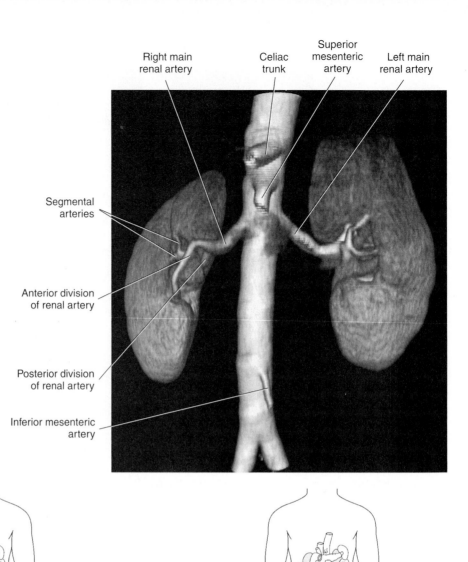

Right main renal artery

Celiac trunk

Superior mesenteric artery

Left main renal artery

Segmental arteries

Anterior division of renal artery

Posterior division of renal artery

Inferior mesenteric artery

Figure 7.143
CTA of renal arteries. *SMA*, Superior mesenteric artery.

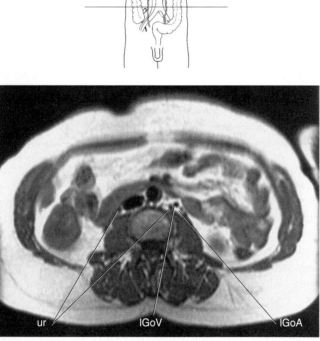

ur   lGoV   lGoA

Figure 7.144
Axial, T1-weighted MR scan of abdomen and gonadal arteries and veins.

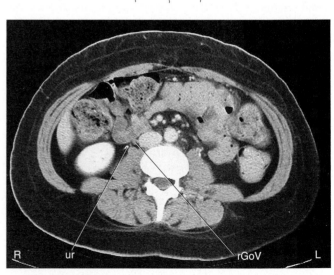

R   ur   rGoV   L

Figure 7.145
Axial CT scan of abdomen and gonadal arteries and veins.

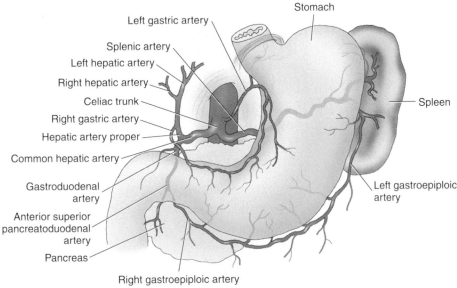

Figure 7.146
Anterior view of celiac trunk and branches.

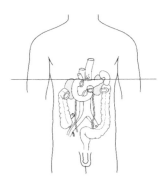

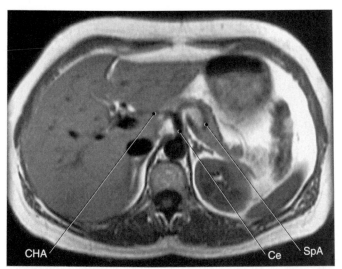

Figure 7.147
Axial, T1-weighted MR scan of abdomen with celiac trunk.

KEY: **ur,** Ureters; **lGoV,** gonadal vein; **lGoA,** gonadal artery; **rGoV,** right gonadal vein; **CHA,** common hepatic artery; **Ce,** celiac axis; **SpA,** splenic artery.

Unpaired Visceral Branches

CELIAC TRUNK   The celiac trunk is a very short vessel that leaves the anterior wall of the aorta just after the aorta passes through the diaphragm. The short celiac trunk divides into three branches: left gastric, common hepatic, and splenic arteries (Figures 7.146 through 7.148). Variations of the celiac trunk are not rare; occasionally the hepatic artery will branch from the superior mesenteric artery.

The **left gastric** artery courses superiorly and leftward within the lesser omentum to supply the cardiac region of the stomach then passes along the lesser curvature toward the pylorus, giving off esophageal and gastric branches to supply the abdominal esophagus and adjacent anterior and posterior walls of the body of the stomach. The left gastric artery continues toward the right to anastomose with the right gastric artery, which is a branch of the hepatic artery (Figures 7.146 and 7.149 through 7.152).

The **common hepatic artery** crosses to the right toward the superior aspect of the duodenum and divides into the **hepatic artery proper** and the **gastroduodenal artery** (Figures 7.146 through 7.148 and 7.151 and 7.152). The hepatic artery proper ascends obliquely to the right in the hepatoduodenal ligament, adjacent to the portal vein and common bile duct, and divides near the porta hepatis into the **right** and **left hepatic** branches and usually gives off the **right gastric artery** (Figures 7.146, 7.151, and 7.152). The right hepatic branch dispatches the **cystic artery** to the gallbladder and divides into the anterior and posterior segmental arteries to supply the segments of the right and caudate lobes of the liver. The left branch also gives off an artery to the caudate lobe, as well as medial and lateral segmental arteries to supply the segments of the left lobe and the intermediate branch to the quadrate lobe. The **right gastric artery,** which can also come from the

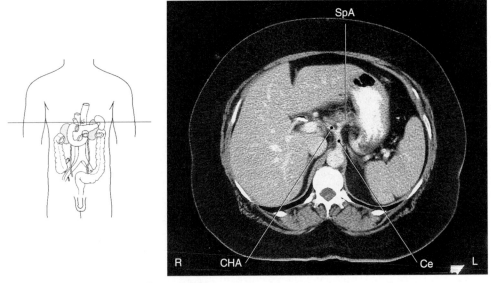

Figure 7.148
Axial CT scan of abdomen with celiac trunk.

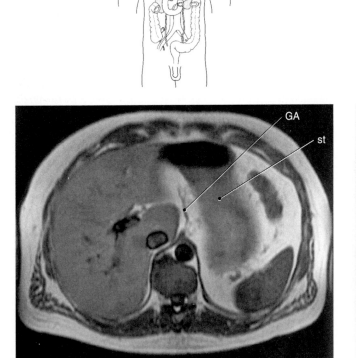

Figure 7.149
Axial, T1-weighted MR scan of abdomen with gastric artery.

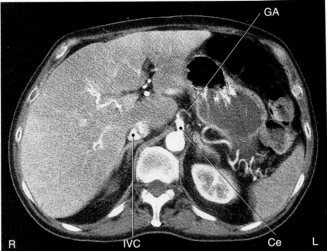

Figure 7.150
Axial CT scan of abdomen with gastric artery.

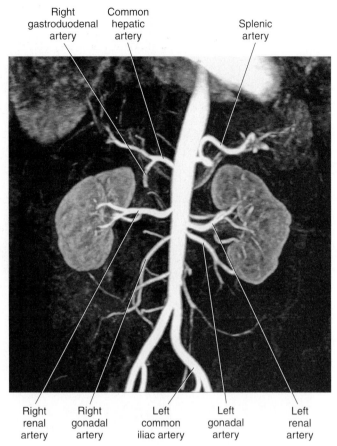

Right
gastroduodenal
artery

Common
hepatic
artery

Splenic
artery

Right
renal
artery

Right
gonadal
artery

Left
common
iliac artery

Left
gonadal
artery

Left
renal
artery

Figure 7.151
MR angiogram of celiac trunk.

common hepatic or gastroduodenal arteries, supplies the lower part of the lesser curvature of the stomach and anastomoses with the left gastric artery within the lesser curvature of the stomach (Figures 7.146 and 7.151). The **gastroduodenal artery** descends behind the pylorus to give off many branches, including the **anterior and posterior superior pancreatico-duodenal arteries,** which supply the superior part of the duodenum and head of the pancreas, and the **right gastro-epiploic (gastro-omental) artery.** The right gastroepiploic artery passes in the greater omentum, anastomoses with the left gastroepiploic artery on the inferior surface of the greater curvature, and dispatches numerous gastric branches to the anterior and posterior walls of the pyloric and body portions of the stomach (Figures 7.146, and 7.151 through 7.153).

The **splenic (lienal) artery** is the largest branch of the celiac trunk and passes to the left behind the stomach and along the upper border of the pancreas, within the splenorenal ligament, to the hilum of the spleen. At the point where the splenic artery courses near the border of the pancreas, it gives off numerous **pancreatic branches** that supply the body and tail of the pancreas, including the **dorsal, great,** and **caudal pancreatic arteries** (Figure 7.154). Just before the splenic artery terminates into numerous splenic branches, it gives rise to the **left gastroepiploic (gastro-omental) artery,** which gives off epiploic and gastric branches to the greater omentum and anterior and posterior walls of the fundus of the stomach (Figures 7.146 and 7.151 through 7.156).

KEY: **SpA,** splenic artery; **CHA,** common hepatic artery; **Ce,** celiac axis; **GA,** left gastric artery; **st,** stomach; **IVC,** inferior vena cava.

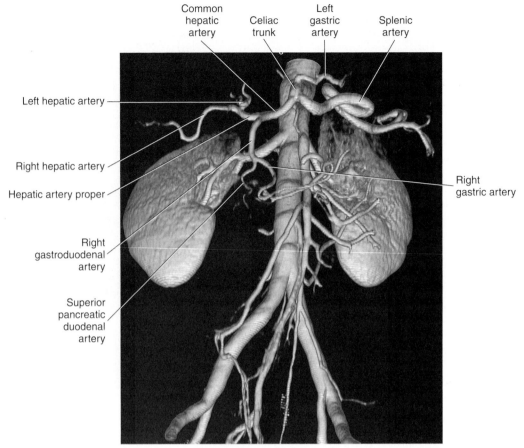

Common hepatic artery

Celiac trunk

Left gastric artery

Splenic artery

Left hepatic artery

Right hepatic artery

Hepatic artery proper

Right gastric artery

Right gastroduodenal artery

Superior pancreatic duodenal artery

Figure 7.152
CT angiogram of celiac trunk.

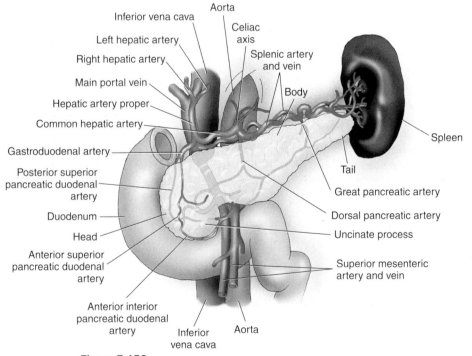

Inferior vena cava

Aorta

Celiac axis

Left hepatic artery

Right hepatic artery

Splenic artery and vein

Main portal vein

Body

Hepatic artery proper

Common hepatic artery

Spleen

Gastroduodenal artery

Posterior superior pancreatic duodenal artery

Tail

Duodenum

Great pancreatic artery

Head

Dorsal pancreatic artery

Anterior superior pancreatic duodenal artery

Uncinate process

Superior mesenteric artery and vein

Anterior interior pancreatic duodenal artery

Inferior vena cava

Aorta

Figure 7.153
Anterior view of hepatic artery, common bile duct, and portal vein.

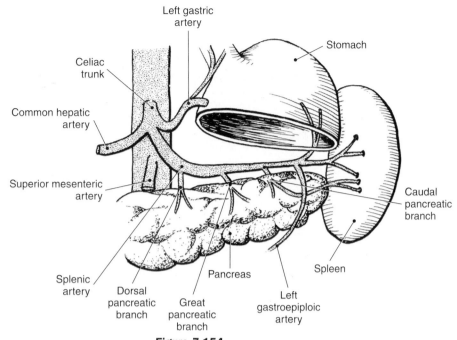

Left gastric
artery

Stomach

Celiac
trunk

Common hepatic
artery

Superior mesenteric
artery

Caudal
pancreatic
branch

Splenic
artery

Dorsal
pancreatic
branch

Great
pancreatic
branch

Pancreas

Left
gastroepiploic
artery

Spleen

Figure 7.154
Anterior view of splenic artery.

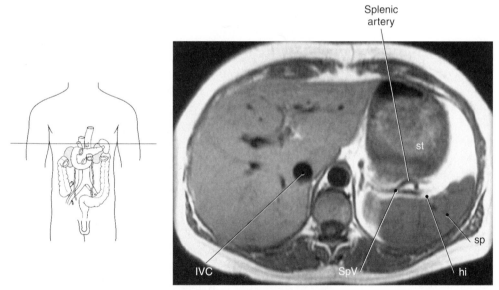

Splenic
artery

st

IVC

SpV

hi

sp

Figure 7.155
Axial, T1-weighted MR scan of splenic artery.

KEY: IVC, Inferior vena cava; **SpV,** splenic vein; **hi,** hilum; **sp,** spleen; **st,** stomach.

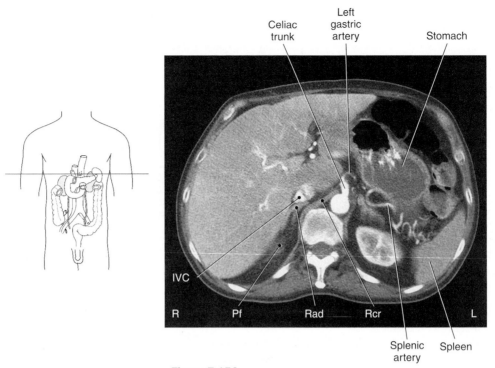

Figure 7.156
Axial CT scan of splenic artery.

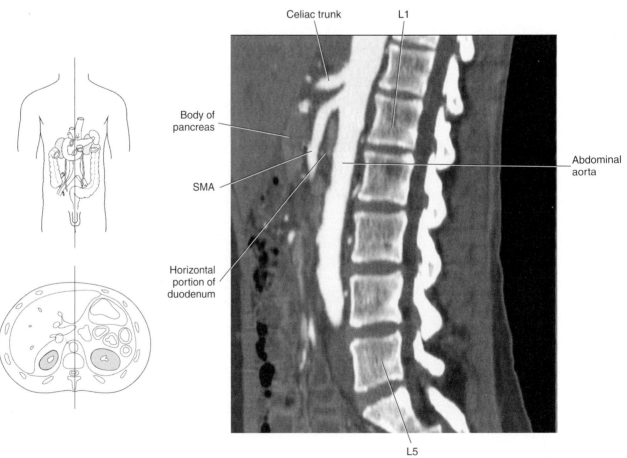

Figure 7.157
Sagittal CT reformat of superior mesenteric artery.

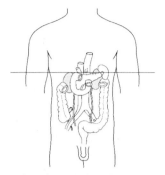

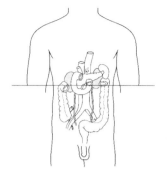

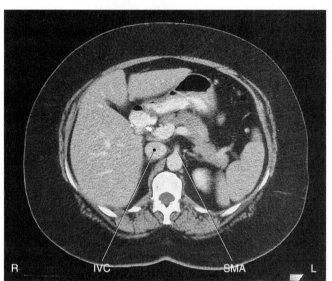

Figure 7.158
Axial CT scan with superior mesenteric artery.

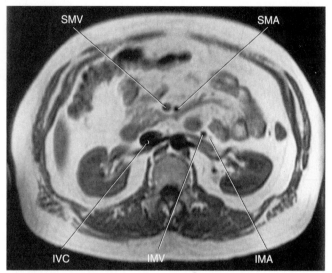

Figure 7.159
Axial, T1-weighted MR scan of superior mesenteric vessels.

SUPERIOR MESENTERIC ARTERY   The large superior mesenteric artery branches just below the celiac trunk at approximately the level of L1 (Figures 7.134, 7.157, and 7.158). It descends behind the body of the pancreas, then over the horizontal portion of the duodenum to course in the mesentery to the ileum (Figures 7.157, 7.159, and 7.160). The artery supplies the head of the pancreas and the majority of the small and large intestines. Branches of the **superior mesenteric artery** include the inferior pancreaticoduodenal artery, jejunal arteries, ileal arteries, middle colic artery, right colic artery, and ileocolic artery (Figure 7.161). The **inferior pancreaticoduodenal artery** extends to the head of the pancreas and duodenum, then divides into the posterior ramus anastomosing with the posterior superior pancreaticoduodenal artery and the anterior ramus, which anastomoses with the anterior superior pancreaticoduodenal artery. The **jejunal** and **ileal arteries** extend to supply the jejunum and ileum, except the end segment near the cecum. The **middle colic artery** reaches the transverse colon and the **right colic artery** passes to the ascending colon. The **ileocolic artery** courses behind the peritoneum across the right ureter into the right iliac fossa and divides to supply a portion of the ascending colon, the cecum, vermiform appendix, and terminal portion of the ileum (Figures 7.162 and 7.163).

KEY: IVC, Inferior vena cava; **Pf,** perirenal fat; **Rad,** right adrenal gland; **Rcr,** right crus; **SMA,** superior mesenteric artery; **SMV,** superior mesenteric vein; **IMV,** inferior mesenteric vein; **IMA,** inferior mesenteric vein.

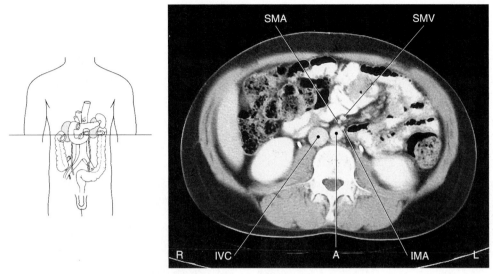

Figure 7.160
Axial CT scan of inferior mesenteric vessels.

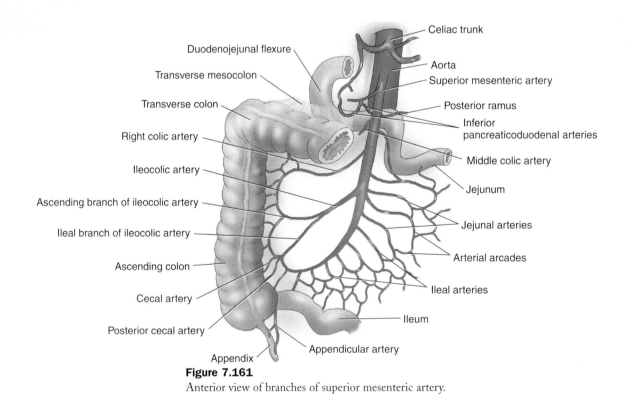

Figure 7.161
Anterior view of branches of superior mesenteric artery.

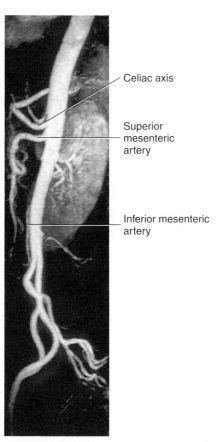

Figure 7.162
Sagittal MR angiogram of superior mesenteric artery.

Celiac axis

Superior
mesenteric
artery

Inferior mesenteric
artery

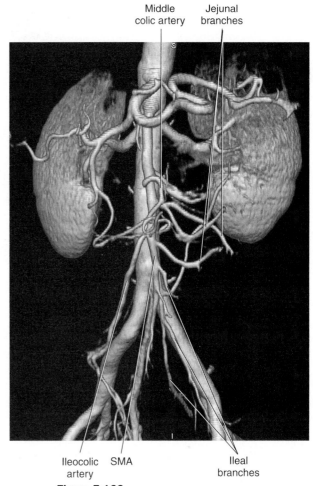

Middle
colic artery

Jejunal
branches

Ileocolic
artery

SMA

Ileal
branches

Figure 7.163
CT angiogram of superior mesenteric artery.

KEY: SMA, Superior mesenteric artery; **SMV,** superior mesenteric vein; **IVC,** inferior vena cava; **A,** aorta; **IMA,** inferior mesenteric vein.

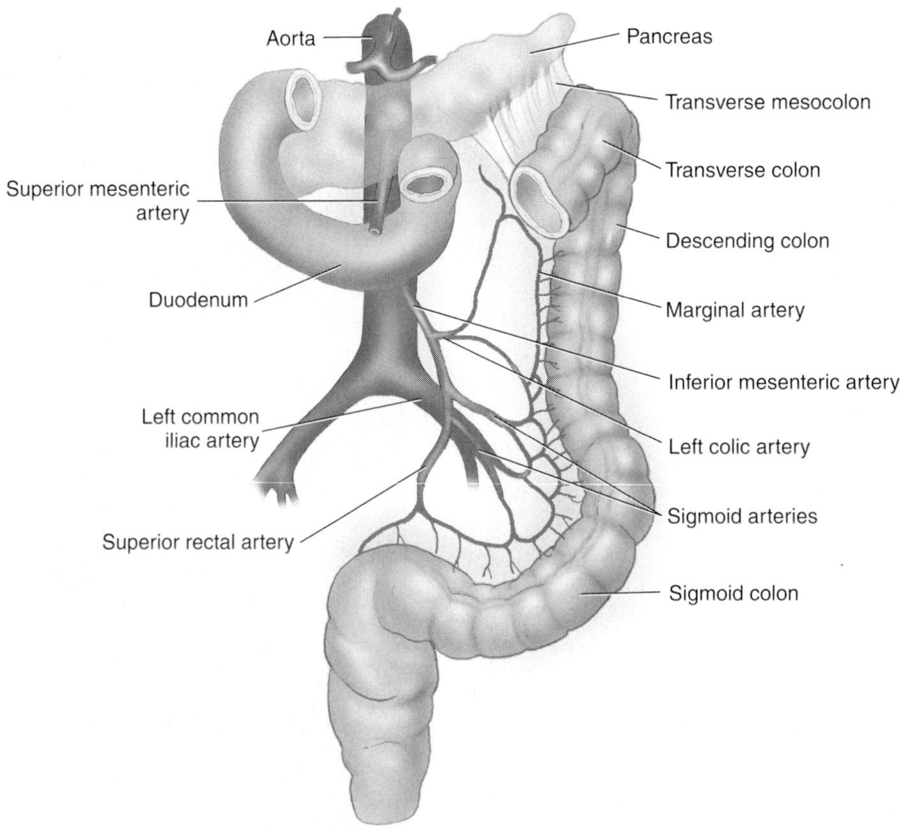

Figure 7.164
Anterior view of inferior mesenteric artery.

INFERIOR MESENTERIC ARTERY   The inferior mesenteric artery arises 3 to 4 cm above the bifurcation of the aorta at approximately the level of L3-L4. It descends in front of the abdominal aorta and then to the left, where it gives off the left colic artery, sigmoid arteries, and the superior rectal arteries (Figures 7.159, 7.160, and 7.164). The **left colic artery** is a retroperitoneal structure that passes along the posterior body wall on the anterior surface of the left psoas and quadratus lumborum muscles. It bifurcates into ascending and descending branches that supply the walls of the left third of the transverse colon and the entire descending colon. The **sigmoid branches** (2 or 3) course within the mesentery to supply branches to the terminal descending colon and to the sigmoid colon. The **superior rectal artery** crosses the common iliac artery and vein as it descends to branch and supply the rectum (Figures 7.165 through 7.166).

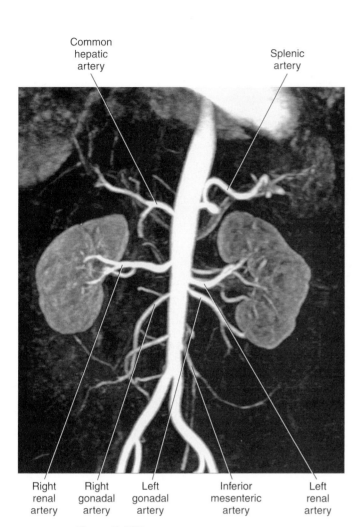

Common
hepatic
artery

Splenic
artery

Right
renal
artery

Right
gonadal
artery

Left
gonadal
artery

Inferior
mesenteric
artery

Left
renal
artery

Figure 7.165
MR angiogram of inferior mesenteric artery.

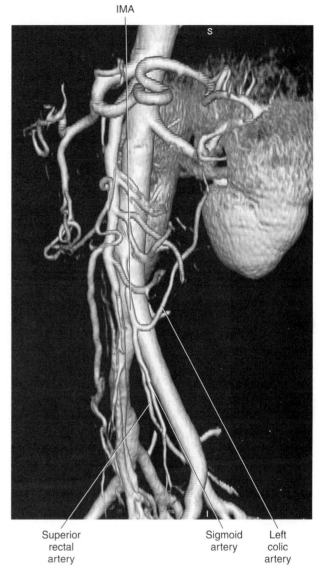

IMA

S

Superior
rectal
artery

Sigmoid
artery

Left
colic
artery

Figure 7.166
CT angiogram of inferior mesenteric artery (IMA).

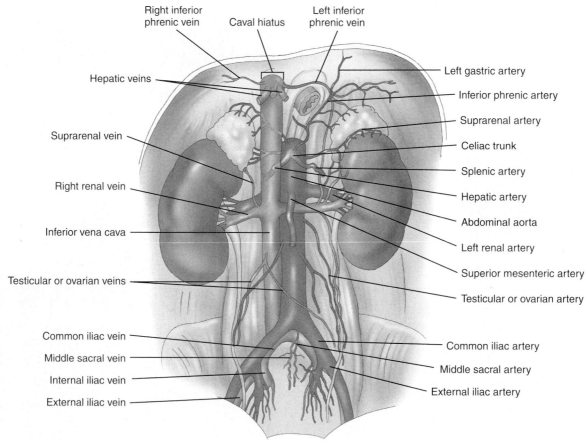

Figure 7.167
Anterior view of abdominal aorta and inferior vena cava.

INFERIOR VENA CAVA AND TRIBUTARIES

The **IVC** is the largest vein of the body (Figure 7.167). It carries blood to the heart from the lower limbs, pelvic organs and the abdominal viscera, and abdominal wall. The IVC is formed by the union of the common iliac veins at approximately the level of L5. It courses superiorly through the retroperitoneum along the anterior aspect of the vertebral column and to the right of the aorta (Figures 7.159 and 7.160). As the IVC ascends the abdominal cavity, it passes the posterior surface of the liver and pierces the diaphragm at the caval hiatus to enter the right atrium of the heart. The IVC receives many tributaries throughout its course in the abdomen that include the inferior phrenic, lumbar, right gonadal, renal, right suprarenal, and hepatic veins (Figure 7.167).

Inferior Phrenic Veins

The inferior phrenic veins extend from the inferior surface of the diaphragm. The **left inferior phrenic vein** is often doubled and drains into either the left suprarenal vein or to the left renal vein. The **right inferior phrenic vein** drains directly into the inferior vena cava (Figure 7.167).

Lumbar Veins

The **lumbar veins** consist of four pairs of vessels that collect blood from the posterior abdominal wall from the level of L1 to L4 (Figures 7.168 through 7.170). They receive veins from the vertebral plexuses and then travel horizontally along the transverse processes deep to the psoas muscles. The lumbar veins on the left are typically longer than those on the right because they must cross over the vertebral column to drain into the IVC. The arrangement of these veins varies, with some entering the lateral walls of the IVC and others emptying into the common iliac vein or are united on each side by a vertical connecting vein termed the **ascending lumbar vein.** Typically, the right ascending lumbar vein continues as the azygos vein and the left ascending lumbar vein continues as the hemiazygos vein. Additionally, a diminutive median sacral vein may accompany the median sacral artery. It typically drains into the left common iliac vein but may also drain into the junction of the common iliac veins (Figure 7.167).

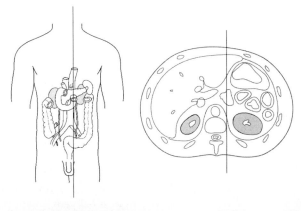

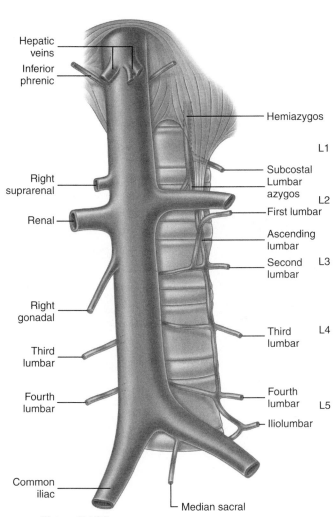

Figure 7.168
Anterior view of inferior vena cava and lumbar veins.

Hepatic veins
Inferior phrenic
Hemiazygos
L1
Right suprarenal
Subcostal
Lumbar azygos
L2
Renal
First lumbar
Ascending lumbar
Second lumbar
L3
Right gonadal
Third lumbar
L4
Third lumbar
Fourth lumbar
Fourth lumbar
L5
Iliolumbar
Common iliac
Median sacral

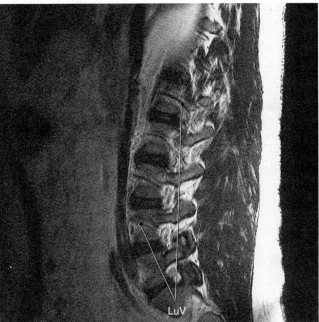

Figure 7.169
Sagittal, T1-weighted MR scan with lumbar veins.

LuV

KEY: LuV, Lumbar veins.

Gonadal Veins

The gonadal veins, ovarian in females and testicular in males, ascend the abdomen along the psoas muscle, anterior to the ureters. The **right gonadal vein** enters the anterolateral wall of the IVC just below the opening for the right renal vein, whereas the **left gonadal vein** empties into the left renal vein (Figures 7.144, 7.145, and 7.167).

Renal Veins

Blood leaves the kidney by way of **interlobular veins** that carry blood from the renal cortex to the **arcuate veins,** which carry blood from the medulla to the interlobar veins. The **interlobar veins** join to form the renal vein at the renal hilum (Figure 7.141). The **renal veins** pass anterior to the renal arteries to empty into the IVC at about the level of L2. The **left renal vein** passes posterior to the superior mesenteric artery and anterior to the aorta on its route from the left kidney to enter the left lateral wall of the IVC. It receives the left gonadal vein, left inferior phrenic vein, and generally the left suprarenal vein. The shorter **right renal vein** is typically lower than the left renal vein as it travels its short course to enter the right lateral wall of the IVC (Figures 7.167, 7.171, and 7.172).

Suprarenal Veins

The **right suprarenal vein** courses from the medial side of the right suprarenal gland to empty directly into the IVC. The **left suprarenal vein** courses from the inferior pole of the left suprarenal gland to empty directly into the left renal vein or left inferior phrenic vein (Figures 7.167 and 7.168).

Hepatic Veins

The three short **hepatic veins (right, middle, left)** begin as smaller vessels that collect blood from the liver parenchyma. The hepatic veins course from the inferior aspect of the liver to the superior aspect of the liver, where they empty into the IVC just below the diaphragm. In general, the right and left hepatic veins drain the right and left lobes of the liver, respectively, whereas the middle hepatic vein drains the medial segment of the left lobe and the anterior portions of the right (see Liver section, Figures 7.61, 7.62, and 7.167).

KEY: pa, Pancreas; **GB,** gallbladder; **duo,** duodenum; **IVC,** inferior vena cava; **SMV,** superior mesenteric vein; **LRV,** left renal vein; **RRV,** right renal vein; **A,** aorta.

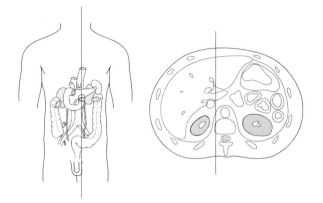

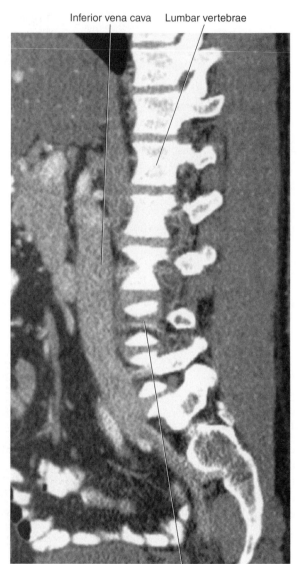

Inferior vena cava   Lumbar vertebrae

Lumbar veins

Figure 7.170
Sagittal CT reformat with lumbar veins. *SMA,* Superior mesenteric artery.

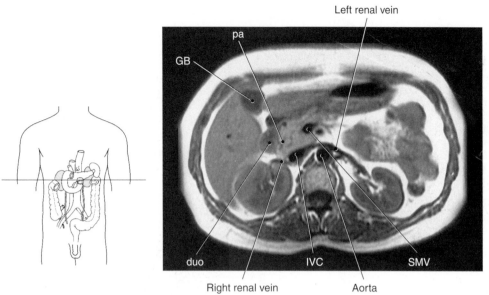

Figure 7.171
Axial, T1-weighted MR scan with renal veins.

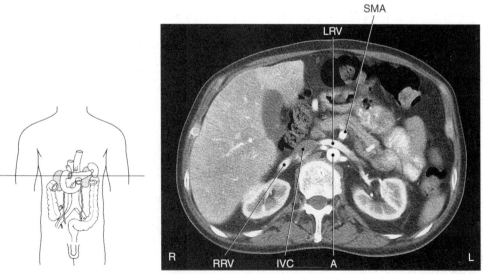

Figure 7.172
Axial CT scan with renal veins.

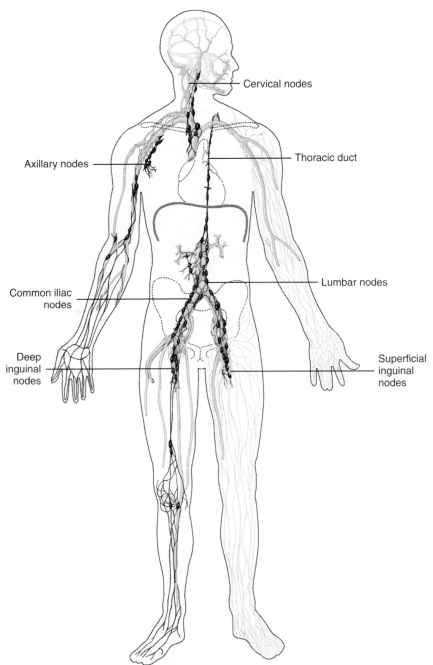

Figure 7.173
Anterior view of lymphatic system.

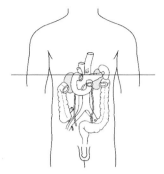

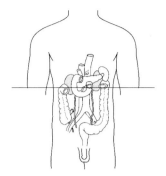

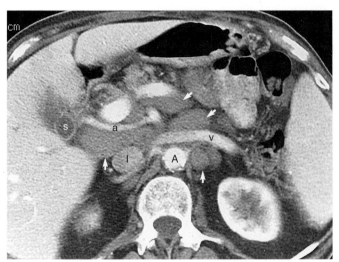

Figure 7.174
Axial CT scan of upper abdomen with enlarged lymph nodes *(arrows)*.

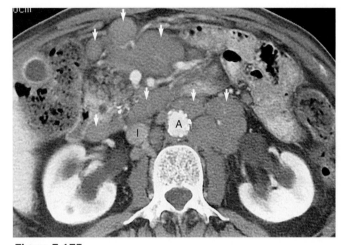

Figure 7.175
Axial CT scan of abdomen with enlarged lymph nodes *(arrows)* in small bowel mesentery.

LYMPH NODES

Many lymph nodes exist within the abdominal cavity. Abdominal lymph nodes occur in chains along the main branches of the arteries of the intestine and abdominal aorta. Most abdominal lymph nodes appear as small oblong soft tissue masses oriented parallel to their accompanying vessels and may be difficult to visualize in cross section unless they are enlarged as a result of an abnormality. Typically, lymph nodes are considered enlarged if their short axis diameter is greater than 1 cm. **Abdominoaortic nodal groups** surround the aorta and IVC and **visceral lymph nodes** drain adjacent organs that include the mesenteric hepatic, splenic, and pancreatico-duodenal nodal groups. Lymph from the abdominal cavity empties into the lumbar trunk, which drains lymph from the legs, lower abdominal wall, and the pelvic organs; and the intestinal trunk, which drains organs located within the abdominal cavity. These trunks then join the **thoracic duct** and ultimately enter the venous system (Figures 7.173 through 7.175).

KEY: **s,** gallbladder; **a,** hepatic artery; **I,** inferior vena cava; **A,** aorta; **v,** splenic vein.

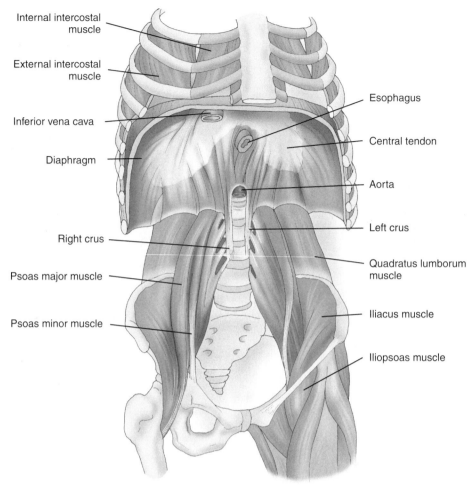

Figure 7.176
Anterior view of psoas and quadratus lumborum muscles.

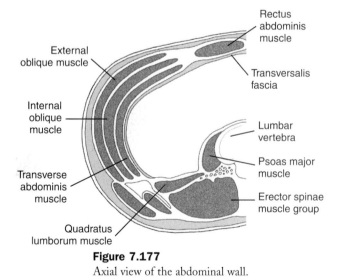

Figure 7.177
Axial view of the abdominal wall.

MUSCLES OF THE ABDOMINAL WALL

The **abdominal wall** is formed superiorly by the **diaphragm** and is inferiorly continuous with the pelvic cavity at the pelvic inlet. Posteriorly, the abdominal wall is formed by the five lumbar vertebrae, twelfth pair of ribs, upper portion of the pelvis, quadratus lumborum muscles, and psoas muscles (Figure 7.176). The **quadratus lumborum muscle** forms a large portion of the posterior abdominal wall. It extends from the iliac crest to the inferior border of the twelfth rib and transverse processes of the lumbar vertebrae to aid in lateral flexion of the vertebral column. The large **psoas muscles** extend along the lateral surfaces of the lumbar vertebrae to insert on the lesser trochanter of the femur and act to flex the thigh and trunk (Figures 7.177 through 7.180). Anteriorly, the abdominal wall is formed by the lower portion of the thoracic cage and by layers of muscles that include the rectus abdominis, external

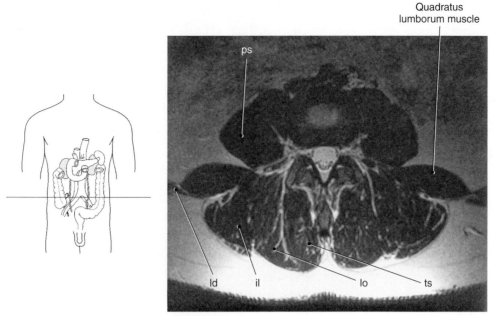

Figure 7.178
Axial, T1-weighted MR scan of psoas and quadratus lumborum muscles.

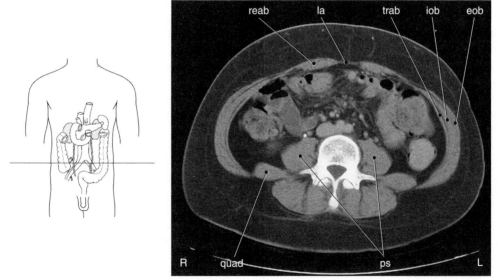

Figure 7.179
Axial CT scan of psoas and quadratus lumborum muscles.

KEY: ps, psoas muscles; **ld,** latissimus dorsi; **il,** iliocostalis muscle; **lo,** longissimus muscle; **ts,** transversospinal muscles; **reab,** rectus abdominis; **la,** linea alba; **trab,** transverse abdominis; **iob,** internal oblique; **eob,** external oblique; **quad,** quadratus lumborum.

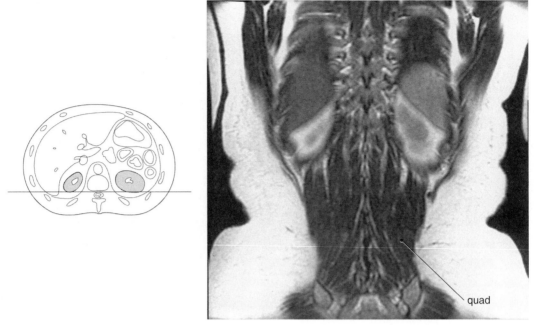

Figure 7.180
Coronal, T1-weighted MR scan of quadratus lumborum muscle.

oblique, internal oblique, and transversus abdominis (Figures 7.181 and 7.182). The paired **rectus abdominis muscles,** visualized on the anterior surface of the abdomen and pelvis, originate from the pubic symphysis and extend vertically to the xiphoid process and costal cartilage of the fifth, sixth, and seventh ribs. They function to flex the lumbar vertebrae and support the abdomen (Figures 7.177 and 7.179). The anterior surface of the rectus muscle is crossed by three tendinous intersections that course transversely, forming individual muscle bellies that can contract separately (Figure 7.181). A longitudinal band of fibers that forms a central anterior attachment for the muscle layers of the abdomen is the **linea alba,** which extends from the xiphoid process of the sternum to the pubic symphysis. The linea alba is formed, at the midline, by the interlacing of fibers from the rectus abdominis and oblique muscles (Figures 7.178, 7.179, and 7.182). The **external** and **internal oblique** muscles are located on the outer lateral portion of the abdomen and extend from the cartilages of the lower ribs to the level of the iliac crest (Figures 7.177, 7.179,

and 7.181 through 7.183). The oblique muscles work together to flex and rotate the vertebral column and compress the abdominal viscera. The external oblique is the most extensive of the three broad abdominal muscles and contains a triangular opening, the superficial inguinal ring, that allows for the passage of the spermatic cord or round ligament of the uterus (Figure 7.181). The **inguinal ligament** is a fibrous band formed by the thickened inferior border of the aponeurosis of the external oblique muscle. It extends from the anterior superior iliac spine to the pubic tubercle and gives origin to the lowermost fibers of the internal oblique and transversus abdominis muscles (Figure 7.182). The **transversus abdominis** muscle lies deep to the internal oblique muscles. Its fibers extend transversely across the abdomen to provide maximum support for the abdominal viscera. The transversus abdominis muscle extends from the lower six costal cartilages, lumbar fascia, iliac crest, and inguinal ligament to insert into the xiphoid process, linea alba, and pubic symphysis (Figures 7.177, 7.179, and 7.183 and Table 7.3).

KEY: quad, Quadratus lumborum.

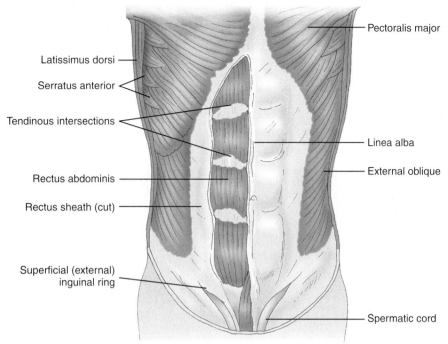

Latissimus dorsi

Serratus anterior

Tendinous intersections

Rectus abdominis

Rectus sheath (cut)

Superficial (external)
inguinal ring

Pectoralis major

Linea alba

External oblique

Spermatic cord

Figure 7.181
Anterior view of muscles of abdominal wall.

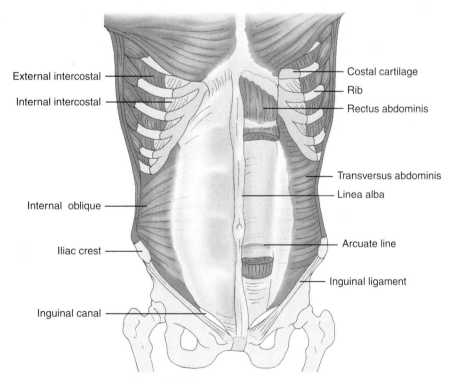

External intercostal

Internal intercostal

Internal oblique

Iliac crest

Inguinal canal

Costal cartilage

Rib

Rectus abdominis

Transversus abdominis

Linea alba

Arcuate line

Inguinal ligament

Figure 7.182
Anterior view of rectus abdominis muscle.

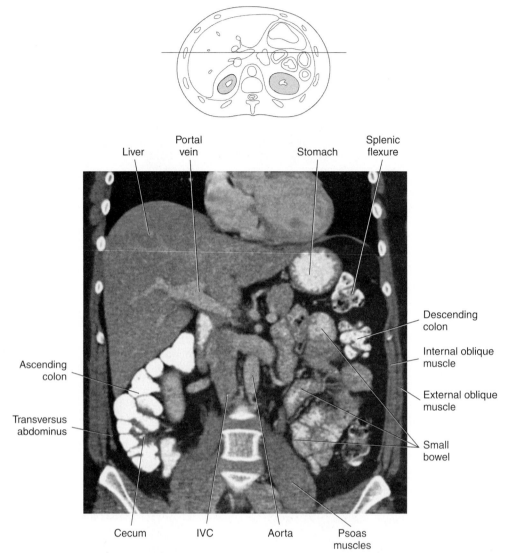

Figure 7.183
Coronal CT reformat of psoas muscles. *IVC*, Inferior vena cana.

TABLE 7-3   **Abdominal Muscles**

MUSCLE	ORIGIN	INSERTION	FUNCTION
Rectus abdominis	Pubic bone near symphysis	Costal cartilage of fifth, sixth, seventh ribs; xiphoid process of sternum	Flexes trunk
External oblique	Lower eight ribs	Linea alba and iliac crest	Compresses abdominal viscera, flexes and rotates spine
Internal oblique	Iliac crest and lumbodorsal fascia	Lower three ribs	Compresses abdominal viscera, flexes and rotates spine
Transversus abdominis	Lower six ribs, iliac crest, and lumbodorsal fascia	Pubic bone and linea alba	Compresses abdominal viscera
Quadratus lumborum	Iliac crest	Twelfth rib and transverse processes of lumbar vertebrae	Flexes spine laterally

PELVIS

"These, gentlemen, are the tuberosities of the ischia, on which man was designed to sit and survey the works of creation.

OLIVER WENDELL HOLMES (1809-1894),
Life and Letters of Oliver Wendell Holmes, *vol. I, Chapter VII*

The pelvis provides structural support for the body and encloses the male and female reproductive organs. Because of its role as a support mechanism for the body, the pelvis has a large amount of musculoskeletal anatomy, which, together with the differences in male and female anatomy, makes this area challenging to learn (Figure 8.1). This chapter demonstrates cross-section anatomy of the following structures:

BONY PELVIS
   Sacrum, Coccyx, and Os Coxae
   Pelvic Inlet and Outlet
   Perineum

MUSCLES
   Extrapelvic Muscles
   Pelvic Wall Muscles
   Pelvic Diaphragm Muscles

VISCERA
   Urinary Bladder
   Rectum
   Female Reproductive Organs
   Male Reproductive Organs

VASCULATURE
   Arteries
   Venous Drainage

LYMPH NODES

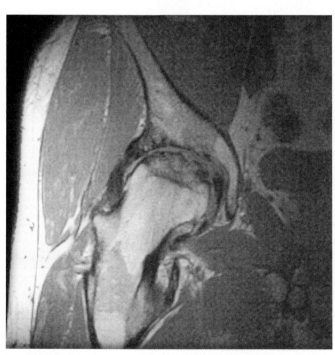

Figure 8.1
Coronal, T1-weighted MR image of right hip demonstrating avascular necrosis involving two thirds of the femoral head.

BONY PELVIS

Sacrum, Coccyx, and Os Coxae

The bony pelvis is formed by the sacrum, coccyx, and two os coxae or innominate bones (Figures 8.2 and 8.3). The **sacrum** is a triangular-shaped bone formed by the fusion of five vertebral segments. The first sacral segment has a prominent ridge located on the anterior surface of the body termed the **sacral promontory,** which acts as a bony landmark separating the abdominal cavity from the pelvic cavity. The transverse processes of the five sacral segments combine to form the **lateral mass (ala),** which articulates with the os coxae at the **sacroiliac joints** (Figures 8.4 and 8.5). The lateral mass contains **sacral foramina** that allow for the passage of sacral nerves (Figure 8.6). Articulating with the fifth sacral segment is the **coccyx,** which consists of three to five small fused bony segments (Figure 8.7).

The **os coxae** are made up of three bones: ilium, pubis, and ischium (Figure 8.8).

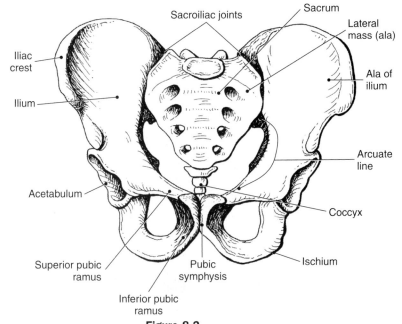

Figure 8.2

Anterior view of pelvis.

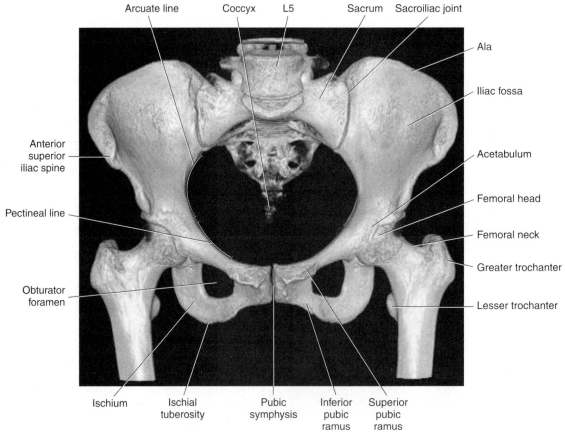

Figure 8.3

3D CT scan of anterior view of pelvis.

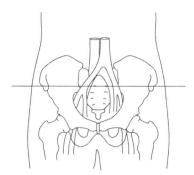

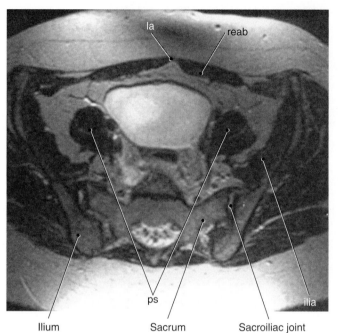

Figure 8.4
Axial, T1-weighted MR scan of ilium and sacroiliac joints.

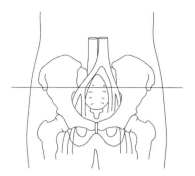

Lateral mass of sacrum

Figure 8.5
Axial CT scan of sacroiliac joints with ala of ilium.

KEY: **la,** Linea alba; **reab,** rectus abdominis; **ilia,** iliacus muscle; **ps,** psoas muscles; **ala,** ala of ilium; **Sljt,** sacroiliac joint; **spro,** sacral promontory; **ili,** iliac fossa; **S,** sacrum; **lm,** lateral mass; **sfor,** sacral foramina.

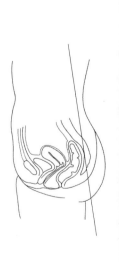

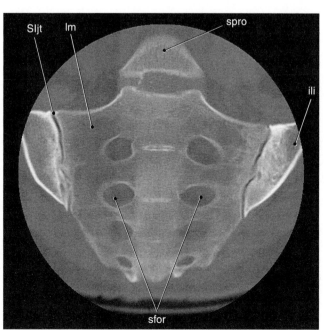

Figure 8.6
Coronal oblique CT scan of sacroiliac joints.

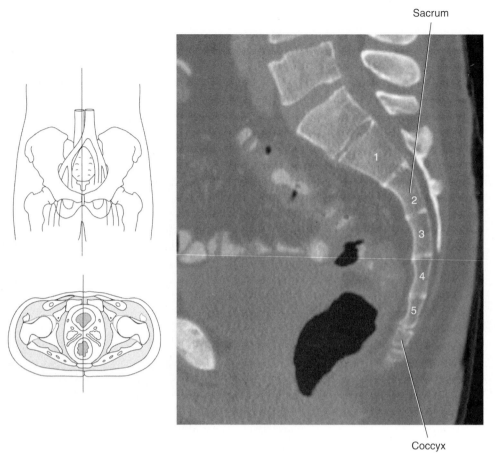

Sacrum

Coccyx

Figure 8.7
Sagittal CT reformat of sacrum and coccyx.

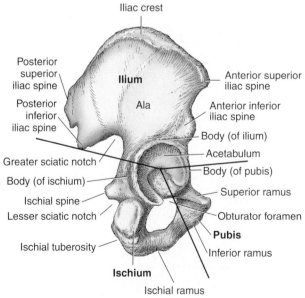

Iliac crest

Posterior superior iliac spine

Ilium

Anterior superior iliac spine

Ala

Posterior inferior iliac spine

Anterior inferior iliac spine

Body (of ilium)

Acetabulum

Greater sciatic notch

Body (of pubis)

Body (of ischium)

Superior ramus

Ischial spine

Obturator foramen

Lesser sciatic notch

Pubis

Ischial tuberosity

Inferior ramus

Ischium

Ischial ramus

Figure 8.8
Lateral aspect of right os coxae with divisions.

ILIUM The ilium, the largest and most superior portion, consists of a body and a large winglike projection called the **ala** (Figure 8.9). The concave, anterior surface of the ala is termed the **iliac fossa,** which is separated from the body by the **arcuate line.** This arch-shaped line, located on the anterior surface of the ilium, forms part of the pelvic brim (Figures 8.10 and 8.11). The superior ridge of the ala is termed the **iliac crest;** it slopes down to give rise to the **superior** and **inferior iliac spines** on both the anterior and posterior surfaces (Figures 8.9 and 8.10). The **body of the ilium** creates the upper portion of the **acetabulum,** which is a deep fossa that articulates with the head of the femur (Figures 8.12 and 8.13).

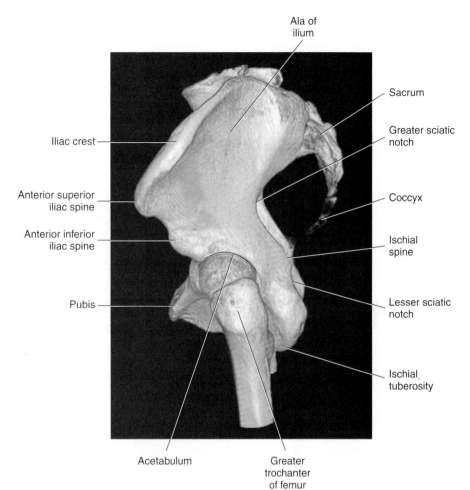

Figure 8.9
3D CT scan of lateral os coxae.

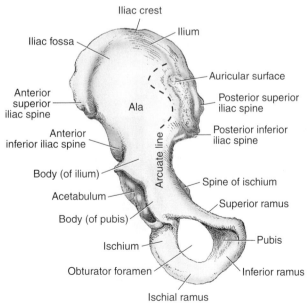

Figure 8.10
Anterior aspect of right os coxae.

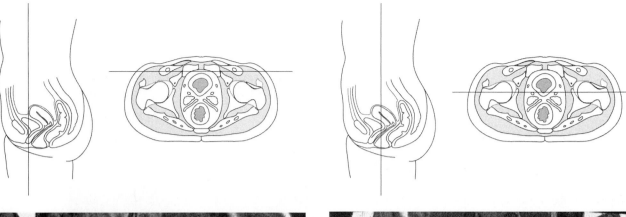

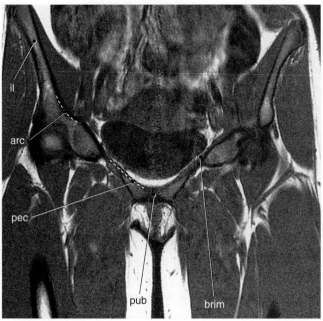

Figure 8.11
Coronal, T1-weighted MR scan of pelvis with pelvic brim.

Figure 8.12
Coronal, T1-weighted MR scan of acetabulum.

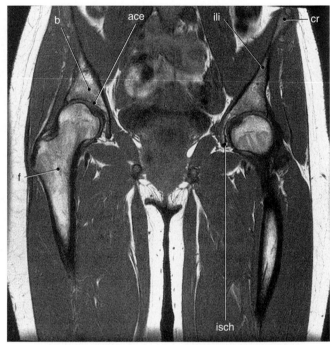

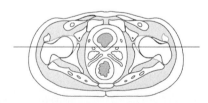

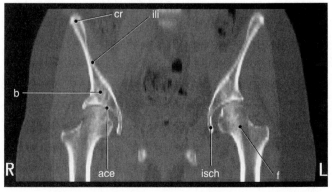

Figure 8.13
Coronal CT reformat of pelvis with acetabulum.

PUBIS   The pubis, or pubic bone, forms the lower anterior portion of the acetabulum and consists of a body and a superior and inferior pubic rami (Figure 8.8). The **bodies** of the two pubic bones meet at the midline to form the **pubic symphysis.** The **superior pubic ramus** projects inferiorly and medially from the acetabulum to the midline of the body (Figures 8.14 and 8.15). Located on the upper surface of the superior pubic ramus is a ridge termed the **pectineal line,** which is continuous with the arcuate line of the ilium, forming the pelvic brim (Figure 8.11). The **inferior pubic ramus** projects inferiorly and laterally from the body to join the ischium at an indistinct point; as a result, the two together are often referred to as the *ischiopubic ramus* (Figure 8.16).

KEY: **pub,** Pubis symphysis; **b,** body of ilium; **gtro,** greater trochanter; **ace,** acetabulum; **spub,** superior pubic ramus; **isch,** ischium; **ispi,** ischial spine; **fh,** femoral head; **ipub,** inferior pubic ramus; **tub,** ischial tuberosity.

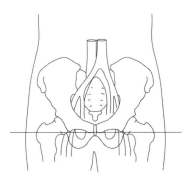
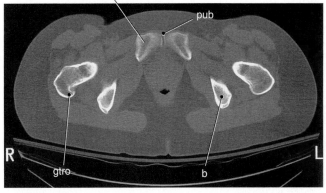

Figure 8.14
Axial CT scan with pubic symphysis and superior pubic ramus.

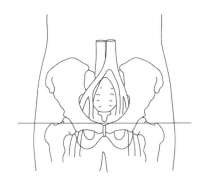
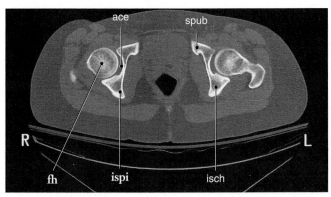

Figure 8.15
Axial CT of acetabulum in superior pubic ramus.

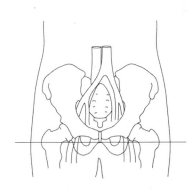
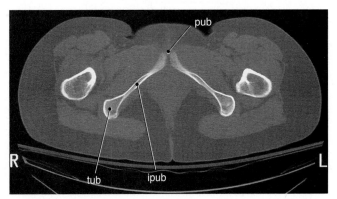

Figure 8.16
Axial CT scan of inferior pubic ramus and ischial tuberosity.

ISCHIUM   The ischium, the inferior portion of the os coxae, like the pubis is composed of a body and two rami. The **body** of the ischium forms the lower posterior portion of the acetabulum (Figures 8.8, 8.10, and 8.13). The **superior ischial ramus** extends posteriorly and inferiorly to a roughened, enlarged area termed the **ischial tuberosity** (Figures 8.9 and 8.16). From the ischial tuberosity, the **inferior ischial ramus** extends anteriorly and medially to join the inferior pubic ramus. The **ischial spine** projects from the superior ischial ramus between two prominent notches on the posterior surface of the os coxae (Figures 8.8 through 8.10, and 8.15). The **greater sciatic notch** extends from the posterior inferior iliac spine to the ischial spine, and the **lesser sciatic notch** extends from the ischial spine to the ischial tuberosity (Figures 8.8 and 8.9). The two notches are spanned by ligaments that create foramina for the passage of nerves and vessels. The union of the pubic rami and ischium surrounds a large opening termed the **obturator foramen,** which is enclosed by the obturator muscles (Figures 8.3 and 8.10).

Pelvic Inlet and Outlet

The pelvis is divided into the false or greater pelvis and the true or lesser pelvis by an oblique plane that extends from the upper anterior margin of the sacrum, along the arcuate line, to the upper margin of the pubic symphysis. The boundary line of this plane is called the **pelvic brim,** which delineates the boundaries of the abdominal and pelvic cavities. The region above the brim is called the **false pelvis,** and the region below the brim is called the **true pelvis,** which can be subdivided by the pelvic diaphragm into the main pelvic cavity and the perineum (Figure 8.17, *A*). The **superior aperture** or **inlet** of the true pelvis is measured in the anteroposterior direction from the sacral promontory to the superior margin or crest of the pubic bone (Figure 8.17, *B*). The **pelvic outlet** or **inferior aperture** is an opening bounded by the inferior edges of the pelvis and is measured from the tip of the coccyx to the inferior margin of the pubic symphysis in the anteroposterior direction and between the ischial tuberosities in the horizontal direction (Figure 8.17, *C*).

Perineum

The **perineum** and its contents cover and partially fill the inferior aperture of the bony pelvis. The bony circumferential boundaries of the perineum are the inner edges of the pelvic outlet and consist of the following surface relationships: anteriorly by the pubic symphysis; laterally by the pubic rami, ischial rami, ischial tuberosities, and sacrotuberous ligaments; and posteriorly by the coccyx (Figure 8.18). The region is divided into two triangles, posterior and anterior, by joining the ischial tuberosities by an imaginary line. The posterior triangle is the **anal triangle,** and the anterior triangle is the **urogenital triangle.** The anal triangle contains the inferior one third of the anal canal and its sphincter muscles, and ischioanal fossae. The urogenital triangle contains the openings of the urethra and vagina in the female and the urethra and root structures of the penis in the male (Figures 8.18 through 8.20).

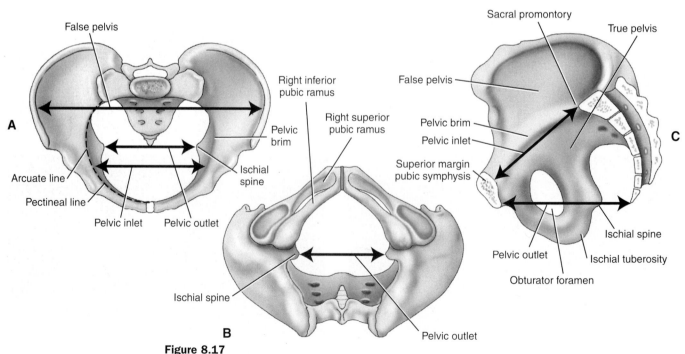

Figure 8.17
Divisions of the pelvis. **A,** Superior view. **B,** Lateral view. **C,** Inferior view.

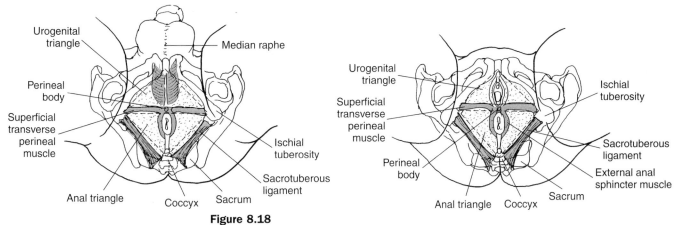

Figure 8.18
Boundaries of the perineum. *Left*, Male. *Right*, Female.

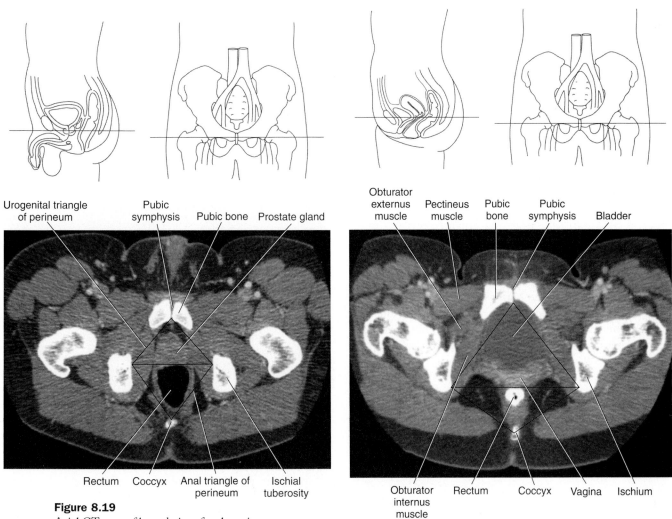

Figure 8.19
Axial CT scan of boundaries of male perineum.

Figure 8.20
Axial CT scan of boundaries of female perineum.

MUSCLES

Multiple muscles are visualized in the pelvis. For ease of description, the major pelvic muscles have been divided into functional groups: extra pelvic, pelvic wall, and pelvic diaphragm.

Extrapelvic Muscles

Several of the muscles visualized in the pelvis are actually abdominal muscles such as the rectus abdominis, psoas, and internal and external oblique muscles. The **rectus abdominis muscles,** visualized on the anterior surface of the abdomen and pelvis, originate from the symphysis pubis and extend to the xiphoid process and the costal cartilage of the fifth, sixth, and seventh ribs. They function to flex the lumbar vertebrae and support the abdomen. The **psoas muscles** extend along the lateral surfaces of the lumbar vertebrae and act to flex the thigh or trunk. The **external** and **internal oblique muscles** are located on the outer lateral portion of the abdomen and span primarily between the cartilages of the lower ribs to the level of the iliac crest. The oblique muscles work together to flex and rotate the vertebral column and compress the abdominal viscera. An inferior band of fibrous connective tissue from the external oblique muscle folds back on itself to form the **inguinal ligament,** which spans the anterior superior iliac spine and the pubic tubercle (Figures 7.176 through 7.182)

> **Indirect inguinal hernias are protrusions of the intestine at the inguinal ring. They account for approximately 80% of all hernias.**

Many of the muscles visualized in the pelvis are considered to be muscles of the hip. The largest of this group are the **gluteus muscles** (maximus, medius, minimus), which function together to abduct, rotate, and extend the thigh. The largest and most superficial is the **gluteus maximus muscle,** which makes up the bulk of the buttocks. The **gluteus medius** and **minimus muscles** are smaller in size, respectively, and are deep to the gluteus maximus muscle (Figures 8.21 through 8.24; see also Chapter 10).

KEY: **reab,** Rectus abdominis; **ilps,** iliopsoas; **gmax,** gluteus maximus; **gmed,** gluteus medius; **gmin,** gluteus minimus; **pir,** piriformis; **ace,** acetabulum.

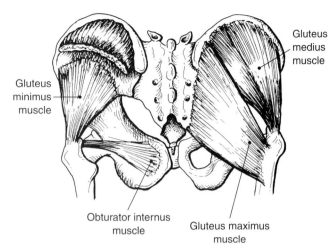

Figure 8.21
Posterior view of gluteus muscle group.

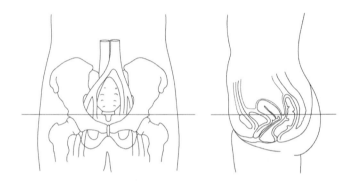

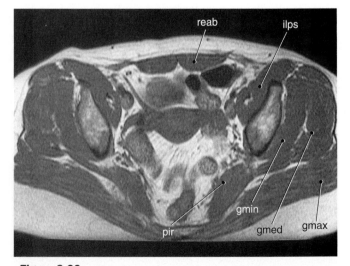

Figure 8.22
Axial, T1-weighted MR scan of pelvis with gluteus muscle group.

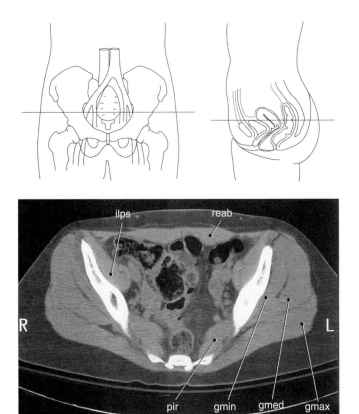

Figure 8.23
Axial CT scan of pelvis with gluteus muscle group.

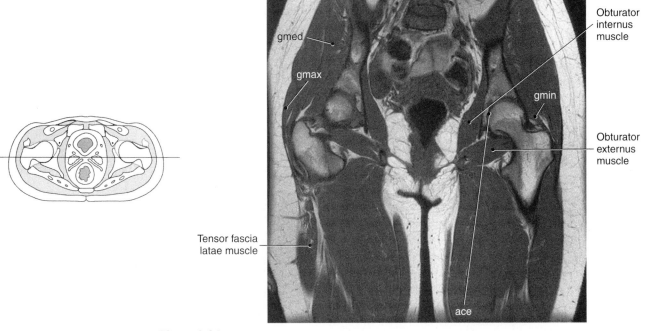

Figure 8.24
Coronal, T1-weighted MR scan of pelvis with gluteus muscle group.

TABLE 8-1   Muscles of the Pelvic Wall and Diaphragm

MUSCLE	ORIGIN	INSERTION	FUNCTION
Piriformis	Ilium and sacrum	Greater trochanter of femur	Laterally rotates and adducts thigh
Obturator internus	Obturator foramen and pubic bone	Greater trochanter of femur (medial surface)	Laterally rotates thigh
Obturator externus	Obturator foramen	Greater trochanter of femur (trochanteric fossa)	Laterally rotates and adducts thigh
Iliacus	Iliac crest and sacrum	Lesser trochanter of femur (tendon fused with that of psoas muscle)	Flexes hip
Levator ani	Symphysis pubis and ischial spine	Coccyx	Supports pelvic viscera, flexes coccyx, elevates and retracts anus
Coccygeus	Ischial spine	Sacrum and coccyx	Assists in support of pelvic floor and flexes coccyx

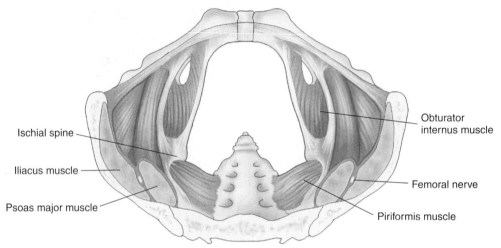

Figure 8.25
Pelvic cavity viewed from above.

Pelvic Wall Muscles

The muscles of the pelvic wall include the piriformis, obturator internus and externus, and iliacus muscles. The **piriformis muscle,** which acts to rotate the thigh laterally, originates from the ilium and the sacrum and passes through the greater sciatic notch to insert on the greater trochanter of the femur. Also functioning to rotate the thigh laterally is the **obturator internus muscle.** This fan-shaped muscle extends from the pubic bone and obturator foramen to pass through the lesser sciatic notch and attaches to the greater trochanter of the femur. Inserting on the greater trochanter just below the obturator internus muscle is the **obturator externus muscle.** This strong muscle originates on the obturator foramen, aiding in adduction and rotation of the thigh. Extending from the iliac crest and sacrum is the triangular-shaped **iliacus muscle.** As the iliacus muscle spans the iliac fossa it is joined by the psoas muscle to form the **iliopsoas muscle,** which extends to insert on the lesser trochanter of the femur. The iliopsoas muscle is the most important muscle for flexing the leg, which makes walking possible (Figures 8.25 through 8.30 and Table 8.1; see also Chapter 10).

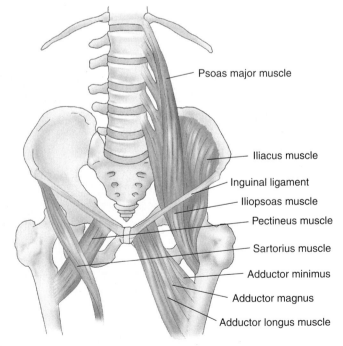

Figure 8.26
Anterior view of muscles of pelvic wall.

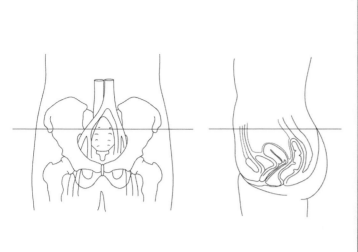

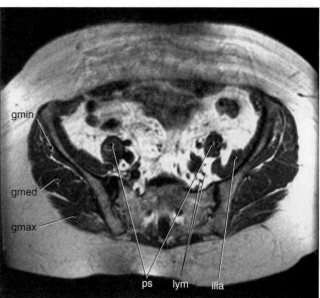

Figure 8.27
Axial, T1-weighted MR scan of pelvis with iliacus muscle.

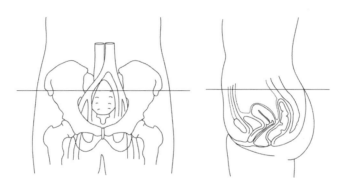

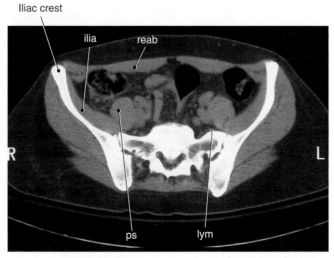

Figure 8.28
Axial CT scan of pelvis with iliacus muscle.

KEY: **gmin,** Gluteus minimus; **gmed,** gluteus medius; **gmax,** gluteus maximus; **ps,** psoas muscle; **lym,** lymph nodes; **ilia,** iliacus; **reab,** rectus abdominis.

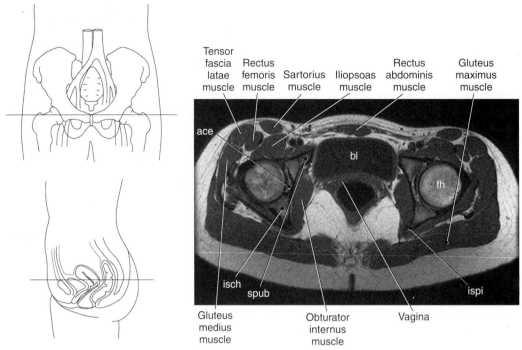

Figure 8.29

Axial, T1-weighted MR scan of female pelvis with iliopsoas muscle.

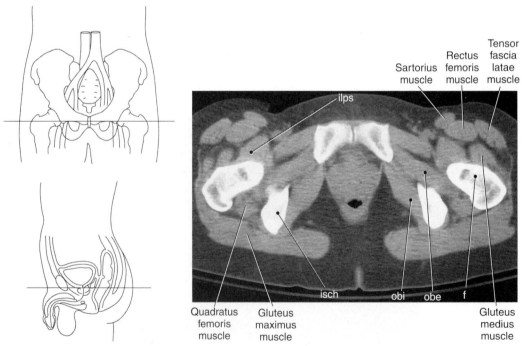

Figure 8.30

Axial CT scan of male pelvis with iliopsoas muscle.

KEY: ace, Acetabulum; **bl,** bladder; **fh,** femoral head; **ipsi,** ischial spine; **spub,** superior pubic ramus; **isch,** ischium; **ilps,** iliopsoas; **f,** femur; **obe,** obturator externus; **obi,** obturator internus.

Pelvic Diaphragm Muscles

The funnel-shaped pelvic diaphragm is a layer of muscles and fascia that forms the greatest majority of the pelvic floor. The primary muscles of the pelvic diaphragm are the levator ani and coccygeus muscles. The two **levator ani** muscles are the largest and most important muscles of the pelvic floor, originating from the symphysis pubis and ischial spines to form winglike arches that attach to the coccyx. The levator ani muscle can be subdivided into the pubococcygeus, puborectalis, and iliococcygeus muscles. The two **coccygeus muscles** form the posterior portion of the pelvic floor, arising from the ischial spines and fanning out to attach to the lower sacrum and coccyx. Together, the levator ani and coccygeus muscles provide support for the pelvic contents (Figures 8.31 through 8.38 and Table 8.1).

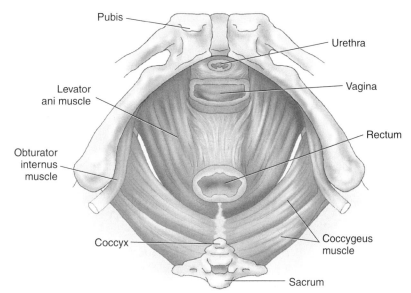

Figure 8.31
Inferior view of pelvic diaphragm muscles, female pelvis.

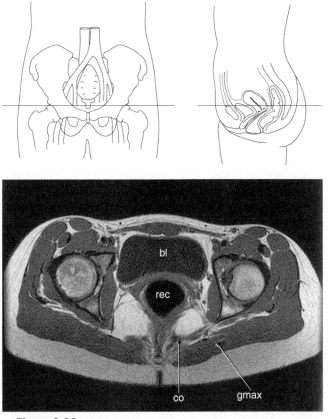

Figure 8.32
Axial, T1-weighted MR scan of pelvis with coccygeus muscles.

KEY: bl, Bladder; **rec,** rectum; **co,** coccygeus; **gmax,** gluteus maximus.

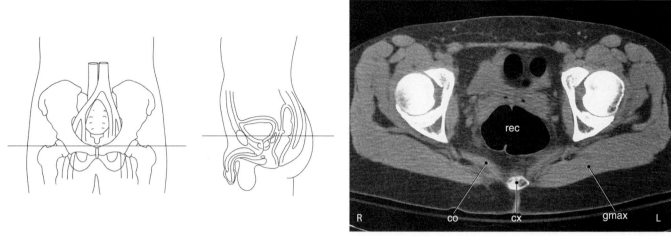

Figure 8.33
Axial CT scan of pelvis with coccygeus muscles.

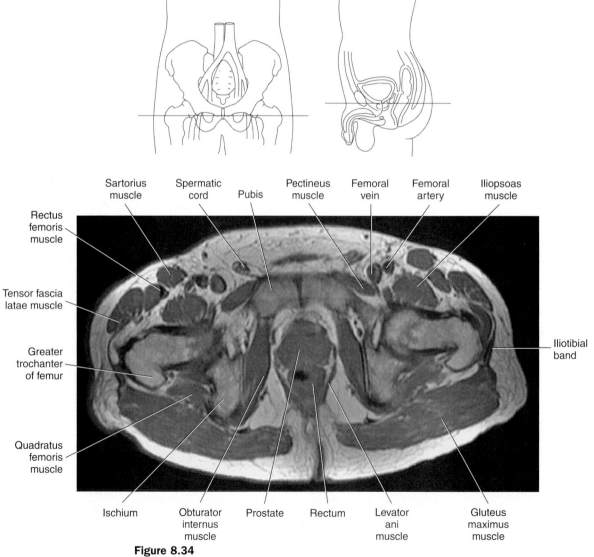

Figure 8.34
Axial, T1-weighted MR scan of male pelvis with levator ani muscles.

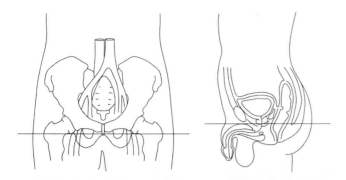

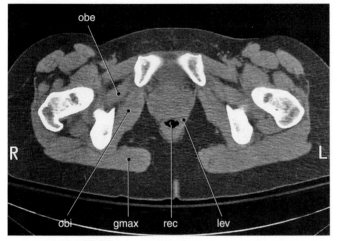

KEY: **rec,** Rectum; **co,** coccygeus; **cx,** coccyx; **gmax,** gluteus maximus; **obe,** obturator externus; **lev,** levator ani; **obi,** obturator internus.

Figure 8.35
Axial CT scan of pelvis with levator ani muscles.

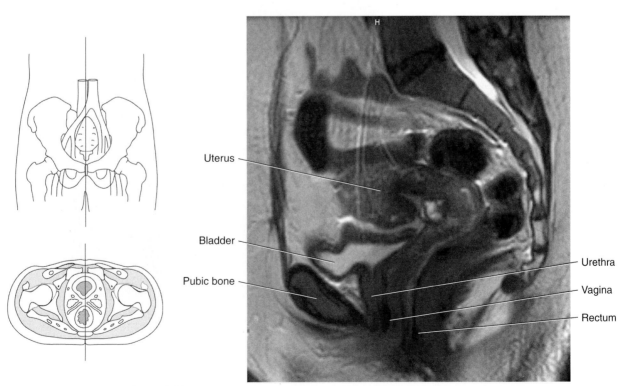

Figure 8.36
Sagittal, T2-weighted MR scan of female pelvis with pelvic diaphragm muscles.

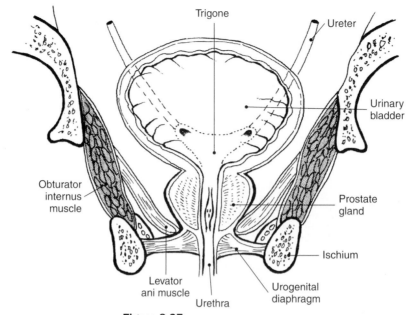

Figure 8.37
Anterior view of levator ani muscles.

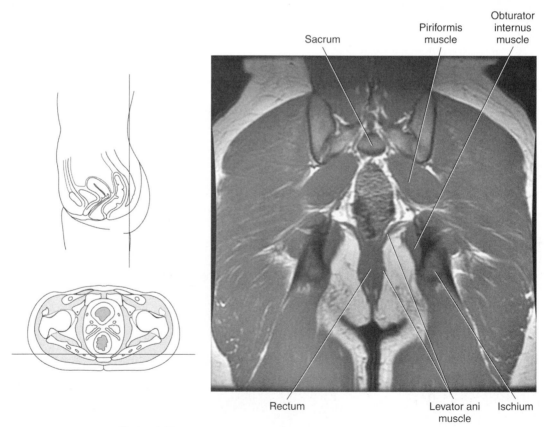

Figure 8.38
Coronal, T1-weighted MR scan of pelvis with levator ani muscles.

VISCERA

The pelvic cavity contains the urinary bladder, rectum, and internal reproductive organs.

Urinary Bladder

The **urinary bladder** is a pyramid-shaped muscular organ that rests on the pelvic floor, immediately posterior to the symphysis pubis (Figures 8.39 through 8.44). It functions as a temporary reservoir for the storage of urine. In a normal adult,

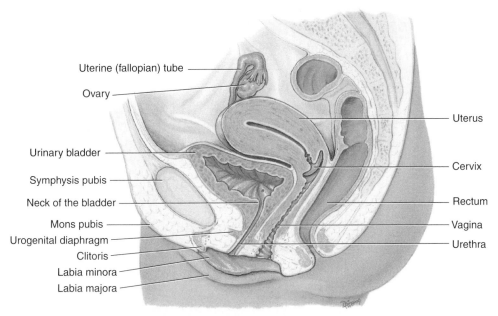

Uterine (fallopian) tube
Ovary
Urinary bladder
Symphysis pubis
Neck of the bladder
Mons pubis
Urogenital diaphragm
Clitoris
Labia minora
Labia majora
Uterus
Cervix
Rectum
Vagina
Urethra

Figure 8.39
Lateral view of female pelvis.

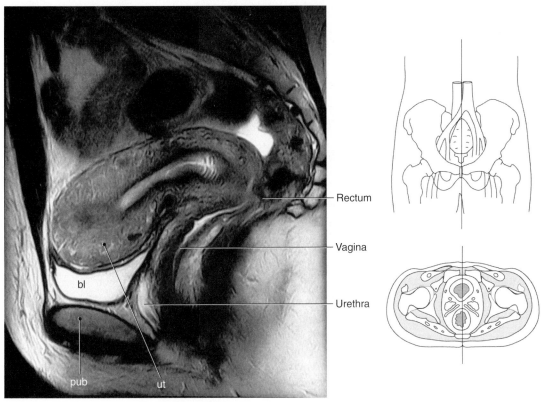

Rectum
Vagina
Urethra
bl
pub
ut

Figure 8.40
Sagittal, T2-weighted MR scan of female pelvis.

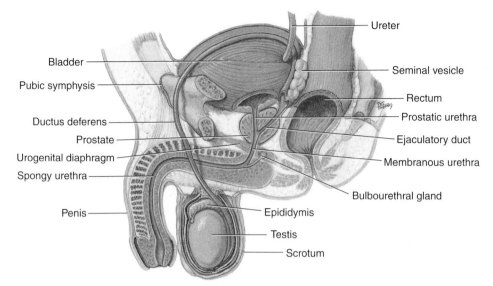

Figure 8.41
Lateral view of male pelvis.

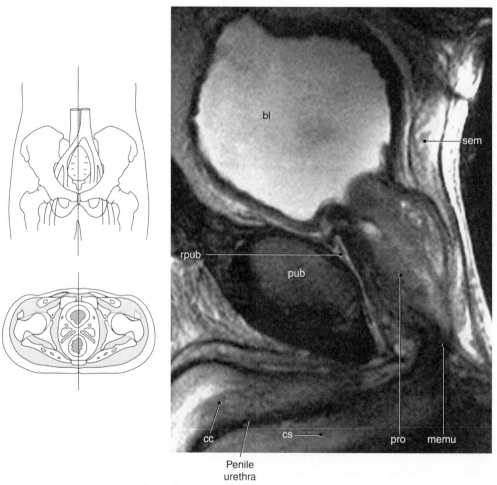

Figure 8.42
Sagittal, T2-weighted MR scan of male pelvis.

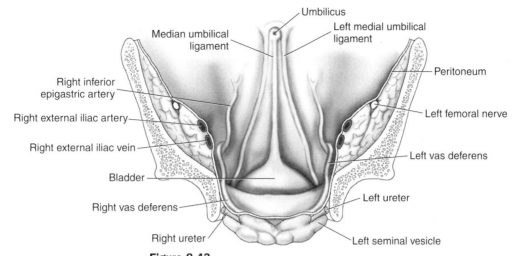

Figure 8.43
Anterior view of urinary bladder and ligaments.

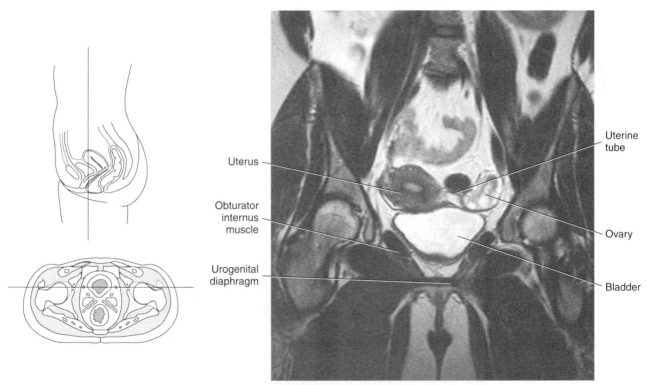

Figure 8.44
Coronal, T2-weighted MR scan of female pelvis with urinary bladder.

KEY: bl, Bladder; **sem,** seminal vesicle; **pub,** pubic symphysis; **rpub,** retropubic space; **cc,** corpora cavernosum; **cs,** corpus spongiosum; **pro,** prostate gland; **memu,** membranous urethra.

it takes approximately 250 to 250 mL of urine to accumulate before the urge to urinate is triggered. However, the bladder has the potential storage capacity of approximately 750 mL. When empty, the bladder has four surfaces (superior, posterior, and two inferolateral) and four angles (anterior, inferior, and two posterolateral). The **superior surface** (body) of the bladder is covered by peritoneum, allowing loops of ileum and sigmoid colon to rest on it. The **posterior surface** is referred to as the fundus or base of the bladder. This surface is closely related to the anterior wall of the vagina in the female and to the rectum in the male. The two **inferolateral surfaces** face inferior, lateral, and anterior and are in contact with the fascia covering the levator ani muscles (Figure 8.37). As urine is collected in the bladder, the superior and inferolateral surfaces distend accordingly while the posterior surface remains relatively fixed. The **inferior angle** is a funnel-shaped narrowing formed by

the convergence of the inferolateral and posterior surfaces and is called the **neck of the bladder,** which is continuous with the urethra (Figure 8.39). The bladder neck contains the muscular **internal urethral sphincter,** which provides for involuntary control over the release of urine from the bladder. The two **posterolateral angles** mark the point where the ureters enter the bladder. The **anterior angle** is formed by the convergence of the superior and inferolateral surfaces and is referred to as the **apex** of the bladder. The bladder is anchored to the pelvis by peritoneal ligaments. The apex is attached to the anterior abdominal wall by the **median umbilical ligament,** which is the remains of the fetal urachus (obliterated umbilical artery). Two **lateral (medial) umbilical ligaments** from the body of the bladder ascend along with the median umbilical ligament to the umbilicus (Figures 8.43 and 8.44). The fibrous cords of these ligaments represent the obliterated remains of the two

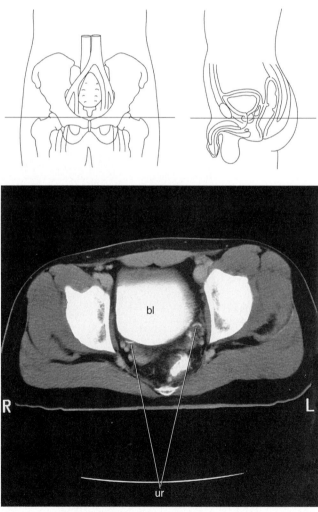

Figure 8.45
Axial CT scan of pelvis with urinary bladder.

umbilical arteries that provided blood to the placenta during fetal development. The bladder neck is held in place by the **puboprostatic ligament** in males and the **pubovesical ligament** in females. Three openings in the floor of the bladder form a triangular area called the **trigone** (Figure 8.37). Two of the openings are created by the ureters. The pelvic portions of the ureters run anterior to the internal iliac arteries and enter the posterolateral surface of the bladder at an oblique angle (Figure 8.45). The third opening is located in the apex of the trigone and is formed by the entrance to the urethra (Figures 8.44 and 8.46).

The **urethra** in both genders passes through the **urogenital diaphragm,** which contains the **urethral sphincter muscle** responsible for the voluntary closure of the bladder.

The **female urethra** is a short (3-4 cm) muscular tube that drains urine from the bladder. It descends inferiorly and anteriorly while embedded in the anterior vaginal wall and terminates at the **external urethral opening** located between the clitoris and vagina (Figures 8.39 and 8.40). The **male urethra** is much longer (18-20 cm) and extends from the inferior portion of the bladder to the tip of the penis (Figures 8.41, 8.42, and 8.46). It can be subdivided into three regions: prostatic urethra, membranous urethra, and penile urethra. The **prostatic urethra** passes through the middle of the prostate gland. The **membranous urethra** is the shortest and narrowest portion of the urethra and is the portion that penetrates the external urethral sphincter. The **penile urethra** is the longest portion, extending from the external urethral sphincter to the tip of the penis (Figures 8.41 and 8.42). The male urethra has the dual function to drain urine from the bladder and to receive secretions from the prostatic and ejaculatory ducts and the ducts of the bulbourethral glands.

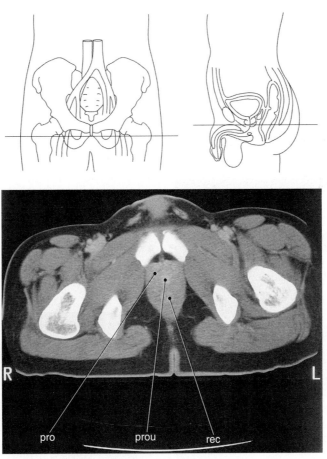

Figure 8.46
Axial CT scan of pelvis with male urethra.

KEY: bl, Bladder; **ur,** ureter; **pro,** prostate gland; **prou,** prostatic urethra; **rec,** rectum.

Rectum

The rectum is the terminal part of the large intestine extending from S3 to the tip of the coccyx, approximately 15 cm. It follows the anteroposterior curve of the sacrum and coccyx (**sacral flexure**) and ends by turning inferiorly and anteriorly (**perineal flexure**) to become the anal canal, which ends at the anus (Figures 8.39 through 8.42). Between the two flexures is a fold of tissue called the **transverse rectal fold (Kohlrausch's fold)** located 5 to 8 cm from the anus (Figure 8.47). It serves as a topographic landmark during a rectal exam marking the posterior side of the prostate in males and the vault of the vagina in females. The upper third of the rectum, the **rectal ampulla,** has considerable distensibility. As fecal material collects in this area, it triggers the urge to defecate. The **anal canal** is the distal portion of the rectum and contains small longitudinal folds called **rectal** or **anal columns.** The **anus** marks the exit of the anal canal and is under involuntary control by the **internal anal sphincter,** a circular muscle layer within the rectal wall. The **external anal sphincter** consists of a ring of skeletal muscle fibers and is under voluntary control (Figures 8.47 through 8.49).

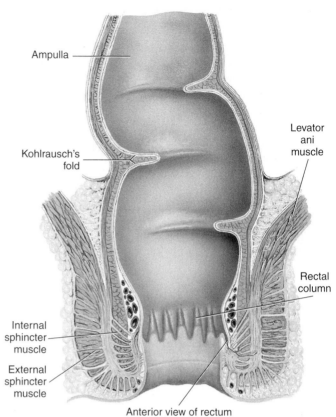

Figure 8.47
Anterior view of rectum.

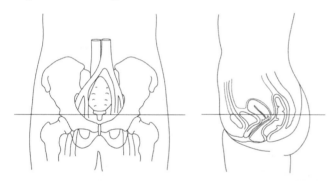

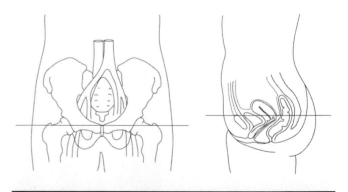

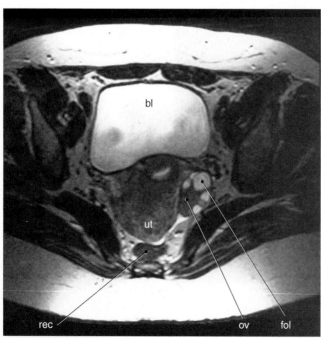

Figure 8.48
Axial, T2-weighted MR scan of pelvis with rectum.

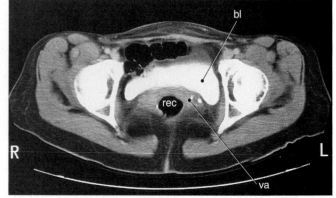

Figure 8.49
Axial CT scan of pelvis with rectum.

Female Reproductive Organs

The female reproductive system is responsible for producing sex hormones and ova and functions to protect and support a developing embryo. The principal organs of the female reproductive system are located within the pelvic cavity and include the uterus, ovaries, uterine tubes, and vagina (Figures 8.50 and 8.51).

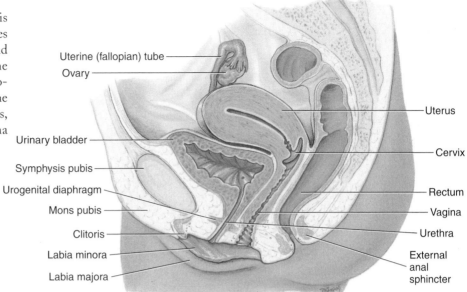

Figure 8.50
Lateral view of female pelvis.

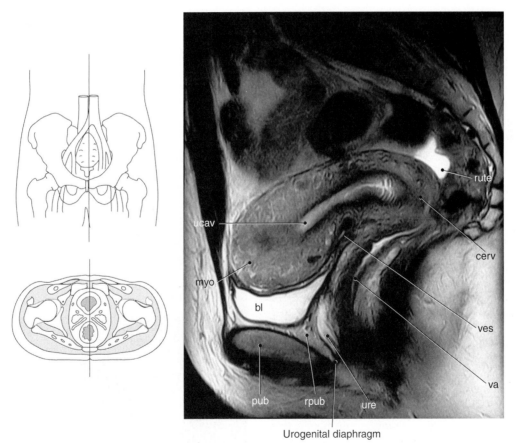

Figure 8.51
Sagittal, T2-weighted MR scan of female reproductive system.

KEY: ut, Uterus; **rec,** rectum; **ov,** ovaries; **fol,** follicular cyst; **bl,** bladder; **va,** vagina; **rute,** rectouterine pouch; **cerv,** cervix; **ves,** vesicouterine pouch; **ure,** urethra; **rpub,** retropubic space; **pub,** pubic symphysis; **myo,** myometrium; **ucav,** uterine cavity.

454

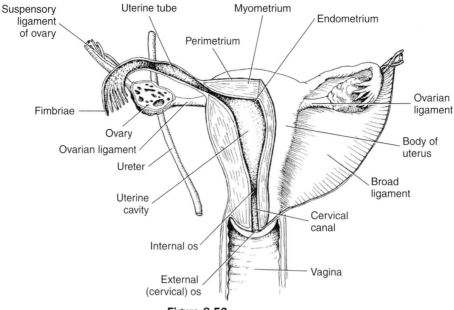

Suspensory
ligament
of ovary

Uterine tube

Myometrium

Endometrium

Perimetrium

Fimbriae

Ovary

Ovarian ligament

Ureter

Uterine
cavity

Internal os

External
(cervical) os

Ovarian
ligament

Body of
uterus

Broad
ligament

Cervical
canal

Vagina

Figure 8.52
Anterior view of uterus.

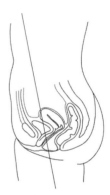

UTERUS The **uterus** is a pear-shaped muscular organ
located in the anterior portion of the pelvic cavity between the
bladder and the rectum (Figures 8.50 and 8.51). The uterus
can be subdivided into two anatomic regions: body and cervix.
The **body** is the largest division, comprising the upper two
thirds of the uterus. The rounded superior portion of the body
is called the **fundus,** which is located just superior to the
region where the uterine tubes enter the uterus. The lateral
borders of the fundus contain the **cornua,** where the uterine
tubes attach to the uterus. The narrow inferior third of the
uterus is called the **cervix,** which communicates with the
vagina. The narrow lumen within the cervix, called the **cervical
canal,** is a conduit between the uterine cavity superiorly via
the **internal os** and opens inferiorly into the vagina via the
external os (Figure 8.52). The most common position of the
uterus is with the body projecting superiorly and anteriorly
over the bladder, with the fundus adjacent to the anterior
abdominal wall and the cervix directed inferior and posteriorly
into the vaginal vault. The wall of the uterus is composed of
three layers: the **endometrium** is the inner glandular tissue
lining the inner wall; the **myometrium** is the middle, muscular
layer and the thickest component of the uterine wall; and the
perimetrium is the outer layer consisting of a serous membrane that covers the fundus and posterior surface of the
uterus. The endometrium is lined by a mucous membrane that
is continuous with the inner lining of the vagina and uterine
tubes. The thick myometrial layer is highly vascular and is
responsible for the main contractive force during childbirth.
The perimetrium is formed by peritoneum and is firmly
attached to the myometrium. The uterus is the reproductive
organ responsible for protecting and nourishing the fetus
during development (Figures 8.50 through 8.55).

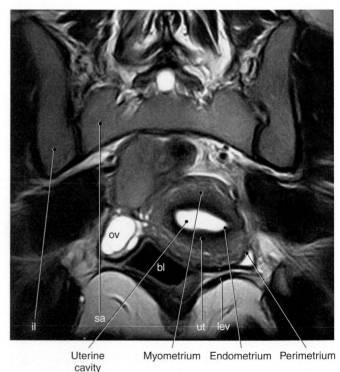

Uterine
cavity

Myometrium Endometrium Perimetrium

Figure 8.53
Coronal, T2-weighted MR scan of female bladder.

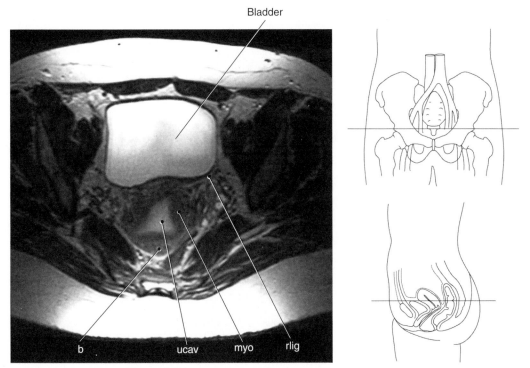

Figure 8.54
Axial, T2-weighted MR scan of pelvis with body of uterus.

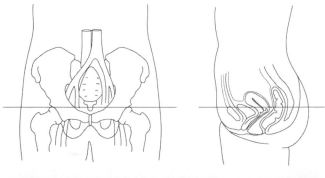

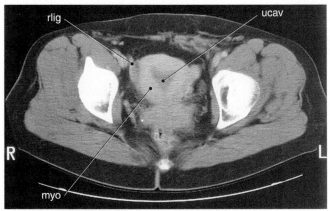

Figure 8.55
Axial CT scan of pelvis with body of uterus.

KEY: ov, Ovaries; **bl,** bladder; **il,** ilium; **sa,** sacrum; **ut,** uterus; **lev,** levator ani; **b,** body of uterus; **ucav,** uterine cavity; **myo,** myometrium; **rlig,** round ligament.

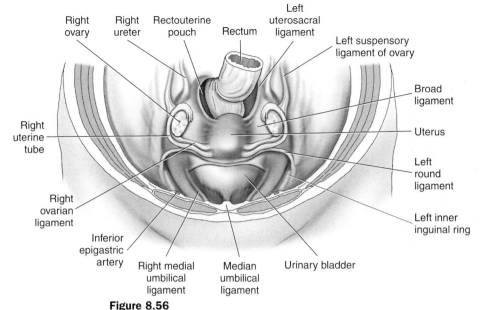

Figure 8.56
Anterior view of female pelvis with peritoneal ligaments.

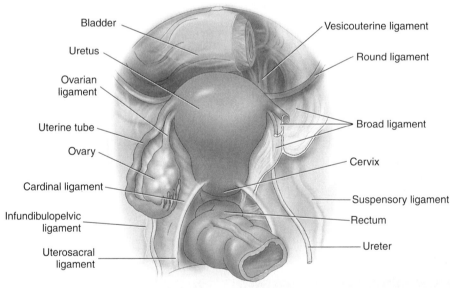

Figure 8.57
Superior view of female pelvis with ligaments.

SUSPENSORY LIGAMENTS OF THE UTERUS   The uterus is stabilized by several pair of suspensory ligaments formed by peritoneum. The **round ligaments** extend laterally from the uterine cornu to the inner inguinal ring, through the inguinal canal, and anchor to the labia majora (Figures 8.54 and 8.55). They help keep the body flexed anteriorly (anteversion) and help to prevent posterior movement of the uterus (Figures 8.56 and 8.57). The **uterosacral ligaments** extend from the lateral walls of the cervix to the anterior surface of the sacrum, preventing forward movement of the uterus (Figure 8.58). The **lateral cervical (cardinal) ligaments** extend like a fan from the lateral walls of the cervix and vagina and anchor into the fascia of the wall of the lesser pelvis. They help suspend the uterus above the bladder and help to prevent downward displacement of the uterus. Additional support is provided by the muscles and fascia of the pelvic floor (Figures 8.59 through 8.61).

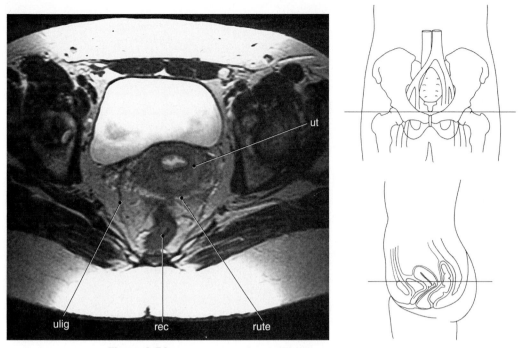

Figure 8.58
Axial, T2-weighted MR scan of pelvis with uterosacral ligaments.

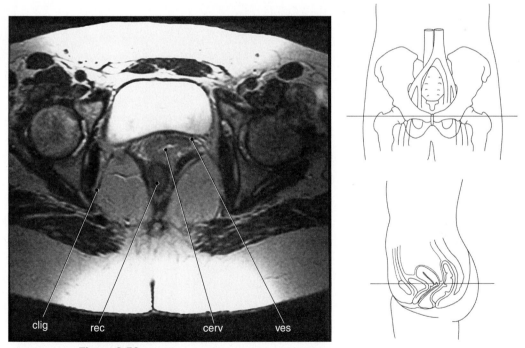

Figure 8.59
Axial, T2-weighted MR scan of pelvis with lateral cervical (cardinal) ligaments.

KEY: **ut,** Uterus; **rute,** rectouterine pouch; **rec,** rectum; **ulig,** uterosacral ligament; **clig,** cardinal ligament; **cerv,** cervix; **ves,** vesicouterine pouch.

458

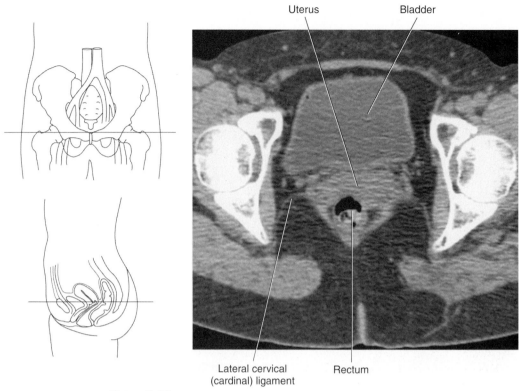

Uterus   Bladder

Lateral cervical
(cardinal) ligament   Rectum

Figure 8.60
Axial CT scan of pelvis with lateral cervical (cardinal) ligaments.

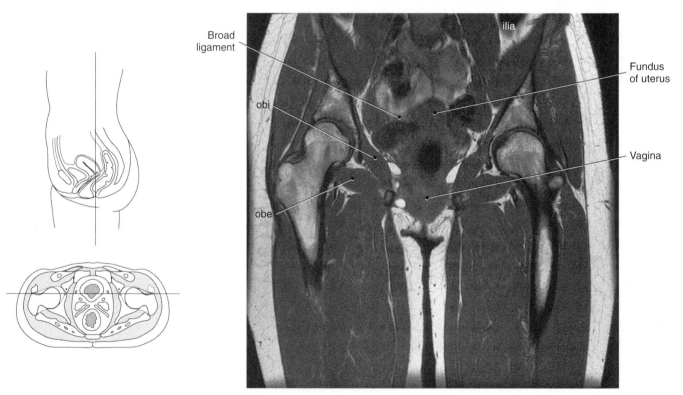

Broad
ligament

ilia

obi

Fundus
of uterus

obe

Vagina

Figure 8.61
Coronal, T1-weighted MR scan of female pelvis.

KEY: **obi,** Obturator internus; **obe,** obturator externus; **ilia,** iliacus muscle.

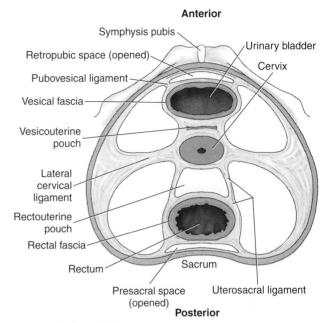

Figure 8.63
Superior view of pelvic spaces of female pelvis.

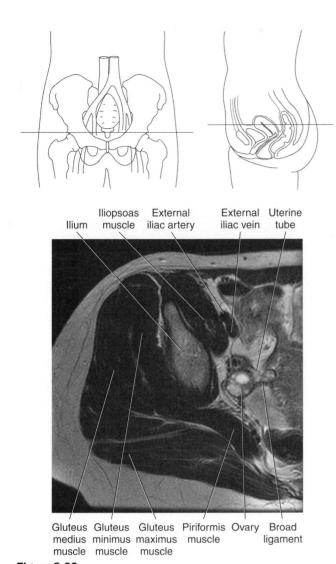

Figure 8.62
Axial, T2-weighted MR scan of female pelvis with broad ligament.

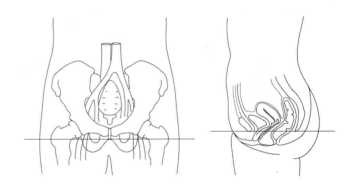

PELVIC SPACES A peritoneal fold called the **broad ligament** encloses the ovaries, uterine tubes, and uterus (Figures 8.57 and 8.62). The broad ligament extends from the sides of the uterus to the walls and floor of the pelvis, preventing side-to-side movement of the uterus and dividing the pelvis into anterior and posterior pouches. The anterior **vesicouterine pouch** is located between the uterus and the posterior wall of the bladder, whereas the posterior **rectouterine pouch (pouch of Douglas)** lies between the uterus and rectum (Figures 8.58, 8.59, and 8.63). The pelvic spaces are common areas for the accumulation of fluid within the pelvis. Another space in the pelvis is the **retropubic space,** located between the pubic bones and the bladder and containing extraperitoneal fat and connective tissue for the expansion of the bladder (Figures 8.63 and 8.64).

KEY: **pub,** Pubic symphysis; **gtro,** greater trochanter; **b,** body of ischium.

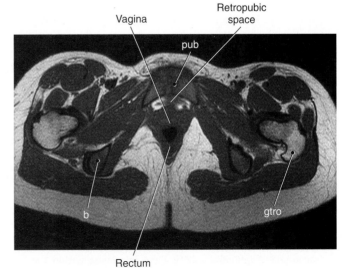

Figure 8.64
Axial, T1-weighted MR scan of pelvis with vagina.

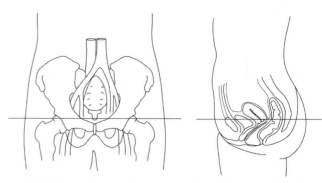

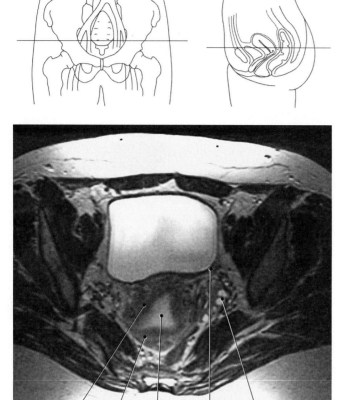

Figure 8.65
Axial, T2-weighted MR scan of pelvis with ovaries.

myo   b   ucav   rlig   ov

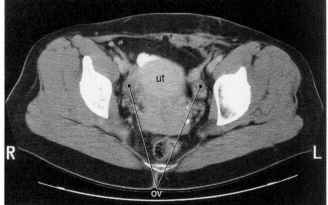

Figure 8.66
Axial CT scan of pelvis with ovaries.

KEY: myo, Myometrium; **b,** body of uterus; **ucav,** uterine cavity; **rlig,** round ligament; **ov,** ovaries; **ut,** uterus.

OVARIES The paired **ovaries** are small almond-shaped organs located on either side of the uterus (Figures 8.65 through 8.67). They lie in a depression on the lateral walls of the pelvis and are held in place by the ovarian and suspensory ligaments (Figure 8.57). The cordlike **ovarian ligament** attaches the inferior aspect of the ovaries to the lateral surface of the uterus and uterine tubes (Figure 8.52). The **suspensory ligament** attaches the superior aspect of the ovaries to the lateral sides of the pelvic wall and contains the ovarian vessels (Figures 8.56 and 8.57). The ovaries are responsible for the production of **ova** and the production and secretion of estrogens and progesterone. **Estrogens** are responsible for the development

and maintenance of female characteristics and reproductive organs. **Progesterone** is responsible for the uterine changes in preparation of pregnancy, such as thickening of the uterine lining and decreasing contractions by uterine muscle.

UTERINE TUBES The **uterine (fallopian) tubes** are slender, muscular tubes (approximately 8-20 cm long) extending laterally from the body of the uterus to the peritoneum near the ovaries (Figure 8.57). They are supported by the broad ligament and at their distal end expand to form a funnel-shaped **infundibulum.** The infundibulum has numerous 1- to 2-cm fingerlike projections called **fimbriae** that spread loosely over the surface of the ovaries. During ovulation, the fimbriae trap the ovum and sweep it into the uterine tubes. The proximal portion of the uterine tubes opens into the uterus, and the distal portion opens directly into the peritoneal cavity, immediately superior to the ovaries, thereby providing a direct route for pathogens to enter the pelvic cavity. The uterine tubes provide a method of transport for ova to reach the uterus from the ovaries.

A follicular cyst represents the mature oocyte and its surrounding follicular cavity. Fluid increases within the cavity as the oocyte matures.

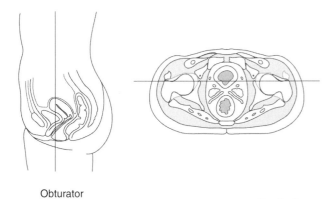

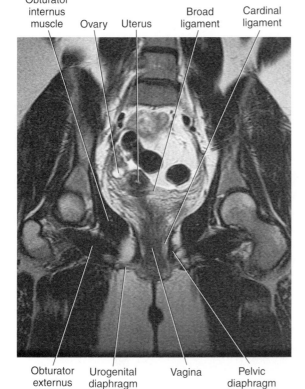

Obturator internus muscle · Ovary · Uterus · Broad ligament · Cardinal ligament

Obturator externus muscle · Urogenital diaphragm · Vagina · Pelvic diaphragm

Figure 8.67
Coronal, T2-weighted MR scan of pelvis with vagina.

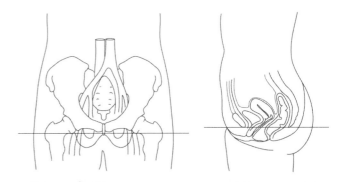

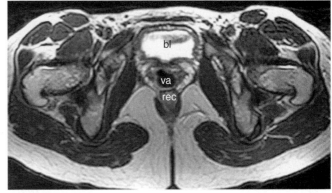

bl
va
rec

Figure 8.68
Axial, T2-weighted MR scan of female pelvis with vagina.

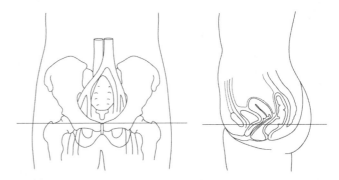

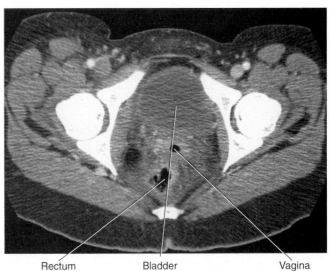

Rectum · Bladder · Vagina

Figure 8.69
Axial CT scan of pelvis with vagina.

VAGINA   The **vagina** is an 8- to 10-cm muscular tube extending anteroinferiorly from the cervix of the uterus to the external vaginal orifice. The **vaginal vault** or **fornix** is the upper vaginal area surrounding the cervical os like a ring and is commonly divided into **anterior** and **posterior fornices.** The vagina is located between the bladder and the rectum and functions as a receptacle for sperm and as the lower portion of the birth canal (Figures 8.52 and 8.67 through 8.69).

KEY: **bl,** Bladder; **va,** vagina; **rec,** rectum.

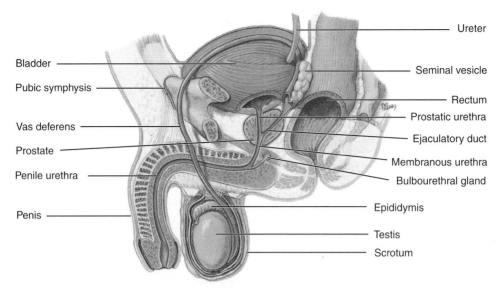

Figure 8.70
Lateral view of male pelvis.

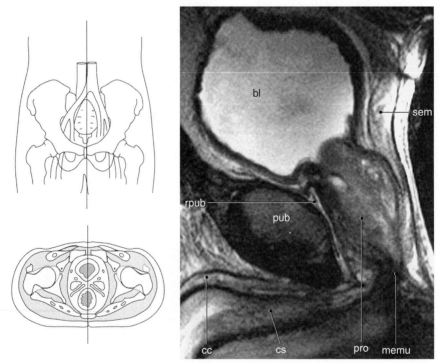

Figure 8.71
Sagittal, T2-weighted MR scan of male pelvis.

Male Reproductive Organs

The principal structures of the male reproductive system are the testis, epididymis, vas deferens, ejaculatory duct, seminal vesicle, prostate gland, bulbourethral gland, and penis. All these structures, except the testes and penis, are located within the pelvic cavity (Figures 8.70 and 8.71).

KEY: **bl**, Bladder; **sem**, seminal vesicle; **rpub**, retropubic space; **pub**, pubic symphysis; **cc**, corpora cavernosum; **cs**, corpus spongiosum; **pro**, prostate gland; **memu**, membranous urethra.

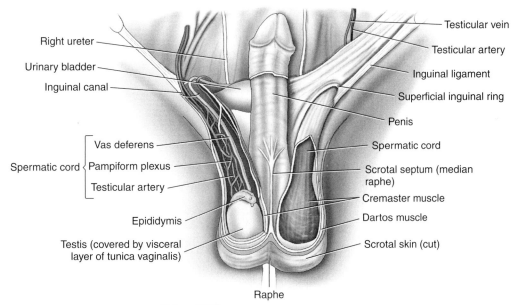

Figure 8.72
Coronal view of male reproductive system.

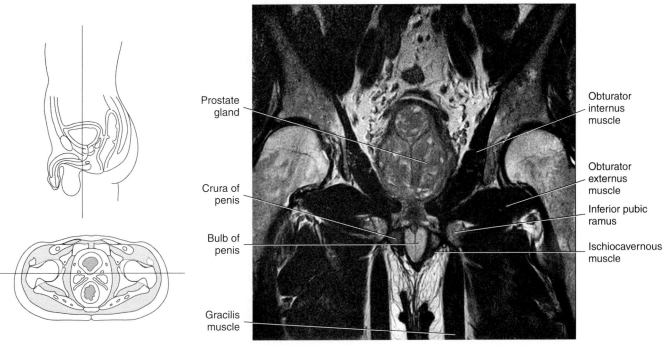

Figure 8.73
Coronal, T2-weighted MR scan of male reproductive system.

SCROTUM The **scrotum** is a musculotendinous pouch that encloses the testis, epididymis, and lower portions of the spermatic cord. It is composed of three fascial layers and a connective tissue layer embedded with smooth muscle fibers called the **dartos tunica.** Internally, the dartos tunic forms a septum that divides the scrotum into right and left compartments **(median raphe),** each containing a testis (Figures 8.72 and 8.73). The scrotum facilitates sperm formation by distending the testes outside the peritoneum in a cooler environment, in effect regulating the temperature of the testes. In cold temperatures the dartos tunica responds by constricting and pulling the testis closer to the body. This gives the scrotum its wrinkled appearance.

TESTES AND EPIDIDYMIS The paired **testes** are suspended in the fleshy, pouchlike scrotal sacs. Each testis is an ovoid organ that produces sperm and male sex hormones. The outer fibrous covering of the testes is the **tunica albuginea,** which also projects into each organ to create wedge-shaped lobules. Each testis is made up of several hundred lobules, with each lobule containing 1 to 4 seminiferous tubules, approximately 800 seminferous tubules in total. The seminiferous tubules leave their respective lobule and converge in an area called the **rete testis.** From here, about 15 to 20 ductules leave the rete testis to enter the head of the epididymis. The **epididymis** is a tightly coiled tubular structure located on the superoposterior surface of each testis. The **head** of the epididymis is located on the upper pole of each testis, whereas the **body** courses along the posterior surface to the **tail,** which is located under the lower pole of each testis. Sperm are transmitted from the testis to the **epididymis,** where they are stored as they undergo the final stages of maturation (Figures 8.70 and 8.75 through 8.78).

KEY: bl, Bladder; **rec,** rectum; **pub,** pubic symphysis; **pe,** penis; **pro,** prostate gland; **te,** testes; **ep,** epididymis.

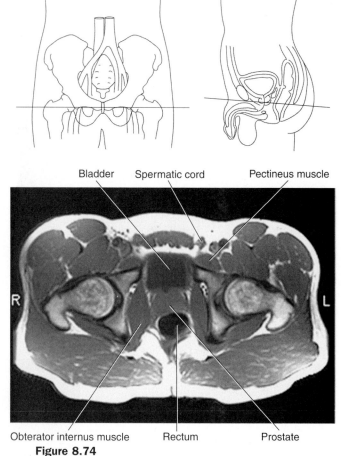

Figure 8.74
Axial, T1-weighted MR scan of male reproductive system.

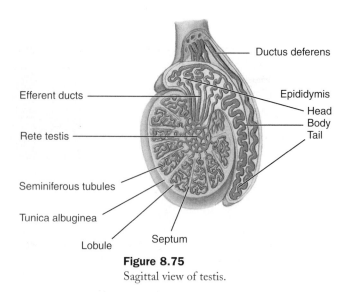

Figure 8.75
Sagittal view of testis.

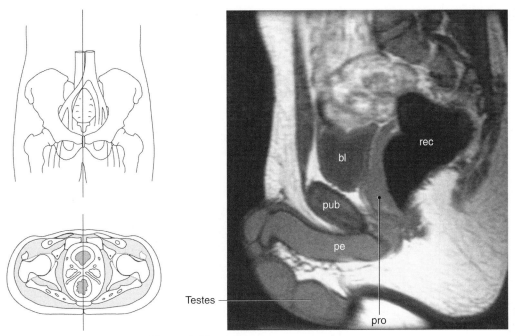

Figure 8.76
Sagittal, T1-weighted MR scan of male pelvis.

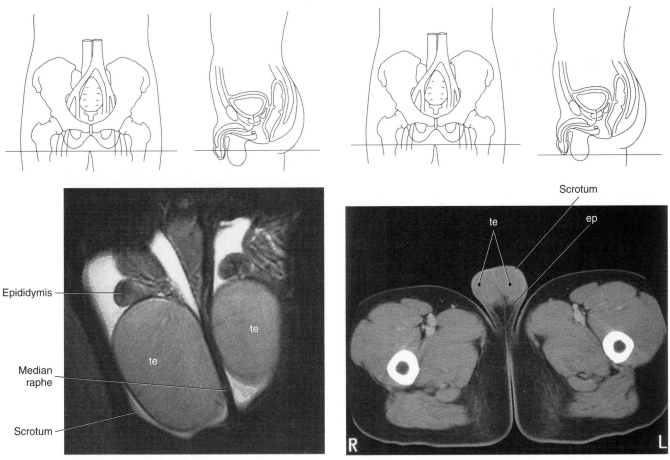

Figure 8.77
Axial, T2-weighted MR scan of pelvis with testis.

Figure 8.78
Axial CT scan of pelvis with testis.

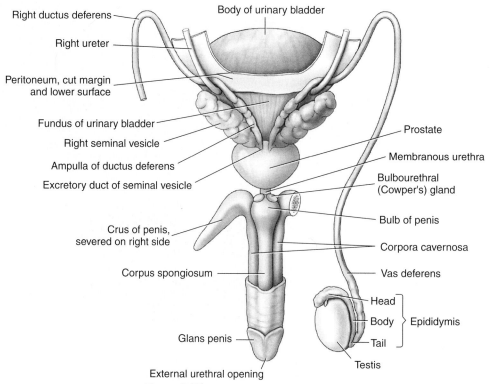

Right ductus deferens

Right ureter

Peritoneum, cut margin and lower surface

Fundus of urinary bladder

Right seminal vesicle

Ampulla of ductus deferens

Excretory duct of seminal vesicle

Body of urinary bladder

Prostate

Membranous urethra

Bulbourethral (Cowper's) gland

Bulb of penis

Crus of penis, severed on right side

Corpus spongiosum

Corpora cavernosa

Vas deferens

Head

Body } Epididymis

Tail

Glans penis

Testis

External urethral opening

Figure 8.79
Coronal view of male reproductive system.

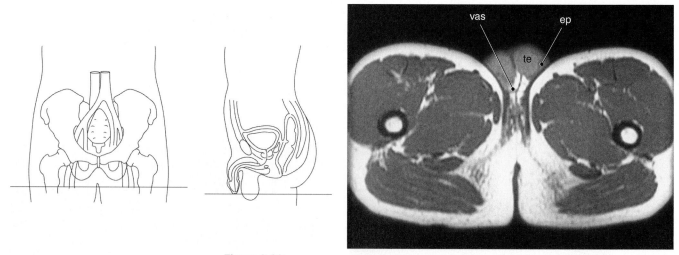

vas   ep

te

Figure 8.80
Axial, T1-weighted MR scan of pelvis with testes.

KEY: vas, Vas deferens; **te,** testes; **ep,** epididymis.

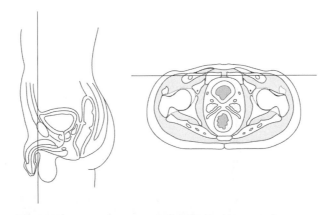

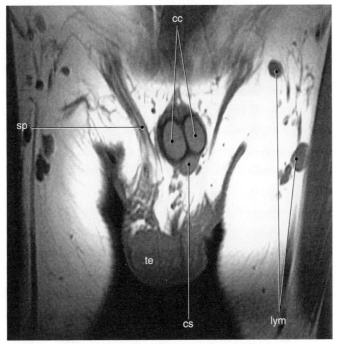

Figure 8.81
Coronal, T1-weighted MR scan of pelvis with spermatic cord.

VAS DEFERENS (DUCTUS) AND EJACULATORY DUCT   As a continuation from the tail of the epididymis, the **vas deferens** is a long muscular tube that ascends in the posterior portion of the spermatic cord and traverses the inguinal canal, exiting at the deep inguinal ring. It then leaves the spermatic cord, passing along the lateral pelvic wall over the ureter to the posterior surface of the bladder, where it broadens and becomes the **ampulla** of the vas deferens. Near its proximal end it joins with the duct of the seminal vesicle to form the **ejaculatory duct,** which empties into the prostatic urethra. Each vas deferens, along with a testicular artery and vein, is surrounded by the tough connective tissue and muscle of the paired **spermatic cords.** The spermatic cords begin at the inguinal ring and exit through the inguinal ligament to descend into the scrotum (Figures 8.74 and 8.79 through 8.83).

SEMINAL VESICLES   The **seminal vesicles** are paired accessory glands consisting of coiled tubes that form two pouches, lateral to the vas deferens, on the posterior inferior surface of the bladder. They lie superior to the prostate gland and produce fructose and a coagulating enzyme for the seminal fluid that mixes with sperm before ejaculation (Figures 8.70, 8.79, and 8.84 through 8.88).

KEY: sp, Spermatic cord; **cc,** corpora cavernosum; **te,** testes; **cs,** corpus spongiosum; **lym,** lymph nodes.

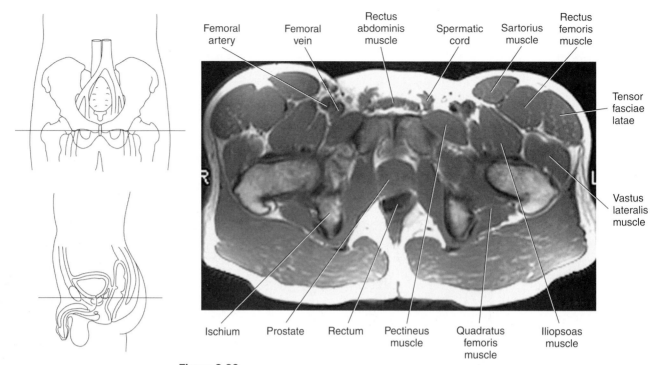

Femoral artery — Femoral vein — Rectus abdominis muscle — Spermatic cord — Sartorius muscle — Rectus femoris muscle — Tensor fasciae latae — Vastus lateralis muscle

Ischium — Prostate — Rectum — Pectineus muscle — Quadratus femoris muscle — Iliopsoas muscle

Figure 8.82
Axial, T1-weighted MR scan of male pelvis with spermatic cord.

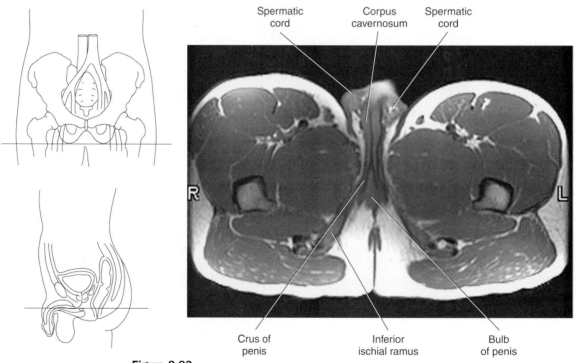

Spermatic cord — Corpus cavernosum — Spermatic cord

Crus of penis — Inferior ischial ramus — Bulb of penis

Figure 8.83
Axial, T1-weighted MR scan of male pelvis with spermatic cord and penis.

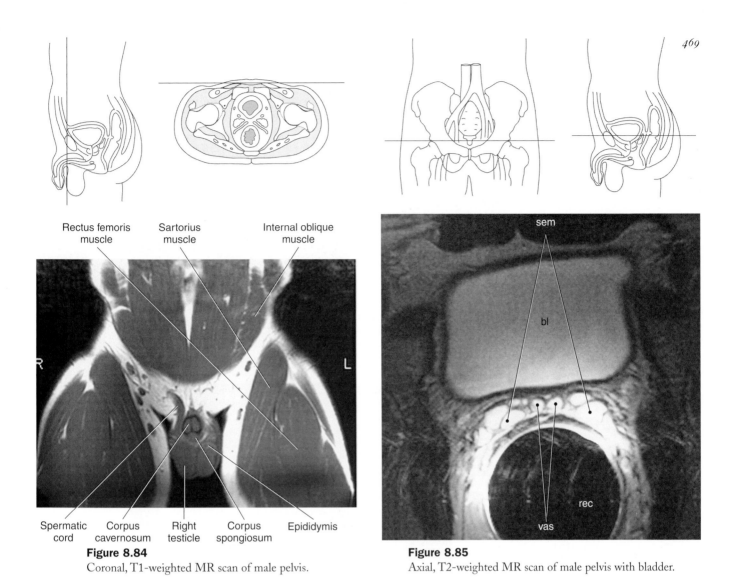

Figure 8.84
Coronal, T1-weighted MR scan of male pelvis.

Figure 8.85
Axial, T2-weighted MR scan of male pelvis with bladder.

KEY: **sem,** Seminal vesicle; **bl,** bladder; **vas,** vas deferens; **rec,** rectum.

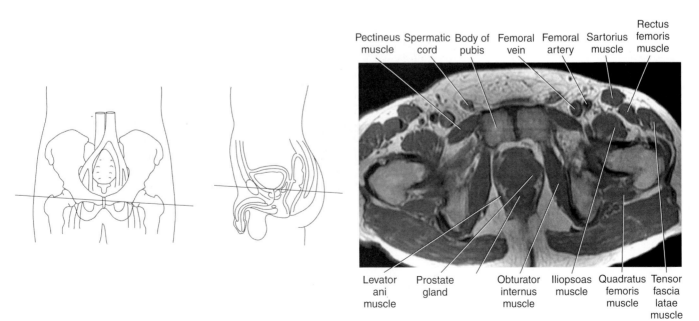

Figure 8.86
Axial, T1-weighted MR scan of male pelvis.

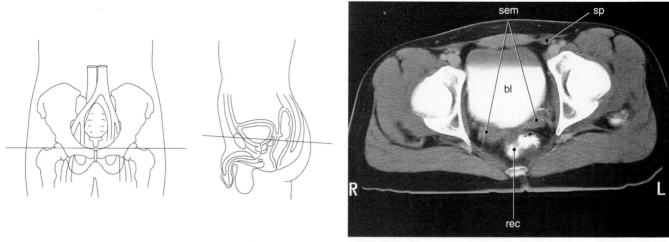

Figure 8.87
Axial CT scan of pelvis with seminal vesicles.

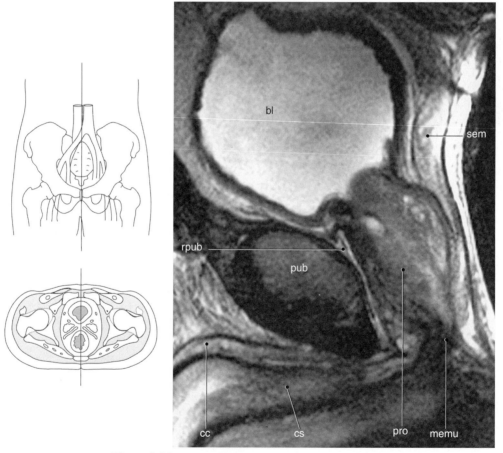

Figure 8.88
Sagittal, T2-weighted MR scan of pelvis with prostate gland.

KEY: sem, Seminal vesicle; **sp,** spermatic cord; **bl,** bladder; **rec,** rectum; **rpub,** retropubic space; **pub,** pubic symphysis; **cc,** corpora cavernosum; **cs,** corpus spongiosum; **pro,** prostate gland; **memu,** membranous urethra.

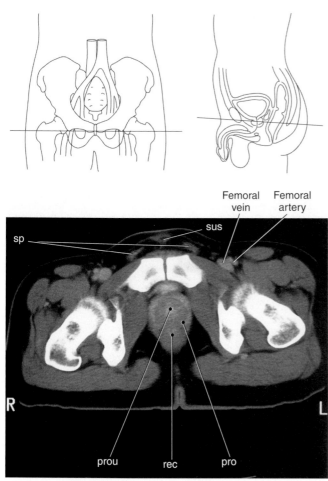

Femoral vein   Femoral artery

Figure 8.89
Axial CT scan of pelvis with prostate gland.

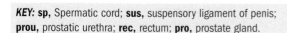

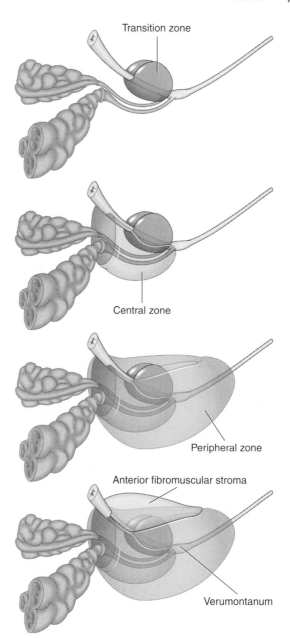

Transition zone

Central zone

Peripheral zone

Anterior fibromuscular stroma

Verumontanum

Figure 8.90
Zonal anatomy of prostate.

PROSTATE GLAND   The **prostate gland** is the largest accessory gland of the male reproductive system. It secretes a thin, slightly alkaline fluid that forms a portion of the seminal fluid. The prostate gland is located inferior to the bladder and surrounds the prosthetic urethra, which courses through the anterior portion of the gland (Figures 8.70, 8.88, and 8.89). The prostate has a base adjacent to the neck of the bladder and an apex that is in contact with the urogenital diaphragm. The prostate gland is composed of glandular and fibromuscular tissue and surrounded by a fibrous capsule. It can be divided into two lateral lobes, a middle lobe, and an anterior fibromuscular portion. The ejaculatory ducts, which are extensions of the seminal vesicles, descend within the central zone of the gland and open into the prostatic urethra at the verumontanum. The **verumontanum** is a longitudinal mucosal fold that forms an elliptical segment of the prostatic urethra, marking the point where the ejaculatory ducts enter the urethra. The glandular tissue comprises two thirds of the prostate's parenchymal tissue and in sectional imaging can be divided into zonal anatomy. The four main regions are the central, peripheral, transition, and periurethral zones (Figures 8.90 through 8.92). The **central zone** is located at the base of the prostate between the peripheral and transition zones and accounts for approximately 25% of the glandular tissue. It surrounds the ejaculatory ducts, then narrows to an apex at the verumontanum. The **peripheral zone** is the larger of the zones, comprising approximately 70%

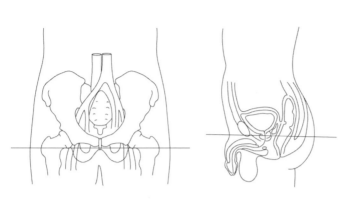

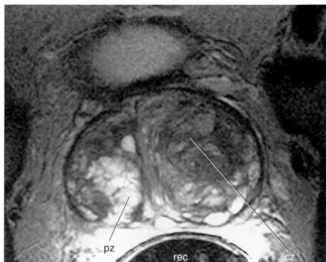

Figure 8.91
Axial, T2-weighted MR scan of pelvis with prostate gland and zones.

of the glandular tissue. It extends from the base to the apex along the posterior or rectal surface of the gland and surrounds the distal urethra. The peripheral zone is separated from the central and transition zones by the surgical capsule. The **transition zone** forms only 5% of the glandular tissue. It consists of two small lobules that are located lateral to the proximal urethra between the verumontanum and the neck of the bladder. This is the portion of the glandular tissue that enlarges due to benign prostatic hypertrophy. The periurethral zone comprises less than 1% of the glandular tissue. It is found embedded along the smooth muscular wall of the urethra. The **anterior fibromuscular area** is devoid of glandular tissue and is composed of fibrous and muscular elements. As it extends laterally and posteriorly, it thins to form the fibrous capsule that surrounds the prostate gland.

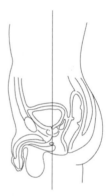

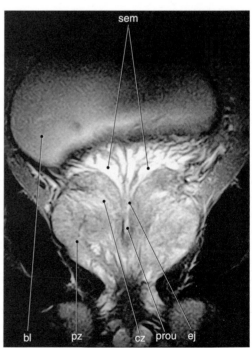

Cancer of the prostate gland is the second most common type of cancer in men, occurring with increasing frequency after the age of 55 years.

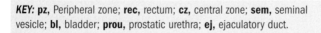

KEY: pz, Peripheral zone; **rec,** rectum; **cz,** central zone; **sem,** seminal vesicle; **bl,** bladder; **prou,** prostatic urethra; **ej,** ejaculatory duct.

Figure 8.92
Coronal, T2-weighted MR scan of prostate gland.

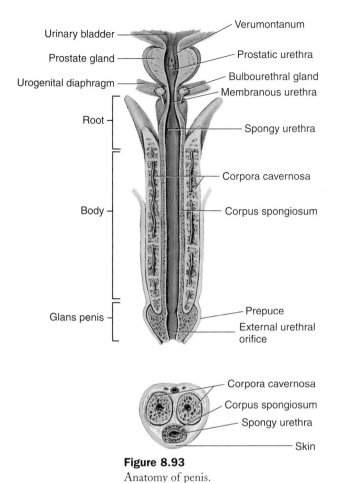

Figure 8.93
Anatomy of penis.

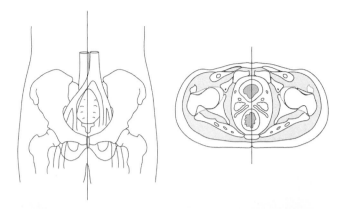

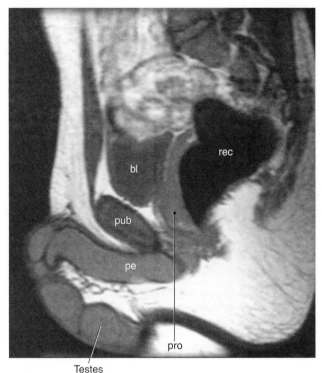

Figure 8.94
Sagittal, T2-weighted MR scan of male pelvis.

BULBOURETHRAL GLANDS   The two small, **bulbourethral glands (Cowper's glands)** lie posterolateral to the membranous urethra, embedded in the urogenital diaphragm. These glands secrete an alkaline fluid into the membranous urethra that forms a portion of the seminal fluid (Figure 8.93).

PENIS   The **penis,** the external reproductive organ, is attached to the pubic arch via suspensory ligaments. It has two parts: the **root,** which is attached to the pubic arch, and the **body,** which remains free. Three cylindric masses of erectile tissue compose the root of the penis: two corpora cavernosa and the corpus spongiosum. The **corpora cavernosa** consists of a network of collagen fibers and spaces that become enlarged when filled with blood, contributing to an erection. The **corpus spongiosum** consists mostly of a dense venous plexus and contributes to an erection. The two corpora cavernosa form the upper surface, whereas the corpus spongiosum forms the undersurface and contains the greater part of the urethra. At the root of the penis the corpora cavernosa forms the **crura,** which attach along the ischiopubic ramus. The corpus spongiosum forms the **bulb** of the penis that is located between the two crura and is firmly attached to the inferior aspect of the urogenital diaphragm. The distal end of the cylindric masses forms the **glans penis,** which surrounds the external urethral meatus (Figures 8.93 through 8.97).

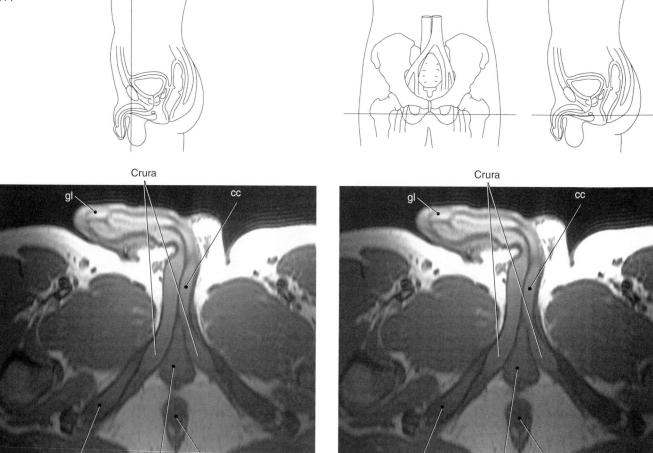

Figure 8.95
Coronal, T1-weighted MR scan of pelvis and penis.

Figure 8.96
Axial, T1-weighted MR scan of pelvis and penis.

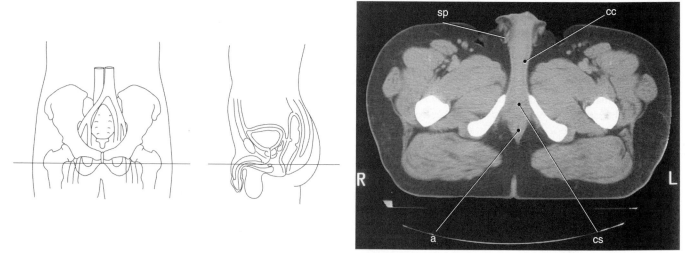

Figure 8.97
Axial CT scan of pelvis and penis.

KEY: cc, Corpora cavernosum; **te,** testes; **cs,** corpus spongiosum; **gl,** glans of penis; **ipub,** inferior pubic ramus; **bulb,** bulb of penis; **rec,** rectum; **sp,** spermatic cord; **a,** anus.

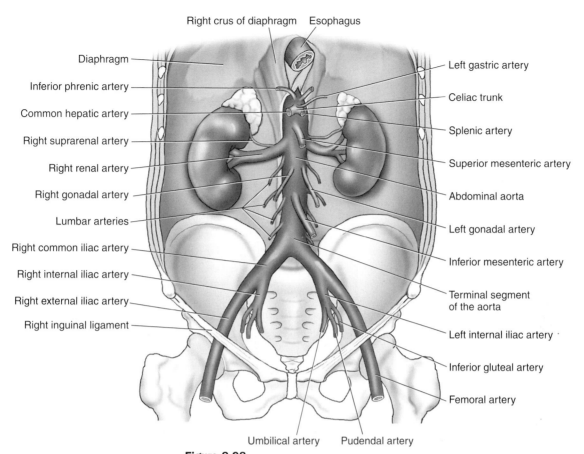

Right crus of diaphragm   Esophagus

Diaphragm

Inferior phrenic artery

Common hepatic artery

Right suprarenal artery

Right renal artery

Right gonadal artery

Lumbar arteries

Right common iliac artery

Right internal iliac artery

Right external iliac artery

Right inguinal ligament

Left gastric artery

Celiac trunk

Splenic artery

Superior mesenteric artery

Abdominal aorta

Left gonadal artery

Inferior mesenteric artery

Terminal segment of the aorta

Left internal iliac artery

Inferior gluteal artery

Femoral artery

Umbilical artery   Pudendal artery

Figure 8.98
Anterior view of abdominal aorta and vessels.

VASCULATURE

Arteries

The descending aorta bifurcates at the level of the fourth lumbar vertebra into the right and left **common iliac arteries** (Figures 8.98 and 8.99). Each common iliac artery bifurcates at the upper margin of the sacroiliac joint into the internal and external iliac arteries (Figure 8.100). The smaller **internal iliac artery** extends posteromedially into the pelvis just medial to the external iliac vein and branches into an anterior trunk and a posterior trunk. The **anterior trunk of the internal iliac artery** supplies blood to the perineum, gluteal region, and pelvic viscera. Branches of the anterior trunk of the internal iliac artery include the **obturator, umbilical, inferior vesical** in males, **uterine** and **vaginal** in females, **middle rectal, internal**

pudendal, and **inferior gluteal arteries** (Figure 8.101). The **posterior trunk of the internal iliac artery** supplies blood to the posterior and lateral walls of the pelvis, iliac crest, and gluteal region. Branches of the posterior trunk include the **iliolumbar, lateral sacral,** and **superior gluteal arteries.** The large **external iliac artery** does not enter the true pelvis but extends along the pelvic brim to exit the iliac fossa and course under the inguinal ligament to supply the leg. The external iliac artery becomes the femoral artery at approximately the level of the anterior superior iliac spine. Branches of the external iliac artery include the **inferior epigastric artery,** which supplies blood to the muscles and skin of the anterior abdominal wall, and the **deep circumflex iliac artery,** which supplies blood to the lateral abdominal muscles (Figures 8.102 through 8.112 and Table 8.2).

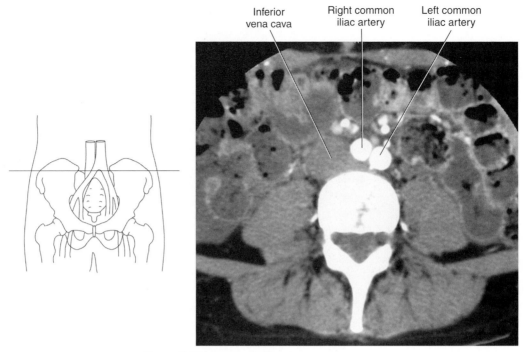

Figure 8.99
Axial CT scan of pelvis with common iliac vessels.

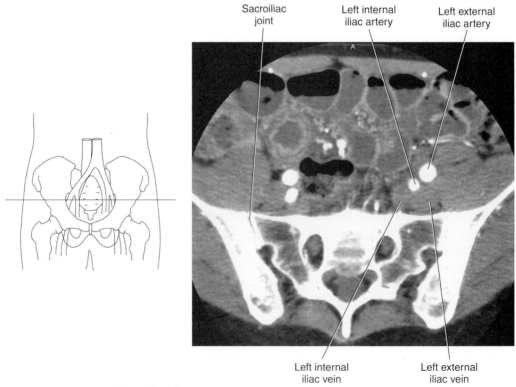

Figure 8.100
Axial CT scan of pelvis with internal and external iliac vessels.

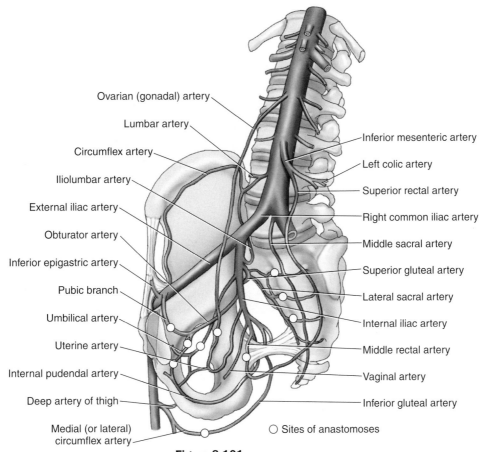

Ovarian (gonadal) artery

Lumbar artery

Circumflex artery

Iliolumbar artery

External iliac artery

Obturator artery

Inferior epigastric artery

Pubic branch

Umbilical artery

Uterine artery

Internal pudendal artery

Deep artery of thigh

Medial (or lateral)
circumflex artery

Inferior mesenteric artery

Left colic artery

Superior rectal artery

Right common iliac artery

Middle sacral artery

Superior gluteal artery

Lateral sacral artery

Internal iliac artery

Middle rectal artery

Vaginal artery

Inferior gluteal artery

○ Sites of anastomoses

Figure 8.101
Anterior view of iliac arteries.

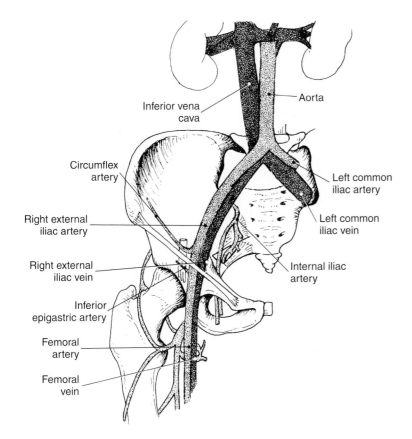

Circumflex
artery

Right external
iliac artery

Right external
iliac vein

Inferior
epigastric artery

Femoral
artery

Femoral
vein

Inferior vena
cava

Aorta

Left common
iliac artery

Left common
iliac vein

Internal iliac
artery

Figure 8.102
Anterior view of inferior vena cava and abdominal aorta.

478

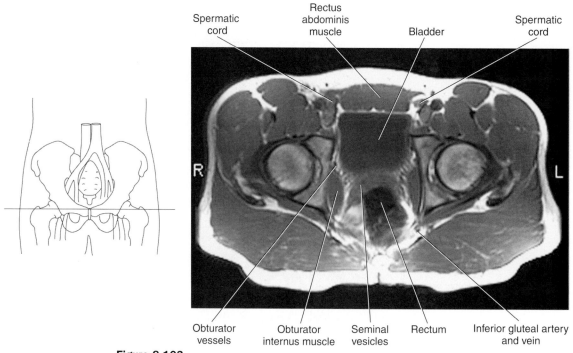

Figure 8.103

Axial, T1-weighted MR scan of male pelvis with inferior gluteal vessels.

Spermatic cord | Rectus abdominis muscle | Bladder | Spermatic cord

Obturator vessels | Obturator internus muscle | Seminal vesicles | Rectum | Inferior gluteal artery and vein

R | L

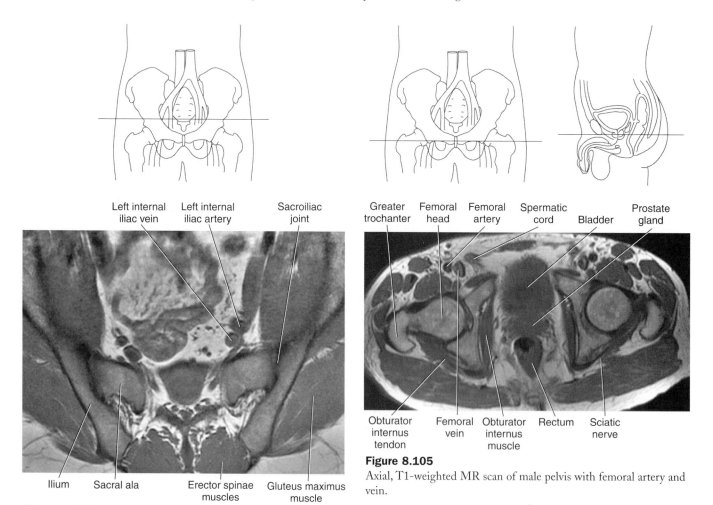

Left internal iliac vein | Left internal iliac artery | Sacroiliac joint

Ilium | Sacral ala | Erector spinae muscles | Gluteus maximus muscle

Figure 8.104

Axial, T1-weighted MR scan of male pelvis with internal iliac vessels.

Greater trochanter | Femoral head | Femoral artery | Spermatic cord | Bladder | Prostate gland

Obturator internus tendon | Femoral vein | Obturator internus muscle | Rectum | Sciatic nerve

Figure 8.105

Axial, T1-weighted MR scan of male pelvis with femoral artery and vein.

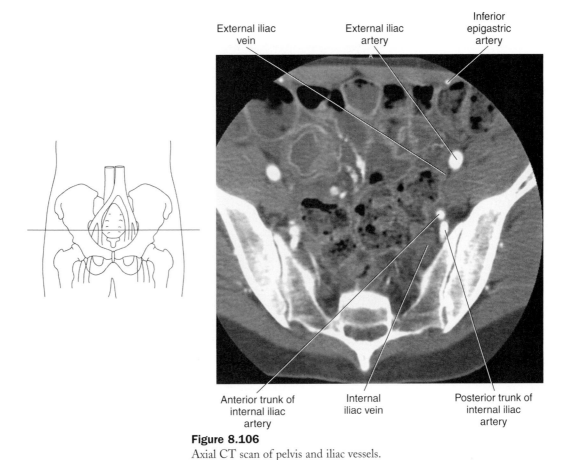

External iliac vein

External iliac artery

Inferior epigastric artery

Anterior trunk of internal iliac artery

Internal iliac vein

Posterior trunk of internal iliac artery

Figure 8.106
Axial CT scan of pelvis and iliac vessels.

Obturator artery

Femoral vein

Femoral artery

Internal pudendal artery

Inferior gluteal artery

Rectal artery

Figure 8.107
Axial CT scan of pelvis with internal pudendal artery.

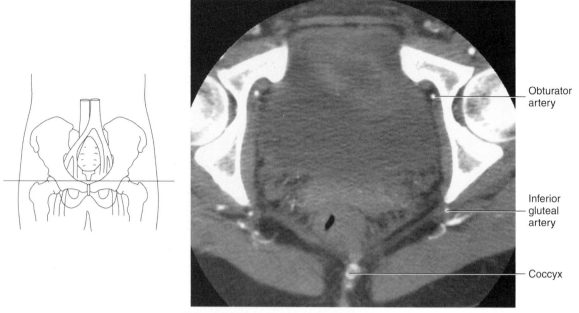

Obturator
artery

Inferior
gluteal
artery

Coccyx

Figure 8.108
Axial CT scan of pelvis with obturator artery.

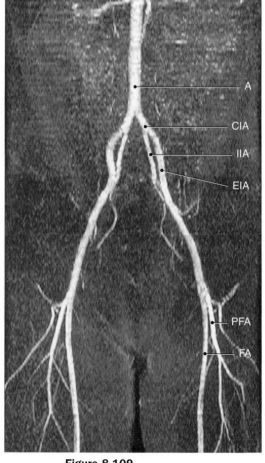

A

CIA

IIA

EIA

PFA

FA

Figure 8.109
MR angiogram of iliac vessels.

KEY: **A,** Aorta; **CIA,** common iliac artery; **IIA,** internal iliac artery;
EIA, external iliac artery; **PFA,** profunda femoris artery; **FA,** femoral
artery.

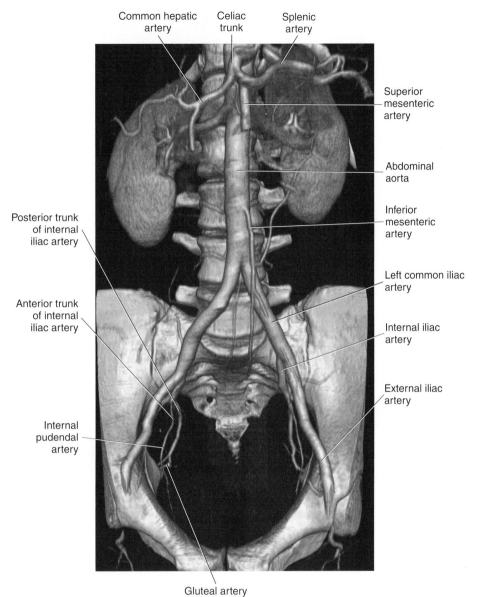

Common hepatic
artery

Celiac
trunk

Splenic
artery

Superior
mesenteric
artery

Abdominal
aorta

Inferior
mesenteric
artery

Posterior trunk
of internal
iliac artery

Anterior trunk
of internal
iliac artery

Internal
pudendal
artery

Left common iliac
artery

Internal iliac
artery

External iliac
artery

Gluteal artery

Figure 8.110
Coronal CT angiogram of iliac vessels.

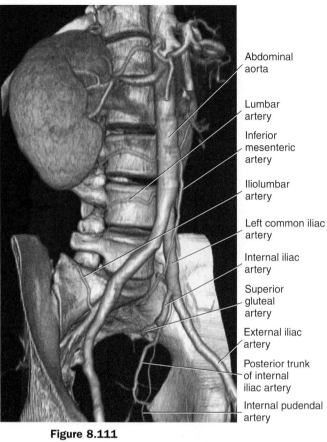

Figure 8.111
Coronal oblique CT angiogram of iliac vessels.

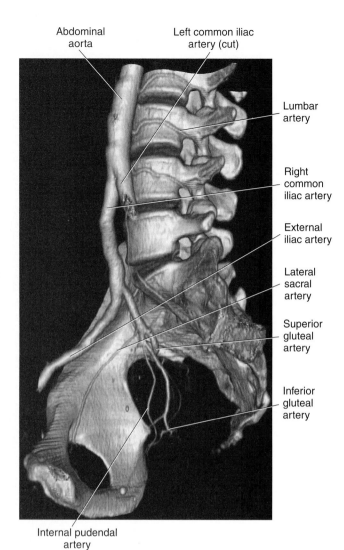

Figure 8.112
Sagittal CT angiogram of iliac vessels.

TABLE 8-2   Branches of the Internal and External Iliac Arteries

ARTERIAL BRANCH	STRUCTURES SUPPLIED
Anterior Branch of Internal Iliac	
Obturator artery	Medial thigh
Umbilical artery	Superior bladder, vas deferens
Uterine artery	Uterus, cervix, and vagina
Vaginal artery	Vagina, posteroinferior bladder, pelvic part of urethra
Inferior vesicle artery	Prostate, seminal vesicles, and posteroinferior part of the bladder
Middle rectal artery	Distal end of rectum, prostate, and seminal vesicles or vagina.
Internal pudendal artery	Anal canal and perineum
Inferior gluteal artery	Muscles and skin of the buttock and posterior surface of the thigh
Posterior Branch of Internal Iliac	
Iliolumbar artery	Psoas, iliacus, quadratus lumborum, and gluteal muscles, cauda equina
Lateral sacral artery	Spinal meninges, roots of the sacral nerves, and muscles and skin of dorsal sacrum
Superior gluteal artery	Obturator internus, piriformis, and gluteus muscles
Branches of External Iliac Artery	
Inferior epigastric artery	Ascend abdomen to anastomose with internal thoracic vessels to supply the anterior abdominal wall
Deep circumflex iliac artery	Ascend abdomen to anastomose with internal thoracic vessels to supply the lateral aspect of the anterior abdominal wall

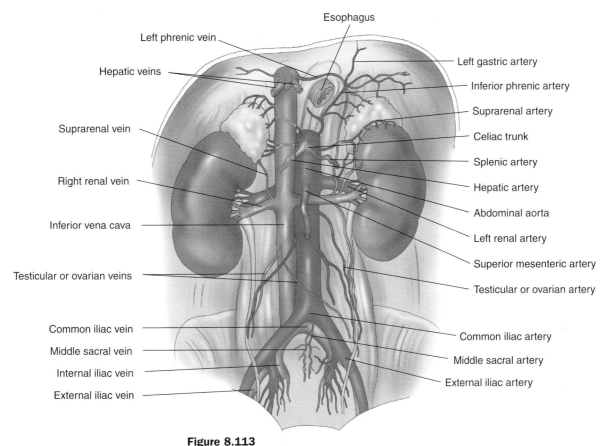

Figure 8.113
Anterior view of inferior vena cava and tributaries.

Venous Drainage

Venous drainage of the pelvis follows a pattern similar to that of the arterial supply. Mainly the **internal iliac veins** and their tributaries drain the pelvis (Figure 8.113). However, there is some drainage through the **superior rectal, median sacral, and gonadal veins.** The internal iliac vein ascends the pelvis medial to the internal iliac artery as it returns blood from the pelvic viscera. Tributaries of the internal iliac vein are similar to that of the branches of the internal iliac artery with some differences, such as the umbilical vein, which usually obliterates to form the ligamentum teres, and the iliolumbar vein that usually drains into the common iliac vein. In addition, **venous plexuses** are formed by the veins in the pelvis and unite to drain mainly into the internal iliac vein (Figure 8.114).

These plexuses include the uterine, vaginal, prostatic, vesical, and rectal. The **external iliac veins,** extensions of the femoral veins, return blood from the legs. Typically, both external iliac veins course medial to their respective external iliac artery, then change to a posterior position as they ascend to join the common iliac vein at approximately the level of the sacroiliac joint. The **common iliac vein** arises posterior to the common iliac artery from the junction of the internal and external iliac veins. The **inferior vena cava** is formed at the level of L5, just a little to the right of the midline, by the union of the common iliac veins. From this level it continues to ascend the abdomen to the right of the abdominal aorta (Figures 8.99, 8.100, and 8.102 through 8.107).

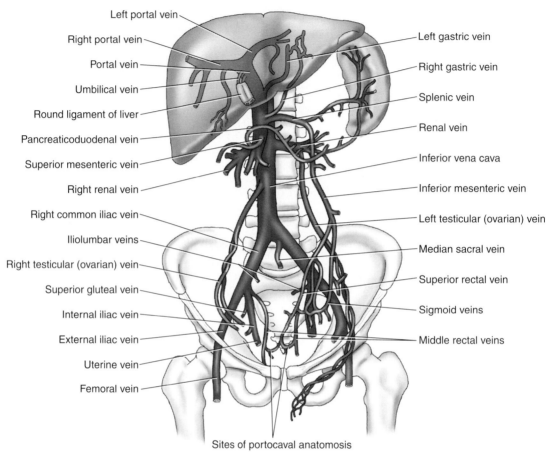

Left portal vein

Right portal vein

Portal vein

Umbilical vein

Round ligament of liver

Pancreaticoduodenal vein

Superior mesenteric vein

Right renal vein

Right common iliac vein

Iliolumbar veins

Right testicular (ovarian) vein

Superior gluteal vein

Internal iliac vein

External iliac vein

Uterine vein

Femoral vein

Left gastric vein

Right gastric vein

Splenic vein

Renal vein

Inferior vena cava

Inferior mesenteric vein

Left testicular (ovarian) vein

Median sacral vein

Superior rectal vein

Sigmoid veins

Middle rectal veins

Sites of portocaval anatomosis

Figure 8.114

Veins of the pelvis.

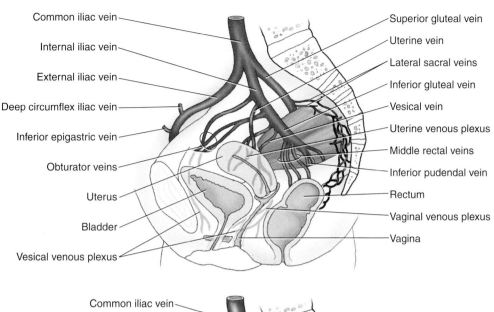

Common iliac vein
Internal iliac vein
External iliac vein
Deep circumflex iliac vein
Inferior epigastric vein
Obturator veins
Uterus
Bladder
Vesical venous plexus

Superior gluteal vein
Uterine vein
Lateral sacral veins
Inferior gluteal vein
Vesical vein
Uterine venous plexus
Middle rectal veins
Inferior pudendal vein
Rectum
Vaginal venous plexus
Vagina

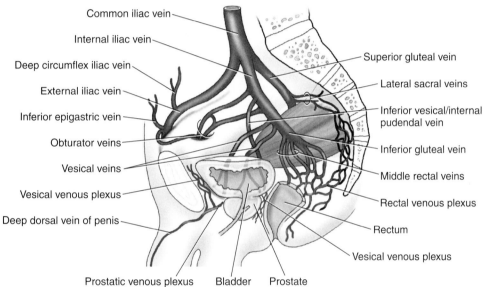

Common iliac vein
Internal iliac vein
Deep circumflex iliac vein
External iliac vein
Inferior epigastric vein
Obturator veins
Vesical veins
Vesical venous plexus
Deep dorsal vein of penis

Superior gluteal vein
Lateral sacral veins
Inferior vesical/internal pudendal vein
Inferior gluteal vein
Middle rectal veins
Rectal venous plexus
Rectum
Vesical venous plexus

Prostatic venous plexus   Bladder   Prostate

Figure 8.114, cont'd
Veins of the pelvis. *Top,* Female. *Bottom,* Male.

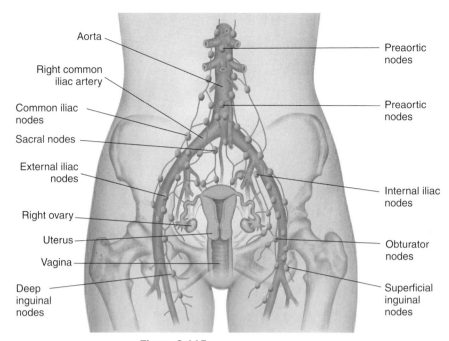

Figure 8.115
Anterior view of pelvic lymph nodes.

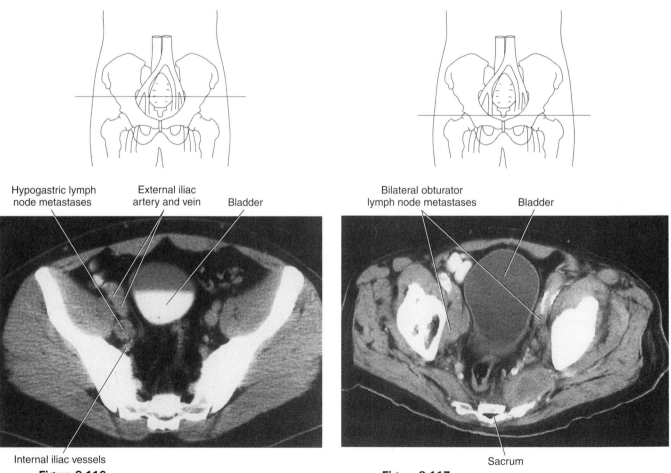

Figure 8.116
Axial CT scan of pelvis with enlarged lymph nodes.

Figure 8.117
Axial CT scan of pelvis with enlarged lymph nodes.

LYMPH NODES

Pelvic lymph nodes include nodal chains or groups that accompany their corresponding vessels and inguinal nodal groups. Those nodal groups that correspond to pelvic vessels include the common iliac, internal iliac, external iliac, and sacral nodal groups (Figure 8.115). The **common iliac lymph nodes** form two groups along the surface of the common iliac artery: a lateral group and a median group. The **lateral common iliac group** receives lymph from the lower limb and pelvis via the external and internal iliac lymph nodes. The **median common iliac group** receives lymph directly from the pelvic viscera and indirectly through the internal iliac and sacral lymph nodes. The **obturator nodes** that course along the midportion of the obturator internus muscle are included in the medial common iliac group. The **external iliac lymph nodes** lie on the external iliac vessels and drain lymph from the lower limb, abdominal wall, bladder, and prostate in males or uterus and vagina in females. The **internal iliac lymph nodes** surround the internal iliac vessels and their branches. They receive lymph from all the pelvic viscera, deep parts of the perineum, and gluteal and thigh regions. **Sacral lymph nodes** lie along the median and lateral sacral arteries. They receive lymph from the posterior pelvic wall, rectum, neck of the bladder, and prostate or cervix. The **inguinal lymph nodes** drain lymph from the lower limb, perineum, anterior abdominal wall as far superiorly as the umbilicus, gluteal region, and parts of the anal canal. They can be divided into the superficial inguinal lymph nodes that are situated distal to the inguinal ligament in the subcutaneous tissue anterior and medial to common femoral vessels. The deep inguinal lymph nodes are fewer in number and are situated medial to the femoral vessels at the approximate level of the ischial tuberosity. Pelvic lymph nodes are considered pathologically enlarged when they exceed 10 mm in the short axis (Figures 8.116 through 8.118).

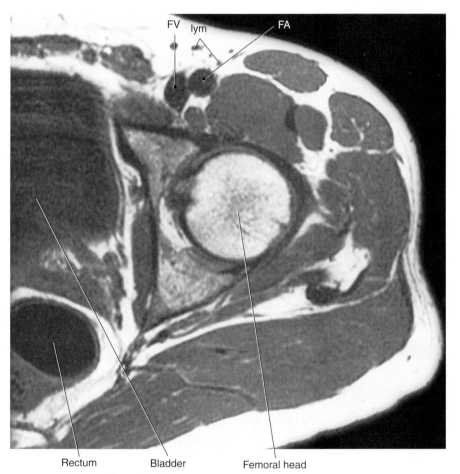

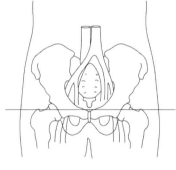

Figure 8.118
Axial, T1-weighted MR scan of pelvis with femoral artery and vein and inguinal lymph nodes.

KEY: FV, Femoral vein; **lym,** lymph nodes; **FA,** femoral artery.

CHAPTER 9

UPPER EXTREMITY

It is sometimes on one's weakest limbs that one must lean in order to keep going.

JEAN ROSTAND
Substance of Man

The intricate anatomy of the musculoskeletal system can make identification of the joint anatomy challenging (Figure 9.1). A basic knowledge of the anatomy and kinesiology of these areas increases the ability to identify pathology or injury that may occur.

SHOULDER
  Bony Anatomy
  Labrum and Ligaments
  Articular Joint Capsule
  Bursae
  Muscles and Tendons

ELBOW
  Bony Anatomy
  Ligaments
  Muscles of the Forearm

WRIST AND HAND
  Bony Anatomy
  Joints
  Ligaments and Fascia
  Muscles and Tendons

NEUROVASCULATURE
  Arterial Supply
  Venous Drainage

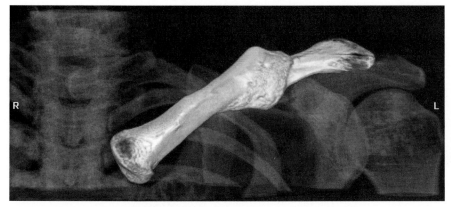

Figure 9.1
3D CT—healing fracture of the clavicle.

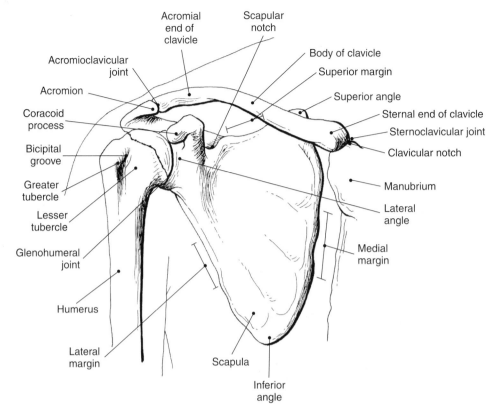

Figure 9.2
Anterior view of shoulder girdle.

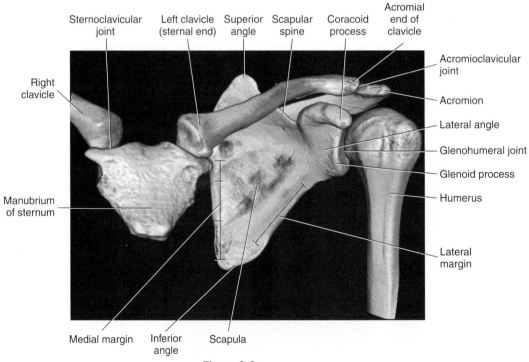

Figure 9.3
3D CT of shoulder girdle.

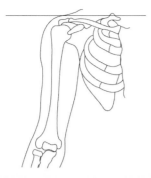

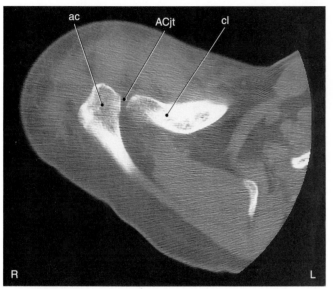

Figure 9.4
Axial CT scan of shoulder with acromioclavicular joint.

SHOULDER

Bony Anatomy

The bony anatomy that comprises the shoulder girdle includes the clavicle, scapula, and humerus (Figures 9.2 and 9.3).

CLAVICLE   The clavicle connects the upper limb to the trunk of the body and provides attachments for several muscles and ligaments. The clavicle is a long, slender S-shaped bone located anteriorly that extends transversely from the sternum to the acromion of the scapula. The widened **sternal end** of the clavicle articulates with the clavicular notch of the sternal manubrium to form the **sternoclavicular (SC) joint,** and its flattened **acromial end** articulates with the acromial process of the scapula to form the **acromioclavicular (AC) joint.** The medial two thirds of the body of the clavicle are convex anteriorly, whereas the lateral one third is flattened and concave anteriorly (Figures 9.2 through 9.6).

KEY: **ac,** Acromion; **ACjt,** acromioclavicular joint; **cl,** clavicle.

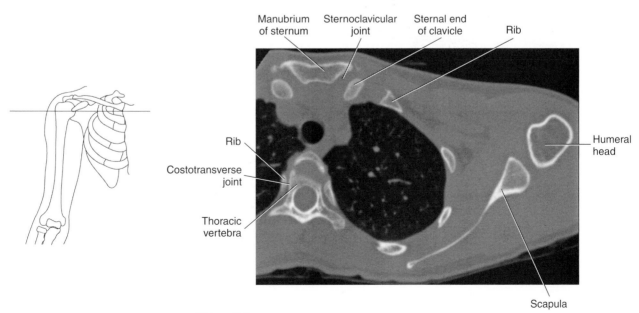

Figure 9.5
Axial CT scan of shoulder with sternoclavicular joint.

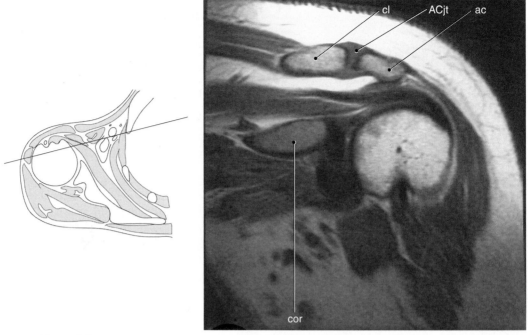

Figure 9.6
Coronal oblique, T1-weighted MR scan of shoulder with acromioclavicular joint.

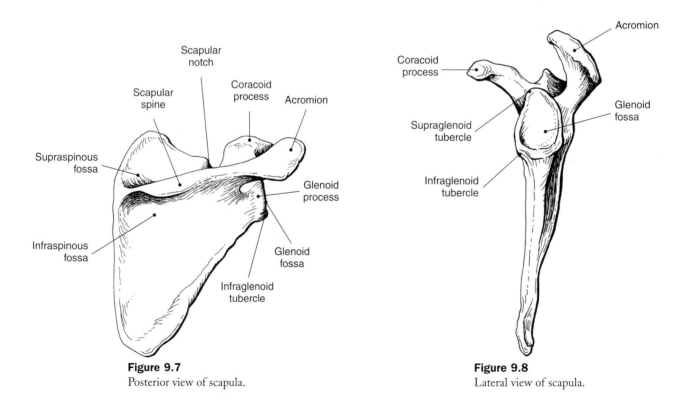

Figure 9.7
Posterior view of scapula.

Figure 9.8
Lateral view of scapula.

KEY: cl, Clavicle; **ACjt,** acromioclavicular joint; **ac,** acromion; **cor,** coracoid process.

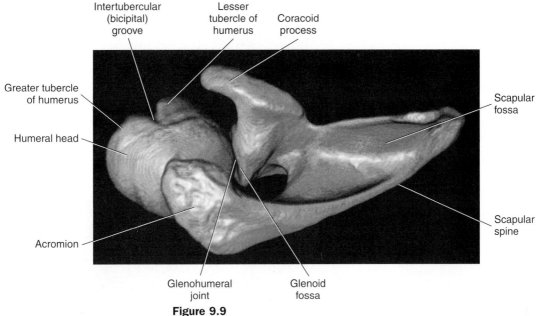

Intertubercular (bicipital) groove

Lesser tubercle of humerus

Coracoid process

Greater tubercle of humerus

Humeral head

Scapular fossa

Acromion

Scapular spine

Glenohumeral joint

Glenoid fossa

Figure 9.9
3D CT scan of superior aspect of scapula.

SCAPULA The scapula is a triangular-shaped flat bone that forms the posterior portion of the shoulder girdle. It has a medial margin, a lateral margin, and a superior margin. The margins are separated by the superior, inferior, and lateral angles (Figures 9.2 and 9.3). The anterior surface of the scapula, **subscapular fossa,** is flat and slightly concave. The posterior surface of the scapula is divided by the scapular spine into a smaller **supraspinous fossa,** and a larger **infraspinous fossa** (Figure 9.7). Four projections of the scapula provide attachment sites for the muscles and ligaments contributing to the shoulder girdle. These include the **scapular spine, acromion, coracoid process,** and **glenoid process** (Figures 9.7 through 9.10). The scapular spine arises from the upper third of the posterior surface of the scapula and extends obliquely and laterally to give rise to a flattened process termed the **acromion.** Located on the anterolateral surface of the scapula is a beaklike process termed the **coracoid process,** which arises just medial to the glenoid process and functions to protect the shoulder joint, which lies beneath it. The coracoid process is an attachment site for the pectoralis minor, short head of the biceps brachii, and the coracobrachialis muscles. The **scapular notch** is located just medial to the coracoid process, on the superior margin of the scapula and allows for the passage of the suprascapular nerve (Figure 9.2). The **glenoid process,** the largest of the projections, forms the lateral angle of the scapula and ends in a depression called the **glenoid fossa (glenoid cavity)** (Figures 9.7 through 9.9). There are two tubercles associated with the glenoid fossa, an upper **supraglenoid tubercle** and a lower **infraglenoid tubercle,** which serve as attachment sites for the biceps brachii and triceps brachii (Figure 9.8). The shallow articular surface of the glenoid fossa joins with the relatively large articular surface of the humeral head to create the freely moving **glenohumeral joint** (Figures 9.2, 9.3, 9.11, and 9.12).

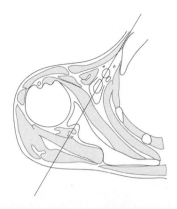

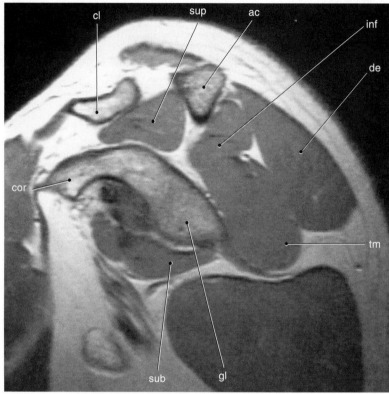

Figure 9.10
Sagittal oblique, T1-weighted MR scan of shoulder.

KEY: cor, Coracoid process; **cl,** clavicle; **sup,** supraspinatus; **ac,** acromion; **inf,** infraspinatus; **de,** deltoid; **tm,** teres minor; **gl,** glenoid; **sub,** subscapularis; **h,** humerus; **grt,** greater tubercle; **sc,** scapula; **glf,** glenoid fossa; **hh,** humeral head.

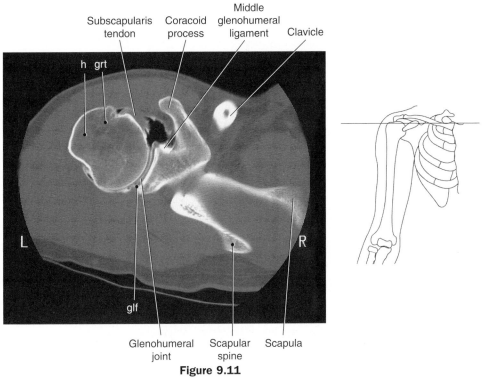

Figure 9.11
Axial CT scan of shoulder, midjoint.

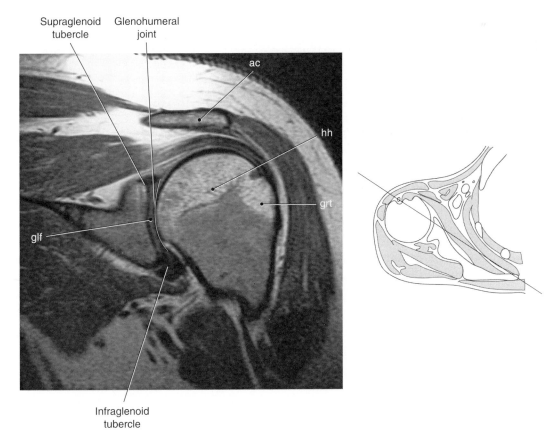

Figure 9.12
Coronal oblique, T1-weighted MR scan of shoulder, midjoint.

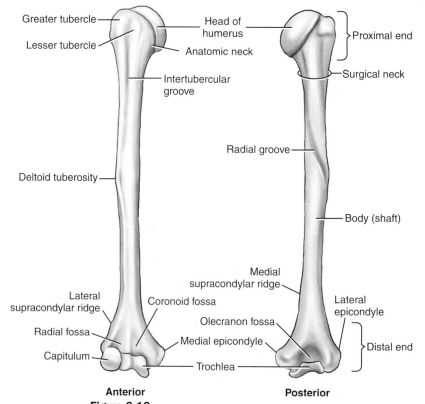

Figure 9.13

Humerus. *Left*, Anterior view. *Right*, Posterior view.

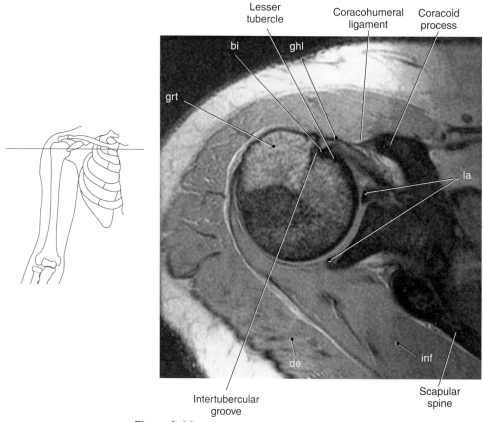

Figure 9.14

Axial, T1-weighted MR scan of shoulder, midjoint.

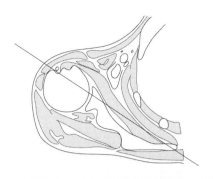

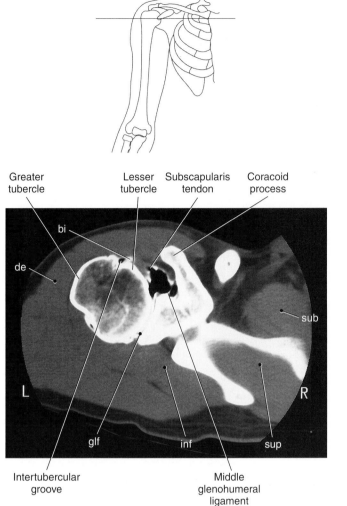

Greater tubercle Lesser tubercle Subscapularis tendon Coracoid process

bi

de

sub

L   R

glf   inf   sup

Intertubercular groove   Middle glenohumeral ligament

Figure 9.15
Axial CT scan with shoulder, midjoint.

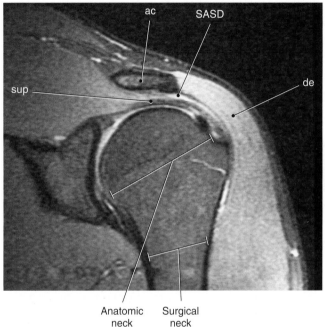

ac   SASD

sup   de

Anatomic neck   Surgical neck

Figure 9.16
Coronal oblique, T2-weighted MR scan of shoulder with subacromial-subdeltoid bursa.

HUMERUS The humerus is a long bone that articulates with the scapula superiorly and the radius and ulna inferiorly. It consists of a body or shaft, a lower end (distal end), and an upper (proximal) end (Figure 9.13). The proximal end is formed by the head of the humerus. Two tubercles project from the **humeral head** to provide attachment sites for tendons and ligaments. The **lesser tubercle** is located on the anterior surface of the humeral head, whereas the **greater tubercle** is located on the lateral surface of the humeral head (Figures 9.12 through 9.15). The tubercles are separated by the **intertubercular** **(bicipital) groove,** which is bounded by the crests of the lesser and greater tubercles as it descends the humerus (Figures 9.9 and 9.13 through 9.15). The humerus has two necks, the more proximal **anatomic neck** and the **surgical neck,** located inferior to the tubercles just distal to the humeral head (Figures 9.13 and 9.16). In the middle of the body or shaft of the humerus, on the anterior surface, is the roughened area of the **deltoid tuberosity** that gives attachment for the deltoid muscle (Figure 9.13).

KEY: **grt,** Greater tubercle; **bi,** biceps tendon; **ghl,** glenohumeral ligament; **la,** labrum; **inf,** infraspinatus; **de,** deltoid; **sub,** subscapularis; **sup,** supraspinatus tendon; **glf,** glenoid fossa; **ac,** acromion; **SASD,** subacromial-subdeltoid bursa.

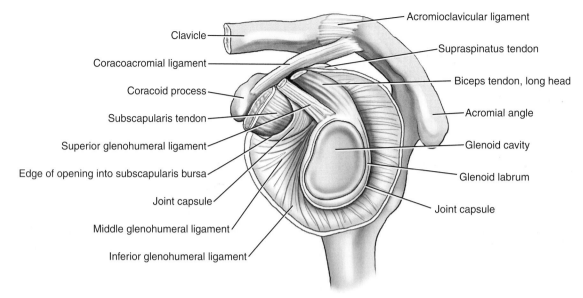

Figure 9.17
Lateral view of glenohumeral ligaments and glenoid labrum.

Labrum and Ligaments

The edge of the glenoid fossa is surrounded by a fibro-cartilaginous ring termed the **glenoid labrum (glenoid lip)** (Figure 9.17). The glenoid labrum is a fold of the articular capsule, which functions to deepen the articular surface of the glenoid fossa. Superiorly, the labrum blends with the long head of the biceps brachii muscle. In cross section it appears triangular (Figure 9.18). The three **glenohumeral ligaments** (superior middle, and inferior) are thickenings of the fibrous capsule that surrounds the shoulder joint; they contributes to the formation of the glenoid labrum (Figures 9.17 and 9.19). They extend from the supraglenoid tubercle of the scapula to the lesser tubercle of the humerus. Also aiding in strengthening the fibrous capsule is the **coracohumeral ligament** that passes from the lateral side of the coracoid process of the scapula to the anatomic neck of the humerus (Figure 9.19). The **coraco-acromial ligament** is another important ligament located on the anterior portion of the shoulder. As this ligament joins the coracoid process and acromion, it forms a strong bridge, termed the **coracoacromial arch,** which protects the humeral head and rotator cuff tendons from direct trauma and prevents displacement of the humeral head superiorly (Figures 9.17 and 9.19). The **coracoclavicular ligaments** help to maintain the position of the clavicle, in relation to the acromion, by spanning the distance between the clavicle and coracoid process of the scapula (Figure 9.19). The **acromioclavicular ligament,** at the acromioclavicular joint, provides support for the superior surface of the shoulder (Figures 9.17 and 9.19). The **transverse humeral ligament** is a broad band of connective tissue passing from the greater tubercle to the lesser tubercle of the humerus, forming a bridge over the intertubercular groove for protection of the long head of the biceps tendon (Figure 9.19). The ligaments of the shoulder are demonstrated in Figures 9.20 through 9.30.

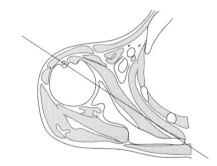

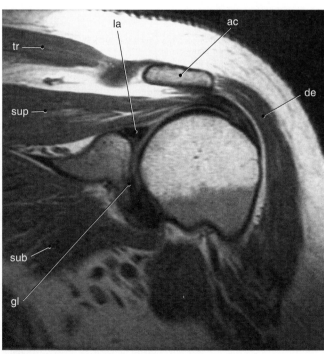

Figure 9.18
Coronal oblique, T1-weighted MR scan of shoulder with glenoid labrum.

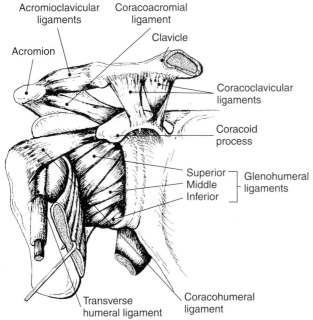

Acromioclavicular ligaments
Coracoacromial ligament
Clavicle
Acromion
Coracoclavicular ligaments
Coracoid process
Superior Middle Inferior ⎤ Glenohumeral ⎦ ligaments
Transverse humeral ligament
Coracohumeral ligament

Figure 9.19
Anterior view of shoulder ligaments.

KEY: **tr,** Trapezius; **la,** labrum; **ac,** acromion; **de,** deltoid; **gl,** glenoid; **sub,** subscapularis; **sup,** supraspinatus.

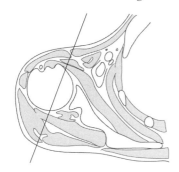

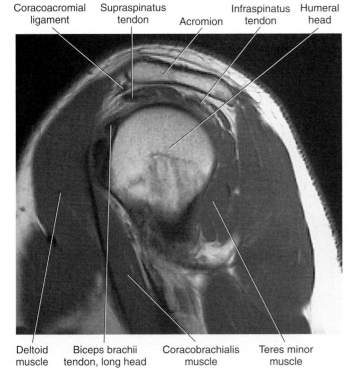

Coracoacromial ligament
Supraspinatus tendon
Acromion
Infraspinatus tendon
Humeral head

Deltoid muscle
Biceps brachii tendon, long head
Coracobrachialis muscle
Teres minor muscle

Figure 9.20
Sagittal oblique, T1-weighted MR scan of shoulder.

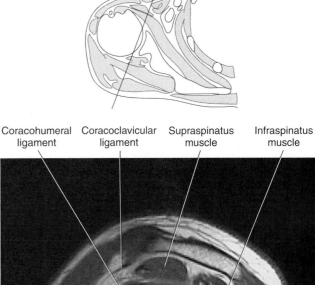

Coracohumeral ligament
Coracoclavicular ligament
Supraspinatus muscle
Infraspinatus muscle

Subscapularis muscle
Coracobrachialis muscle
Teres major muscle
Teres minor muscle
Deltoid muscle

Figure 9.21
Sagittal oblique, T1-weighted MR scan of shoulder.

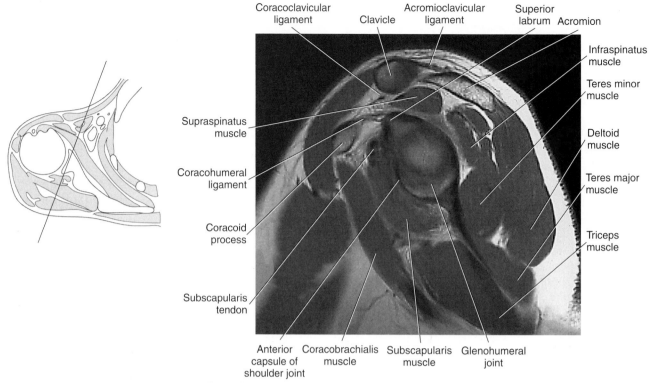

Figure 9.22
Sagittal oblique, T1-weighted MR scan of shoulder.

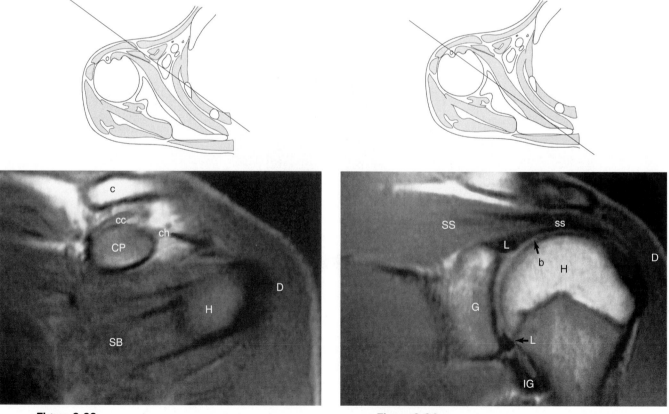

Figure 9.23
Coronal oblique, T1-weighted MR scan of shoulder.

Figure 9.24
Coronal oblique, T1-weighted MR scan of shoulder.

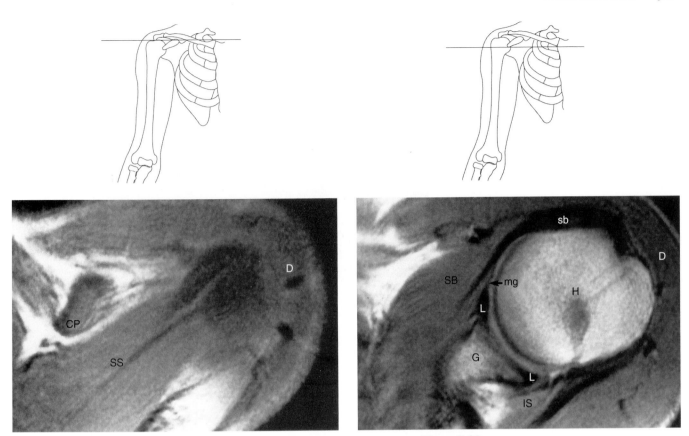

Figure 9.25
Axial, T1-weighted MR scan of shoulder.

Figure 9.26
Axial, T1-weighted MR scan of shoulder.

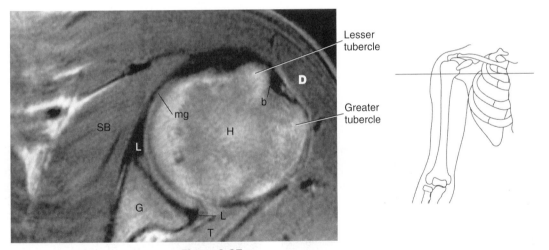

Figure 9.27
Axial, T1-weighted MR scan of shoulder.

KEY: c, Clavicle; **cc,** coracoclavicular ligament; **CP,** coracoid process; **ch,** coracohumeral ligament;
D, deltoid muscle; **H,** humeral head; **SB,** subscapularis muscle; **SS,** supraspinatus muscle;
G, glenoid fossa; **L,** labrum; **ss,** supraspinatus tendon; **b,** tendon of long head of biceps muscle;
IG, inferior glenohumeral ligament; **mg,** middle glenohumeral ligament; **sb,** subscapularis tendon;
T, teres minor muscle; **IS,** infraspinotus muscle.

502

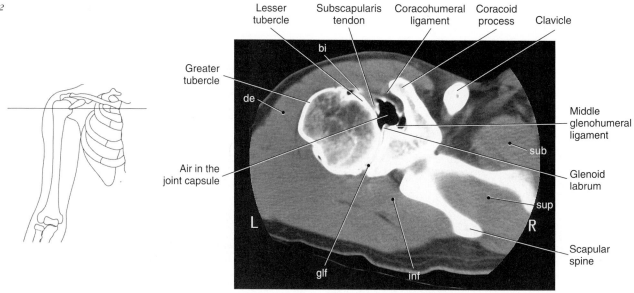

Figure 9.28
Axial CT scan of shoulder.

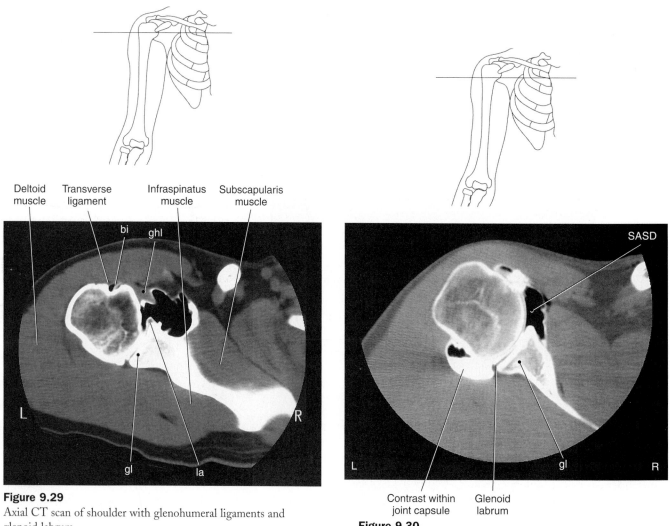

Figure 9.29
Axial CT scan of shoulder with glenohumeral ligaments and
glenoid labrum.

Figure 9.30
Axial CT scan of shoulder with subacromial-subdeltoid bursa.

KEY: **de,** Deltoid; **bi,** biceps tendon; **sub,** subscapularis; **sup,** supraspinatus;
inf, infraspinatus; **glf,** glenoid fossa; **ghl,** glenohumeral ligament; **la,** labrum; **gl,** glenoid;
SASD, subacromial-subdeltoid bursa.

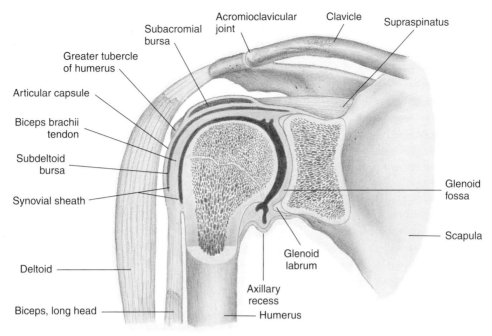

Figure 9.31
Anterior cross section of shoulder joint.

Articular Joint Capsule

The **articular joint capsule** completely encloses the shoulder joint and is quite thin and loose to allow for extreme freedom of movement. When the arm is adducted, the capsule sags to form a pouchlike area termed the **axillary recess** (Figure 9.31). The capsule is attached medially to the glenoid fossa of the scapula and laterally to the anatomic neck of the humerus. The capsule is strengthened by several muscles and ligaments, including the rotator cuff muscles and the long head of the triceps brachii muscle, as well as the glenohumeral and coracohumeral ligaments. There are two openings of the joint capsule. The first is to allow for the transition of the long head of the biceps brachii and the second establishes a communication between the joint and the subscapularis bursa. A synovial membrane lines the fibrous capsule and extends from it onto the glenoid labrum and neck of the humerus. The synovial membrane provides a sheath for the tendon of the long head of the biceps brachii muscle, where it passes into the joint cavity through the intertubercular groove, extending as far as the surgical neck of the humerus (Figure 9.31).

Bursae

The tendons and ligaments of the shoulder joint are cushioned by several fluid-filled bursae. Bursae, within the shoulder, reduce friction where large muscles and tendons pass across the joint capsule. Two prominent shoulder bursae include the subacromial-subdeltoid and subscapular bursae (Figure 9.32). The **subacromial-subdeltoid bursa** is the main bursa of the shoulder and the largest bursa within the body. Beginning at the coracoid process, the bursa extends laterally over the superior surface of the supraspinatus and infraspinatus tendon,

Figure 9.32
Anterior view of shoulder with subacromial-subdeltoid bursa.

extends beyond the acromion, and continues beneath the deltoid muscle to the greater tubercle of the humerus. This bursa cushions the rotator cuff muscles and coracoacromial arch (Figure 9.16). The **subscapular bursa** is located between the subscapularis tendon and the scapula and communicates with the synovial cavity through an opening in the joint capsule. This bursa protects the subscapularis tendon where it passes inferior to the coracoid process and over the neck of the scapula (Figure 9.32).

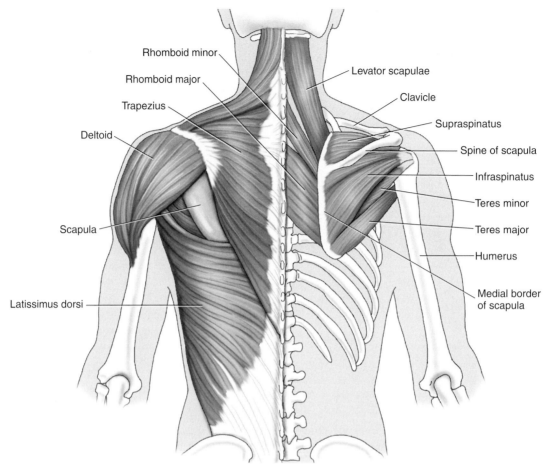

Figure 9.33
Posterior view of trapezius, rhomboid, levator scapula, and latissimus dorsi muscles.

Muscles and Tendons

Numerous muscles and their tendons provide stability for the shoulder joint and movement of the upper arm. These can be separated into four muscle groups: (1) muscles that connect the upper limb to the vertebral column, (2) muscles of the scapula, (3) muscles that connect the upper limb to the anterior thoracic wall, and (4) the muscles of the upper arm.

MUSCLES CONNECTING THE UPPER LIMB TO THE VERTEBRAL COLUMN   Muscles connecting the upper limb to the vertebral column include the following:

Trapezius	Rhomboid major
Levator scapulae	Rhomboid minor
Latissimus dorsi	

Muscles connecting the upper limb to the vertebral column are demonstrated in Figures 9.33 through 9.47 and are described in Table 9.1. The large triangular **trapezius muscle** covers the posterior aspect of the neck and superior half of the trunk (Figure 9.33). It connects the upper limb to the cranium via the external occipital protuberance and to the vertebral column via the spinous processes of C7-T12. The trapezius muscle functions to stabilize the scapula as well as elevate, retract, and depress the scapula. The **levator scapulae muscle** lies deep in the neck and functions to elevate and rotate the scapula.

It extends from the transverse processes of C1-C4 to the superior angle and medial border of the scapula above its spine (Figure 9.33). The **latissimus dorsi** muscle covers the inferior portion of the back as it extends from the spinous processes of the inferior six thoracic vertebrae, iliac crest, and inferior three or four ribs to the distal end of the intertubercular groove of the humerus. The latissimus dorsi medially rotates, extends, and adducts the humerus. The **rhomboid muscles, major** and **minor,** lie deep to the trapezius muscle. The rhomboid major is wider than the rhomboid minor. They parallel each other as they span from the ligamentum nuchae and spinous processes of C7-T5 to the medial border of the scapula. They function to retract the scapula and fix the scapula to the thoracic wall (Figures 9.33 through 9.47).

> The majority of rotator cuff lesions are a result of chronic impingement of the supraspinatus tendon against the acromial arch. The most susceptible area is approximately 1 cm from the insertion site of the supraspinatus tendon. This location is commonly referred to as the *critical zone.*

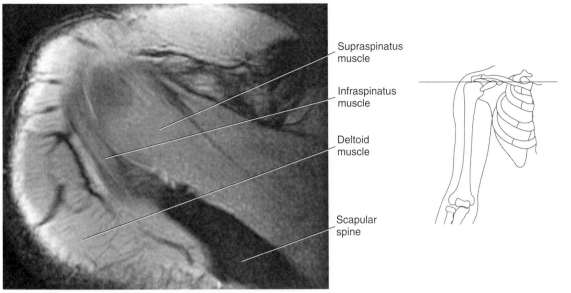

Figure 9.34
Axial, T1-weighted MR scan of shoulder muscles.

Supraspinatus
muscle

Infraspinatus
muscle

Deltoid
muscle

Scapular
spine

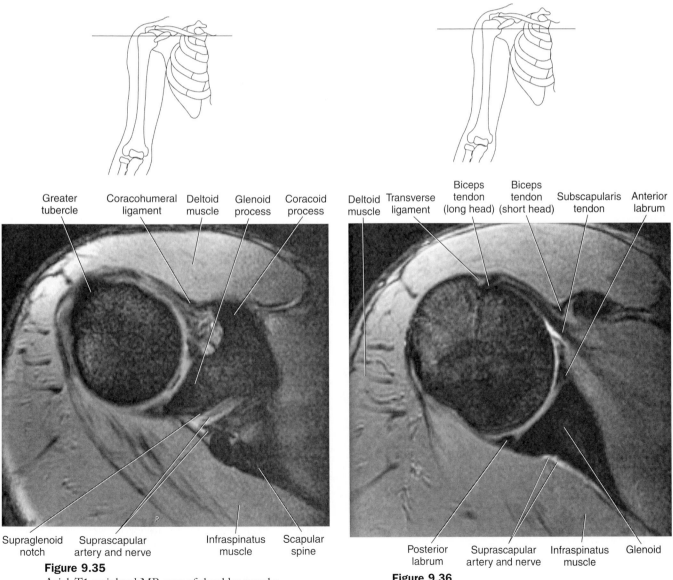

Greater
tubercle

Coracohumeral
ligament

Deltoid
muscle

Glenoid
process

Coracoid
process

Supraglenoid
notch

Suprascapular
artery and nerve

Infraspinatus
muscle

Scapular
spine

Figure 9.35
Axial, T1-weighted MR scan of shoulder muscles.

Deltoid
muscle

Transverse
ligament

Biceps
tendon
(long head)

Biceps
tendon
(short head)

Subscapularis
tendon

Anterior
labrum

Posterior
labrum

Suprascapular
artery and nerve

Infraspinatus
muscle

Glenoid

Figure 9.36
Axial, T1-weighted MR scan of shoulder muscles.

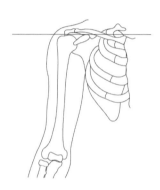

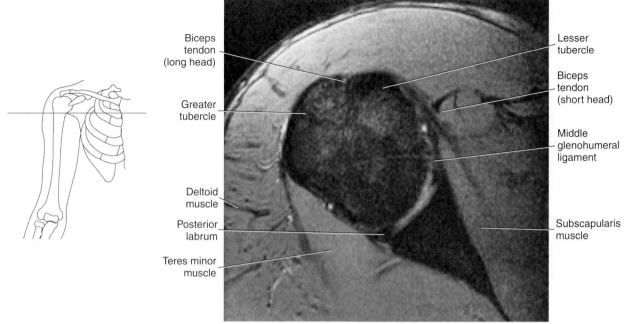

Figure 9.37
Axial, T1-weighted MR scan of shoulder muscles.

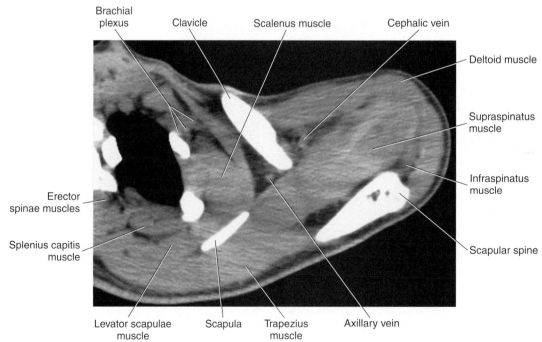

Figure 9.38
Axial CT scan of shoulder with shoulder muscles.

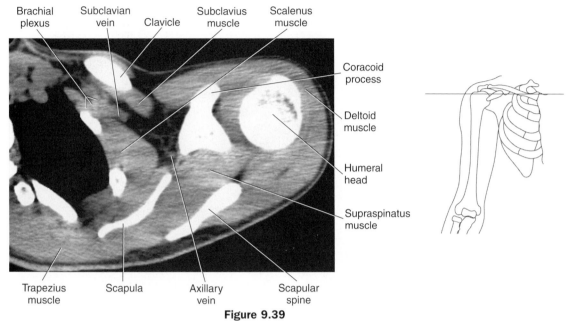

Brachial plexus | Subclavian vein | Clavicle | Subclavius muscle | Scalenus muscle

Coracoid process

Deltoid muscle

Humeral head

Supraspinatus muscle

Trapezius muscle | Scapula | Axillary vein | Scapular spine

Figure 9.39
Axial CT scan of shoulder.

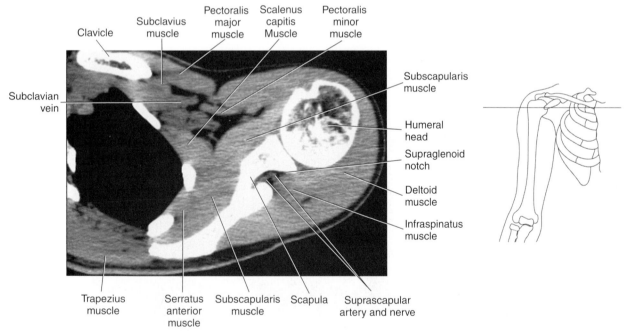

Clavicle | Subclavius muscle | Pectoralis major muscle | Scalenus capitis Muscle | Pectoralis minor muscle

Subscapularis muscle

Subclavian vein

Humeral head

Supraglenoid notch

Deltoid muscle

Infraspinatus muscle

Trapezius muscle | Serratus anterior muscle | Subscapularis muscle | Scapula | Suprascapular artery and nerve

Figure 9.40
Axial CT scan of shoulder.

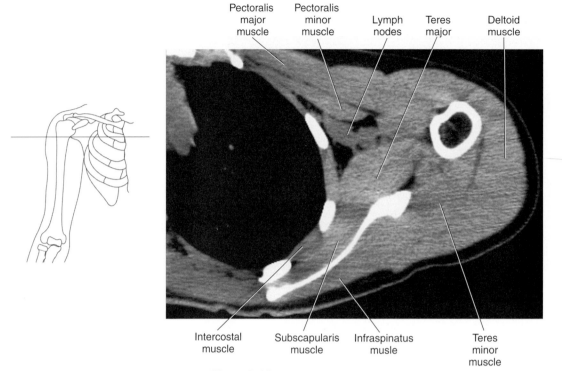

Figure 9.41
Axial CT scan of shoulder.

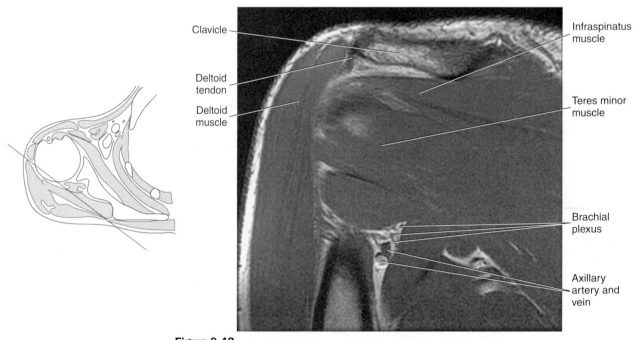

Figure 9.42
Coronal oblique, T1-weighted MR scan of shoulder muscles.

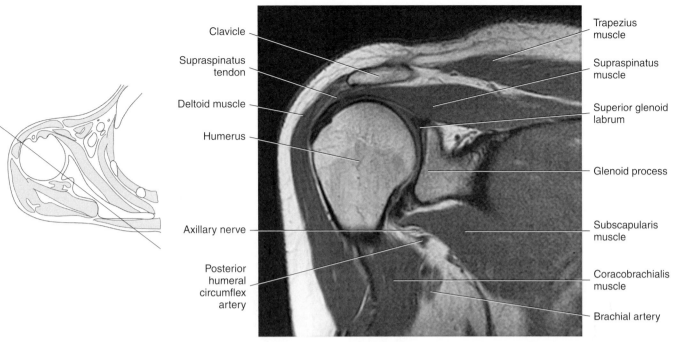

Figure 9.43
Coronal oblique, T1-weighted MR scan of shoulder muscles.

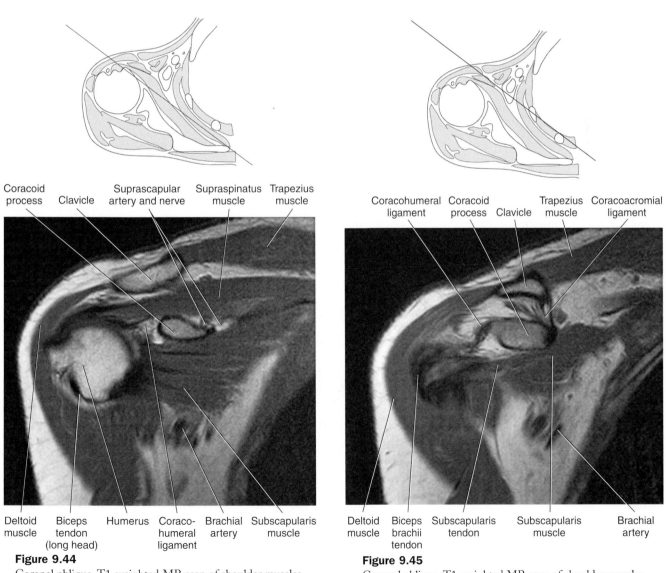

Figure 9.44
Coronal oblique, T1-weighted MR scan of shoulder muscles.

Figure 9.45
Coronal oblique, T1-weighted MR scan of shoulder muscles.

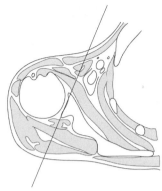

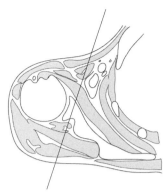

Coraco-humeral ligament Coraco-clavicular ligament Supra-spinatus tendon Acromio-clavicular joint Supra-spinatus muscle Acromion Infra-spinatus tendon

Coraco-humeral ligament Sub-scapularis tendon Superior labrum Acromio-clavicular ligament Supra-spinatus muscle Infra-spinatus muscle

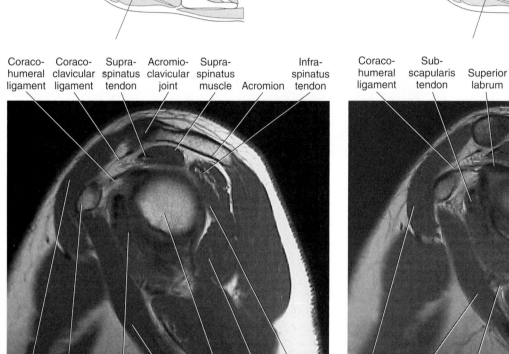

Deltoid muscle Coracoid process Subscapularis muscle Coraco-brachialis muscle Humerus Teres minor muscle Infra-spinatus muscle

Deltoid muscle Coraco-brachialis muscle Brachial plexus Teres minor muscle Triceps muscle Teres major muscle Deltoid muscle

Figure 9.46
Sagittal oblique, T1-weighted MR scan of shoulder muscles.

Figure 9.47
Sagittal oblique, T1-weighted MR scan of shoulder muscles.

TABLE 9-1   Muscles Connecting the Upper Limb to the Vertebral Column

MUSCLE	ORIGIN	INSERTION	PRIMARY ACTIONS
Trapezius	External occipital protuberance, ligamentum nuchae, spinous processes of C7-T12	Clavicle and spine and acromion of the scapula	Stabilizes, elevates, retracts, and depresses scapula
Levator scapula	Transverse processes of C1-C4	Superior angle and medial border of scapula	Elevates scapula
Latissimus dorsi	Spinous process of T6-T12, iliac crest, and inferior three or four ribs	Intertubercular groove of the humerus	Extends, medially rotates, and adducts the humerus
Rhomboid major	Ligamentum nuchae and spinous processes of C7-T1	Medial border of scapula	Retracts scapula and fixes scapula to thoracic wall
Rhomboid minor	Spinous processes of T2-T5	Medial border of scapula	Retracts scapula and fixes scapula to thoracic wall.

TABLE 9-2   Scapular Muscles

MUSCLE	PROXIMAL/MEDIAL ATTACHMENT	DISTAL/LATERAL ATTACHMENT	PRIMARY ACTION
Deltoid	Clavicle, acromion, and spine of scapula	Deltoid tuberosity of humerus	Flexes, medial rotates abductor, extensor, and lateral rotator of humerus
Teres major	Inferior angle of scapula	Intertubercular groove of humerus	Adducts and medially rotates humerus
Teres minor	Axillary border of scapula	Greater tubercle of humerus	Laterally rotates humerus, stabilizes glenohumeral joint
Supraspinatus	Supraspinous fossa of scapula	Greater tubercle of humerus	Abducts humerus and stabilizes glenohumeral joint
Infraspinatus	Infraspinous fossa of scapula	Greater tubercle of humerus	Laterally rotates humerus and stabilizes glenohumeral joint
Subscapularis	Subscapular fossa of scapula	Lesser tubercle of humerus	Medially rotates humerus and stabilizes glenohumeral joint

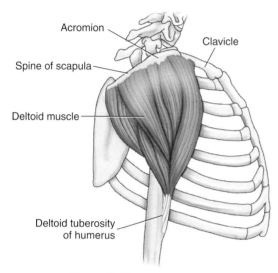

Figure 9.48
Lateral view of deltoid muscle.

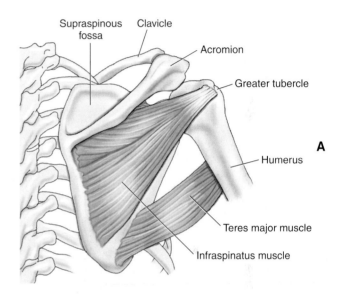

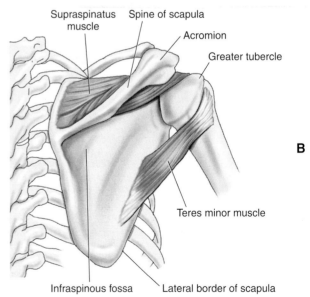

Figure 9.49
A, Posterior view of teres major and infraspinatus muscles.
B, Posterior view of supraspinatus and teres minor muscles.

MUSCLES OF THE SCAPULA   Muscles of the scapula include the following:

Deltoid muscle
Teres major
Teres minor
Supraspinatus
Infraspinatus
Subscapularis

Muscles of the scapula are described in Table 9.2 and demonstrated in Figures 9.34 through 9.52. The large **deltoid muscle** originates on the clavicle, acromion, and scapular spine to blanket the shoulder joint as it extends to insert on the deltoid tuberosity of the humerus. This powerful muscle forms the rounded contour of the shoulder and functions primarily to abduct the arm (Figure 9.48). The **teres major muscle** is a flat rectangular muscle that adducts and medially rotates the arm. It extends from the inferior angle of the scapula to the medial aspect or lip of the intertubercular groove of the humerus (Figure 9.49, *A*). The four remaining muscles, **supraspinatus,**

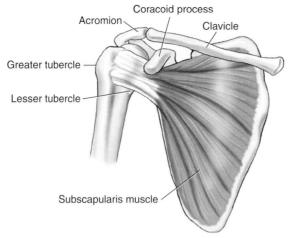

Figure 9.50
Anterior view of subscapularis muscle.

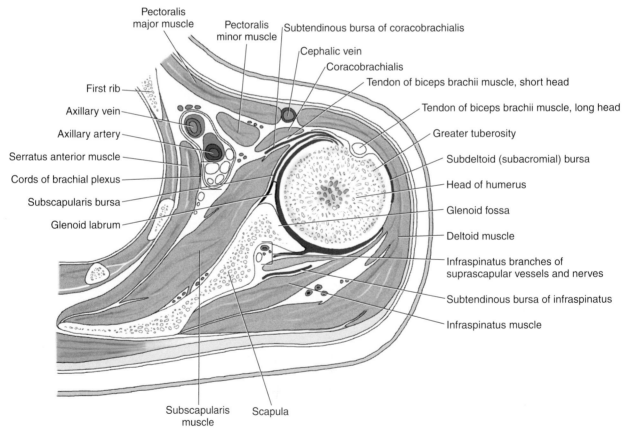

Figure 9.51
Axial view of shoulder muscles.

infraspinatus, teres minor, and **subscapularis,** closely surround the scapula and compose the **rotator cuff** (Figures 9.49 through 9.52). The rotator cuff provides dynamic stability to the shoulder joint and allows for adduction, abduction, and rotation of the humerus. The supraspinatus, infraspinatus, and teres minor muscles are located on the posterior aspect of the scapula. The tendons of these muscles insert on the greater tubercle of the humerus. The **supraspinatus muscle** lies in the supraspinous fossa of the scapula and helps to abduct the arm. The tendon of the supraspinatus muscle is the most frequently injured tendon of the rotator cuff because of possible impingement as it extends under the acromioclavicular joint and continues over the humeral head (Figure 9.49, *B*). The **infraspinatus muscle** is a triangular muscle that lies below the scapular spine in the infraspinous fossa. It acts to laterally rotate the arm (Figure 9.49, *A*). Lying along the inferior border of the infraspinatus muscle is the elongated **teres minor muscle,** which also acts to laterally rotate the arm (Figure 9.49, *B*). The **subscapularis muscle** is the only muscle of the rotator cuff located on the anterior surface of the scapula; its tendon inserts on the lesser tubercle of the humerus (Figures 9.50 through 9.52). The subscapularis muscle acts to medially rotate the humerus. See sequential images through the shoulder (Figures 9.34 through 9.47).

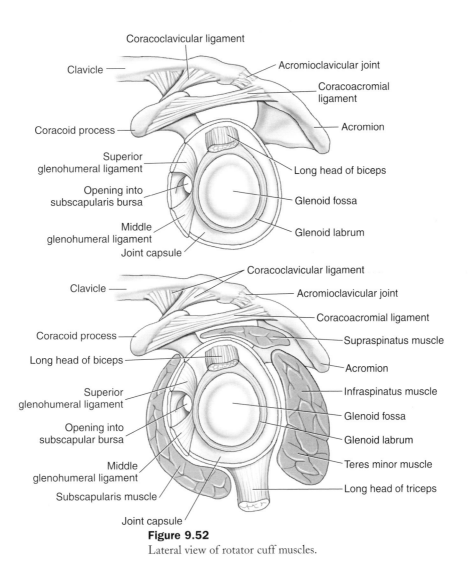

Figure 9.52
Lateral view of rotator cuff muscles.

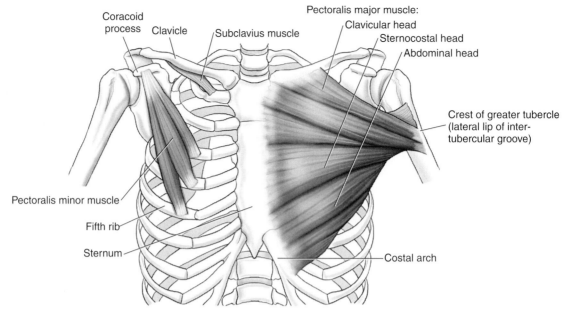

Figure 9.53
Anterior view of pectoralis and subclavius muscles.

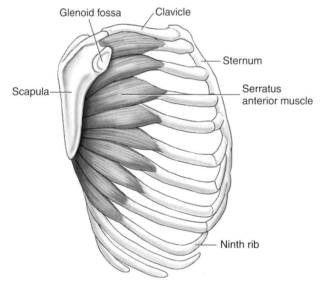

Figure 9.54
Anterior view of serratus anterior muscle.

TABLE 9-3	Muscles Connecting the Upper Extremity to the Anterior and Lateral Thoracic Wall		
MUSCLE	PROXIMAL/MEDIAL ATTACHMENT	DISTAL/LATERAL ATTACHMENT	PRIMARY ACTION
Pectoralis major	Clavicular head—medial half of clavicle. Manubrium and body of sternum, six upper costal cartilages	Lateral lip intertubercular groove of humerus	Adducts and medially rotates humerus. Flexion of the arm
Pectoralis minor	Anterior surface of third-fifth ribs	Coracoid process of the scapula	Depresses and downwardly rotates scapula. Assists in scapular protraction and stabilizes scapula
Serratus anterior	Angles of superior eighth or ninth ribs	Medial border of scapula	Rotates, stabilizes, and protracts scapula
Subclavius	First rib and cartilage	Inferior surface of the clavicle	Stabilizes the clavicle and depresses the shoulder

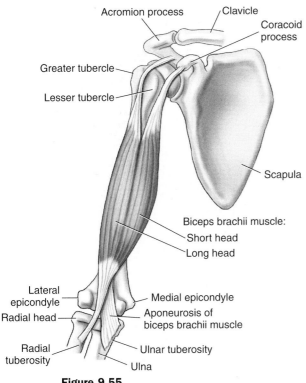

Figure 9.55
Anterior view of biceps brachii muscle.

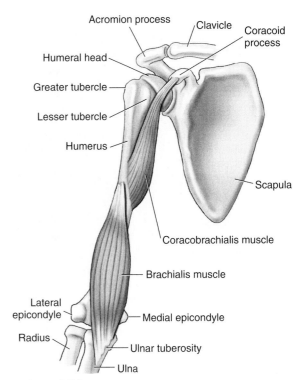

Figure 9.56
Anterior view of coracobrachialis and brachialis muscles.

MUSCLES CONNECTING THE UPPER EXTREMITY TO THE ANTERIOR AND LATERAL THORACIC WALLS Muscles connecting the upper extremity to the anterior and lateral thoracic walls include the following:

Pectoralis major
Subclavius
Pectoralis minor
Serratus anterior

Muscles connecting the upper extremity to the anterior and lateral thoracic walls are demonstrated in Figures 9.34 through 9.47, 9.53, and 9.54 and described in Table 9.3. The **pectoralis muscles (major and minor),** located on the anterior surface of the chest, primarily aid in the movement of the upper limb (Figure 9.53). The large fan-shaped **pectoralis major** muscle covers the superior part of the thorax as it spans from the sternum, clavicle, and cartilaginous attachments of the upper six ribs to the lateral aspect or lip of the intertubercular groove of the humerus. Its primary functions are to adduct, medially rotate, flex, and extend the humerus and to assist in forced inspiration. The smaller triangular-shaped **pectoralis minor** lies beneath the pectoralis major muscle and acts to depress the scapula and assist the serratus anterior muscle in pulling the scapula forward (Figure 9.53). The **serratus (sawlike) anterior muscle** is visualized on the lateral border of the thorax. It extends from the first rib through eighth rib to the medial border of the scapula. The primary action of the serratus anterior muscle is to protract and

stabilize the scapula (Figure 9.54). The **subclavius,** a small triangular-shaped muscle that spans between the first rib and clavicle, acts to stabilize the clavicle and depress the shoulder (Figure 9.53).

MUSCLES OF THE UPPER ARM The muscles of the upper arm can be divided into ventral and dorsal groups according to their position. The ventral group contains the biceps brachii, brachialis, and coracobrachialis muscle, and the dorsal group consists of the triceps brachii and anconeus muscles. These muscles are demonstrated in Figures 9.55 through 9.69 and described in Table 9.4.

VENTRAL GROUP The **biceps brachii muscle** is located on the anterior surface of the humerus and acts as a strong flexor of the forearm. The biceps brachii muscle is so named "biceps" because of its two expanded heads of proximal attachment (long and short). The **tendon of the long head** arises from the supraglenoid tubercle and courses through the intertubercular (bicipital) groove to merge with the tendon from the short head. The **short head** of the biceps brachii muscle originates from the coracoid process and joins with the long head to create the biceps brachii muscle, which terminates in two tendons. The stronger tendon inserts on the radial tuberosity, and the other tendon creates the **bicipital aponeurosis,** which radiates into the fascia of the forearm (Figure 9.55).

The **brachialis muscle** originates from the anterior surface of the distal humerus and covers the anterior surface of the elbow joint before inserting on a roughened area of the proximal

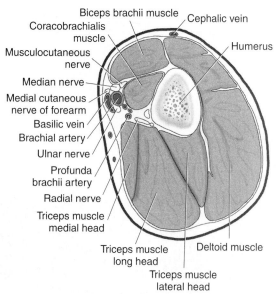

Figure 9.57
Axial view of humerus, proximal one third.

Figure 9.58
Axial view of humerus, midhumerus.

and anterior surface of the ulna termed the *ulnar tuberosity* and the *coronoid process*. The brachialis muscle is considered to be the most important flexor muscle of the elbow joint (Figure 9.56). The **coracobrachialis** is a long, narrow muscle located in the superomedial aspect of the arm. It arises from the coracoid process along with the short head of the biceps brachii and extends to insert on the medial surface of the humerus. The primary action of the coracobrachialis muscle is to assist with flexion and adduction of the arm, but it also helps hold the head of the humerus within the joint capsule (Figures 9.56 through 9.67).

DORSAL GROUP   The **triceps brachii muscle** is located on the posterior surface of the humerus and is the main extensor of the forearm. Its name *triceps* is associated with three heads of proximal attachment (long, lateral, and medial). The **long head** of the triceps originates from the infraglenoid tubercle of the scapula, the **medial head** originates from the entire dorsal surface of the humerus distal to the radial groove, and the **lateral head** arises from the dorsal surface and lateral intermuscular septum of the humerus. All three heads join in a common tendon that inserts on the olecranon process of the ulna and the posterior joint capsule (Figure 9.68). The small, triangular **anconeus muscle** originates on the lateral epicondyle and crosses obliquely to insert on the dorsal surface of the olecranon process, close to the tendon of the triceps brachii (Figure 9.69). It assists the triceps brachii in extension and also provides dynamic joint stability to the lateral joint capsule. For images of the upper arm, see Figures 9.57 through 9.67.

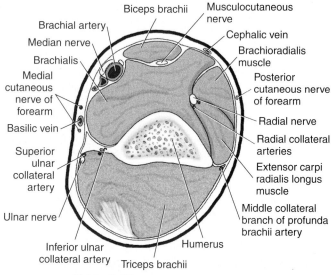

Figure 9.59
Axial view of humerus, distal one third.

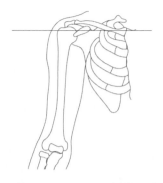

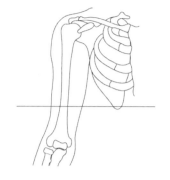

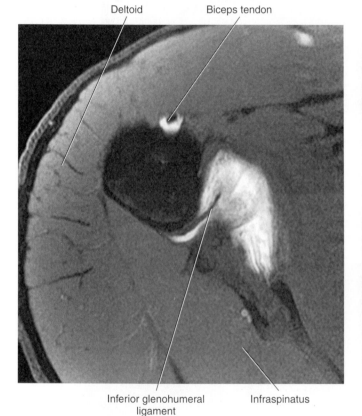

Deltoid   Biceps tendon

Inferior glenohumeral   Infraspinatus
ligament

Figure 9.60
Axial, MR arthrogram of shoulder.

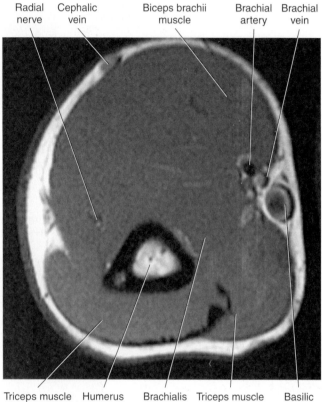

Radial   Cephalic   Biceps brachii   Brachial   Brachial
nerve   vein   muscle   artery   vein

Triceps muscle Humerus   Brachialis   Triceps muscle   Basilic
(lateral head)   muscle   (long head)   vein

Figure 9.61
Axial, T1-weighted MR scan of midhumerus.

TABLE 9-4   Muscles of the Upper Arm

MUSCLE	PROXIMAL ATTACHMENT	DISTAL ATTACHMENT	PRIMARY ACTION
Biceps brachii	Long head—supraglenoid tubercle of scapula Short head—coracoid process of scapula	Radial tuberosity	Supinates and flexes forearm
Brachialis	Distal humerus	Ulnar tuberosity and coronoid process	Flexion of elbow joint
Coracobrachialis	Coracoid process of scapula	Middle third medial surface of humerus	Assists to flex and adduct the arm
Triceps brachii	Long head—infraglenoid tubercle of scapula Medial head—posterior surface of humerus below radial groove Lateral head—posterior surface of humerus below greater tubercle	Proximal end of olecranon process of the ulna	Chief extensor of forearm, long head steadies head of humerus if abducted
Anconeus	Lateral epicondyle of humerus	Olecranon process of the ulna	Assists triceps brachii in extension of elbow

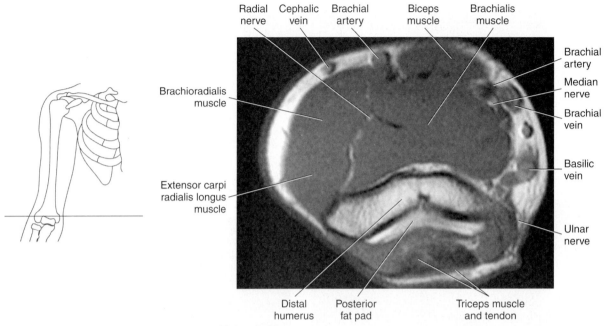

Figure 9.62
Axial, TI-weighted MR scan of distal humerus.

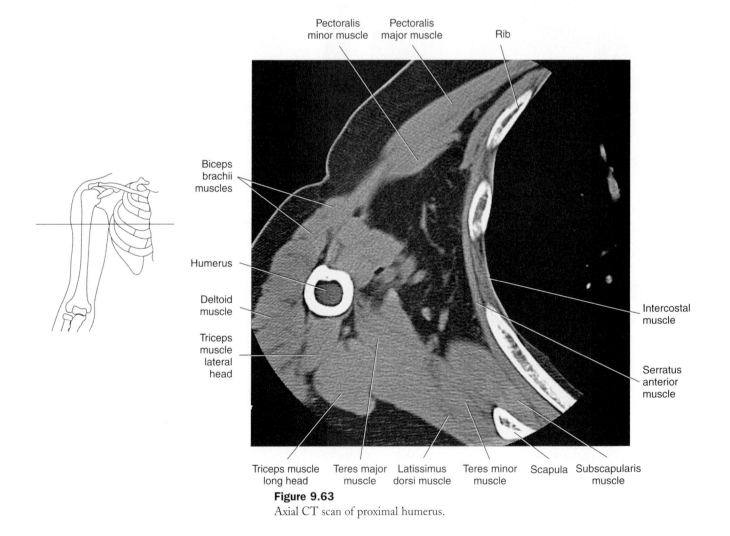

Figure 9.63
Axial CT scan of proximal humerus.

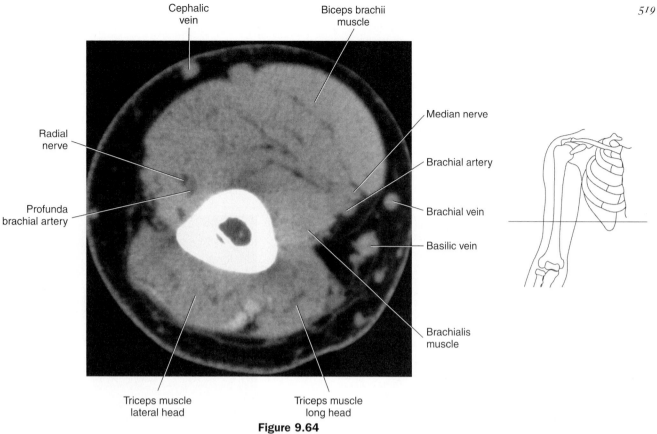

Cephalic
vein

Biceps brachii
muscle

Radial
nerve

Profunda
brachial artery

Median nerve

Brachial artery

Brachial vein

Basilic vein

Brachialis
muscle

Triceps muscle
lateral head

Triceps muscle
long head

Figure 9.64
Axial CT scan of upper arm.

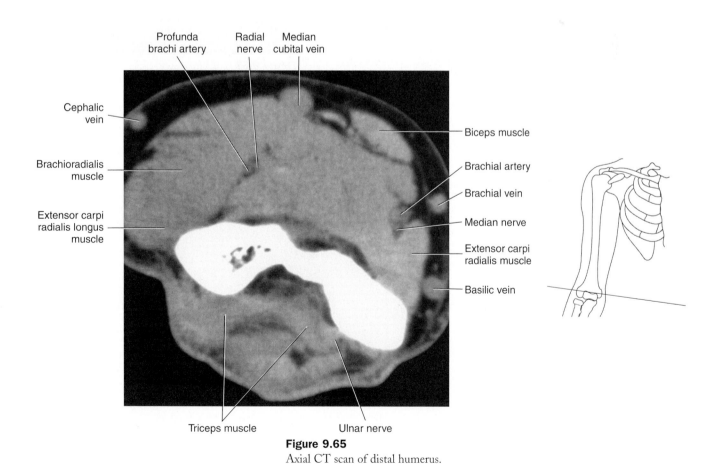

Profunda
brachi artery

Radial
nerve

Median
cubital vein

Cephalic
vein

Brachioradialis
muscle

Extensor carpi
radialis longus
muscle

Biceps muscle

Brachial artery

Brachial vein

Median nerve

Extensor carpi
radialis muscle

Basilic vein

Triceps muscle

Ulnar nerve

Figure 9.65
Axial CT scan of distal humerus.

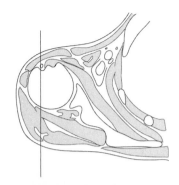

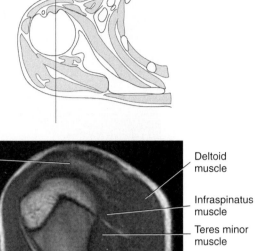

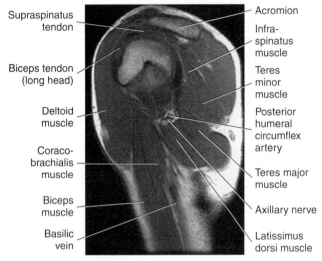

Supraspinatus tendon

Biceps tendon (long head)

Deltoid muscle

Coracobrachialis muscle

Biceps muscle

Basilic vein

Acromion

Infraspinatus muscle

Teres minor muscle

Posterior humeral circumflex artery

Teres major muscle

Axillary nerve

Latissimus dorsi muscle

Figure 9.66
Sagittal oblique, MR arthrogram of shoulder.

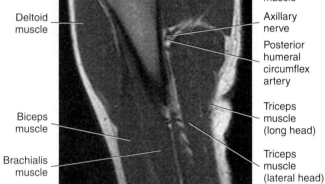

Supraspinatus tendon

Deltoid muscle

Biceps muscle

Brachialis muscle

Deltoid muscle

Infraspinatus muscle

Teres minor muscle

Axillary nerve

Posterior humeral circumflex artery

Triceps muscle (long head)

Triceps muscle (lateral head)

Figure 9.67
Sagittal oblique, MR arthrogram of shoulder.

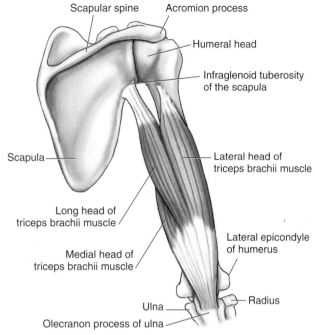

Scapular spine

Acromion process

Humeral head

Infraglenoid tuberosity
of the scapula

Scapula

Lateral head of
triceps brachii muscle

Long head of
triceps brachii muscle

Medial head of
triceps brachii muscle

Lateral epicondyle
of humerus

Radius

Ulna

Olecranon process of ulna

Figure 9.68

Posterior view of triceps brachii muscle.

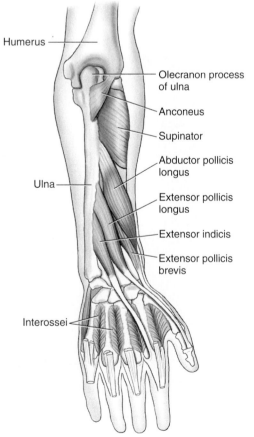

Humerus

Olecranon process
of ulna

Anconeus

Supinator

Abductor pollicis
longus

Ulna

Extensor pollicis
longus

Extensor indicis

Extensor pollicis
brevis

Interossei

Figure 9.69

Posterior view of anconeus muscle.

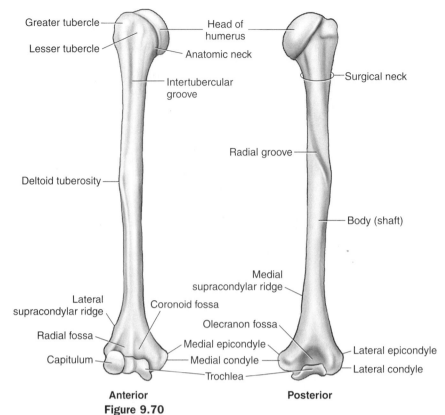

Greater tubercle

Lesser tubercle

Head of humerus

Anatomic neck

Intertubercular groove

Surgical neck

Radial groove

Deltoid tuberosity

Body (shaft)

Medial supracondylar ridge

Lateral supracondylar ridge

Coronoid fossa

Olecranon fossa

Radial fossa

Medial epicondyle

Lateral epicondyle

Capitulum

Medial condyle

Lateral condyle

Trochlea

Anterior

Posterior

Figure 9.70

Humerus. *Left,* Anterior view. *Right,* Posterior view.

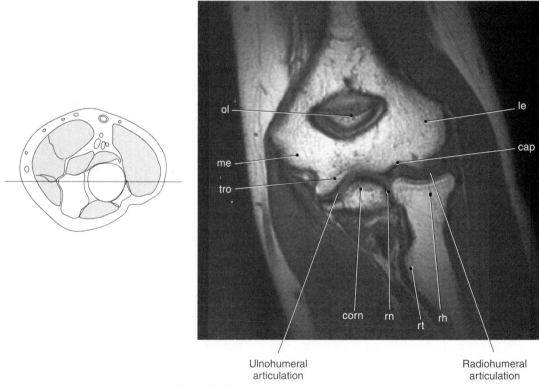

ol

le

cap

me

tro

corn   rn   rt   rh

Ulnohumeral articulation

Radiohumeral articulation

Figure 9.71

Coronal T1-weighted MR scan of elbow.

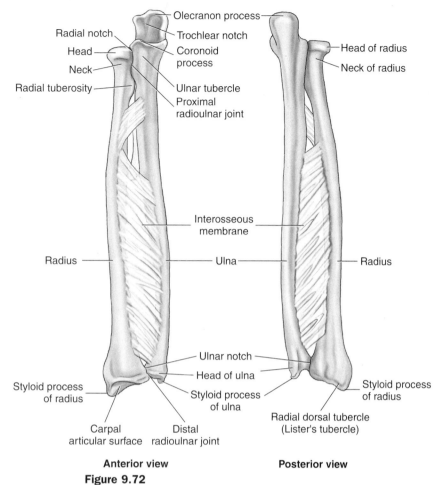

Figure 9.72
Radius and ulna. *Left,* Anterior view. *Right,* Posterior view.

ELBOW

The elbow is a complex hinge-pivot joint created by the articulations of the humerus, radius, and ulna. All three articulations communicate with each other within a single joint capsule. The radius and ulna are the bones of the forearm, with the radius located on the lateral side. The **radioulnar** and **radiohumeral** articulations create the pivot joint that aids in supination and pronation of the elbow. The radiohumeral and **ulnohumeral** articulations form the hinge joint that allows for flexion and extension (Figures 9.70 through 9.73).

Bony Anatomy

DISTAL HUMERUS   The distal portion of the humerus has two distinct prominences termed the **medial** and **lateral condyles,** with associated **epicondyles,** that provide attachment sites for tendons and ligaments (Figure 9.70). The medial epicondyle serves as the site of origin for the common flexor tendon,

pronator teres muscle, and medial collateral ligament, whereas the lateral epicondyle serves as the attachment site for the common extensor tendon, supinator muscle, and lateral collateral ligament. Just lateral to the medial epicondyle along its posterior surface is a shallow groove containing the ulnar nerve. Two depressions located on the distal humerus are the anterior **coronoid fossa** and the deep posterior **olecranon fossa.** These depressions accommodate the coronoid and olecranon processes of the proximal ulna (Figures 9.70, 9.71, and 9.73). The distal humerus has two cartilage-covered articular surfaces—the capitellum and the trochlea for articulation with the radius and ulna (Figure 9.71). The lateral of the two surfaces is the **capitellum,** a rounded projection that articulates with the concave surface of the radial head. The **trochlea** is more medial and has the appearance of an hourglass if viewed in the horizontal plane. The shape of the trochlea helps keep the ulna in position during flexion between the distal humerus and proximal radius (Figure 9.73).

KEY: ol, Olecranon fossa; **me,** medial epicondyle; **tro,** trochlea; **le,** lateral epicondyle; **cap,** capitellum; **rh,** radial head; **rt,** radial tuberosity; **rn,** radial notch; **corn,** coronoid process.

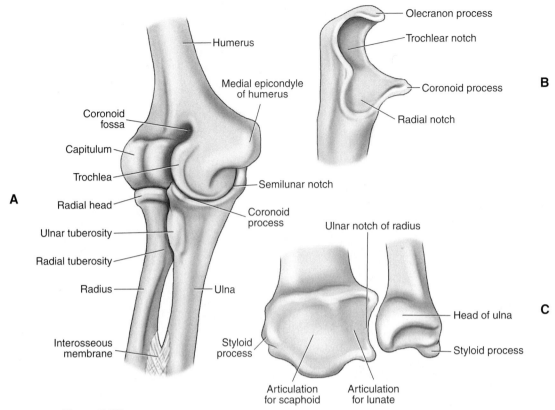

Figure 9.73
Anatomy of the elbow and distal forearm. **A,** Elbow in medial view. **B,** Proximal ulna in lateral view. **C,** Distal radius and ulna.

RADIUS: PROXIMAL RADIUS   The radius is a long, slender bone with a proximal portion that consists of the radial head, neck, and tuberosity. The **radial head** has a flat cartilage-covered depression or **fossa** (fovea of the radius) that articulates with the capitellum of the humerus. In addition, the articular circumference of the radial head articulates against the radial notch of the ulna during supination and pronation. The radial head is attached to the body of the radius by the narrow **radial neck.** Located at the distal portion of the neck on the medial side of the radius is a roughened projection termed the **radial tuberosity.** The radial tuberosity serves as the attachment point for the biceps brachii muscle (Figures 9.72 through 9.74).

Because of its superficial location, the ulnar nerve is the most frequently injured nerve of the body.

DISTAL RADIUS   The broadened distal end of the radius includes the cartilage-covered carpal articular surface, the ulnar notch, and the radial styloid process. The **carpal articular surface** articulates with the scaphoid and lunate bones of the wrist. The **ulnar notch** articulates with the ulna, and the **styloid process** serves as an attachment site for the extensor pollicis longus and extensor carpi radialis tendons. The dorsal surface of the radius contains several grooves that serve as passages for the extensor tendons. Along with the grooves,

a prominent ridge is located on the dorsal surface termed the **radial dorsal tubercle,** or **Lister's tubercle,** a common site for the formation of bony spurs (Figure 9.72).

ULNA: PROXIMAL ULNA   The ulna is located medial within the forearm. The proximal ulna consists of the olecranon and coronoid processes and the trochlear and radial notches. The superficial dorsal surface is formed by the hook-shaped **olecranon process,** which is the attachment site for the triceps brachii. The **trochlear notch** is a half-moon–shaped concave articular surface that curves around the trochlea of the humerus. This articulation allows for flexion and extension of the elbow. Located on the anterior portion of the distal end of the trochlear notch is a small beaklike process called the **coronoid process.** Just distal and lateral to the coronoid process is a flattened depression called the **radial notch.** It is covered by articular cartilage for articulation with the radial head. Immediately distal to the coronoid process is a roughened bony surface termed the **ulnar tuberosity.** The tendon of the brachialis muscle inserts on both the coronoid process and the ulnar tuberosity (Figures 9.72, 9.73, 9.75, and 9.76).

KEY: **bi,** Biceps; **br,** brachialis; **cap,** capitellum; **brd,** brachioradialis; **rh,** radial head; **su,** supinator; **tr,** triceps; **ol,** olecranon fossa; **tro,** trochlea; **corn,** coronoid process; **le,** lateral epicondyle; **u,** ulna; **me,** medial epicondyle.

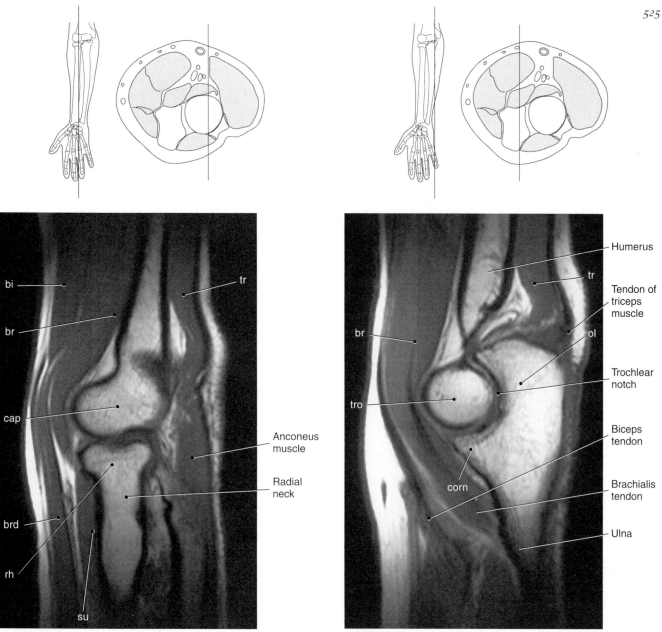

Figure 9.74
Sagittal, T1-weighted MR scan of elbow with proximal radius.

bi
tr
br
cap
Anconeus
muscle
Radial
neck
brd
rh
su

Figure 9.75
Sagittal, T1-weighted MR scan of elbow with proximal ulna.

Humerus
tr
Tendon of
triceps
muscle
br
ol
Trochlear
notch
tro
Biceps
tendon
corn
Brachialis
tendon
Ulna

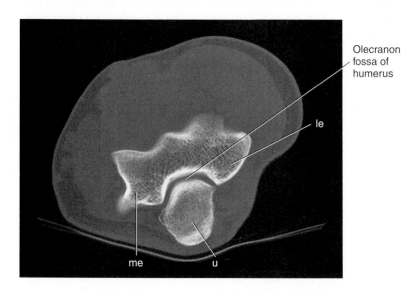

Olecranon
fossa of
humerus
le
me
u

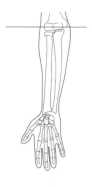

Figure 9.76
Axial CT scan of elbow joint.

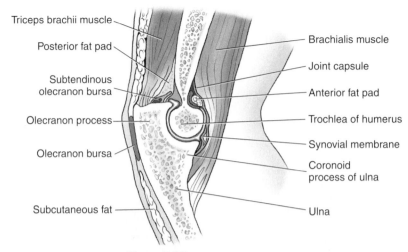

Triceps brachii muscle

Posterior fat pad

Subtendinous olecranon bursa

Olecranon process

Olecranon bursa

Subcutaneous fat

Brachialis muscle

Joint capsule

Anterior fat pad

Trochlea of humerus

Synovial membrane

Coronoid process of ulna

Ulna

Figure 9.77
Lateral view of elbow at midjoint.

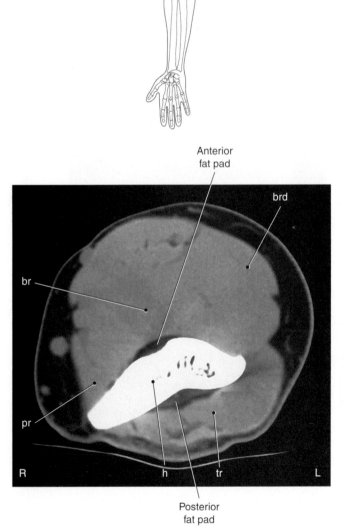

Anterior fat pad

brd

br

pr

h   tr

R   L

Posterior fat pad

Figure 9.78
Axial CT scan of elbow with fat pads.

ULNA: DISTAL ULNA   The smaller, distal end of the ulna has two prominent projections. The larger, rounded projection is an articular eminence termed the *head of the ulna*. It articulates with the ulnar notch of the radius and the triangular fibrocartilage complex. The small conical projection on the medial surface is called the *ulnar styloid process,* which serves as the attachment site for the ulnar collateral ligament of the wrist. Another structure that is important in stabilizing and strengthening the connection between the radius and ulna is the **interosseous membrane,** a strong fibrous sheath stretching between the interosseous borders of both bones (Figure 9.72, *A* and *B*).

JOINT CAPSULE AND FAT PADS   The entire elbow joint is surrounded by a relatively loose joint capsule that allows for the movements of flexion and extension. The joint capsule is weaker anteriorly and posteriorly but is reinforced medially and laterally by the strong radial and ulnar collateral ligaments (discussed in the next section). Located within the olecranon and coronoid fossas are fat pads that fill the space between the synovial membrane and joint capsule (Figures 9.77 and 9.78). The fat pads help cushion the area where the olecranon and coronoid processes move during flexion and extension of the elbow. There are two clinically important bursae located in the elbow: the olecranon bursa and the distal bicipitoradial bursa. The **olecranon bursa** is located within the subcutaneous tissue overlying the olecranon process (Figure 9.77). The distal **bicipitoradial** bursa lies between the insertion of the biceps tendon and the humerus.

KEY: **brd,** Brachioradialis; **tr,** triceps; **h,** humerus; **pr,** pronator teres; **br,** brachialis.

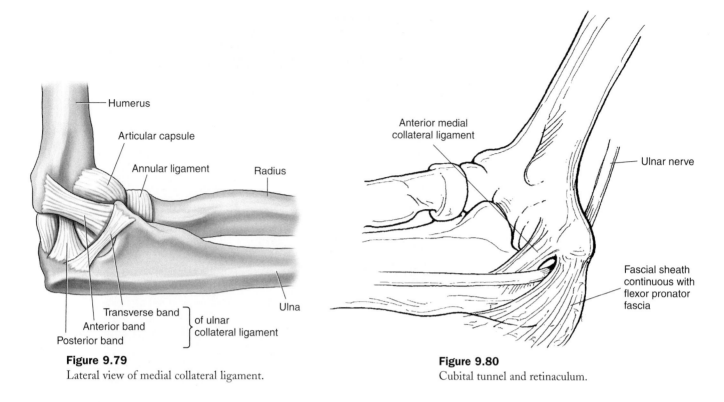

Figure 9.79
Lateral view of medial collateral ligament.

Figure 9.80
Cubital tunnel and retinaculum.

Ligaments

The stability of the elbow joint primarily depends on the collateral ligaments that are woven into the lateral portions of the joint capsule. The **ulnar collateral ligament (medial collateral ligament)** consists of three components: an anterior band, a posterior band, and a transverse band (ligament of Cooper) (Figures 9.79 through 9.82). The anterior band, which is the strongest, extends from the medial epicondyle of the humerus to the medial aspect of the coronoid process. The posterior band originates along with the anterior band from the medial epicondyle of the humerus and inserts on the medial aspect of the olecranon process, forming a triangular plate. The weaker transverse band stretches between the medial surfaces of the coronoid and olecranon processes to unite the anterior and posterior bands. Reinforcing the lateral side is the triangular **radial collateral ligament (lateral collateral ligament).** The radial collateral ligament originates from the lateral epicondyle of the humerus, adjacent to and beneath the common extensor tendons, and spreads distally to insert on the annular ligament and the anterior and posterior margins of the radial notch of the ulna (Figures 9.81 and 9.83). The **annular ligament** forms a fibrous ring that encircles the radial head, with a narrow portion that tightens around the radial neck to prevent inferior displacement of the radius (Figures 9.79 and 9.83 through 9.85). The annular ligament is considered a key structure in the proximal radioulnar joint, allowing the head of the radius to rotate freely. Just distal to the annular ligament is the **quadrate ligament,** a small band of tissue that passes from the radial notch of the ulna to the neck of the radius to provide stability to the joint during supination and pronation.

528

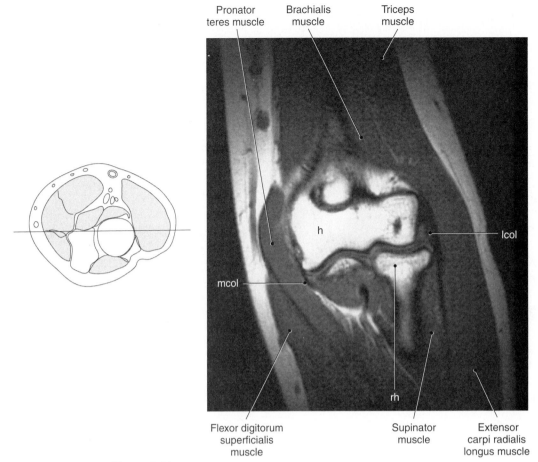

Pronator
teres muscle

Brachialis
muscle

Triceps
muscle

h

lcol

mcol

rh

Flexor digitorum
superficialis
muscle

Supinator
muscle

Extensor
carpi radialis
longus muscle

Figure 9.81
Coronal, T1-weighted MR scan of elbow with collateral ligaments.

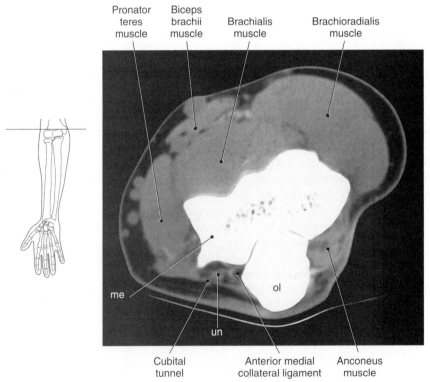

Pronator
teres
muscle

Biceps
brachii
muscle

Brachialis
muscle

Brachioradialis
muscle

me

ol

un

Cubital
tunnel

Anterior medial
collateral ligament

Anconeus
muscle

Figure 9.82
Axial CT scan with ulnar nerve and cubital tunnel.

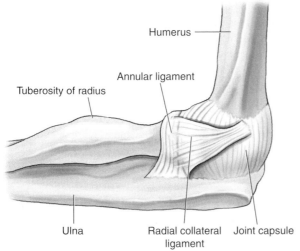

Humerus

Annular ligament

Tuberosity of radius

Ulna

Radial collateral ligament

Joint capsule

Figure 9.83
Lateral view of lateral collateral ligament.

KEY: **mcol,** Medial collateral ligament; **h,** humerus; **lcol,** lateral collateral ligament; **rh,** radial head; **ol,** olecranon fossa; **un,** ulnar nerve; **me,** medial epicondyle; **anl,** annular ligament; **rn,** radial notch.

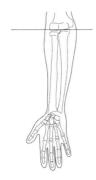

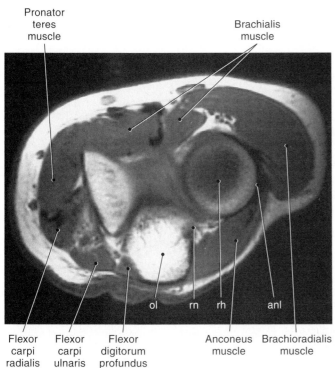

Pronator teres muscle

Brachialis muscle

Flexor carpi radialis muscle

Flexor carpi ulnaris muscle

Flexor digitorum profundus muscle

ol   rn   rh   anl

Anconeus muscle

Brachioradialis muscle

Figure 9.84
Axial, T1-weighted MR scan of elbow with annular ligament.

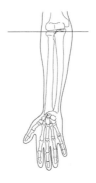

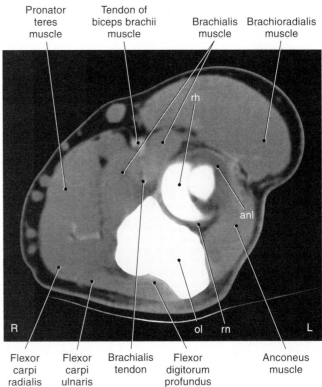

Pronator teres muscle

Tendon of biceps brachii muscle

Brachialis muscle

Brachioradialis muscle

rh

anl

R   ol   rn   L

Flexor carpi radialis muscle

Flexor carpi ulnaris muscle

Brachialis tendon

Flexor digitorum profundus muscle

Anconeus muscle

Figure 9.85
Axial CT scan of elbow with annular ligament.

Muscles of the Forearm

One method to classify the muscles of the forearm is to use the radius, ulna, and interosseous membrane to divide them into a ventral group (the flexors) and a dorsal group (the extensors). The two groups can be further divided into superficial and deep muscles. The muscles of the forearm are described in Table 9.5.

VENTRAL GROUP—SUPERFICIAL MUSCLES

Pronator teres
Flexor carpi radialis
Palmaris longus
Flexor carpi ulnaris
Flexor digitorum superficialis

All five of the superficial muscles in the ventral group have an origin from the common flexor tendon off the medial epicondyle of the humerus. These muscles are demonstrated in Figures 9.86 through 9.98.

TABLE 9-5   Muscles of the Forearm

MUSCLE	ORIGIN	INSERTION	PRIMARY ACTIONS
Ventral-Superficial Group			
Pronator teres	Humeral head—medial epicondyle Ulnar head—near coronoid process of ulna	Lateral surface of radius, midshaft	Pronates and flexes forearm
Flexor carpi radialis	Medial epicondyle of humerus (common origin)	Base of second metacarpal	Flexes and abducts hand
Palmaris longus		Distal half of flexor retinaculum	Flexes hand
Flexor carpi ulnaris	Humeral head—common flexor tendon Ulnar head—olecranon process	Humeral head—distal half of flexor retinaculum Ulnar head—pisiform, hook of hamate, fifth metacarpal	Flexes and adducts hand
Flexor digitorum superficialis	Humeral head—common flexor tendon Ulnar head—coronoid process Radial head—anterior surface of proximal half of radius	Lateral sides of middle phalanges of second-fifth fingers	Flexes middle and proximal phalanges of second-fifth fingers
Ventral-Deep Group			
Flexor digitorum profundus	Anterior surface of proximal ulna	Bases of distal phalanges of fourth or fifth finger	Flexes distal phalanges of fourth or fifth finger at distal interphalangeal joint
Flexor pollicis longus	Anterior surface of radius and interosseous membrane	Base of distal phalanx of thumb	Flexes phalanges of thumb
Pronator quadratus	Anterior and radial aspect of distal ulna	Anterior surface of distal radius	Pronates forearm
Dorsal-Superficial Group			
Brachioradialis	Proximal two thirds of supraepicondylar ridge of humerus	Distal radius, proximal to styloid process on lateral surface	Weak forearm flexion
Extensor carpi radialis longus	Lateral supraepicondylar ridge of humerus	Dorsal aspect base of second metacarpal	Extend and abduct hand at wrist joint
Extensor carpi radialis brevis		Dorsal aspect of base of third metacarpal	Extend and abduct hand at wrist joint
Extensor digitorum	Lateral epicondyle of humerus (common origin)	Extensor expansions of second-fifth fingers	Extends second-fifth fingers at metacarpophalangeal joints
Extensor digiti minimi		Extensor expansion of fifth finger	Extends fifth finger at metacarpophalangeal joint
Extensor carpi ulnaris		Dorsal aspect of base of fifth metacarpal	Extends and adducts hand at wrist joint
Dorsal-Deep Group			
Abductor pollicis longus	Posterior surface of proximal ulna, radius, and interosseous membrane	Base of first metacarpal	Abducts thumb and extends thumb at carpometacarpal joint
Extensor pollicis brevis	Posterior surface of distal third of radius and interosseous membrane	Dorsal aspect of base of proximal phalanx of thumb	Extends proximal phalanx of thumb at metacarpophalangeal joint
Extensor pollicis longus	Posterior surface of middle third of ulna and interosseous membrane	Dorsal aspect of base of distal phalanx of thumb	Extends distal phalanx of thumb at interphalangeal joint
Extensor indicis	Posterior surface distal third of ulna and interosseous membrane	Extensor expansion of second finger	Extends second finger
Supinator	Lateral epicondyle of humerus; radial and collateral ligaments; supinator fossa; crest of ulna	Lateral, posterior, and anterior surface of proximal third of radius	Supinates forearm

The **pronator teres muscle** has two heads of origin. Its humeral head originates from the common flexor tendon, whereas the ulnar head originates near the coronoid process of the ulna. The pronator teres muscle courses obliquely before inserting on the lateral surface of the radius at midshaft. It works in conjunction with the pronator quadratus muscle to pronate the forearm (Figure 9.86).

The **flexor carpi radialis muscle** originates from the common flexor tendon and is located medial to the pronator teres. Its tendon passes through the carpal tunnel before inserting on the palmar surface of the base of the second metacarpal. Its actions include flexion and radial deviation of the hand at the wrist joint (Figure 9.86).

The **palmaris longus muscle** originates from the common flexor tendon and passes superficial to the flexor retinaculum to merge with the palmar aponeurosis. It acts to flex the hand and tighten the palmar aponeurosis (Figure 9.86).

The **flexor carpi ulnaris muscle** is the most medial of the superficial muscles located in the anterior compartment of the forearm. It has two heads: The humeral head originates from the common flexor tendon, and the ulnar head originates from the olecranon process. It inserts onto the pisiform, hook of the hamate, and fifth metacarpal and acts to flex and adduct (ulnar deviation) the hand at the wrist joint (Figure 9.86).

The **flexor digitorum superficialis muscle** is the largest muscle of the superficial muscles in the forearm. It arises from three heads: the humeral head from the common flexor tendon, the ulnar head from the coronoid process, and the radial head from the anterior surface of the proximal half of the radius. Just before reaching the flexor retinaculum, the muscle divides into four tendons that share a common synovial sheath through the carpal tunnel. After passing under the flexor retinaculum, the tendons insert on the lateral sides of the middle phalanges of the second to fifth digits. The flexor digitorum superficialis is a strong flexor of the middle and proximal phalanges of the second through fifth digits (Figure 9.86).

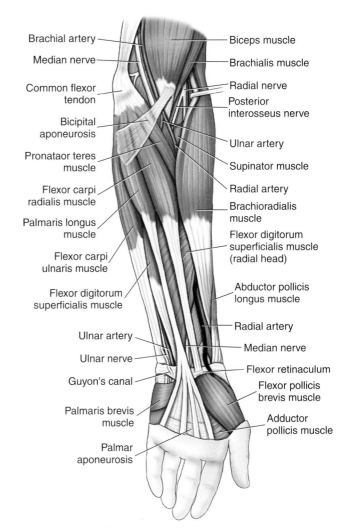

Figure 9.86
Anterior view of superficial flexor muscles of forearm.

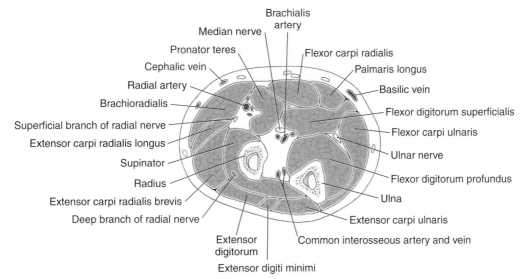

Figure 9.87
Axial view of forearm, proximal one third.

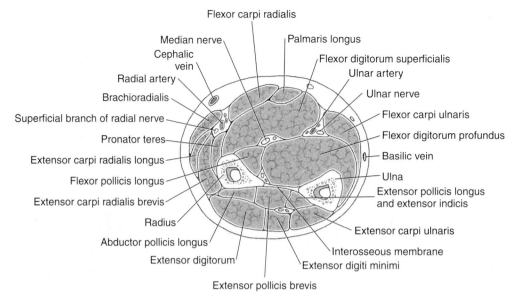

Flexor carpi radialis
Median nerve
Palmaris longus
Cephalic vein
Flexor digitorum superficialis
Radial artery
Ulnar artery
Brachioradialis
Ulnar nerve
Superficial branch of radial nerve
Flexor carpi ulnaris
Pronator teres
Flexor digitorum profundus
Extensor carpi radialis longus
Basilic vein
Flexor pollicis longus
Ulna
Extensor carpi radialis brevis
Extensor pollicis longus and extensor indicis
Radius
Extensor carpi ulnaris
Abductor pollicis longus
Interosseous membrane
Extensor digitorum
Extensor digiti minimi
Extensor pollicis brevis

Figure 9.88
Axial view of forearm, midforearm.

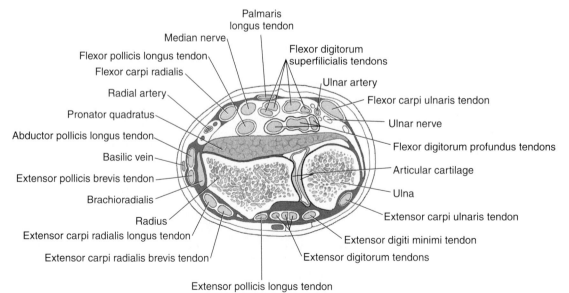

Palmaris longus tendon
Median nerve
Flexor digitorum superfilicialis tendons
Flexor pollicis longus tendon
Flexor carpi radialis
Ulnar artery
Radial artery
Flexor carpi ulnaris tendon
Pronator quadratus
Ulnar nerve
Abductor pollicis longus tendon
Flexor digitorum profundus tendons
Basilic vein
Articular cartilage
Extensor pollicis brevis tendon
Ulna
Brachioradialis
Extensor carpi ulnaris tendon
Radius
Extensor digiti minimi tendon
Extensor carpi radialis longus tendon
Extensor digitorum tendons
Extensor carpi radialis brevis tendon
Extensor pollicis longus tendon

Figure 9.89
Axial view of forearm, distal one third.

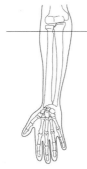
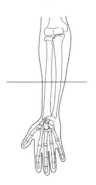

Palmaris longus muscle | Flexor digitorum superficialis muscle | Pronator teres muscle | Median nerve | Brachio-radialis muscle | Radius | Extensor carpi radialis longus muscle

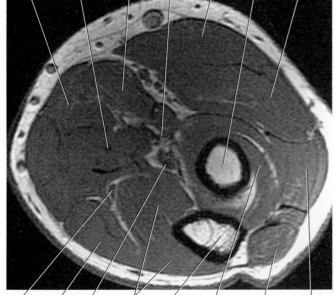

Ulnar nerve | Flexor carpi ulnaris muscle | Ulnar artery | Flexor digitorum profundus muscle | Ulna | Supinator muscle | Anconeus muscle | Extensor radialis brevis muscle

Figure 9.90
Axial, T1-weighted MR scan of forearm muscles.

Flexor carpi ulnaris muscle | Ulnar artery and nerve | Flexor digitorum profundus muscle | Flexor digitorum superficialis muscle | Flexor carpi radialis muscle | Radial artery and nerve | Extensor carpi radialis longus muscle | Cephalic vein

Basilic vein | Extensor pollicis longus muscle | Extensor carpi ulnaris muscle | Abductor pollicis longus muscle | Extensor digiti minimi muscle | Extensor digitorum muscle | Extensor carpi radialis brevis muscle

Figure 9.91
Axial, T1-weighted MR scan of forearm muscles.

Extensor digiti minimi tendon | Extensor digitorum and indicis tendons | Extensor pollicis longus tendon | Lister's tubercle | Extensor carpi radialis brevis tendon

Radius
Extensor carpi ulnaris tendon
Ulna
Flexor digitorum profundus tendons

Flexor carpi ulnaris muscle and tendon

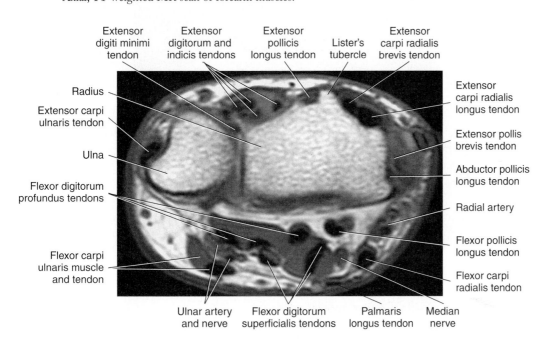

Extensor carpi radialis longus tendon
Extensor pollis brevis tendon
Abductor pollicis longus tendon
Radial artery
Flexor pollicis longus tendon
Flexor carpi radialis tendon

Ulnar artery and nerve | Flexor digitorum superficialis tendons | Palmaris longus tendon | Median nerve

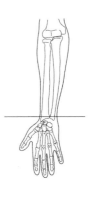

Figure 9.92
Axial, T1-weighted MR scan of distal forearm.

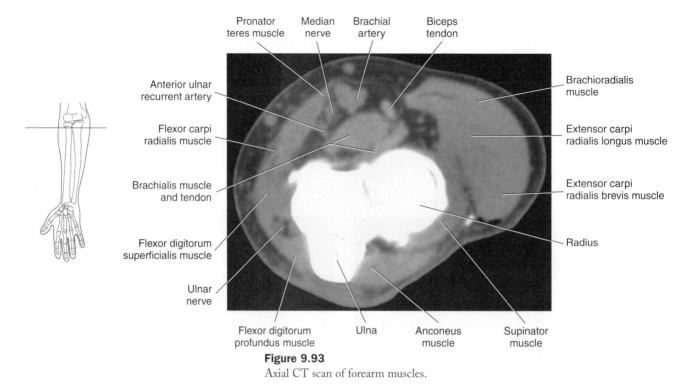

Pronator teres muscle
Median nerve
Brachial artery
Biceps tendon
Brachioradialis muscle
Anterior ulnar recurrent artery
Flexor carpi radialis muscle
Extensor carpi radialis longus muscle
Brachialis muscle and tendon
Extensor carpi radialis brevis muscle
Flexor digitorum superficialis muscle
Radius
Ulnar nerve
Flexor digitorum profundus muscle
Ulna
Anconeus muscle
Supinator muscle

Figure 9.93
Axial CT scan of forearm muscles.

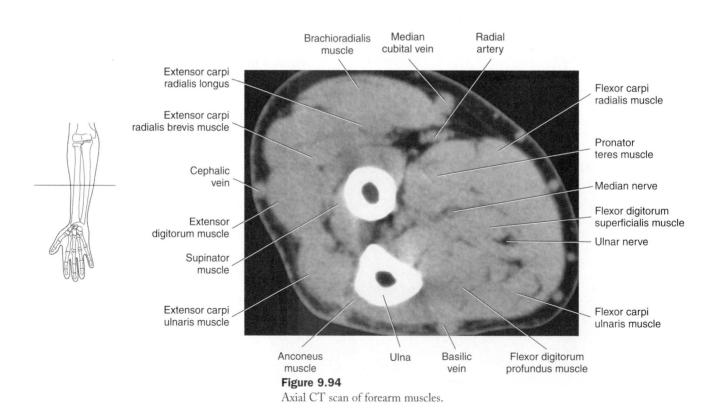

Brachioradialis muscle
Median cubital vein
Radial artery
Extensor carpi radialis longus
Flexor carpi radialis muscle
Extensor carpi radialis brevis muscle
Pronator teres muscle
Cephalic vein
Median nerve
Extensor digitorum muscle
Flexor digitorum superficialis muscle
Supinator muscle
Ulnar nerve
Extensor carpi ulnaris muscle
Flexor carpi ulnaris muscle
Anconeus muscle
Ulna
Basilic vein
Flexor digitorum profundus muscle

Figure 9.94
Axial CT scan of forearm muscles.

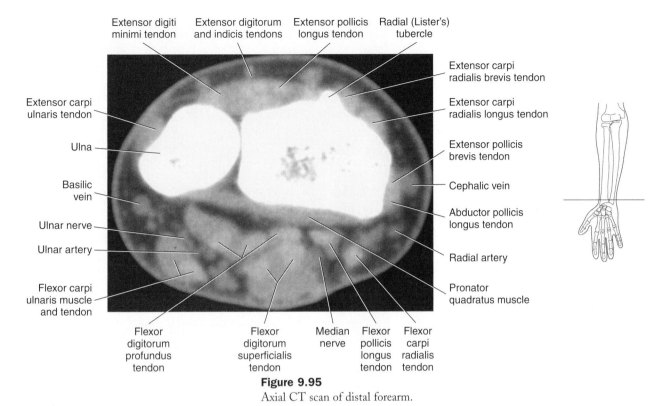

Extensor digiti minimi tendon

Extensor digitorum and indicis tendons

Extensor pollicis longus tendon

Radial (Lister's) tubercle

Extensor carpi radialis brevis tendon

Extensor carpi radialis longus tendon

Extensor pollicis brevis tendon

Cephalic vein

Abductor pollicis longus tendon

Radial artery

Pronator quadratus muscle

Extensor carpi ulnaris tendon

Ulna

Basilic vein

Ulnar nerve

Ulnar artery

Flexor carpi ulnaris muscle and tendon

Flexor digitorum profundus tendon

Flexor digitorum superficialis tendon

Median nerve

Flexor pollicis longus tendon

Flexor carpi radialis tendon

Figure 9.95
Axial CT scan of distal forearm.

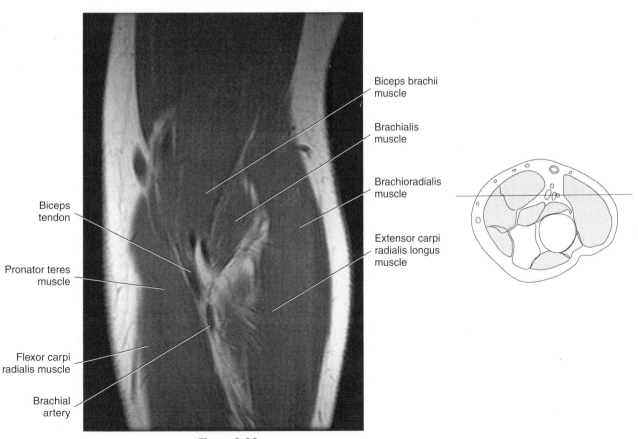

Biceps brachii muscle

Brachialis muscle

Brachioradialis muscle

Extensor carpi radialis longus muscle

Biceps tendon

Pronator teres muscle

Flexor carpi radialis muscle

Brachial artery

Figure 9.96
Coronal, T1-weighted MR scan of forearm muscles.

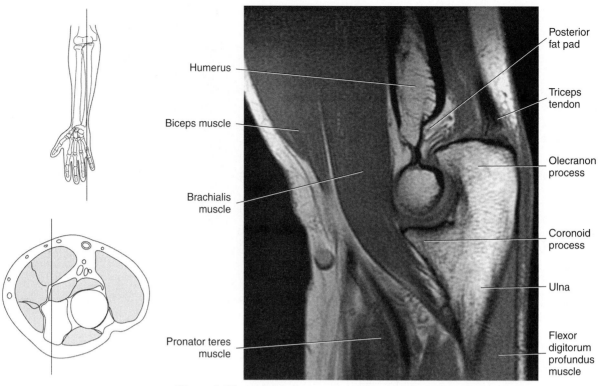

Figure 9.97
Sagittal, T1-weighted MR scan of forearm muscles.

Humerus

Biceps muscle

Brachialis muscle

Pronator teres muscle

Posterior fat pad

Triceps tendon

Olecranon process

Coronoid process

Ulna

Flexor digitorum profundus muscle

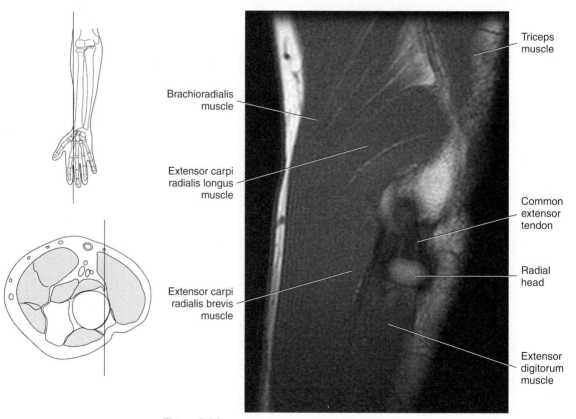

Figure 9.98
Sagittal, T1-weighted MR scan of forearm muscles.

Brachioradialis muscle

Extensor carpi radialis longus muscle

Extensor carpi radialis brevis muscle

Triceps muscle

Common extensor tendon

Radial head

Extensor digitorum muscle

VENTRAL GROUP—DEEP MUSCLES

Flexor digitorum profundus
Flexor pollicis longus
Pronator quadratus

The muscles of the ventral group are demonstrated on Figures 9.97 through 9.99. The **flexor digitorum profundus muscle** is a long, thick muscle responsible for flexing the distal interphalangeal joints of the fingers. It originates from the anterior surface of the proximal ulna and extends medially to the interosseous membrane. Similar to the flexor digitorum superficialis, the flexor digitorum profundus divides into four tendons before reaching the flexor retinaculum. The four tendons pass deep in the carpal tunnel and continue distally to insert on the distal phalanges, where they pair up with the flexor digitorum superficialis to provide flexion of the middle and proximal phalanges of the second through fifth digits (Figure 9.99, *B*).

The **flexor pollicis longus muscle** arises from the anterior surface of the radius and adjacent interosseous membrane and runs lateral to the flexor digitorum profundus to cover the anterior aspect of the radius. After passing through the carpal tunnel, the flexor pollicis longus tendon runs between the flexor pollicis brevis and adductor pollicis brevis muscles to insert on the base of the first distal phalanx (Figure 9.99, *A* and *B*).

The **pronator quadratus,** a quadrangular muscle, is the deepest muscle in the anterior aspect of the forearm. It arises from the anterior and radial aspect of the distal ulna and passes transversely to insert on the anterior surface of the distal radius. The deep fibers of this muscle help bind the radius and ulna together along with the interosseous membrane. The pronator quadratus is the prime mover in pronation of the forearm (Figure 9.99).

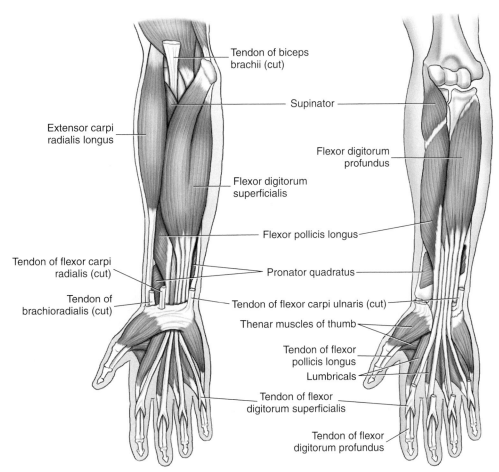

Figure 9.99
Anterior view of forearm muscles. **A,** Superficial muscles. **B,** Deep muscles.

DORSAL GROUP—SUPERFICIAL MUSCLES

- Brachioradialis
- Extensor carpi radialis longus
- Extensor carpi radialis brevis
- Extensor digitorum
- Extensor digiti minimi
- Extensor carpi ulnaris

The muscles of the superficial dorsal group are demonstrated in Figures 9.87 through 9.98 and 9.100. The **brachioradialis** is an extensor muscle lying along the lateral border of the forearm. This large muscle arises from the upper two thirds of the supracondylar ridge of the humerus and attaches distally to the radial styloid process. The brachioradialis flexes the forearm at the elbow and assists with pronation and supination (Figure 9.100).

The **extensor carpi radialis longus muscle** arises just distal to the brachioradialis on the lower third of the supracondylar ridge of the humerus. It runs posterior and deep to the brachioradialis to insert on the base of the second metacarpal. It acts as an extensor and abductor of the hand at the wrist joint (Figure 9.100).

The other superficial muscles (extensor carpi radialis brevis, extensor carpi ulnaris, extensor digitorum, extensor digiti minimi) arise from a common extensor tendon attached to the lateral epicondyle of the humerus. At the level of the elbow they appear as one structure but become more distinct distally as they insert on various structures about the wrist and hand.

The **extensor carpi radialis brevis** has components that arise from the radial collateral and annular ligaments as well as the common extensor tendon. It runs along the dorsal surface of the wrist to insert on the base of the third metacarpal and acts to extend and abduct the hand at the wrist joint (Figure 9.100).

The **extensor digitorum muscle** is the main extensor of the second to fifth digits and occupies much of the posterior surface of the forearm. It arises from the common extensor tendon and divides into four individual tendinous slips just proximal to the wrist. The four tendons run in a single synovial sheath as they pass under the extensor retinaculum. The tendons insert into the extensor expansions of the second through fifth digits, helping to form the extensor hoods (see the section on ligaments of the finger). In addition, small slips of the tendon spread out

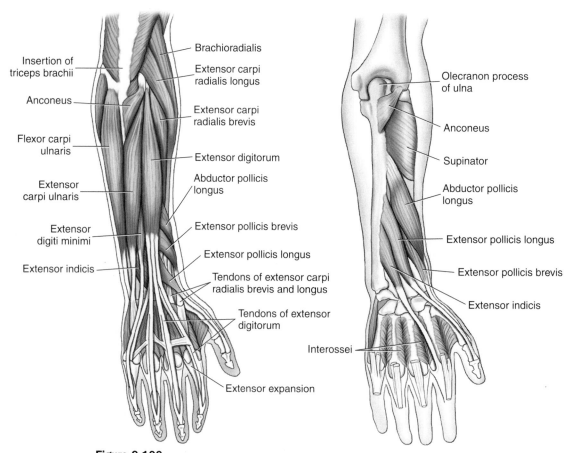

Figure 9.100
Posterior view of forearm muscles. *Left,* Superficial muscles. *Right,* Deep muscles.

and run to the bases of the proximal phalanges and to the capsules of the metacarpophalangeal joints (Figure 9.100). The extensor digitorum muscle extends and spreads the fingers and extends the hand at the wrist joint. The **extensor digiti minimi** muscle arises from the common extensor tendon and passes under the extensor retinaculum in its own synovial compartment. It then divides into two tendinous slips that insert on the proximal phalanx of the fifth digit to help with extension of the little finger (Figure 9.100).

The **extensor carpi ulnaris** is a long, slender muscle that arises from the common extensor tendon and runs along the medial and dorsal side of the ulna to insert on the base of the fifth metacarpal. Its main actions include extension of the hand at the wrist joint and adduction of the hand, resulting in ulnar deviation (Figure 9.100).

DORSAL GROUP—DEEP MUSCLES

Abductor pollicis longus
Extensor pollicis brevis
Extensor pollicis longus
Extensor indicis
Supinator

The deep muscles of the dorsal group consists of four extensors that act on either the first or second digit and includes the supinator muscle. These muscles are demonstrated in Figures 9.87 through 9.98 and 9.100.

The three deep extensors that act on the first digit are the abductor pollicis longus, extensor pollicis brevis, and the extensor pollicis longus muscles. The long, slender **abductor pollicis longus muscle** arises from the dorsal surfaces of the ulna and radius and from the interosseous membrane. It inserts on the base of the first metacarpal to abduct and extend the thumb (Figure 9.100).

The short **extensor pollicis brevis muscle** arises from the dorsal surfaces of the ulna and radius and from the interosseous membrane just distal to the abductor pollicis longus muscle. It inserts on the base of the proximal phalanx of the first digit and works together with the abductor pollicis longus to extend and abduct the thumb (Figure 9.100).

The **extensor pollicis longus muscle** arises from the dorsal surface of the ulna and interosseous membrane just distal to the abductor pollicis longus muscle. After passing through the extensor retinaculum, it crosses over the extensor carpi radialis longus and brevis to insert on the base of the distal phalanx of the first digit. Its main action is to extend the distal phalanx of the first digit, but it can also abduct the hand (Figure 9.100).

The **extensor indicis muscle** arises from the distal third of the dorsal ulna and the interosseous membrane and runs with the extensor digitorum muscle through the extensor retinaculum to insert on the dorsal aponeurosis of the second digit. It functions with the extensor digitorum muscle to extend the index finger, as if pointing (Figure 9.100).

The **supinator muscle** originates from two heads: oblique and transverse. The oblique head originates from the lateral epicondyle and collateral ligament, whereas the transverse head originates from the supinator crest of the ulna. Both heads wrap laterally around the proximal radius to insert on the posterolateral and anterior surfaces of the proximal radius to supinate the forearm (Figure 9.100).

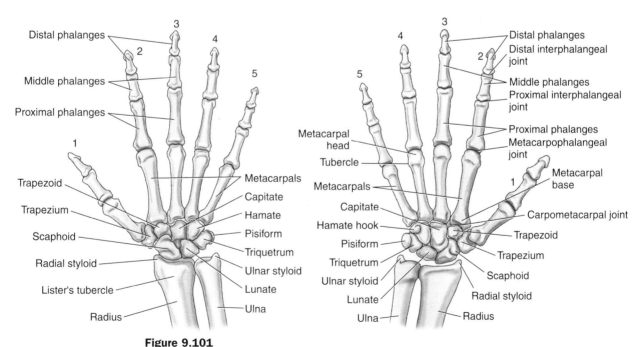

Figure 9.101
Osseous structures of hand and wrist. *Left,* Dorsal view. *Right,* Palmar view.

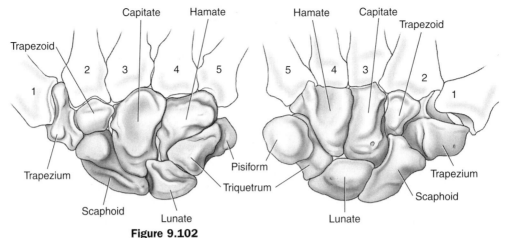

Figure 9.102
Carpal bones. *Left,* Dorsal view. *Right,* Palmar view.

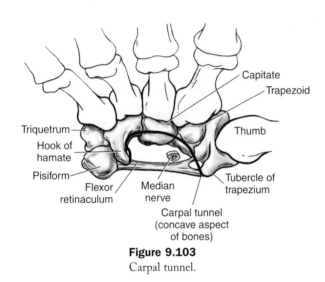

Figure 9.103
Carpal tunnel.

WRIST AND HAND

The complex anatomy of the wrist and hand provides for a multitude of movements unmatched by any other joints of the body.

Bony Anatomy

The bony anatomy of the wrist and hand consists of the distal radius and ulna, 8 carpal bones, 5 metacarpals, and 14 phalanges (Figure 9.101). Both the distal radius and ulna have a conical styloid process that acts as an attachment site for ligaments. The radial styloid process is located on the lateral surface of the radius, whereas the ulnar styloid process is located on the posteromedial side of the ulna. The carpal bones are arranged in proximal and distal rows. Located in the proximal row of carpal bones are the **scaphoid (navicular), lunate (semilunar), triquetral (triquetrum),** and **pisiform** bones. The pisiform is considered a sesamoid bone that is embedded in the tendon of the flexor carpi ulnaris. The distal row consists of the **trapezium (greater multangular), trapezoid (lesser multangular), capitate (os magnum),** and **hamate (unciform)** bones (Figures 9.102 through 9.114). The five **metacarpals** are small tubular bones with a proximal end (base), distal end (head), and shaft (body). The 14 **phalanges** that make up the fingers are short tubular bones. Like the metacarpals, each phalanx consists of a proximal (base), middle (body or diaphysis), and distal (head) portion. Each digit consists of 3 phalanges (proximal, middle, and distal), except for the thumb (first digit), which has only 2 phalanges (proximal and distal). The articulation of the phalanges of the second through fifth digits creates three interphalangeal joints: the **metacarpophalangeal (MCP) joints** classified as condyloid joints, **proximal interphalangeal (PIP),** and **distal interphalangeal (DIP).** The proximal and distal interphalangeal joints are classified as hinge joints (Figure 9.101). The first digit, which consists of 2 phalanges, has just two joints: the MCP joint, classified as a saddle joint, and an interphalangeal joint, classified as a hinge joint (Figure 9.101).

> Compression of the median nerve as it passes through the carpal tunnel is called *carpal tunnel syndrome.* Symptoms include pain and numbness of the fingers supplied by the median nerve.

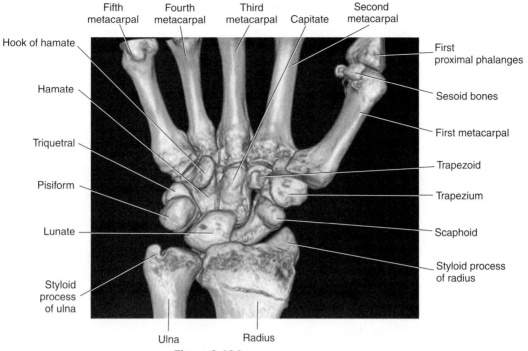

Fifth metacarpal · Fourth metacarpal · Third metacarpal · Capitate · Second metacarpal

Hook of hamate

Hamate

Triquetral

Pisiform

Lunate

Styloid process of ulna

First proximal phalanges

Sesoid bones

First metacarpal

Trapezoid

Trapezium

Scaphoid

Styloid process of radius

Ulna · Radius

Figure 9.104
3D CT scan of palmar aspect of wrist.

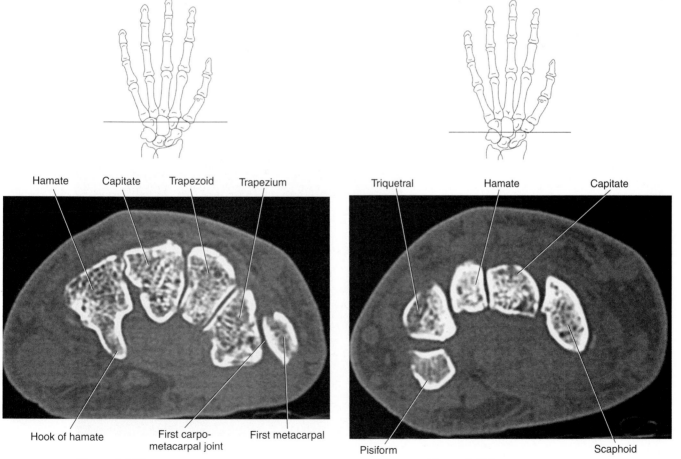

Hamate · Capitate · Trapezoid · Trapezium

Hook of hamate · First carpo-metacarpal joint · First metacarpal

Figure 9.105
Axial CT scan through distal carpals.

Triquetral · Hamate · Capitate

Pisiform · Scaphoid

Figure 9.106
Axial CT scan through midcarpals.

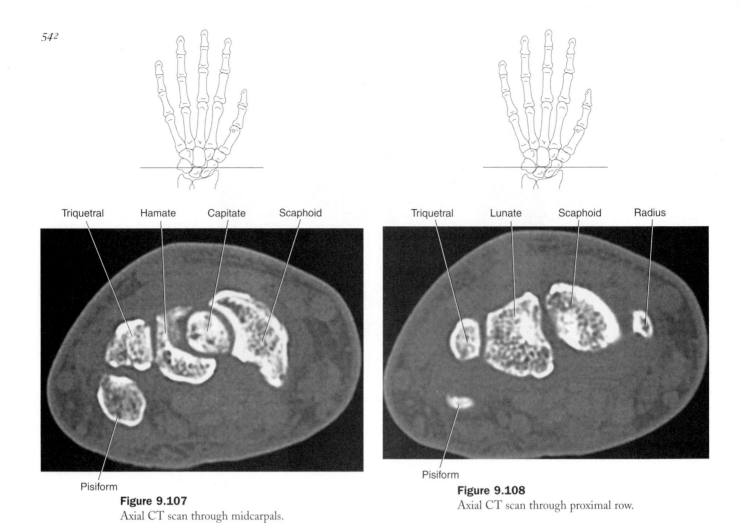

Triquetral   Hamate   Capitate   Scaphoid

Pisiform

Figure 9.107
Axial CT scan through midcarpals.

Triquetral   Lunate   Scaphoid   Radius

Pisiform

Figure 9.108
Axial CT scan through proximal row.

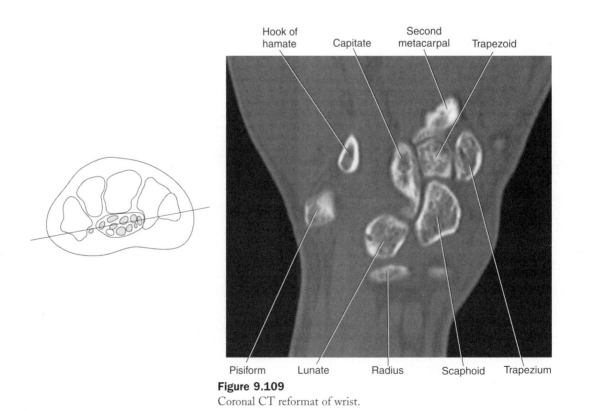

Hook of
hamate   Capitate   Second
metacarpal   Trapezoid

Pisiform   Lunate   Radius   Scaphoid   Trapezium

Figure 9.109
Coronal CT reformat of wrist.

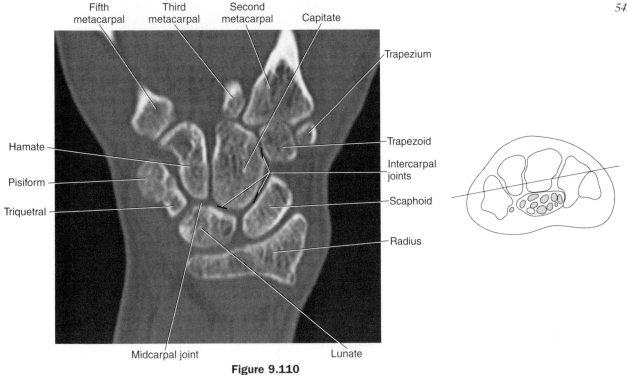

Figure 9.110
Coronal CT reformat of wrist.

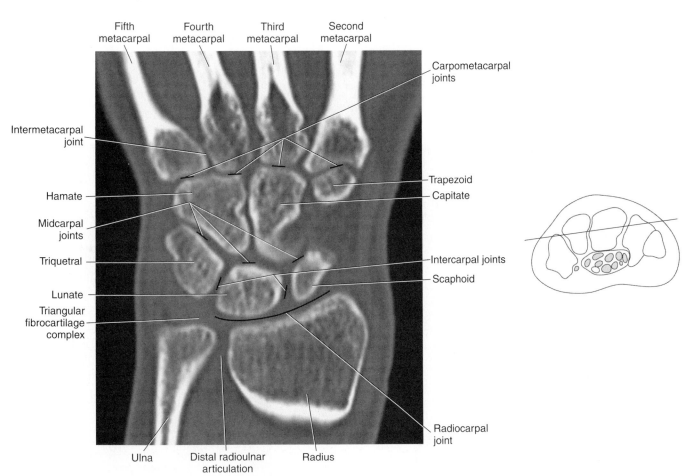

Figure 9.111
Coronal CT reformat of wrist.

544

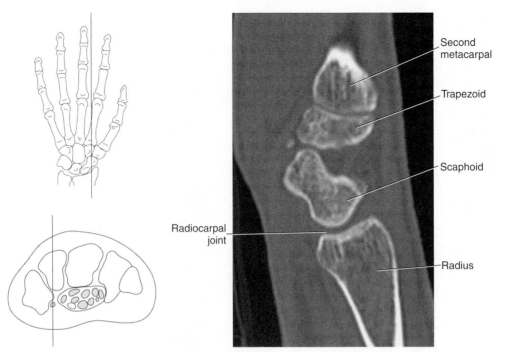

Figure 9.112
Sagittal CT reformat of wrist.

Second metacarpal

Trapezoid

Scaphoid

Radiocarpal joint

Radius

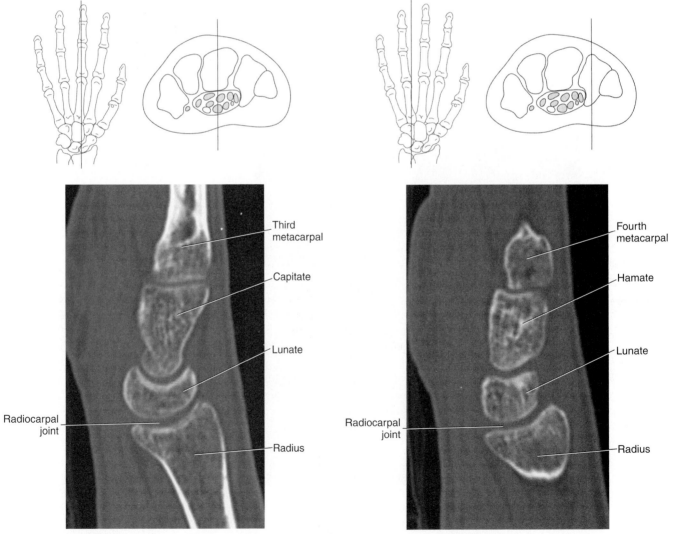

Figure 9.113
Sagittal CT reformat of wrist.

Third metacarpal

Capitate

Lunate

Radiocarpal joint

Radius

Figure 9.114
Sagittal CT reformat of wrist.

Fourth metacarpal

Hamate

Lunate

Radiocarpal joint

Radius

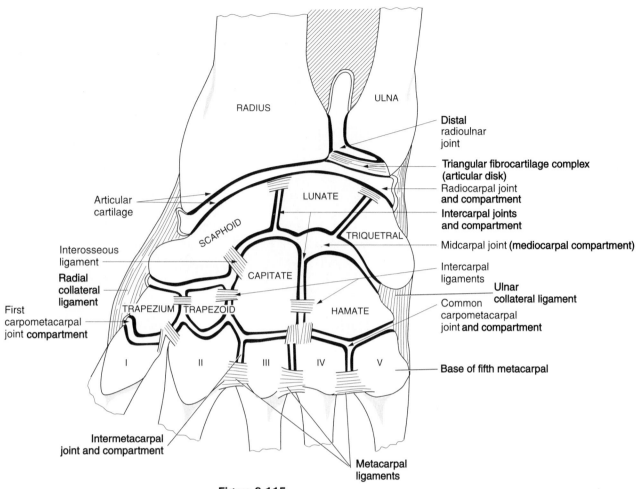

Figure 9.115
Anterior view of cross section of wrist joint.

Joints

The joints of the wrist and hand are quite complex and consist of the following: distal radioulnar articulation, radiocarpal articulation (proximal joint of hand), midcarpal articulation (distal joint of hand), intercarpal articulations (articulations between proximal and distal carpals), carpometacarpal articulations (between carpals and metacarpals), the intermetacarpal articulations (between bases of metacarpals two through five) and the interphalangeal joints (between phalanges of each digit) (Figures 9.111 and 9.115). The **distal radioulnar articulation,** also called the **distal radioulnar joint (DRUJ),** is created when the ulnar notch of the radius moves around the articular circumference of the ulna, providing the movements of supination and pronation. The main stabilizing element of the DRUJ is an articular disk called the **triangular fibrocartilage complex (TFCC).** The TFCC is a fan-shaped band of fibrous tissue that originates on the medial surface of the distal radius and traverses horizontally to insert on the ulnar styloid process (Figures 9.115 and 9.116). It rotates against the distal surface of the ulnar head during pronation and supination

and separates the ulna from the carpal bones. The proximal surface of the **radiocarpal articulation** is formed by the articular carpal surface of the radius and the TFCC, whereas the distal surface is formed by the articular surfaces of the scaphoid, lunate, and triquetrum and the interosseous ligaments connecting them (Figures 9.111 through 9.115). The **midcarpal joint** is formed by the articulations between the proximal and distal carpal rows (Figures 9.110 and 9.115). The articulation between the carpals within each row creates the **intercarpal joints** (Figures 9.111 and 9.115). The **carpometacarpal** joints are formed by the articulations between the carpus and the five metacarpals (Figure 9.111 and 9.115). The carpometacarpal joint of the thumb is an independent joint formed by the articular surfaces of the trapezium and first metacarpal, creating a pure saddle joint. The carpometacarpal articulations of the two to five digits are amphiarthrotic joints with little mobility (Figures 9.105 and 9.115). The **intermetacarpal articulation** exists between the base of the metacarpals and is joined by the palmar and dorsal **metacarpal ligaments** (Figure 9.115).

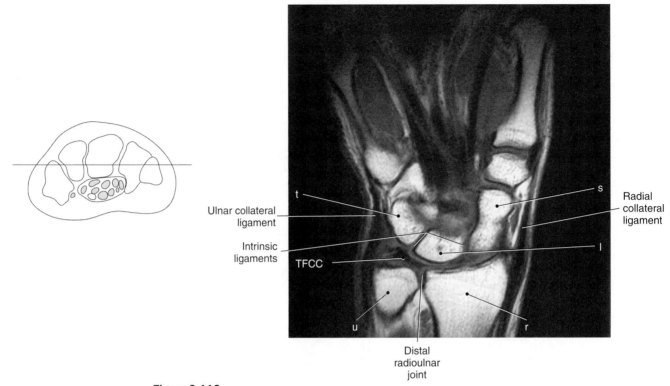

Figure 9.116
Coronal, T1-weighted MR scan of wrist with triangular fibrocartilage complex.

Ligaments and Fascia

Numerous ligaments provide additional stability to the wrist. The **extrinsic ligaments** reinforce the joint cavity surrounding the carpal region and include **palmar** and **dorsal radial carpal ligaments,** the **radial** and **ulnar collateral ligaments,** and the **TFCC** (Figures 9.115 through 9.117). The many articulations between the carpal bones are supported by the **intercarpal ligaments** or **intrinsic ligaments** that connect the carpal bones to each other (Figure 9.115). The configuration of the intrinsic ligaments, metacarpal ligaments, and triangular fibrocartilage complex creates five different joint compartments that can be demonstrated at arthrography: (1) compartment of the first carpometacarpal articulation, (2) common carpo-metacarpal compartment, (3) mediocarpal compartment, (4) intermetacarpal compartment, and (5) radiocarpal compart-ment (Figure 9.115). The **carpal tunnel** is created by the concave arrangement of the carpal bones (Figure 9.103). A thick ligamentous band called the **flexor retinaculum (trans-verse carpal ligament)** stretches across the carpal tunnel to create an enclosure for the passage of tendons and the median nerve (Figures 9.118 through 9.120). The flexor retinaculum inserts medially on the pisiform and hook of the hamate and spans the wrist to insert laterally on the scaphoid and trapezium. In addition to the carpal tunnel, another tunnel called **Guyon's canal** is formed where the ulnar extension of the flexor retinaculum continues over the pisiform and hamate. This

KEY: t, Triquetrum; **TFCC,** triangular fibrocartilage complex; **u,** ulna; **r,** radius; **s,** scaphoid; **l,** lunate; **H,** hamate; **C,** capitate; **Td,** trapezoid; **Tm,** trapezium; **P,** pisiform; **L,** lunate; **S,** scaphoid; **LT,** Lister's tubercle.

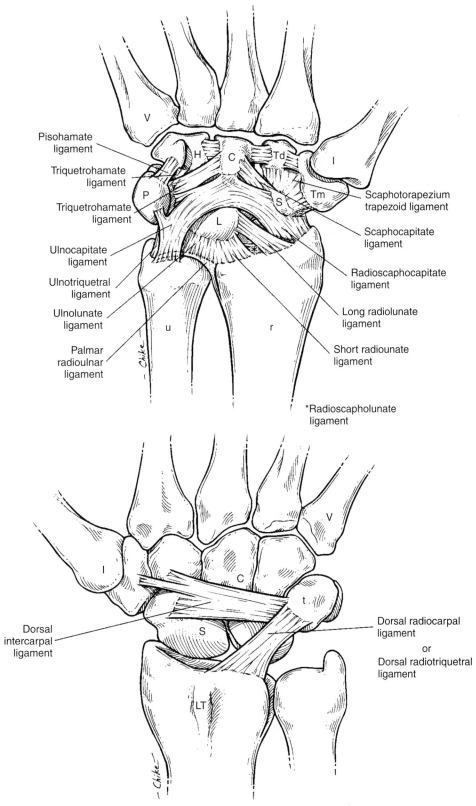

Figure 9.117
Extrinsic ligaments of wrist. *Top*, Palmar view. *Bottom*, Dorsal view.

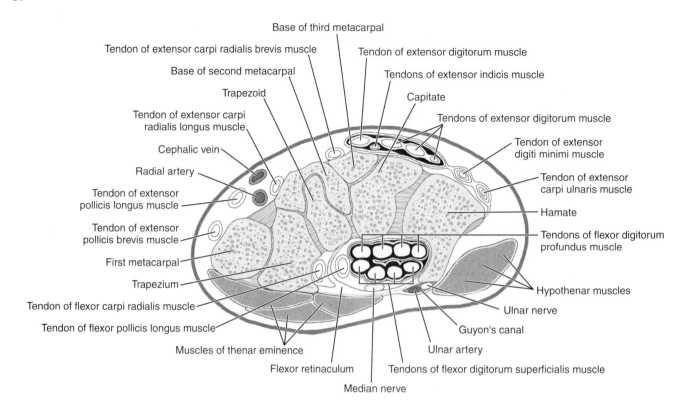

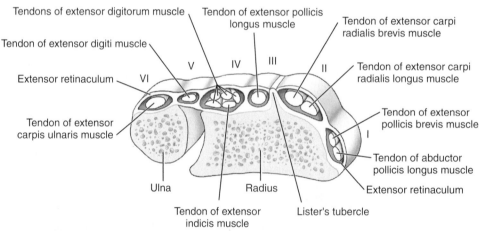

Figure 9.118
Axial view of carpal tunnel and flexor tendons. *Top,* Extensor tendons. *Bottom,* Compartments.

creates a potential site for compression of the ulnar nerve (Figures 9.118, *top,* and 9.119). The **extensor retinaculum (dorsal carpal ligament),** located dorsally, is much thinner. It attaches medially to the ulnar styloid process, triquetrum, and pisiform and laterally to the lateral margin of the radius (Figure 9.120, *left*). Along its course it forms six fibroosseous tunnels for the passage of the synovial sheaths containing the extensor tendons (Figure 9.118, *bottom*).

LIGAMENTS OF THE FINGERS The MCP and interphalangeal joints each have a palmar ligament and two collateral ligaments. The **palmar (volar) ligament** is a thick, dense fibrocartilaginous tissue that covers the palmar surface of the joints. The palmar ligaments run between and are

connected to the collateral ligaments, creating the floor of the interphalangeal and MCP joints. The **deep transverse metacarpal ligament (DTML)** consists of a series of short ligaments that connect the palmar ligaments of the metacarpal heads (Figure 9.123). The DTML prevents separation of the metacarpals. Along the palmar surface of the fingers, the ligamentous structures of the radial and ulnar **collateral ligaments,** radial and ulnar **accessory collateral ligaments,** and palmar plates provide stability for the MCP and interphalangeal joints (Figure 9.121). There is a fibroosseous tunnel along the palmar aspect of each finger for the passage of the flexor tendons. The tunnel is created by well-defined areas of thickening of the tendon sheath and is called the **annular**

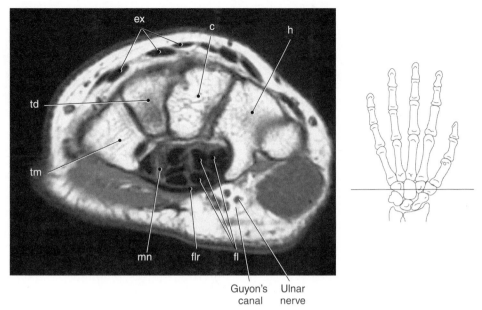

Figure 9.119
Axial, T1-weighted MR scan of wrist with flexor and extensor tendons.

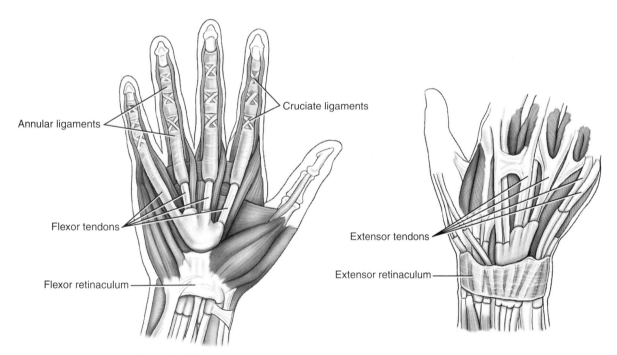

Figure 9.120
Left, Palmar view of flexor tendons. *Right,* Dorsal view of extensor tendons.

KEY: ex, Extensor tendons; **c,** capitate; **h,** hamate; **fl,** flexor tendons; **flr,** flexor retinaculum; **mn,** median nerve; **tm,** trapezium; **td,** trapezoid.

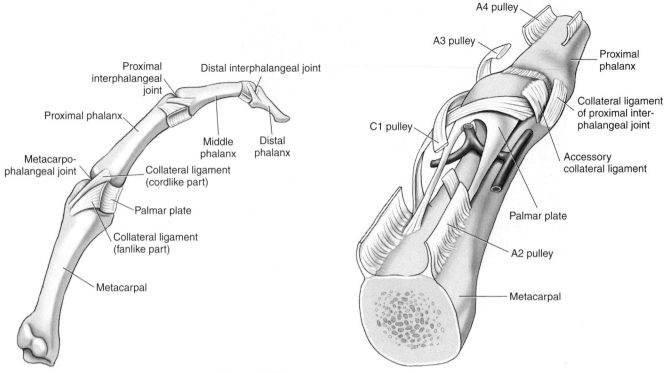

Figure 9.121
Palmar plate. *Left,* Lateral view. *Right,* Anatomy.

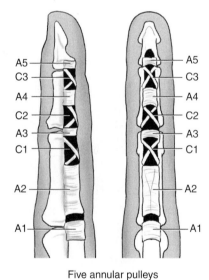

Five annular pulleys
Three cruciate pulleys

Figure 9.122
Annular pulley system. *Left,* Sagittal view. *Right,* Palmar view.

pulley system. It is composed of five **annular pulleys** and three **cruciate pulleys,** which are important structures that prevent the displacement of the tendons during flexion of the fingers (Figure 9.122). The dorsal surface of the hand and fingers contains the **extensor mechanism** or **extensor hood** (Figures 9.123 through 9.126). The extensor hood consists of the digital extensor tendon, extensor hood proper, and insertions of the lumbricals and interossei muscles and serves to maintain the integrity of the extensor tendons along the path of the MCP and interphalangeal joints.

KEY: A, Annular pulley; **C,** cruciate pulley.

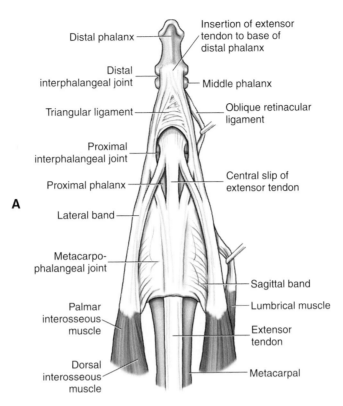

A

Distal phalanx

Insertion of extensor tendon to base of distal phalanx

Distal interphalangeal joint

Middle phalanx

Triangular ligament

Oblique retinacular ligament

Proximal interphalangeal joint

Proximal phalanx

Central slip of extensor tendon

Lateral band

Metacarpo-phalangeal joint

Sagittal band

Lumbrical muscle

Palmar interosseous muscle

Extensor tendon

Dorsal interosseous muscle

Metacarpal

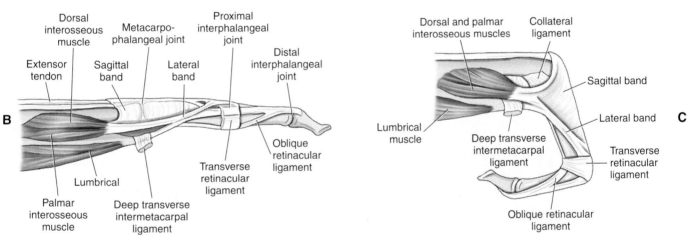

B

Dorsal interosseous muscle

Metacarpo-phalangeal joint

Proximal interphalangeal joint

Distal interphalangeal joint

Extensor tendon

Sagittal band

Lateral band

Oblique retinacular ligament

Lumbrical

Transverse retinacular ligament

Palmar interosseous muscle

Deep transverse intermetacarpal ligament

C

Dorsal and palmar interosseous muscles

Collateral ligament

Sagittal band

Lateral band

Lumbrical muscle

Deep transverse intermetacarpal ligament

Transverse retinacular ligament

Oblique retinacular ligament

Figure 9.123

Extensor mechanism of finger. **A,** Dorsal view. **B,** Lateral view. **C,** Lateral view in flexion.

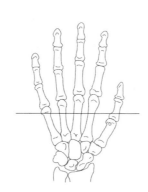

Figure 9.124
Axial view of metacarpophalangeal joint structures.

Extensor tendon
Sagittal band
Main collateral ligament
Accessory collateral ligament
Deep transverse metacarpal ligament
A1 pulley
Flexor tendons
Palmar plate
Lumbrical muscle and tendon
Interosseous tendon
Proximal articular surface of the proximal phalanx

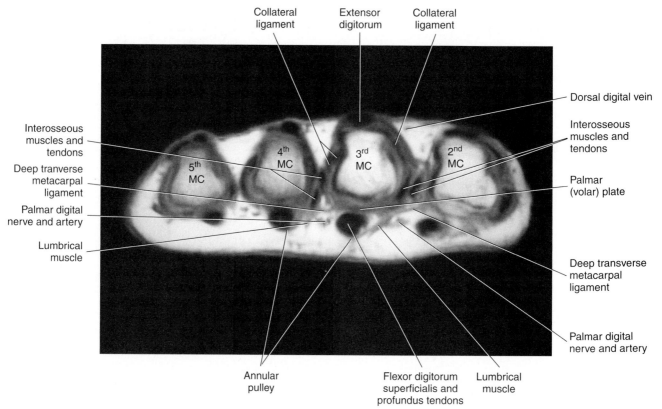

Collateral ligament
Extensor digitorum
Collateral ligament
Dorsal digital vein
Interosseous muscles and tendons
Palmar (volar) plate
Deep transverse metacarpal ligament
Palmar digital nerve and artery
Interosseous muscles and tendons
Deep tranverse metacarpal ligament
Palmar digital nerve and artery
Lumbrical muscle
Annular pulley
Flexor digitorum superficialis and profundus tendons
Lumbrical muscle
5th MC   4th MC   3rd MC   2nd MC

Figure 9.125
Axial MR of finger.

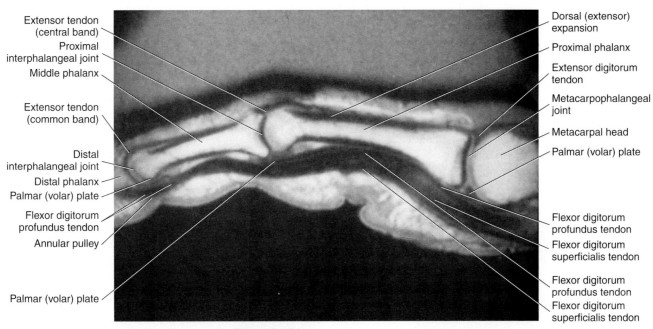

Extensor tendon (central band)

Proximal interphalangeal joint

Middle phalanx

Extensor tendon (common band)

Distal interphalangeal joint

Distal phalanx

Palmar (volar) plate

Flexor digitorum profundus tendon

Annular pulley

Palmar (volar) plate

Dorsal (extensor) expansion

Proximal phalanx

Extensor digitorum tendon

Metacarpophalangeal joint

Metacarpal head

Palmar (volar) plate

Flexor digitorum profundus tendon

Flexor digitorum superficialis tendon

Flexor digitorum profundus tendon

Flexor digitorum superficialis tendon

Figure 9.126
Sagittal, T1-weighted MR scan of finger.

KEY: MC, Metacarpal.

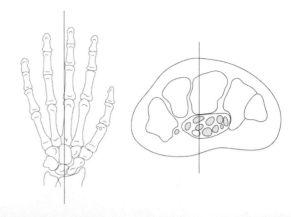

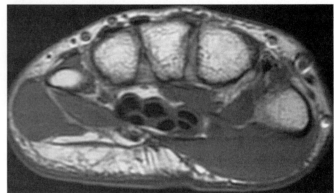

Figure 9.128
Axial, T1-weighted MR scan through hand.

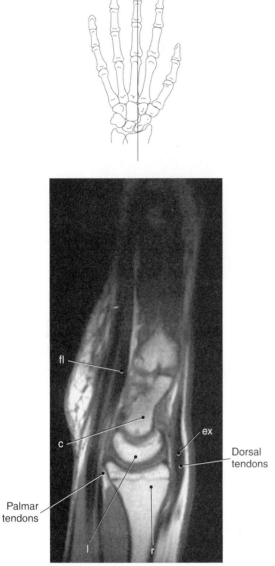

Figure 9.127
Sagittal, T1-weighted MR scan of wrist with flexor and extensor tendons.

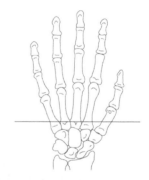

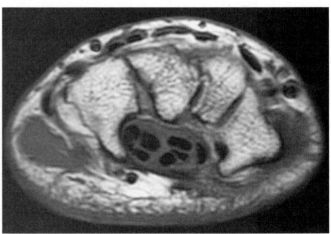

Figure 9.129
Axial, T1-weighted MR scan through wrist.

Muscles and Tendons

The numerous muscles of the forearm become tendinous just before the wrist joint. The many tendons located in the wrist can be divided into **palmar** and **dorsal tendon groups** (Figures 9.120, *A* and *B* and 9.127). The palmar tendon group collectively flexes the fingers and wrist. As this group courses through the carpal tunnel, the tendons appear to be arranged in two discrete rows (Figures 9.118, *A* and 9.119). The tendons of the dorsal tendon group, spanning the superficial surface of the wrist, are considered the extensors of the fingers and wrist (Figures 9.128 through 9.140).

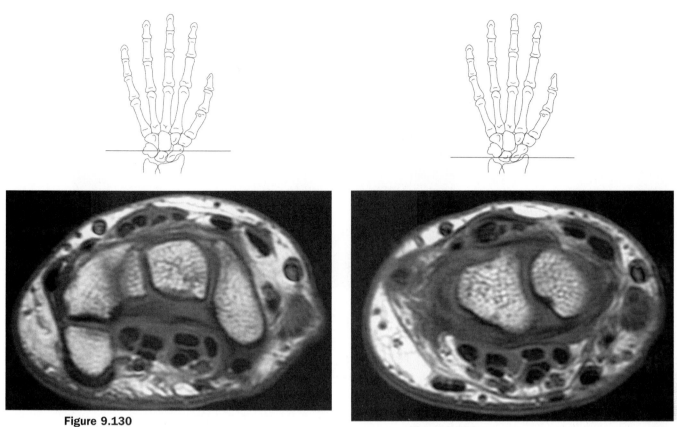

Figure 9.130
Axial, T1-weighted MR scan through wrist.

Figure 9.131
Axial, T1-weighted MR scan through wrist.

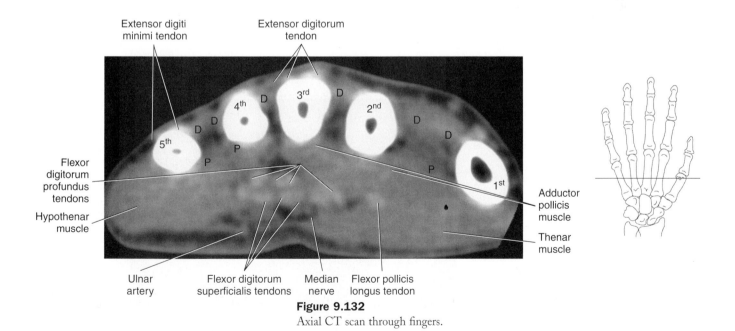

Figure 9.132
Axial CT scan through fingers.

KEY: fl, Flexors; **c,** capitate; **ex,** extensor tendons; **r,** radius; **l,** lunate; **D,** dorsal interosseus muscles; **P,** palmar interosseus muscles.

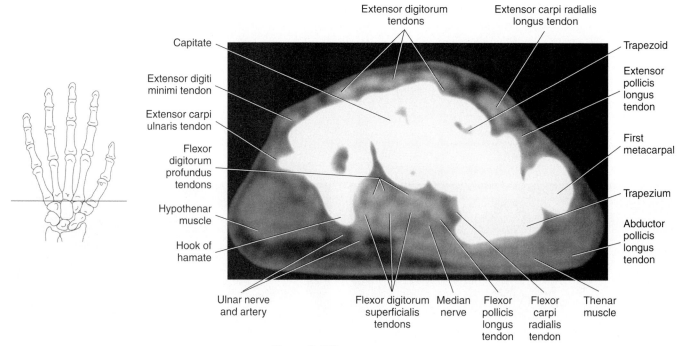

Figure 9.133
Axial CT scan through wrist.

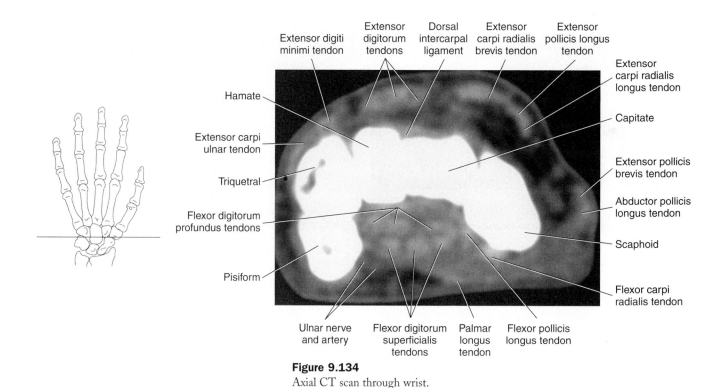

Figure 9.134
Axial CT scan through wrist.

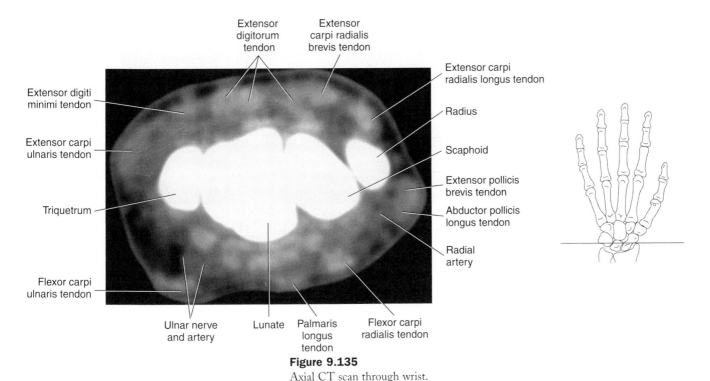

Figure 9.135
Axial CT scan through wrist.

Dorsal interosseous
muscles

Figure 9.136
Axial, T1-weighted MR scan of hand.

The muscles of the hand can be divided into three groups: (1) metacarpal group (muscles of the metacarpals considered to be the central muscles of the hand), (2) thenar group (muscles involving the thumb and creating the thenar eminence on the radial side), (3) hypothenar group (muscles involving the fifth digit and creating the hypothenar eminence on the ulnar side). These muscles are demonstrated in Figures 9.128 through 9.143.

METACARPAL GROUP The **metacarpal muscle group** includes the interossei and lumbrical muscles. There are seven short **interossei muscles** in the metacarpal muscle group: three single-headed muscles located on the palmar surface and four double-headed muscles located on the dorsal surface (Figure 9.141, *A* and *B*). The four **palmar interossei** muscles arise from the first, second, fourth, and fifth metacarpals and insert on the corresponding proximal phalanges, frequently radiating into the corresponding tendons of the dorsal aponeurosis. These muscles are responsible for flexion at the MCP joints and extension at the interphalangeal joints. The **dorsal interossei** arise by two heads from the sides of the five metacarpal bones to insert on the proximal phalanges and radiate onto the dorsal aponeurosis. Like their palmar counterparts, the dorsal interossei flex at the MCP joints and extend at the interphalangeal joints. The four small **lumbrical** muscles arise from the tendons of the flexor digitorum profundus and

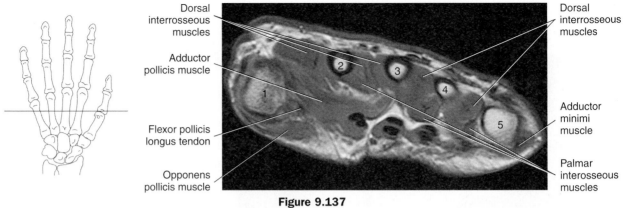

Dorsal interrosseous muscles

Adductor pollicis muscle

Flexor pollicis longus tendon

Opponens pollicis muscle

Dorsal interrosseous muscles

Adductor minimi muscle

Palmar interosseous muscles

Figure 9.137
Axial, T1-weighted MR scan of hand.

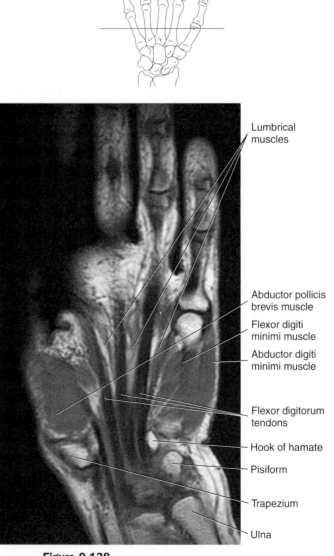

Lumbrical muscles

Abductor pollicis brevis muscle

Flexor digiti minimi muscle

Abductor digiti minimi muscle

Flexor digitorum tendons

Hook of hamate

Pisiform

Trapezium

Ulna

Figure 9.138
Coronal, T1-weighted MR scan of wrist and hand.

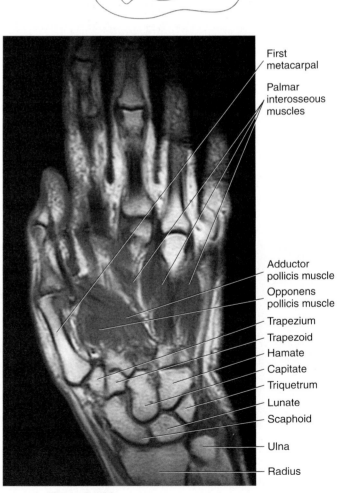

First metacarpal

Palmar interosseous muscles

Adductor pollicis muscle

Opponens pollicis muscle

Trapezium

Trapezoid

Hamate

Capitate

Triquetrum

Lunate

Scaphoid

Ulna

Radius

Figure 9.139
Coronal, T1-weighted MR scan of wrist and hand.

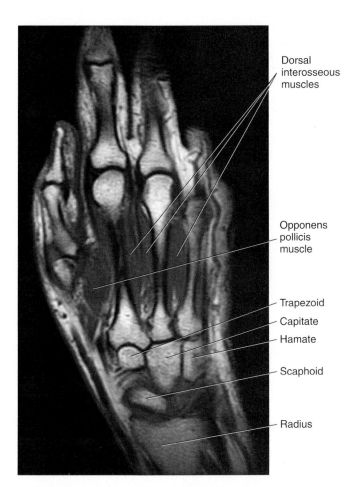

Dorsal interosseous muscles

Opponens pollicis muscle

Trapezoid

Capitate

Hamate

Scaphoid

Radius

Figure 9.140
Coronal, T1-weighted MR scan of wrist and hand.

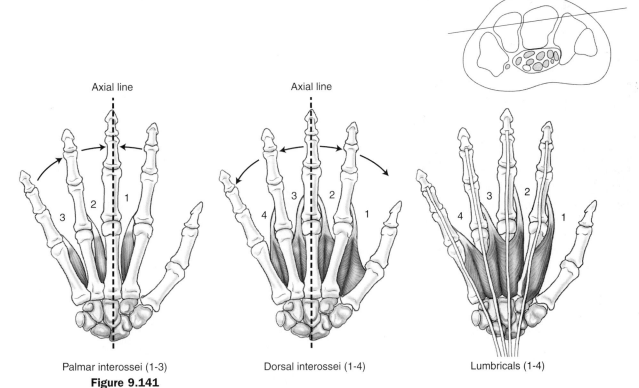

Axial line

Axial line

Palmar interossei (1-3)

Dorsal interossei (1-4)

Lumbricals (1-4)

Figure 9.141
Left, Palmar view of interosseous muscles. *Center,* Dorsal view of interosseous muscles.
Right, Lumbrical muscles.

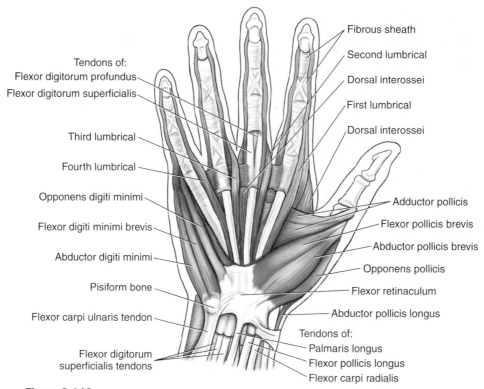

Figure 9.142
Palmar view of flexor pollicis brevis, flexor digiti minimi, abductor pollicis brevis, opponens pollicis, and abdutor digiti minimi muscles.

pass to the radial side of the corresponding finger to insert on the extensor expansion covering the dorsal surface of the finger (Figure 9.142). The lumbricals flex the first phalanges at the MCP joints and extend the second and third phalanges at the interphalangeal joints.

THENAR GROUP   The four muscles of the **thenar group** are the abductor pollicis brevis, flexor pollicis brevis, adductor pollicis, and opponens pollicis. The **abductor pollicis brevis** is a thin, flat superficial muscle arising from the transverse carpal ligament, navicular, and trapezium (Figure 9.143). It runs inferiorly and laterally to insert on the base of the first phalanx of the thumb to abduct the thumb. The **flexor pollicis brevis** has two heads: The superficial or lateral head arises from the flexor retinaculum, and the deep or medial head arises from the trapezium, trapezoid, and capitate. This muscle inserts on the radial and ulnar base of the first phalanx to flex, adduct, and abduct the thumb (Figure 9.143). Frequently, a sesamoid bone can be found in the insertion tendon on the radial side. The **adductor pollicis** also has two heads: The transverse head arises from the dorsal aspect of the third metacarpal, and the

oblique head arises from numerous slips off the capitate, bases of the second and third metacarpals, and the sheath of the flexor carpi radialis tendon. The adductor pollicis inserts onto the base of the first phalanx of the thumb to provide adduction and assist in the opposition and flexion of the thumb (Figures 9.142 and 9.143). The **opponens pollicis** provides the main opposition for the thumb but also assists with adduction. It arises from the trapezium and flexor retinaculum and inserts onto the radial aspect of the first metacarpal (Figures 9.142 and 9.143). These muscles are also demonstrated in sequential Figures 9.128 through 9.140.

HYPOTHENAR GROUP   The hypothenar group consists of three muscles: abductor digiti minimi, flexor digiti minimi brevis, and opponens digiti minimi. The **abductor digiti minimi** muscle arises from the pisiform and the flexor retinaculum to end in a flat tendon that inserts onto the ulnar base of the first phalanx of the little finger (Figures 9.142 and 9.143). The abductor digiti minimi muscle is the main abductor of the little finger. The **flexor digiti minimi brevis** muscle arises from the flexor retinaculum and the hook of the hamate. It fuses

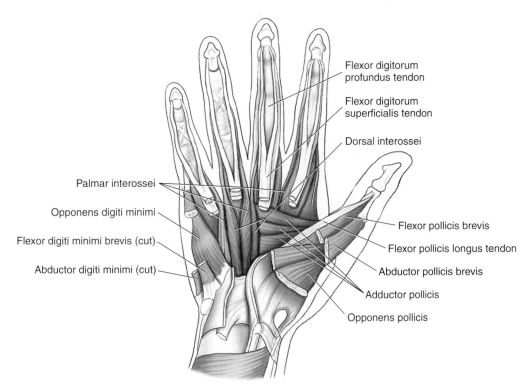

Flexor digitorum
profundus tendon

Flexor digitorum
superficialis tendon

Dorsal interossei

Palmar interossei

Opponens digiti minimi

Flexor digiti minimi brevis (cut)

Abductor digiti minimi (cut)

Flexor pollicis brevis

Flexor pollicis longus tendon

Abductor pollicis brevis

Adductor pollicis

Opponens pollicis

Figure 9.143
Palmar view of adductor pollicis and opponens digiti minimi muscles.

with the tendon of the abductor digiti minimi to insert on the base of the first phalanx of the fifth digit (Figures 9.142 and 9.143). The flexor digiti minimi brevis flexes at the MCP joint. Like the flexor digiti minimi brevis muscle, the **opponens digiti minimi** arises from the hook of the hamate and the flexor retinaculum (Figure 9.143). It inserts on the ulnar surface of the fifth metacarpal to bring the little finger into the position for opposition. For the hand muscles, see Figures 9.128 through 9.140.

NEUROVASCULATURE

The neurovasculature of the upper extremity is composed primarily of the branches of the axillary and brachial arteries, their accompanying deep veins, a system of superficial veins, and the brachial plexus that innervates the upper extremity.

Arterial Supply

SHOULDER   The primary arteries supplying the shoulder region include the axillary and brachial arteries (Figures 9.34 through 9.45 and 9.144, *A*). The **axillary artery** begins at the lateral border of the first rib as a continuation of the subclavian artery. It ends at the inferior border of the teres major muscle, where it passes into the arm and becomes the brachial artery. The axillary artery and its branches supply blood to numerous thoracic and shoulder structures, including the first and second intercostal spaces, axillary lymph nodes, mammary gland in women, and scapular, serratus anterior, pectoral, latissimus dorsi, deltoid, and triceps brachii muscles. The branches of the axillary artery typically include the superior thoracic, thoracoacromial, lateral thoracic, subscapular artery, and anterior and posterior humeral circumflex arteries. The **brachial artery** is the principal arterial supply to the arm. It courses inferiorly on the medial side of the humerus then continues anterior to the cubital fossa of the elbow. The brachial artery is relatively superficial and palpable throughout its course. It accompanies the median nerve, which crosses anterior to the artery in the middle of the arm. During its course, the brachial artery gives rise to numerous muscular branches, which include the profunda brachii, superior ulnar collateral, and inferior ulnar collateral arteries (Figure 9.144, *A*).

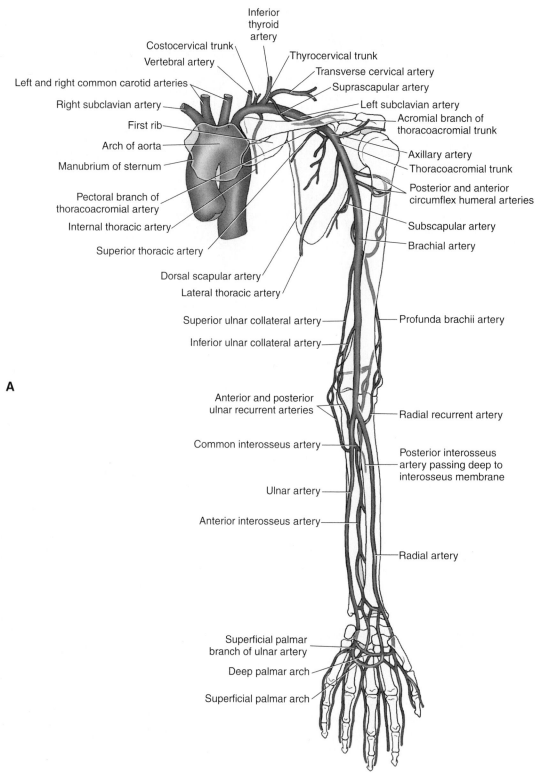

Figure 9.144

A, Anterior view of arteries of the upper extremity.

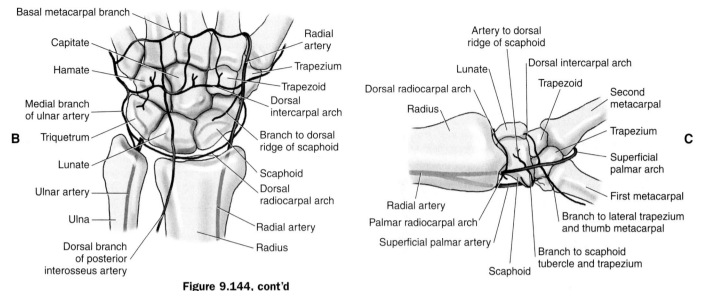

Figure 9.144, cont'd
B, Posterior view of arteries in wrist. **C,** Lateral view of arteries of wrist.

ELBOW The brachial artery divides at the cubital fossa into the radial and ulnar arteries (Figure 9.144, *A*).

The **radial artery** begins at the level of the head of the radius within the anterior compartment of the forearm. It courses beneath the brachioradialis muscle then continues its course just deep to the skin, along the lateral side of the anterior forearm to the wrist. It passes anterior to the radial styloid process to enter the hand. The most proximal branch of the radial artery is the **radial recurrent artery,** which supplies the brachioradialis, supinator, and brachialis muscles and the elbow joint. Within the forearm, the radial artery gives off several direct muscular branches. The **ulnar artery** also gives rise to several branches that supply the elbow and forearm. The first branch of the ulnar artery is the **anterior ulnar recurrent artery,** which supplies the brachialis and pronto teres muscles. It courses just anterior to the medial condyle of the humerus to anastomose with the inferior ulnar collateral branch of the brachial artery. The **posterior ulnar recurrent artery** courses behind the medial epicondyle of the humerus to anastomose with the superior ulnar collateral branch of the brachial artery. It supplies the flexor carpi ulnaris, pronator teres, and anconeus muscles. The **common interosseous artery** branches from the ulnar artery and almost immediately bifurcates into the **anterior** and **posterior interosseous arteries.** These arteries and their branches supply the median nerve, deep flexor and extensor muscles of the forearm, superficial extensor muscles of the forearm, and radius and ulna (Figures 9.57 through 9.67 and 9.87 through 9.98).

WRIST AND HAND The terminal branches of the radial and ulnar arteries form the palmar arches of the wrist and hand. These arches emit branches that serve the wrist, palm, and digits (Figures 9.144 and 9.145). The **palmar carpal arch** or network is formed by the palmar carpal branches from the radial and ulnar arteries, the anterior interosseous artery, also a branch of the ulnar artery, and a recurrent branch from the deep palmar arch. These vessels supply the carpal bones and joints (Figure 9.144, *A* and *C*). The **dorsal carpal arch** or network is formed by dorsal carpal branches of the radial and ulnar arteries. The dorsal carpal arch also receives contributions from the anterior and posterior interosseous arteries. The arch lies close to the dorsal surface of the carpals and gives rise to three dorsal metacarpal arteries and branches that supply the distal regions of the ulna and radius, carpal bones, and intercarpal joints (Figure 9.144, *A* and *C*). The superficial palmar branch of the radial artery anastomoses with the superficial palmar branch of the ulnar artery to form the **superficial palmar arch.** This arch gives rise to three common palmar digital arteries that anastomose with the palmar metacarpal arteries from the deep palmar arch (Figure 9.144, *A* and *C*). The **deep palmar arch** is formed by deep palmar branches of the radial and ulnar arteries and is located approximately 1 cm proximal to the superficial palmar arch. The deep palmar arch also gives rise to a recurrent branch that anastomoses with the palmar carpal branches of the radial and ulnar arteries (Figure 9.144, *A*).

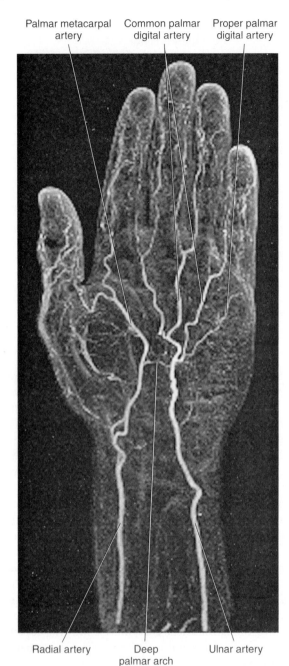

Palmar metacarpal artery   Common palmar digital artery   Proper palmar digital artery

Radial artery   Deep palmar arch   Ulnar artery

Figure 9.145
Anterior view MR angiogram of hand.

Venous Drainage

The veins of the upper extremity are divided into deep and superficial (cutaneous) groups. Numerous anastomoses occur between the groups. The superficial venous system consists of extensive venous networks that are especially well developed within the upper extremity along with their accompanying arteries of the same name. The deep veins are often double and repeatedly anastomose with one another.

SHOULDER   The veins of the upper arm include the brachial, cephalic, and basilic (Figure 9.146). The two deep **brachial veins** ascend the arm, one on either side of the brachial artery. The brachial veins begin in the elbow from the union of the ulnar and radial veins and end in the **axillary vein** near the lower margin of the subscapularis muscle. The two deep brachial veins may join to form one brachial vein during part of their course. The superficial veins of the upper arm include the cephalic and basilic. The **cephalic vein** courses from the radial side of the dorsal venous arch of the hand and then ascends to the midpoint of the forearm, where it curves around to the ventral surface of the forearm and ascends the lateral aspect of the upper arm, along the anterolateral border of the biceps brachii muscle, to open into the axillary vein, just below the clavicle. It drains the superficial parts of the lateral hand and lateral forearm. The **basilic vein** originates from the medial end of the dorsal venous arch of the hand. It then ascends the ulnar side of the forearm, along the medial surface of the biceps brachii muscle, in the upper arm, to form the axillary vein. The basilic vein drains the superficial parts of the medial side of the hand and medial side of the forearm. The large **axillary vein** lies on the medial side of the axillary artery. It extends from the lower border of the teres major muscle to the lateral surface of the first rib to continue as the **subclavian vein.** The axillary vein receives tributaries that correspond to the branches of the axillary artery (Figures 9.34 through 9.47).

ELBOW   The large deep vein of the elbow is the **brachial vein,** which is formed by the union of the **radial** and **ulnar** veins. The superficial veins of the elbow include the cephalic, median cubital, basilica, and intermediate (median) antebrachial veins. The **cephalic vein** courses along the radial side of the elbow and may give rise to the **median cubital vein,** which ascends in an oblique and medial course to create an anastomosis between the basilic and cephalic veins (Figure 9.145). The median cubital vein is a common site for venipuncture. The **basilic vein** courses along the posteromedial aspect of the forearm, crosses the elbow, then takes a deep course in the axilla to joint the brachial vein. The **intermediate (median) antebrachial vein** transports blood from the superficial palmar venous arch and anterior forearm. It ascends the ventral side of the forearm on the ulnar side and typically ends in the basilic vein (Figures 9.147, 9.60 through 9.67, and 9.87 through 9.98).

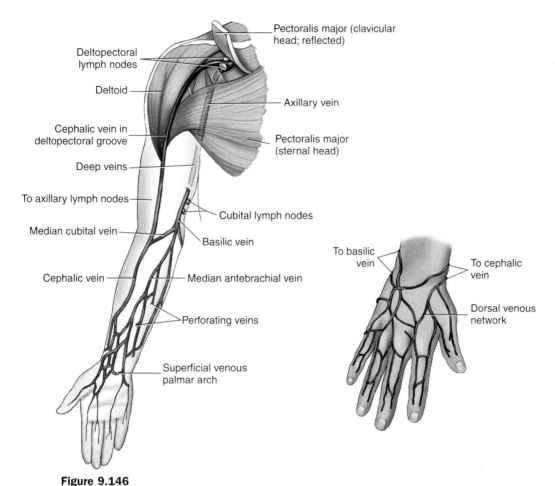

Pectoralis major (clavicular head; reflected)

Deltopectoral lymph nodes

Deltoid

Cephalic vein in deltopectoral groove

Deep veins

To axillary lymph nodes

Median cubital vein

Cephalic vein

Axillary vein

Pectoralis major (sternal head)

Cubital lymph nodes

Basilic vein

Median antebrachial vein

Perforating veins

Superficial venous palmar arch

To basilic vein

To cephalic vein

Dorsal venous network

Figure 9.146

Left, Anterior view of the superficial veins of the upper extremity. *Right,* Posterior view of the superficial veins of the hand.

WRIST AND HAND The superficial venous system forms a network at the dorsum of the hand termed the **dorsal venous network (arch).** It is fed by the subcutaneous dorsal metacarpal veins of the fingers and continues to the distal forearm, where it drains into three major **superficial veins: the cephalic, basilic,** and intermediate (median) antebrachial veins of the forearm. These large superficial veins anastomose frequently as they course superiorly. The **deep** and **superficial palmer venous arches** of the hand empty into the **radial** and **ulnar veins** that then unite to form the **brachial vein** of the arm (Figures 9.89, 9.92 and 9.95, 9.146, and 9.147).

BRACHIAL PLEXUS The **brachial plexus,** also described in Chapter 4, is a large network of nerves that innervate the upper limb (Figures 9.38 and 9.148). It extends from the neck into the axilla. The brachial plexus is formed by the union of the ventral rami of nerves C5-C8 and the greater part of the T1 ventral ramus. The ventral rami from C5 and C6 unite to form a **superior trunk,** the ventral ramus of C7 continues as the **middle trunk,** and the ventral rami of C8 and T1 unite to form an **inferior trunk.** Each of these trunks divides into an anterior and posterior division. The anterior divisions supply the anterior (flexor) parts of the upper limb, and the **posterior**

divisions supply the posterior (extensor) parts of the upper limb. These divisions form three cords (**posterior, lateral,** and **medial**) that continue to divide to form the **median, ulnar, musculocutaneous,** and **radial nerves** (sequential Figures 9.59 through 9.67 and 9.87 through 9.95). These nerves supply the muscles of the forearm and hand. The **median nerve** descends the cubital fossa deep to the median cubital vein. It supplies the pronator teres muscle of the arm and all the superficial and deep flexor muscles of the forearm, except the flexor carpi ulnaris muscle. It gives off an anterior interosseous branch that descends within the forearm to supply the flexor digitorum profundus muscle. The median nerve courses through the carpal tunnel of the wrist, typically superficial to the flexor tendons (Figure 9.147). It supplies flexors of the hand, skin of the wrist, thenar eminence, palm of the hand, and sides of the first three digits and lateral half of the fourth. At the elbow, the **ulnar nerve** passes between the medial epicondyle of the humerus and the olecranon process within the cubital tunnel to enter the medial side of the flexor compartment of the forearm (Figure 9.148). Posterior to the medial epicondyle, the ulnar nerve is superficial and easily palpable. It supplies the flexor carpi ulnaris muscle and the medial side of the flexor

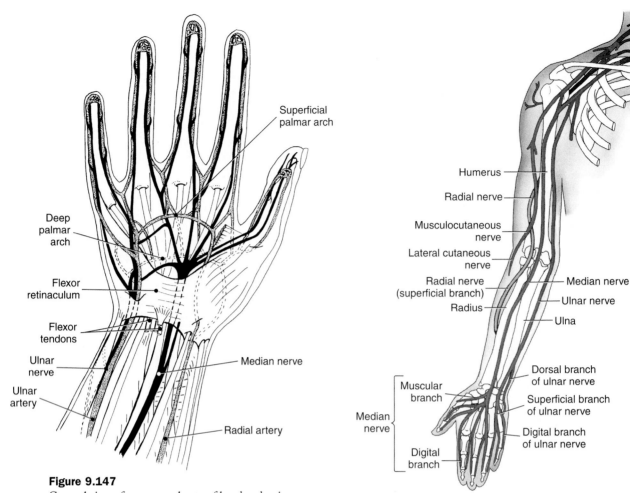

Figure 9.147
Coronal view of neurovasculature of hand and wrist.

Figure 9.148
Anterior view of the brachial plexus.

digitorum profundus muscle in the forearm before entering the hand. The ulnar nerve passes under the flexor retinaculum, along with the ulnar artery, to enter the palmar compartment of the hand (Figure 9.147). At this point, the ulnar nerve divides into superficial and deep terminal branches that supply the ulnar flexors of the hand as well as the skin on the medial side of the palm, medial half of the dorsum of the hand, fifth digit, and medial half of the fourth digit. The **musculo-cutaneous nerve** descends to the lateral side of the arm and elbow to innervate the flexors in the arm and the skin of the forearm, wrist, and thenar region of the hand (Figure 9.146). It emits branches that supply both heads of the biceps brachii muscle, the brachialis muscle, and the elbow joint. It innervates the skin of the dorsal surface of the arm. A continuation of the musculocutaneous nerve is the **lateral cutaneous nerve,** which terminates into cutaneous branches that supply the skin

covering the radial side of the wrist and the thenar eminence. The **radial nerve** is the largest branch of the brachial plexus. It passes inferolaterally around the body of the humerus in the radial groove (Figure 9.146). It continues inferiorly between the brachialis and brachioradialis muscles to the level of the lateral epicondyle of the humerus, where it divides into deep and superficial branches. The deep branches supply all the extensors in the arm and forearm, and the cutaneous branches innervate the skin on the dorsal side of the arm and hand. The superficial branch, the direct continuation of the radial nerve, is entirely sensory. It supplies skin and fascia over the lateral two thirds of the dorsum of the hand, the dorsum of the thumb, and proximal parts of the lateral three and one half digits on their dorsal surfaces (Figures 9.57 through 9.67, 9.87 through 9.98, and 9.146 and 9.147).

LOWER EXTREMITY

And well observe Hippocrates' old rule, the only medicine for the foote is rest.

THOMAS NASH (1567-1601)
Summers' Last Will and Testament

The complex anatomy of the lower extremity joints is responsible for bearing the entire upper body weight and for accommodating the demands of movement placed on this system (Figure 10.1).

HIP
    Bony Anatomy
    Labrum and Ligaments
    Articular Capsule of the Hip Joint
    Muscles of the Hip and Thigh

KNEE AND LOWER LEG
    Bony Anatomy
    Menisci and Ligaments
    Muscles of the Lower Leg

ANKLE AND FOOT
    Bony Anatomy
    Joints
    Fascia, Retinacula, and Ligaments
    Tendons
    Muscles

NEUROVASCULATURE
    Arteries
    Veins
    Nerves

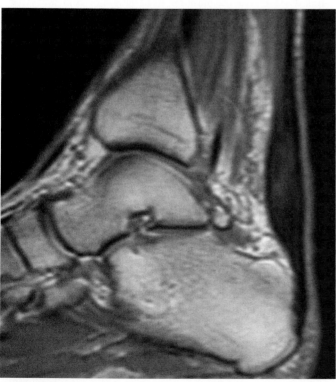

Figure 10.1
Sagittal, T2-weighted MR scan of ankle demonstrating thickening and edema in Achilles tendon.

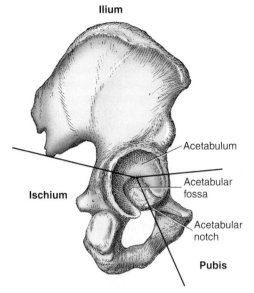

Figure 10.2
Lateral aspect of right hip bone showing its three parts.

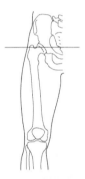

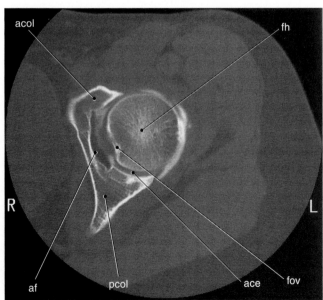

Figure 10.3
Axial CT scan of hip joint.

HIP

The hip provides strength to carry the weight of the body in an erect position. This synovial ball-and-socket joint, created by the articulation of the femoral head to the acetabulum of the pelvis, allows for a wide range of motion.

Bony Anatomy

A cuplike cavity termed the **acetabulum** is created by the three bones of the pelvis: **ilium, ischium,** and **pubis** (Figure 10.2). In axial cross section, this area can be divided into sections known as the **anterior** and **posterior columns** (Figure 10.3). Within the acetabulum is a centrally located, nonarticulating depression called the **acetabular fossa.** It is formed mainly by the ischium and is filled with fat (Figure 10.4). A continuation of the acetabular fossa is the **acetabular notch,** which interrupts the smooth circumference of the acetabular rim below and functions as an attachment site for the transverse acetabular ligament (Figure 10.2).

The **femur** is the longest, heaviest, and strongest bone in the body. The proximal end of the femur consists of a head, a neck, and two large processes: the greater and lesser trochanters (Figures 10.5 and 10.6). On the proximal portion of the femur is the smooth, rounded femoral head. The **femoral head** is covered entirely by articular cartilage, with the exception of a small centrally located pit termed the **fovea capitis.** The fovea capitis is an attachment site for the **ligament of the head of the femur,** also called the **ligamentum teres,** which transmits blood vessels to the femoral head (Figures 10.5 and 10.6). Attaching the head of the femur to the femoral shaft is the **femoral neck.** The neck extends obliquely from the head at an angle of approximately 120 degrees in an inferolateral direction to meet the shaft (Figure 10.5). The result of this angle is increased freedom of movement within the hip joint. At the distal end of the neck are two large bony prominences termed *trochanters* (Figures 10.5 through 10.8). The **greater trochanter** is situated at the junction of the neck with the shaft. The superior portion of the greater trochanter projects above the neck and curves slightly posteriorly and medially (Figures 10.9 and 10.10). The greater trochanter provides attachment for several muscles of the gluteal region. The **lesser trochanter** is at the posteromedial portion of the proximal shaft and gives insertion to the tendon of the psoas major (Figures 10.9 and 10.10). The prominent ridge extending posteriorly between the trochanters at the base of the neck is the **intertrochanteric crest** (Figures 10.9 and 10.11). It provides an attachment site for the ischiofemoral ligament and part of the quadratus femoris tendon. Connecting the trochanters anteriorly is the less prominent ridge termed the **intertrochanteric line,** which provides attachment for the iliofemoral ligament and part of the vastus lateralis tendon (Figures 10.9 and 10.11). On the proximal and posterior end of the femoral shaft is a raised ridge termed the **linea aspera.** Its medial and lateral lips provide attachment sites for muscles of the posterior and

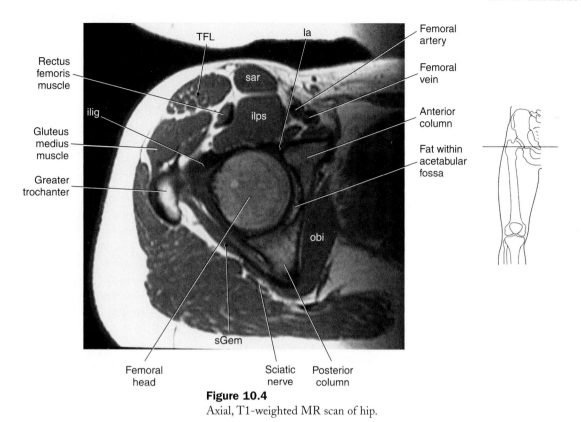

Figure 10.4
Axial, T1-weighted MR scan of hip.

medial compartments of the thigh. The **pectineal line** runs from the medial lip of the linea aspera to the lesser trochanter of the femur (Figures 10.9 and 10.11). It is the insertion site for the tendon of the pectineus muscle. The lateral lip is very rough and runs almost vertically upward to the base of the greater trochanter. The widened portion of the lateral lip, the **gluteal tuberosity,** is an attachment site for the gluteus maximus and adductor magnus muscles (Figures 10.9 and 10.11). The linea aspera extends down to the popliteal surface of the femur.

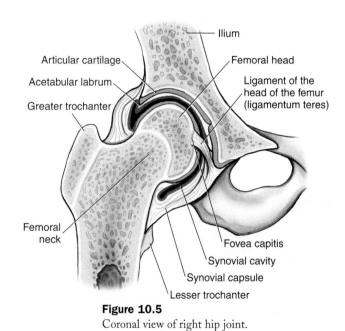

Figure 10.5
Coronal view of right hip joint.

> **Avascular necrosis (AVN) is a major concern following subcapital fractures of the femoral head. Disruption of the arterial supply to the femoral head is the most significant factor leading to AVN.**

KEY: acol, Anterior column; **fh,** femoral head; **fov,** fovea capitus; **ace,** acetabulum; **pcol,** posterior column; **af,** acetabular fossa; **ilig,** iliofemoral ligament; **TFL,** tensor fascia latae; **sar,** sartorius; **ilps,** iliopsoas; **la,** labrum; **obi,** obturator internus; **sGem,** superior gemellus.

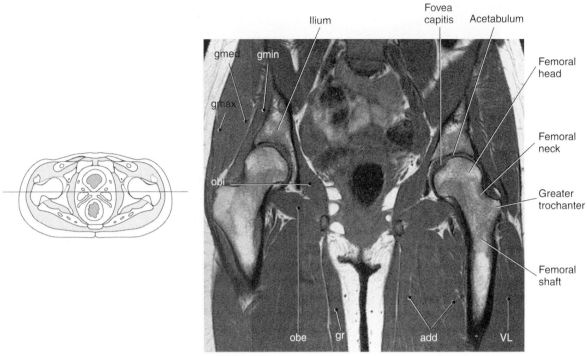

Figure 10.6
Coronal, T1-weighted MR scan of hips.

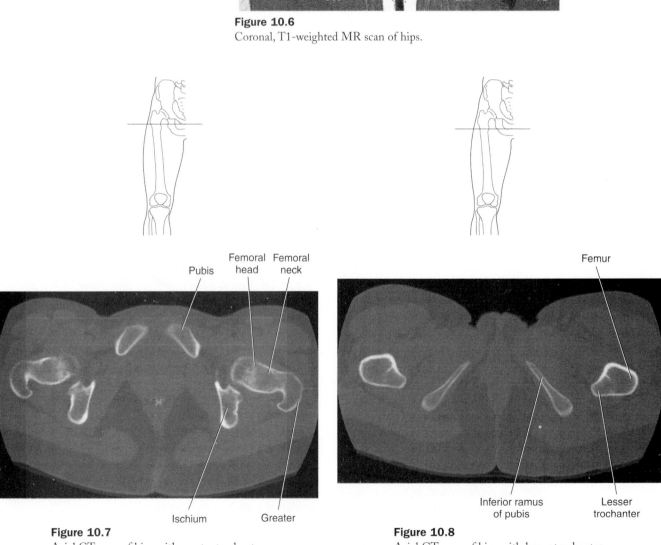

Figure 10.7
Axial CT scan of hips with greater trochanter.

Figure 10.8
Axial CT scan of hips with lesser trochanter.

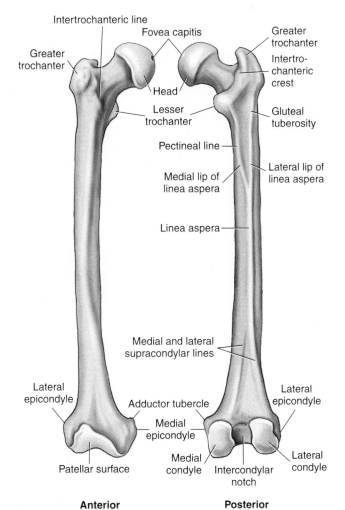

Figure 10.9

Right femur. *Left*, Anterior view. *Right*, Posterior view.

KEY: gmed, Gluteus medius; **gmin,** gluteus minimus; **gmax,** gluteus maximus; **obi,** obturator internus; **obe,** obturator externus; **gr,** gracilis; **add,** adductors; **VL,** vastus lateralis.

572

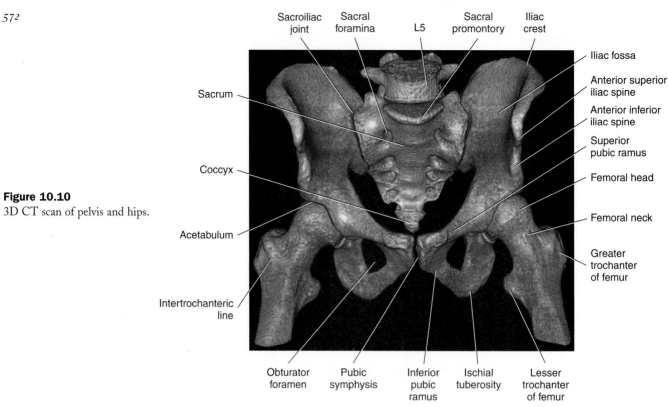

Sacroiliac joint — Sacral foramina — L5 — Sacral promontory — Iliac crest

Sacrum

Coccyx

Acetabulum

Intertrochanteric line

Iliac fossa
Anterior superior iliac spine
Anterior inferior iliac spine
Superior pubic ramus
Femoral head
Femoral neck
Greater trochanter of femur

Obturator foramen — Pubic symphysis — Inferior pubic ramus — Ischial tuberosity — Lesser trochanter of femur

Figure 10.10
3D CT scan of pelvis and hips.

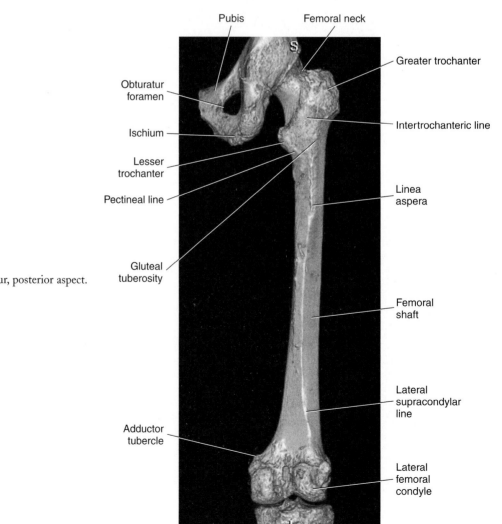

Pubis — Femoral neck

Obturatur foramen

Ischium

Lesser trochanter

Pectineal line

Gluteal tuberosity

Adductor tubercle

Greater trochanter

Intertrochanteric line

Linea aspera

Femoral shaft

Lateral supracondylar line

Lateral femoral condyle

Figure 10.11
3D CT scan of right femur, posterior aspect.

Labrum and Ligaments

The femoral head is held to the acetabulum by several major ligaments. The acetabular labrum, transverse acetabular ligament, iliofemoral ligament, ischiofemoral ligament, pubofemoral ligament, and ligamentum teres are demonstrated in Figures 10.12 through 10.20. The **acetabular labrum,** or **cotyloid ligament,** creates a fibrocartilaginous rim attached to the margin of the acetabulum. This labrum closely surrounds the femoral head, aiding to hold it in place by deepening the acetabular fossa, which adds increased stability to the joint (Figure 10.12). The inferior margin of the acetabulum is incomplete and is reinforced by the **transverse acetabular**

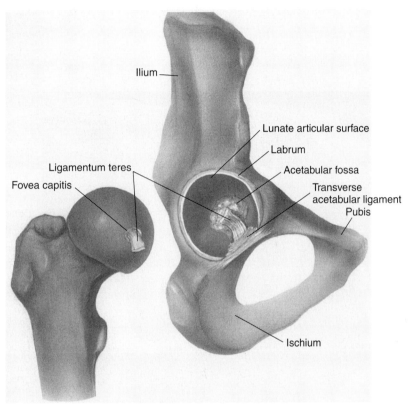

Figure 10.12
Femoral acetabulum and labrum.

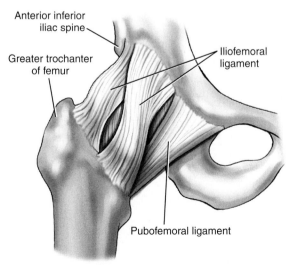

Figure 10.13
Anterior view of right hip joint capsule.

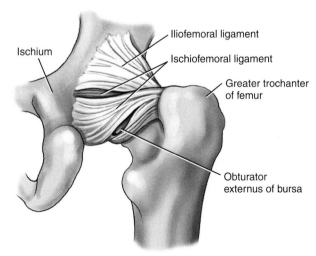

Figure 10.14
Posterior view of right hip joint capsule.

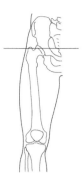

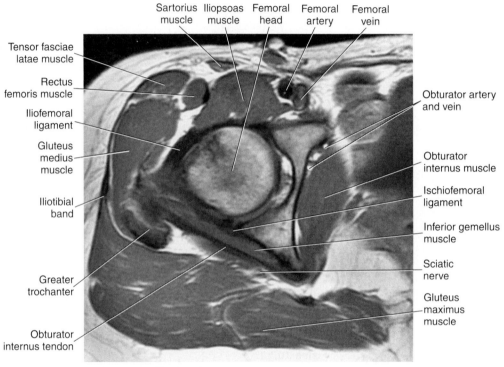

Sartorius muscle Iliopsoas muscle Femoral head Femoral artery Femoral vein

Tensor fasciae latae muscle

Rectus femoris muscle

Iliofemoral ligament

Gluteus medius muscle

Iliotibial band

Greater trochanter

Obturator internus tendon

Obturator artery and vein

Obturator internus muscle

Ischiofemoral ligament

Inferior gemellus muscle

Sciatic nerve

Gluteus maximus muscle

Figure 10.15
Axial, T1-weighted MR scan of hips with ligaments and labrum.

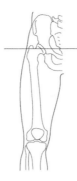

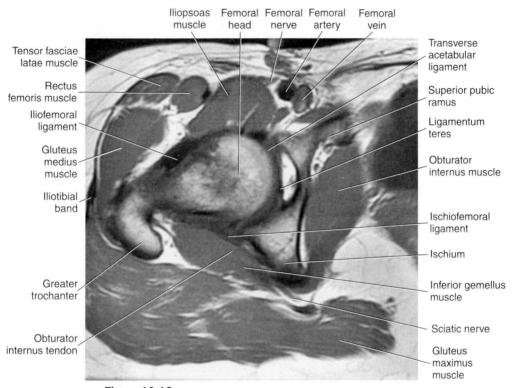

Figure 10.16
Axial, T1-weighted MR scan of hips with ligaments and labrum.

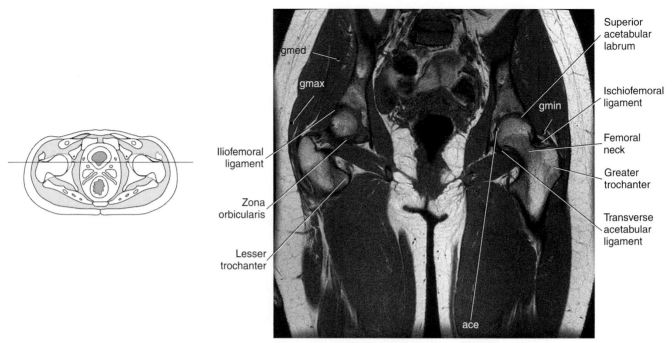

Figure 10.17
Coronal, T1-weighted MR scan of hips with ligaments and labrum.

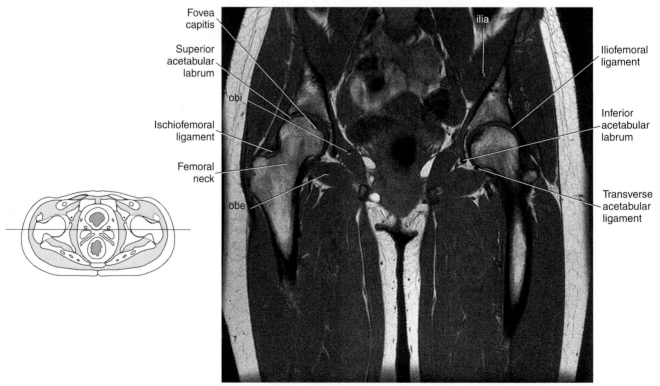

Figure 10.18
Coronal, T1-weighted MR scan of hips with ligaments and labrum.

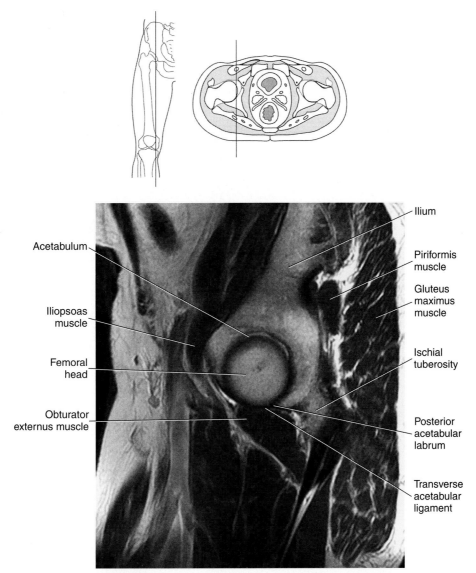

Figure 10.19
Sagittal, T1-weighted MR scan of hips with ligaments and labrum.

ligament, a portion of the acetabular labrum, which spans the acetabular notch on the inferior edge of the acetabulum (Figure 10.12). As the transverse ligament abridges the acetabular notch, it transforms it into the **acetabular foramen,** which allows nerves and blood vessels to pass to and from the hip joint through this foramen. The **iliofemoral ligament** is among the strongest of the body, with many stabilizing functions as it spans from the anterior inferior iliac spine and rim of the acetabulum to insert on the intertrochanteric line of the femur (Figures 10.13 and 10.14). A primary function of this ligament is to provide a thick reinforcement to the anterior part of the hip joint. The **ischiofemoral** and **pubofemoral**

KEY: gmed, Gluteus medius; **gmax,** gluteus maximus; **gmin,** gluteus minimus; **ace,** acetabulum; **obi,** obturator internus; **obe,** obturator externus; **ilia,** iliacus.

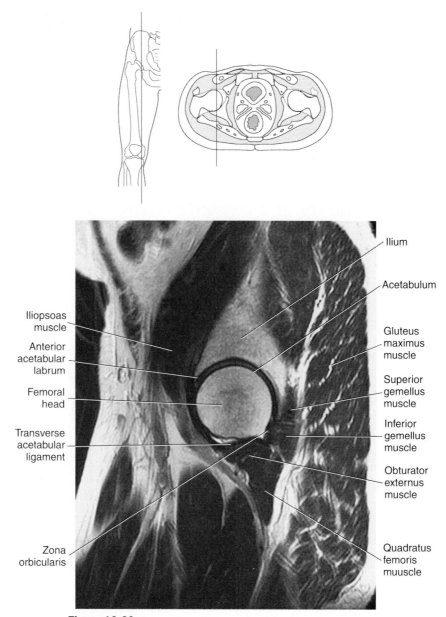

Figure 10.20
Sagittal, T1-weighted MR scan of hips with ligaments and labrum.

ligaments, though difficult to distinguish, present a spiral configuration of femoral attachment (Figures 10.13 and 10.14). The ischiofemoral ligament arises from the ischium and courses in a spiral above the femoral neck to insert on the posterior femoral neck, whereas the pubofemoral ligament arises from the superior pubic ramus to radiate and insert onto the iliofemoral ligament and intertrochanteric line. The spiral configuration of these two ligaments is unique to humans and ensures the stability and function while controlling the overall position of the lower limb. The **ligamentum teres** is a somewhat flattened band that extends from the fovea capitis of the femoral head to attach to the rim of the acetabular notch as well as blend with the transverse ligament (Figure 10.12). This ligament contains the artery to the head of the femur. The ligamentum teres has little influence as a ligament but can assist to prevent dislocation of the hip. Ligaments of the hip are identified in Figures 10.15 through 10.20.

TABLE 10-1   Muscles of the Gluteal Region

MUSCLE	PROXIMAL INSERTION	DISTAL INSERTION	ACTION
Gluteus maximus	Ilium, sacrum, coccyx	Gluteal tuberosity of greater trochanter	Extensor of the hip and maintains erect position of the body
Gluteus medius	Iliac crest	Greater trochanter	Abducts and medially rotates the thigh
Gluteus minimus	Gluteal surface of ilium	Greater trochanter	Abducts and medially rotates the thigh
Piriformis	Sacrum	Greater trochanter	Lateral rotation and abduction of the thigh
Obturator internus	Obturator foramen	Greater trochanter	Lateral rotation and abduction of the thigh
Obturator externus	Obturator foramen	Greater trochanter	Lateral rotation of the thigh
Superior gemellus	Ischial spine	Greater trochanter	Lateral rotation and abduction of the thigh
Inferior gemellus	Ischial tuberosity	Greater trochanter	Lateral rotation and abduction of the thigh
Quadratus femoris	Ischial tuberosity	Intertrochanteric crest	Lateral rotation of the thigh

Articular Capsule of the Hip Joint

The **fibrous capsule** of the hip is strong and dense. It forms a sleeve that encloses the hip joint and most of the neck of the femur. Proximally, it is attached to the edge of the acetabulum, just distal to the acetabular labrum, and to the transverse ligament. Distally, the fibrous capsule is attached to the neck of the femur anteriorly to the intertrochanteric line and the root of the greater trochanter, and posteriorly to the neck, just proximal to the intertrochanteric crest. The capsule consists of two sets of fibers: circular and longitudinal. The circular fibers are deep and form the **orbicular zone (zona orbicularis),** a sling or collar around the femoral neck that constricts the capsule and helps to hold the femoral head in the acetabulum. Extending upward from the femoral neck are the longitudinal fibers, termed **retinacula,** that are most abundant at the superoanterior portion of the capsule. The retinacula contain blood vessels that supply the head and neck of the femur. They are reinforced by distinct bands or accessory ligaments, including the iliofemoral, pubofemoral, and ischiofemoral ligaments (Figures 10.13 through 10.20).

The **synovial capsule** of the hip joint lines the internal surface of the fibrous capsule. The synovial capsule forms a sleeve for the ligamentum teres, lines the acetabular fossa, and covers the fatty pad in the acetabular notch (Figure 10.5). It is attached to the edges of the acetabular fossa and to the transverse acetabular ligament. The synovial capsule protrudes inferior to the fibrous capsule on the posterior aspect and forms the obturator externus bursa, which protects the tendon of the obturator externus muscle (Figure 10.14).

Muscles of the Hip and Thigh

A complex arrangement of muscles around the hip joint and thigh produces the movements of the hip. They are described in this section as gluteal muscles and muscles of the thigh and are illustrated in Figures 10.20 through 10.29 and Table 10.1. The muscles of the gluteal region and thigh muscles may be separated into compartments by thickened sheets of deep fascia called *fascial septa*, thus allowing muscles of the lower

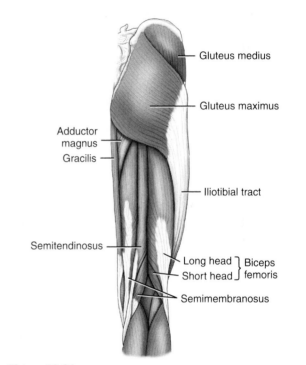

Figure 10.21
Posterior view of superficial muscles of the right hip and thigh.

extremity to be classified according to specific compartments in which they are located, such as gluteal, medial, and posterior compartments of the thigh.

MUSCLES OF THE GLUTEAL COMPARTMENT   The superficial gluteus muscles include the gluteus maximus, gluteus medius, and gluteus minimus. The **gluteus maximus muscle** is the largest and most superficial of the gluteal muscle group. It is very powerful, is situated on the posterior aspect of the hip joint, acts primarily as an extensor of the hip, and is responsible for maintaining the erect position. The gluteus maximus originates from the ilium, sacrum, and coccyx to insert just distal to the gluteal tuberosity of the greater trochanter (Figures 10.21 through 10.29). The **gluteus medius muscle** is

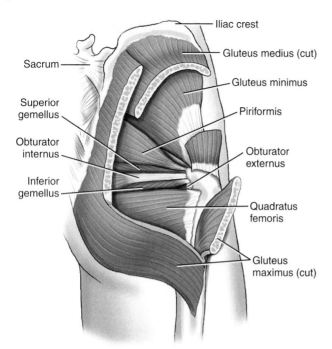

Figure 10.22
Posterior view of deep muscles of right hip and thigh.

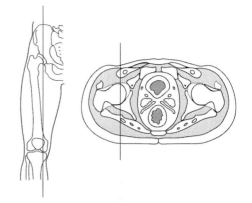

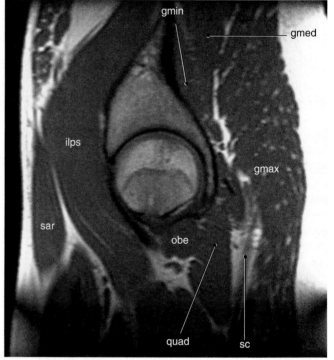

Figure 10.23
Sagittal, T1-weighted, MR scan of hip with muscles.

located on the lateral and upper part of the buttock. It originates from the iliac crest, just lateral to the gluteus maximus muscle, and is partially covered by the gluteus maximus along its medial one third. The gluteus medius is fan shaped as it spans from the iliac crest to insert on the superolateral aspect of the greater trochanter of the femur (Figures 10.22 through 10.29). The **gluteus minimus muscle** is the smallest of the gluteal muscles. It is triangular and completely covered by the gluteus medius. The upper attachment of the gluteus minimus is from the gluteal surface of the ilium, just inferior to that of the gluteus medius. Its tendon attaches to the anterosuperior aspect of the greater trochanter of the femur (Figures 10.22 through 10.29). The gluteus medius and minimus muscles act to abduct and medially rotate the thigh. The deep group of muscles, within the gluteal region, includes the piriformis, obturator internus, obturator externus, gemellus, and quadratus femoris, which are mainly lateral rotators of the thigh at the hip joint and act to stabilize the hip joint. The **piriformis muscle** originates from the inner surface of the sacrum between the sacral foramina. It passes laterally and anteriorly through the greater sciatic foramen to attach to the superior boundary of the greater trochanter of the femur (Figures 10.22, 10.25, and 10.28). The actions of the piriformis muscle include lateral rotation and abduction of the thigh. The **obturator internus muscle** is a thick fan-shaped muscle that like the piriformis muscle originates from the pelvis. It originates from the inner border of the obturator foramen then leaves the pelvis though the lesser sciatic foramen to reach its attachment to the greater trochanter of the femur (Figures 10.22, 10.26, and 10.29). Its primary actions are the same as those of the piriformis muscle:

KEY: gmin, Gluteus minimus; **gmed,** gluteus medius; **ilps,** iliopsoas; **gmax,** gluteus maximus; **sar,** sartorius; **obe,** obturator externus; **quad,** quadratus femoris; **sc,** sciatic nerve.

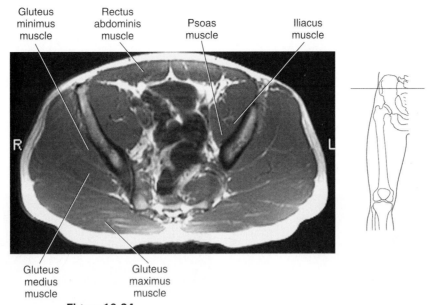

Gluteus minimus muscle
Rectus abdominis muscle
Psoas muscle
Iliacus muscle

R   L

Gluteus medius muscle
Gluteus maximus muscle

Figure 10.24
Axial, T1-weighted MR scan of gluteal region with psoas muscle.

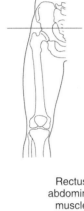

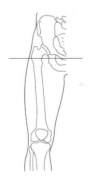

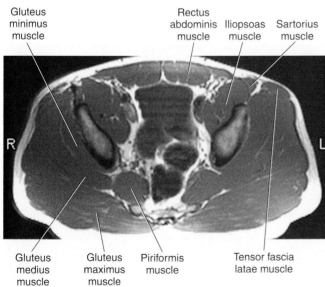

Gluteus minimus muscle
Rectus abdominis muscle
Iliopsoas muscle
Sartorius muscle

R   L

Gluteus medius muscle
Gluteus maximus muscle
Piriformis muscle
Tensor fascia latae muscle

Figure 10.25
Axial, T1-weighted MR scan of gluteal region with piriformis muscle.

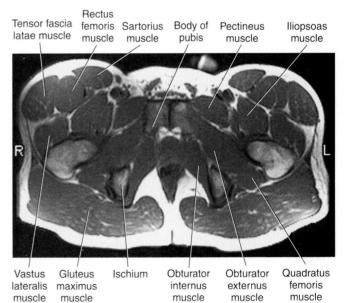

Tensor fascia latae muscle
Rectus femoris muscle
Sartorius muscle
Body of pubis
Pectineus muscle
Iliopsoas muscle

R   L

Vastus lateralis muscle
Gluteus maximus muscle
Ischium
Obturator internus muscle
Obturator externus muscle
Quadratus femoris muscle

Figure 10.26
Axial, T1-weighted MR scan of gluteal region with obturator muscles.

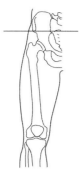

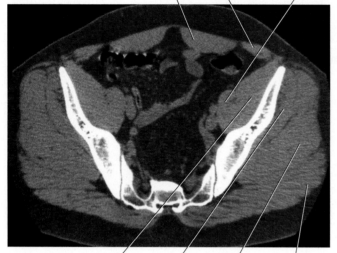

Rectus abdominus muscle   External oblique muscle   Psoas muscle

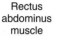

Iliacus muscle   Gluteus minimus muscle   Gluteus medius muscle   Gluteus maximus muscle

Figure 10.27
Axial CT scan of gluteal region with psoas muscle.

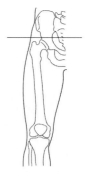

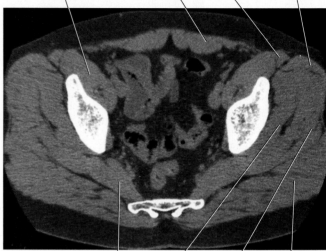

Iliopsoas muscle   Rectus abdominus muscle   Sartorius muscle   Tensor fascia latae muscle

Piriformis muscle   Gluteus minimus muscle   Gluteus medius muscle   Gluteus maximus muscle

Figure 10.28
Axial CT scan of gluteal region with piriformis muscle.

KEY: obe, Obturator externus; **obi,** obturator internus; **gmax,** gluteus maximus; **rec,** rectum; **lev,** levator ani.

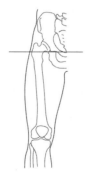

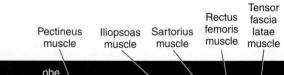

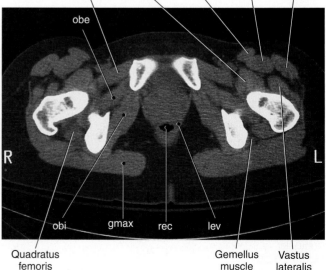

Pectineus muscle   Iliopsoas muscle   Sartorius muscle   Rectus femoris muscle   Tensor fascia latae muscle

obe

R   L

obi   gmax   rec   lev

Quadratus femoris muscle   Gemellus muscle   Vastus lateralis muscle

Figure 10.29
Axial CT scan of gluteal region with obturator muscles.

lateral rotation and abduction of the thigh. The **obturator externus muscle** arises from the outer border of the obturator foramen in the pelvis to essentially mirror the obturator internus muscle. It courses laterally around the posterior side of the neck of the femur to insert into the medial side of the greater trochanter and acts to laterally rotate the thigh (Figures 10.6, 10.22, 10.26, and 10.29). The two **gemellus muscles** (superior and inferior) are located along the superior and inferior boundaries of the obturator internus muscle and tendon (Figures 10.6 and 10.22). The **superior gemellus muscle** arises from the ischial spine, whereas the **inferior gemellus muscle** arises from the ischial tuberosity. Both muscles join with the tendon of the obturator internus muscle to insert into the medial surface of the greater trochanter (Figures 10.6, 10.22, and 10.29). The gemellus muscles also act to laterally rotate and abduct the thigh. The rectangular-shaped **quadratus femoris muscle** is located inferior to the obturator internus and gemellus muscles. It arises from the lateral border of the ischial tuberosity then courses laterally to insert on the intertrochanteric crest of the femur. The primary action of the quadratus femoris muscle is lateral rotation of the thigh (Figures 10.22, 10.23, 10.26, and 10.29). The muscles

of the gluteal compartment are identified in Figures 10.21 through 10.29 and their functions are given in Table 10.1.

MUSCLES OF THE ANTERIOR THIGH COMPARTMENT
The muscles in the anterior compartment of the thigh act both to flex the hip joint and extend the knee joint. They include the iliopsoas muscle of the pelvis and the sartorius, quadriceps femoris, and tensor fasciae latae of the leg. These muscles are demonstrated in Figures 10.30 through 10.45 and described in Table 10.2. The powerful **iliopsoas muscle** is composed of the psoas major and iliacus muscles (Figures 10.27, 10.28, and 10.30). The **psoas major muscle** arises from the transverse processes of the lumbar vertebrae and courses inferiorly within the pelvis. It exits the pelvis as it courses under the inguinal ligament to enter the anterior compartment of the thigh. The tendon of the psoas major joins with the tendon of the iliacus muscle to pass anterior to the hip joint capsule and attach to the lesser trochanter of the femur. The **iliacus muscle** arises from the iliac fossa and courses along the lateral side of the psoas major muscle in the pelvis. These muscles act conjointly in flexing the thigh at the hip and stabilizing the hip joint. The **sartorius muscle** is known as the longest muscle in the body; it extends from the anterior superior iliac spine to the medial

TABLE 10-2   Muscles of the Thigh

MUSCLE	PROXIMAL INSERTION	DISTAL INSERTION	ACTION
Anterior Thigh			
Psoas major	Transverse processes of lumbar vertebrae	Lesser trochanter	Flexes the thigh at hip and stabilizes the hip joint
Iliacus	Iliac fossa	Lesser trochanter	Flexes the thigh at hip and stabilizes the hip joint
Sartorius	Anterior superior iliac spine	Medial surface of tibia	Flexes, abducts, and laterally rotates the thigh
Tensor fascia latae	Anterior superior iliac spine and iliac crest	Iliotibial tract	Abducts, medially rotates, and flexes the thigh and helps to maintain extension of the knee
Quadriceps femoris			
Rectus femoris	Anterior inferior iliac spine	Patellar ligament	Extends the leg at knee joint and flexes the hip joint
Vastus lateralis	Greater trochanter and lateral lip of linea aspera	Patellar ligament	Extends leg at knee joint
Vastus medialis	Intertrochanteric line and medial lip of linea aspera	Patellar ligament	Extends leg at knee joint
Vastus intermedius	Anterior and lateral surfaces femoral body	Patellar ligament	Extends leg at knee joint
Medial Thigh			
Gracilis	Inferior pubic ramus	Anterior surface of tibia	Adducts thigh, flexes leg, and rotates thigh medially
Pectineus	Pectineal line of pubis	Medial lip of linea aspera	Adducts and flex the thigh
Adductor longus	Pubic bone	Middle third of linea aspera	Adducts the thigh
Adductor brevis	Pubic bone	Superior linea aspera	Adducts the thigh
Adductor magnus	Pubic bone	Linea aspera and adductor tubercle of medial condyle of knee	Adducts the thigh
Posterior Thigh			
Hamstrings			
Semitendinosus	Ischial tuberosity	Anterior tibia, medial side	Extend the thigh, flex and medially rotate the leg, and extend the trunk when hip and knee are flexed
Semimembranosus	Ischial tuberosity	Medial condyle of tibia, posterior aspect	Extend the thigh, flex and medially rotate the leg, and extend the trunk when hip and knee are flexed
Biceps femoris		Lateral surface of fibular head	Flex the leg at the knee and laterally rotate the leg when hip is flexed
Long head	Ischial tuberosity		
Short head	Lateral lip of linea aspera		

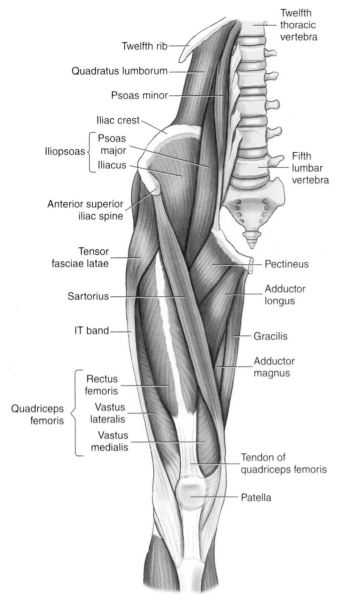

Figure 10.30
Anterior view of superficial muscles of right hip and thigh. *IT band,*
Iliotibial band.

trochanter and lateral lip of the linea aspera of the femur, the vastus medialis from the intertrochanteric line and medial lip of the linea aspera of the femur, and the vastus intermedius from the anterior and lateral surfaces of the body of the femur. All the parts of the quadriceps femoris act to extend the leg at the knee joint and through the actions of the rectus femoris, flex the hip joint. The **tensor fascia latae muscle** lies on the lateral side of the thigh, enclosed between two layers of the fascia. It is a short, thick, teardrop-shaped muscle located on the outer front corner of the ilium. As its name implies, it tightens the lateral fascia, thereby enabling the thigh muscles to act with increased power. It abducts, medially rotates, and flexes the thigh and helps to keep the knee extended. It originates from the anterior superior iliac spine and anterior part of the iliac crest and ends where the muscle inserts in the iliotibial tract (Figures 10.25, 10.26, 10.28, 10.29, and 10.30 through 10.42). The iliotibial tract, also called the *iliotibial band* or *IT band,* is a long, wide band of fascia that lies over the muscles on the outer surface of the thigh. This band is a thickening of the normal fascia that surrounds the entire leg. It arises from tendinous fibers of the tensor fascia latae and the gluteus maximus muscles. Acting almost like a ligament, this tendon helps mainly to stabilize the knee joint but also acts in flexing and extending the knee. It extends downward to insert on the lateral condyle of the tibia (Figures 10.30 through 10.42).

The muscles of the anterior thigh compartment are identified in Figures 10.30 through 10.45, and their functions are given in Table 10.2.

MUSCLES OF THE MEDIAL THIGH COMPARTMENT
Adduction is the primary action of the medial thigh muscles. These muscles include the gracilis, pectineus, adductor longus, adductor brevis, and adductor magnus muscles, which are demonstrated in Figures 10.30 through 10.47 and described in Table 10.2. The long straplike **gracilis muscle** lies along the medial side of the thigh and knee. The gracilis muscle extends from the inferior ramus of the pubis and is the only medial thigh group to cross the knee joint as it inserts onto the anterior surface of the tibia just inferior to the medial condyle. In addition to adducting the thigh, the gracilis muscle acts to flex the leg and helps to rotate the thigh medially. Arising from the pectineal line of the pubis is the short, flat **pectineus muscle.** It lies medial to the psoas major muscle in the superior thigh, then narrows as it courses inferiorly to insert on the medial lip of the linea aspera, at the pectineal line, distal to the lesser trochanter of the femur (Figures 10.29 and 10.30). It acts to adduct and flex the thigh. The adductor muscle group, as named, acts to adduct the thigh and is composed of three muscles, the **adductor longus, adductor brevis,** and **adductor magnus** (Figures 10.30 through 10.45 and 10.47). These muscles originate at the pubic bone and fan out to insert along the length of the medial aspect of the femur. The adductor longus muscle is the most anterior muscle in the adductor group and attaches to the middle third of the linea aspera of the femur. The shorter adductor brevis muscle lies deep to the pectineus and adductor longus muscles. Its distal attachment is

surface of the tibia near the tuberosity (Figures 10.30 through 10.45). It acts to flex, abduct, and laterally rotate the thigh. The biggest muscle in the body is the **quadriceps femoris muscle,** which covers almost all of the anterior surface and sides of the femur. It originates as four heads (**rectus femoris, vastus lateralis, vastus medialis,** and **vastus intermedius**) to create a powerful extensor of the knee (Figures 10.30 through 10.46). The superior ends of the four heads of the quadriceps femoris muscle arise from different locations, but their inferior tendons merge to form the **quadriceps ligament** that courses over the patella and continues as the **patellar ligament** in the knee (Figure 10.30). The rectus femoris originates from the anterior inferior iliac spine, the vastus lateralis from the greater

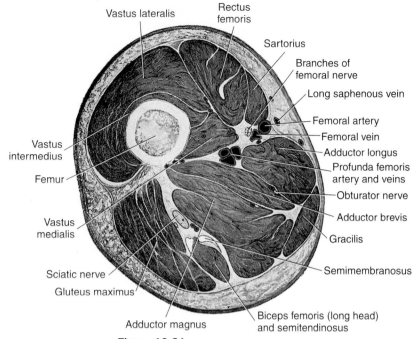

Figure 10.31

Axial view of femur, proximal one third.

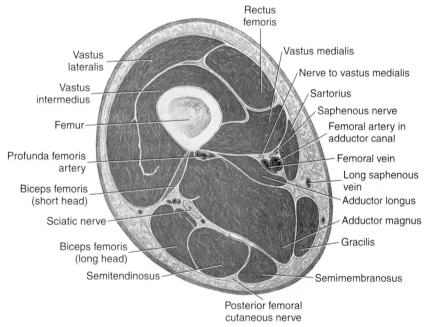

Figure 10.32

Axial view of femur, midthigh.

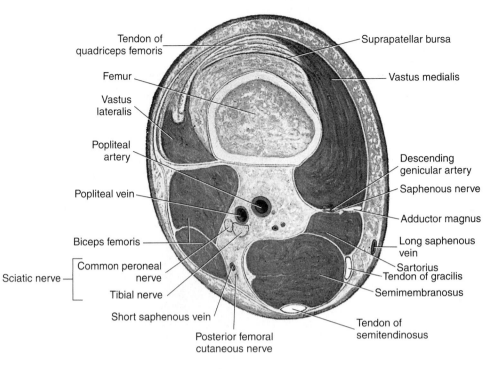

Tendon of quadriceps femoris

Suprapatellar bursa

Femur

Vastus medialis

Vastus lateralis

Popliteal artery

Descending genicular artery

Popliteal vein

Saphenous nerve

Adductor magnus

Biceps femoris

Long saphenous vein

Sartorius

Tendon of gracilis

Semimembranosus

Sciatic nerve — Common peroneal nerve

Tibial nerve

Short saphenous vein

Posterior femoral cutaneous nerve

Tendon of semitendinosus

Figure 10.33
Axial view of femur, distal one third.

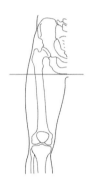

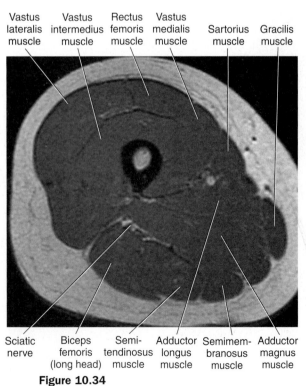

Vastus lateralis muscle

Vastus intermedius muscle

Rectus femoris muscle

Vastus medialis muscle

Sartorius muscle

Gracilis muscle

Sciatic nerve

Biceps femoris (long head)

Semi-tendinosus muscle

Adductor longus muscle

Semimem-branosus muscle

Adductor magnus muscle

Figure 10.34
Axial, T1-weighted MR scan of proximal femur.

Vastus lateralis muscle

Vastus intermedius muscle

Rectus femoris muscle

Biceps femoris (short head)

Vastus medialis muscle

Biceps femoris (long head)

Semi-tendinosus muscle

Semimem-branosus muscle

Adductor magnus muscle

Sartorius muscle

Gracilis muscle

Figure 10.35
Axial, T1-weighted MR scan of mid femur.

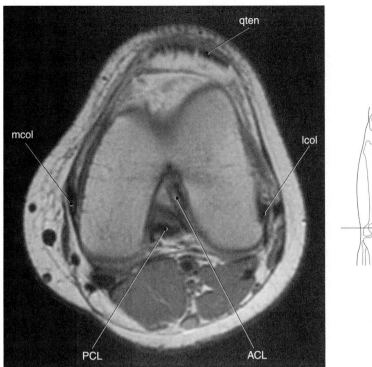

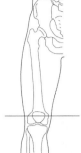

KEY: mcol, Medial collateral ligament; **qten,** quadriceps tendon; **lcol,** lateral collateral ligament; **ACL,** anterior cruciate ligament; **PCL,** posterior cruciate ligament.

Figure 10.36
Axial, T1-weighted MR scan of distal femur.

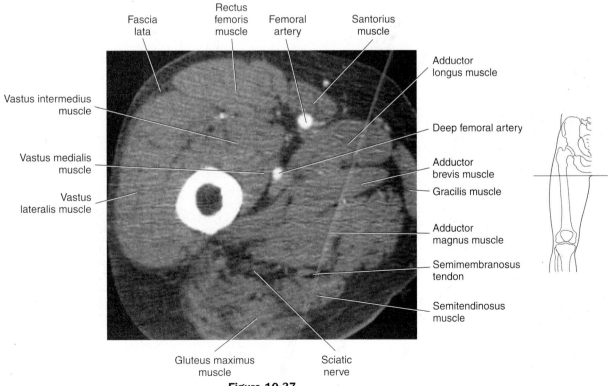

Figure 10.37
Axial CT scan of proximal femur.

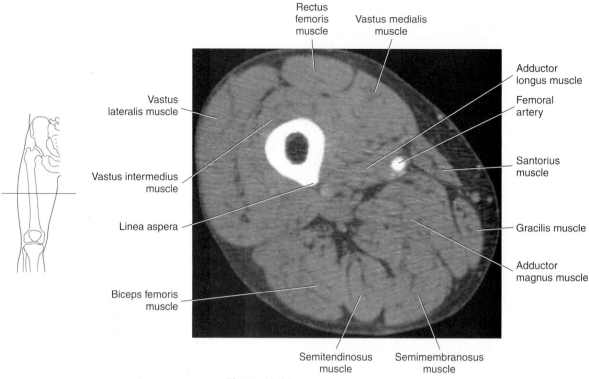

Rectus femoris muscle

Vastus medialis muscle

Vastus lateralis muscle

Vastus intermedius muscle

Linea aspera

Biceps femoris muscle

Adductor longus muscle

Femoral artery

Santorius muscle

Gracilis muscle

Adductor magnus muscle

Semitendinosus muscle

Semimembranosus muscle

Figure 10.38
Axial CT scan of mid femur.

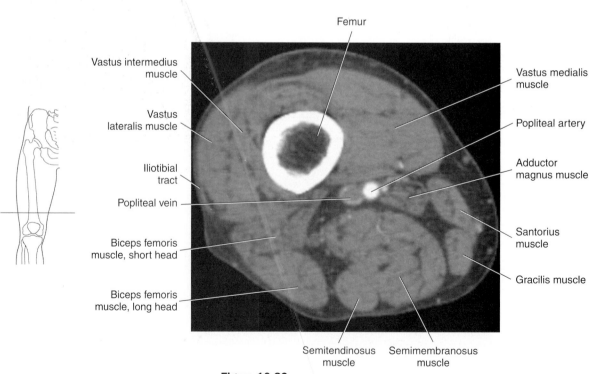

Femur

Vastus intermedius muscle

Vastus lateralis muscle

Iliotibial tract

Popliteal vein

Biceps femoris muscle, short head

Biceps femoris muscle, long head

Vastus medialis muscle

Popliteal artery

Adductor magnus muscle

Santorius muscle

Gracilis muscle

Semitendinosus muscle

Semimembranosus muscle

Figure 10.39
Axial CT scan of distal femur.

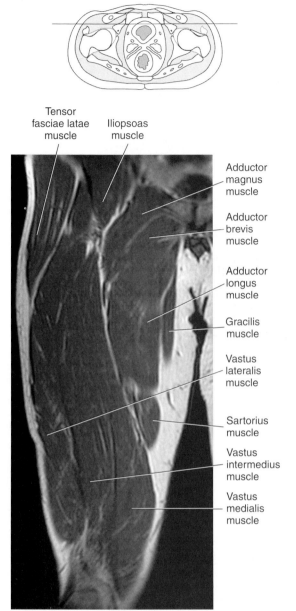

Tensor fasciae latae muscle

Iliopsoas muscle

Adductor magnus muscle

Adductor brevis muscle

Adductor longus muscle

Gracilis muscle

Vastus lateralis muscle

Sartorius muscle

Vastus intermedius muscle

Vastus medialis muscle

Figure 10.40
Coronal, T1-weighted MR scan of hip and thigh muscles.

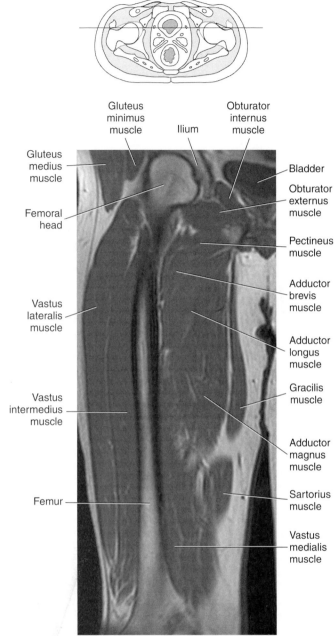

Gluteus minimus muscle

Ilium

Obturator internus muscle

Gluteus medius muscle

Femoral head

Bladder

Obturator externus muscle

Pectineus muscle

Vastus lateralis muscle

Adductor brevis muscle

Adductor longus muscle

Gracilis muscle

Vastus intermedius muscle

Adductor magnus muscle

Sartorius muscle

Femur

Vastus medialis muscle

Figure 10.41
Coronal, T1-weighted MR scan of hip and thigh muscles.

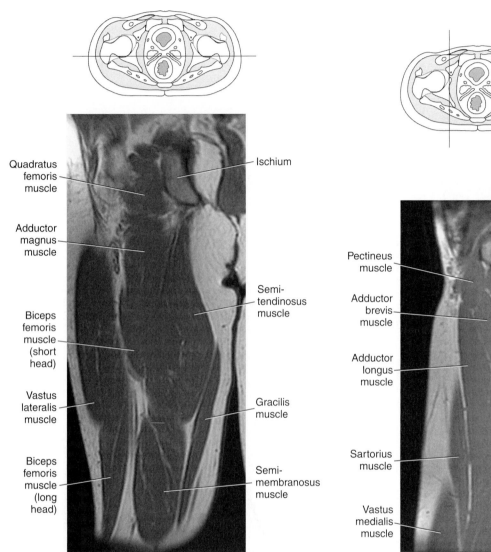

Quadratus femoris muscle

Adductor magnus muscle

Biceps femoris muscle (short head)

Vastus lateralis muscle

Biceps femoris muscle (long head)

Ischium

Semi-tendinosus muscle

Gracilis muscle

Semi-membranosus muscle

Figure 10.42
Coronal, T1-weighted MR scan of hip and thigh muscles.

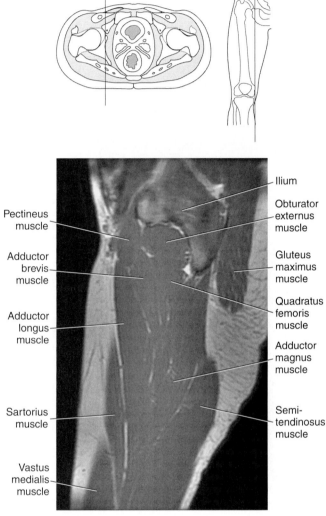

Pectineus muscle

Adductor brevis muscle

Adductor longus muscle

Sartorius muscle

Vastus medialis muscle

Ilium

Obturator externus muscle

Gluteus maximus muscle

Quadratus femoris muscle

Adductor magnus muscle

Semi-tendinosus muscle

Figure 10.43
Sagittal, T1-weighted MR scan of hip and thigh muscles.

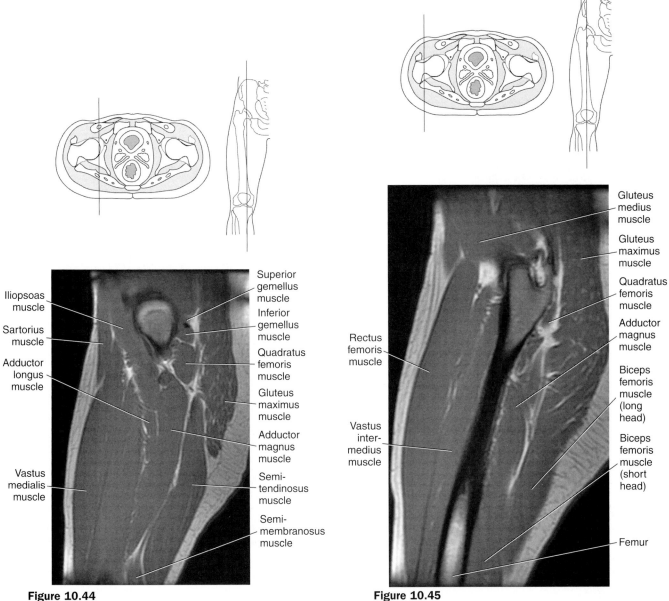

Figure 10.44
Sagittal, T1-weighted MR scan of hip and thigh muscles.

Figure 10.45
Sagittal, T1-weighted MR scan of hip and thigh muscles.

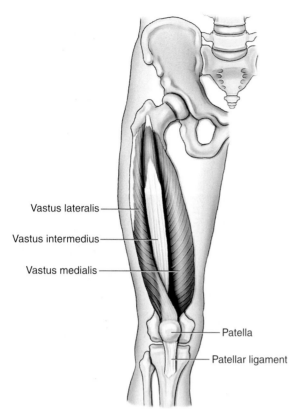

Figure 10.46
Anterior view of quadriceps muscle group.

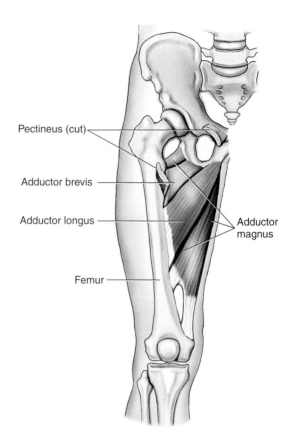

Figure 10.47
Anterior view of adductor muscle group.

between the lesser trochanter and superior end of the linea aspera of the femur. The largest and most medial of the adductor group is the adductor magnus. It is situated posterior to the adductor brevis and adductor longus and anterior to the semitendinosus and semimembranosus muscles. It forms a large triangular sheet of muscle in the thigh and is composed of two parts, an adductor part and a hamstring part. The adductor portion of the adductor magnus has an extensive distal attachment on the linea aspera of the femur, whereas the hamstring part attaches to adductor tubercle on top of the medial condyle of the femur. The muscles of the medial thigh compartment are identified in Figures 10.30 through 10.47, and their functions are given in Table 10.2.

MUSCLES OF THE POSTERIOR THIGH COMPARTMENT
The semitendinosus, semimembranosus, and biceps femoris are collectively known as the **hamstrings** (Figures 10.21 and 10.31 through 10.45). They make up the large mass of muscles that can be palpated on the posterior aspect of the thigh and are involved with extension of the hip, flexion of the knee, and rotation of the flexed knee. The **semitendinosus muscle**

extends from the ischial tuberosity, courses on the medial aspect of the femur, then continues inferiorly around the medial tibial condyle and attaches to the medial side of the anterior tibial surface (Figures 10.21 and 10.31 through 10.39). It, along with the **semimembranosus muscle,** acts to extend the thigh, flex and medially rotate the leg, and extend the trunk when the thigh and leg are flexed. The semimembranosus also originates from the ischial tuberosity but attaches to the posterior part of the medial condyle of the tibia (Figures 10.21 and 10.31 through 10.39). The **biceps femoris,** as named, has two heads (long and short). The long head extends from the ischial tuberosity, whereas the short head extends from the lateral lip of the linea aspera of the femur. The biceps femoris extends inferiorly over the lateral part of the posterior surface of the knee to insert on the lateral surface of the fibular head. It acts to flex the leg at the knee joint and laterally rotate the leg when the leg is flexed. The muscles of the posterior thigh compartment are identified in Figures 10.21 and 10.31 through 10.45, and their functions are given in Table 10.2.

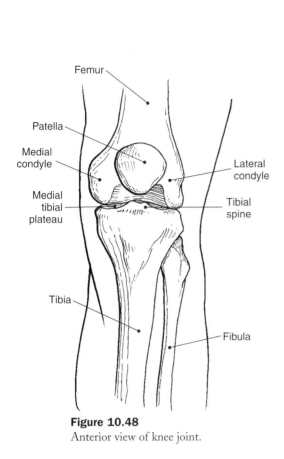

Figure 10.48
Anterior view of knee joint.

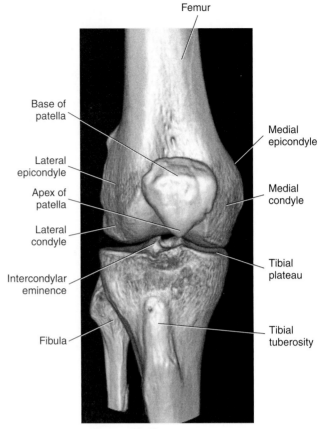

Figure 10.49
3D CT reformat of knee joint.

KNEE AND LOWER LEG

Bony Anatomy

The bones that contribute to the knee joint and lower leg are the femur, tibia, patella, and fibula (Figures 10.48 and 10.49). Cartilage covers the articular surfaces of the femur, tibia, and patella and helps to provide smooth movement within the knee joint.

DISTAL FEMUR   The distal portion of the femur broadens into two articular cartilage–covered projections called the *medial* and *lateral condyles* (Figures 10.50 through 10.54). The **lateral femoral condyle** is wider in front than in back, whereas the **medial femoral condyle** remains more consistent in width. The femoral condyles are connected anteriorly by the smooth **patellar surface** and separated posteriorly by the **intercondylar fossa** (Figure 10.51). On the side of each condyle is a raised edge called the **medial** and **lateral epicondyle** for the attachment of ligaments and muscles (Figures 10.52 and 10.53). A small projection located above the medial epicondyle is the **adductor tubercle,** which serves as an attachment for a portion of the adductor magnus muscle (Figures 10.9 and 10.11). On the posterior surface of the distal femur is a triangular area called the **popliteal surface.** The base of the triangle is located at the **intercondylar line,** which marks the beginning of the intercondylar fossa. The sides of the triangle are formed by the **medial** and **lateral supracondylar lines,** which are continuations of the linea aspera (Figures 10.9 and 10.11).

594

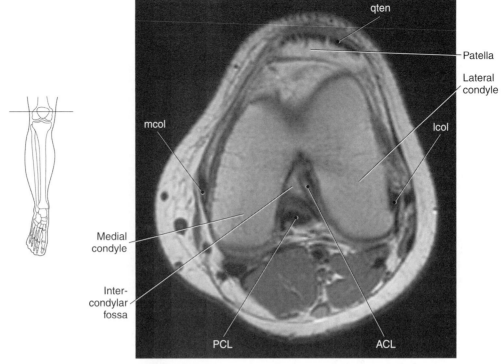

Figure 10.50
Axial, T1-weighted MR scan of distal femur.

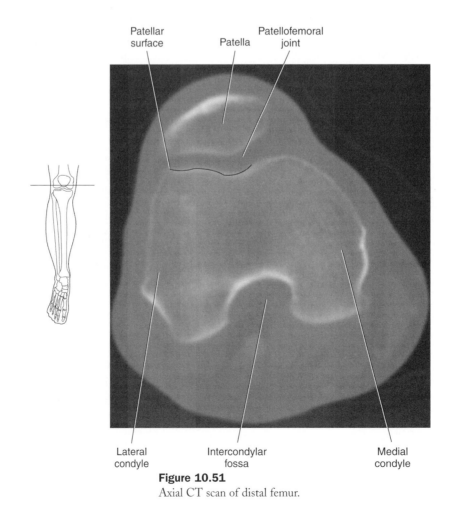

Figure 10.51
Axial CT scan of distal femur.

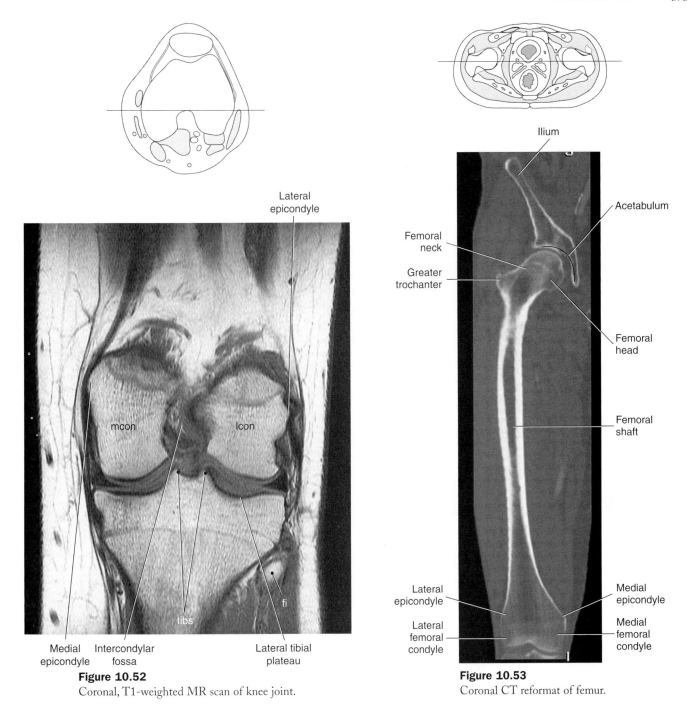

Lateral
epicondyle

mcon

lcon

fi

tibs

Medial   Intercondylar
epicondyle   fossa

Lateral tibial
plateau

Figure 10.52
Coronal, T1-weighted MR scan of knee joint.

Ilium

Acetabulum

Femoral
neck

Greater
trochanter

Femoral
head

Femoral
shaft

Lateral
epicondyle

Medial
epicondyle

Lateral
femoral
condyle

Medial
femoral
condyle

Figure 10.53
Coronal CT reformat of femur.

KEY: **mcol,** Medial collateral ligament; **qten,** quadriceps tendon; **lcol,** lateral collateral ligament; **ACL,** anterior cruciate ligament; **PCL,** posterior cruciate ligament; **mcon,** medial femoral condyle; **lcon,** lateral femoral condyle; **tibs,** tibial spine; **fi,** fibula.

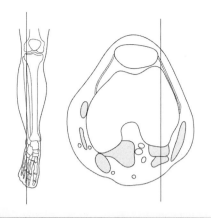

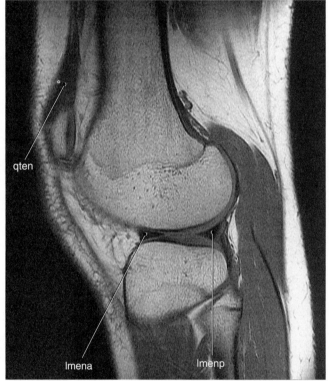

Figure 10.54
Sagittal MR scan of knee with meniscus and ligaments.

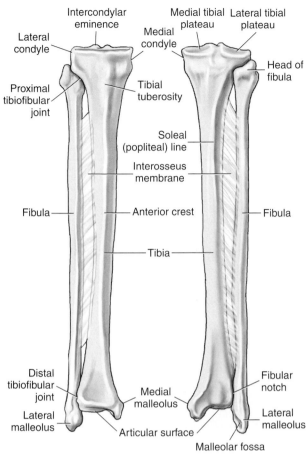

Figure 10.55

Tibia and fibula. *Left,* Anterior view. *Right,* Posterior view.

TIBIA   The **tibia,** also called the *shin bone,* has a widened proximal end that has two cartilaginous projections: the **medial and lateral condyles** (Figure 10.55). The superior articular surface of both condyles has a flattened surface called the **tibial plateaus** for articulation with the femoral condyles (Figures 10.55 through 10.57). The tibial condyles are separated by the **intercondylar eminence (tibial spine),** which ends in two peaks called the **medial** and **lateral intercondylar tubercles;** attachment sites for ligaments (Figures 10.48, 10.49, 10.52, and 10.55). The lateral tibial condyle has a small articular surface called the **articular fibular surface,** which articulates with the head of the fibula (Figures 10.58 and 10.59). The shaft of the tibia is triangular with a sharp anterior edge or crest that contains a bony projection called the **tibial tuberosity** for the attachment of the patellar ligament (Figures 10.60 and 10.61). The **medial margin** of the shaft lies directly beneath the skin and is devoid of muscle, and the **lateral surface** serves as the attachment site for the interosseous membrane. The **posterior surface** has an obliquely oriented bony ridge called the **soleal (popliteal) line,** which gives rise to tendon fibers of the soleus muscle (Figure 10.55). The distal tibia has a flattened articular end with a medial extension that forms the **medial malleolus** (Figures 10.55, 10.62, and 10.63). The posterior surface of the medial malleolus has a small indentation, the **malleolar groove,** for the passage of the tibialis posterior and flexor digitorum longus tendons. On the lateral side of the distal tibia is a shallow indentation called the **fibular notch,** which provides a fibrous attachment with the distal fibula (Figures 10.55 and 10.62).

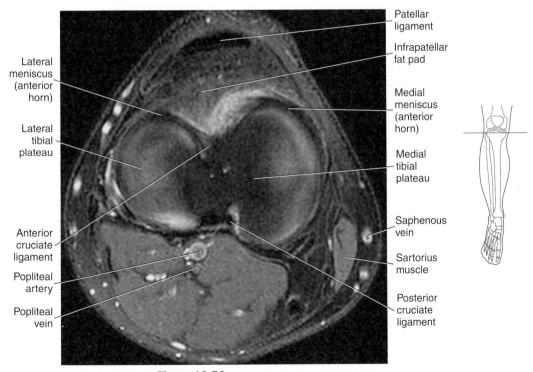

Figure 10.56

Axial, T1-weighted MR scan with tibial plateau.

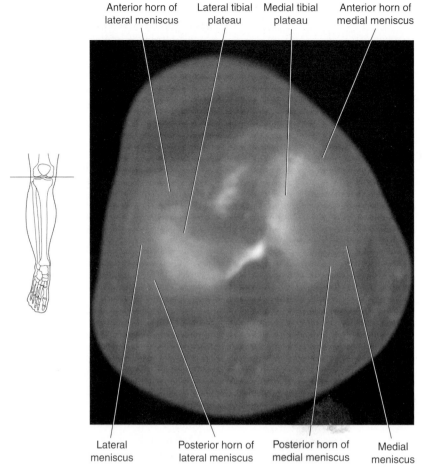

Anterior horn of
lateral meniscus

Lateral tibial
plateau

Medial tibial
plateau

Anterior horn of
medial meniscus

Lateral
meniscus

Posterior horn of
lateral meniscus

Posterior horn of
medial meniscus

Medial
meniscus

Figure 10.57
Axial CT scan with tibial plateau.

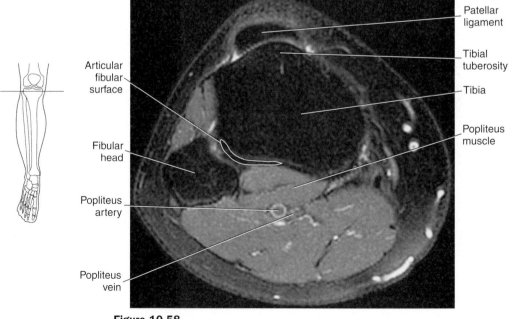

Articular
fibular
surface

Fibular
head

Popliteus
artery

Popliteus
vein

Patellar
ligament

Tibial
tuberosity

Tibia

Popliteus
muscle

Figure 10.58
Axial, T1-weighted MR scan with tibial/fibular articulation.

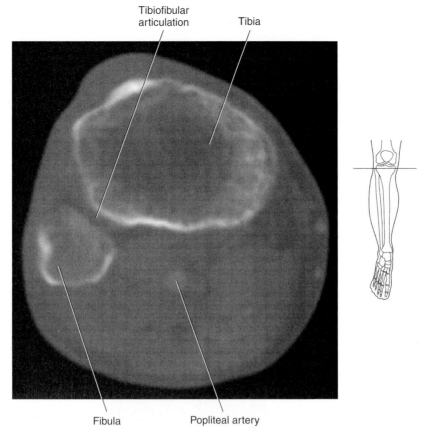

Tibiofibular
articulation

Tibia

Fibula

Popliteal artery

Figure 10.59
Axial CT scan with tibial/fibular articulation.

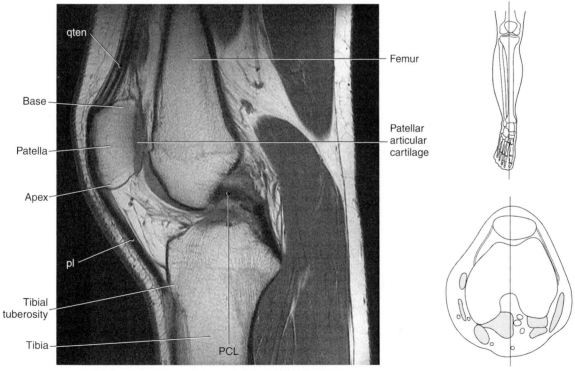

qten

Base

Patella

Apex

pl

Tibial
tuberosity

Tibia

Femur

Patellar
articular
cartilage

PCL

Figure 10.60
Midsagittal, T1-weighted MR scan of tibia.

KEY: **qten,** Quadriceps tendon; **pl,** patellar ligament; **PCL,** posterior cruciate ligament.

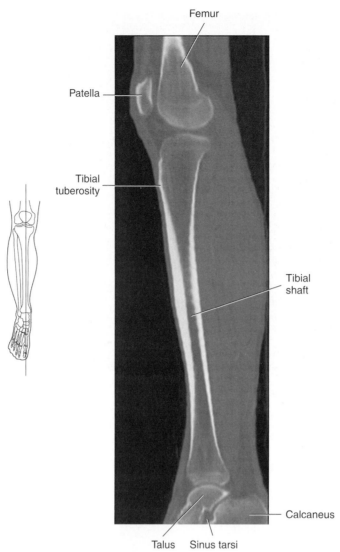

Femur

Patella

Tibial tuberosity

Tibial shaft

Calcaneus

Talus   Sinus tarsi

Figure 10.61
Midsagittal, CT reformat of tibia.

FIBULA   The **fibula** is a long, relatively thin bone that has expanded proximal and distal ends. It is covered by muscles of the lower leg almost along its entire length. The proximal end is the **head of the fibula,** which ends in a sharp superior **apex** and medially has an articular surface for articulation with the lateral condyle of the tibia (Figures 10.55, 10.58, and 10.59). The distal end forms the **lateral malleolus,** which extends farther distally than the medial malleolus of the tibia (Figures 10.62 and 10.63). The medial surface of the lateral malleolus has an **articular facet** that articulates with the talus. Posterior to the malleolar articular surface is a small cavity called the **malleolar fossa,** which is where the posterior talofibular ligament is anchored. On the lateral surface of the lateral malleolus is a groove **(malleolar groove)** for the passage of the peroneus longus and brevis tendons (Figures 10.55, 10.62, and 10.63).

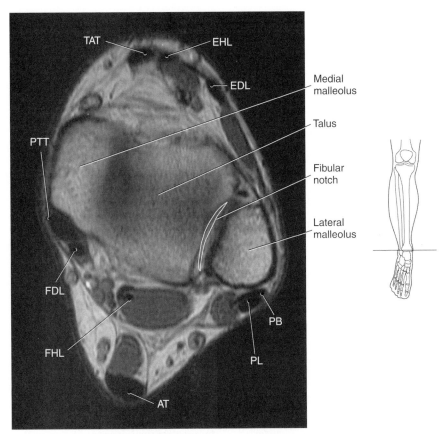

Figure 10.62
Axial, T1-weighted MR scan of ankle with malleoli.

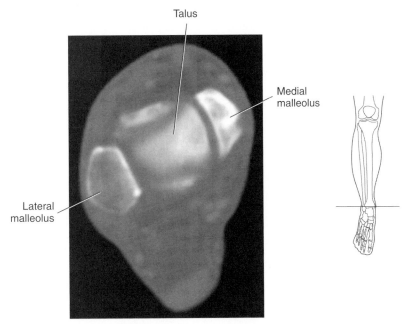

Figure 10.63
Axial CT scan of ankle with malleoli.

Anterior

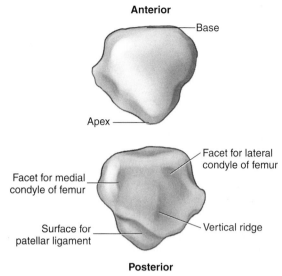

Figure 10.64
Patella. *Top,* Anterior view. *Bottom,* Posterior view.

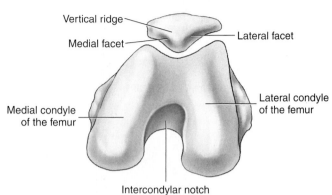

Figure 10.65
Patellofemoral joint with intercondylar notch of femur.

PATELLA AND PATELLOFEMORAL JOINT   The **patella** is the largest sesamoid bone in the body and is embedded within the quadriceps tendon. It is a subcutaneous, flat, triangular bone with the broad **base** facing proximally and the pointed **apex** facing distally (Figure 10.64). The patella has an **anterior** and **posterior surface** and three borders: **superior, medial, and lateral.** The base of the patella has roughened areas for the attachment of the rectus femoris and vastus intermedius muscles, whereas the roughened medial and lateral borders receive attachment for the vastus medialis and lateralis muscles. The posterior surface is covered with the thickest articular cartilage found in the body and is centrally divided by a broad **vertical ridge** into **medial** and **lateral facets.** The larger lateral facet articulates with the lateral femoral condyle and the smaller medial facet articulates with the medial femoral condyle (Figure 10.65). The patella protects the anterior joint surface of the knee and functions to increase the leverage of the quadriceps extensor system (Figures 10.50, 10.51, 10.60, and 10.61).

KNEE JOINT   The **knee** is the largest and one of the most complex joints of the body. The bones that contribute to the knee joint are the femur, tibia, and patella (Figures 10.48 and 10.49). The knee has three separate articulations: two **femorotibial** and a **patellofemoral articulation** within the same synovial membrane. A supporting network of menisci, ligaments, tendons, and muscles functions together in order to meet the demands made on the knee.

Menisci and Ligaments

MENISCI Located between the femoral condyles and tibial plateaus are the paired **menisci** (Figures 10.66 through 10.76). These C-shaped menisci, composed of fibrous connective tissue, cushion the articulation between the femoral condyles and tibial plateaus and are commonly divided into **anterior** and **posterior horns.** On cross section they appear wedge shaped, with a thickened outer margin that flattens medially (Figures 10.67 and 10.68). Their outer margins fuse with the joint capsule, and their anterior and posterior horns attach to the intercondylar eminence of the tibia. The menisci differ in size and shape. The **medial meniscus** is crescent shaped, with the posterior horn being wider than the anterior horn. The medial meniscus is attached to the medial collateral ligament, making it far less mobile than the lateral meniscus. The **lateral meniscus** almost forms a closed ring with anterior and posterior horns of approximately the same width. Two ligaments arise from the posterior horn of the lateral meniscus. The **posterior meniscofemoral ligament (ligament of Wrisberg)** passes behind the posterior cruciate ligament to attach to the medial femoral condyle. The **anterior meniscofemoral ligament (ligament of Humphry)** connects the posterior horn to the medial condyle, passing in front of the posterior cruciate ligament. The two menisci are connected anteriorly by the **transverse ligament** (Figures 10.66 and 10.67).

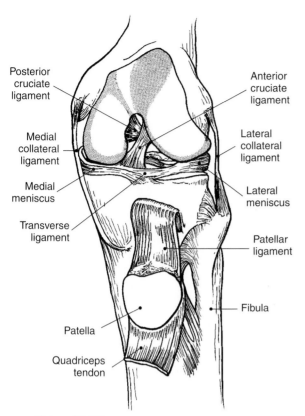

Figure 10.66
Anterior view of meniscus and ligaments of knee.

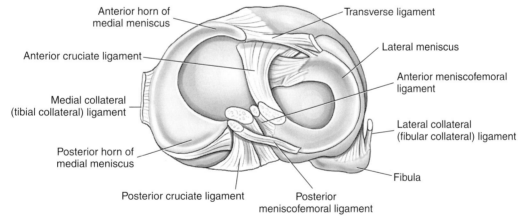

Figure 10.67
Superior view of right knee joint.

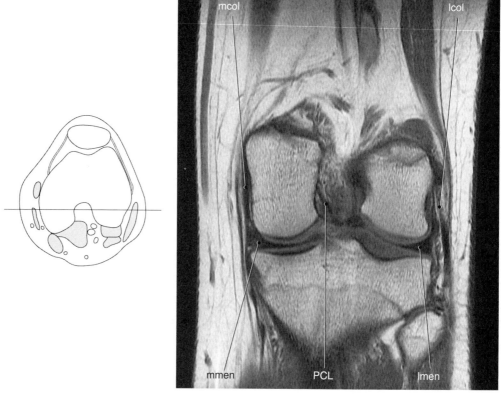

Figure 10.68
Coronal, T1-weighted MR scan of knee with meniscus and ligaments of knee.

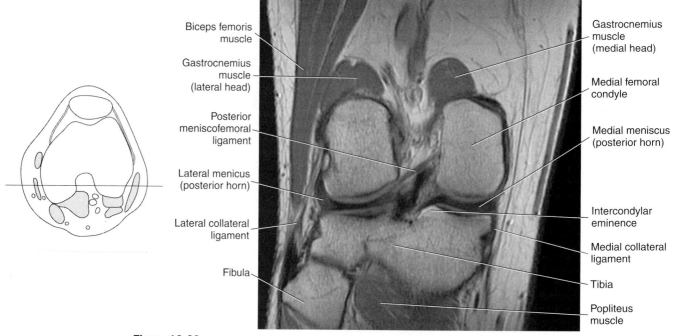

Figure 10.69
Coronal, T1-weighted MR scan of knee with posterior meniscal and arcuate ligaments.

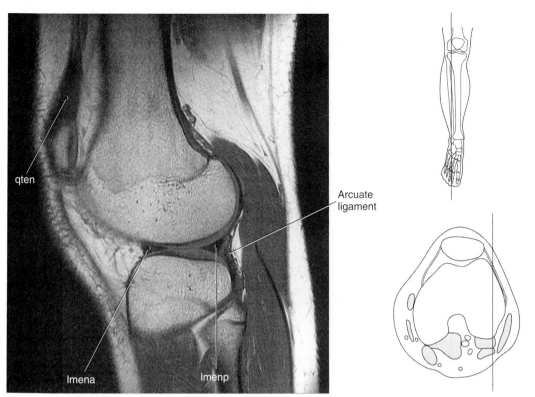

Figure 10.70
Sagittal, T1-weighted MR scan of knee with lateral meniscus and arcuate ligament.

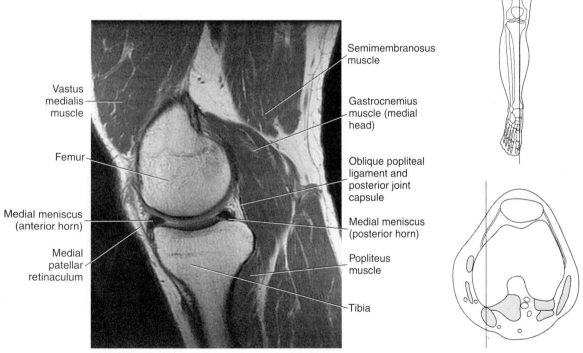

Figure 10.71
Sagittal, T1-weighted MR scan of knee with medial meniscus and retinaculum.

KEY: **mcol**, Medial collateral ligament; **lcol**, lateral collateral ligament; **lmen**, lateral meniscus; **PCL**, posterior cruciate ligament; **mmen**, medial meniscus; **qten**, quadriceps tendon; **lmena**, lateral meniscus, anterior horn; **lmenp**, lateral meniscus, posterior horn.

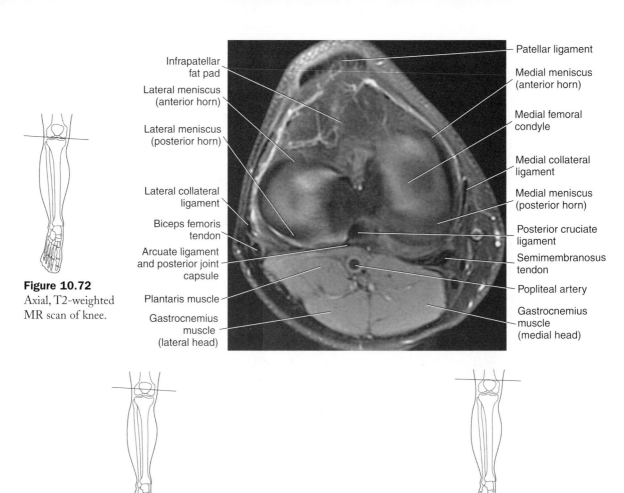

Figure 10.72
Axial, T2-weighted MR scan of knee.

Infrapatellar fat pad
Lateral meniscus (anterior horn)
Lateral meniscus (posterior horn)
Lateral collateral ligament
Biceps femoris tendon
Arcuate ligament and posterior joint capsule
Plantaris muscle
Gastrocnemius muscle (lateral head)

Patellar ligament
Medial meniscus (anterior horn)
Medial femoral condyle
Medial collateral ligament
Medial meniscus (posterior horn)
Posterior cruciate ligament
Semimembranosus tendon
Popliteal artery
Gastrocnemius muscle (medial head)

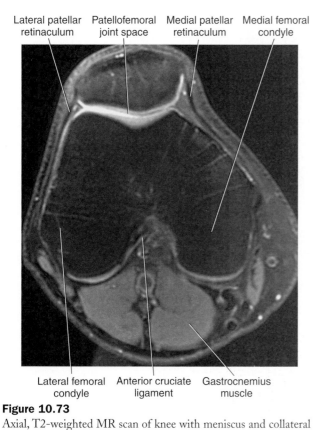

Lateral patellar retinaculum
Patellofemoral joint space
Medial patellar retinaculum
Medial femoral condyle

Lateral femoral condyle
Anterior cruciate ligament
Gastrocnemius muscle

Figure 10.73
Axial, T2-weighted MR scan of knee with meniscus and collateral ligaments.

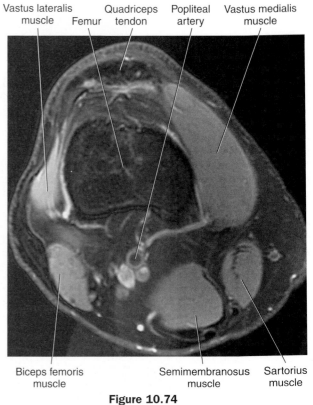

Vastus lateralis muscle
Femur
Quadriceps tendon
Popliteal artery
Vastus medialis muscle

Biceps femoris muscle
Semimembranosus muscle
Sartorius muscle

Figure 10.74
Axial, T2-weighted MR scan of knee.

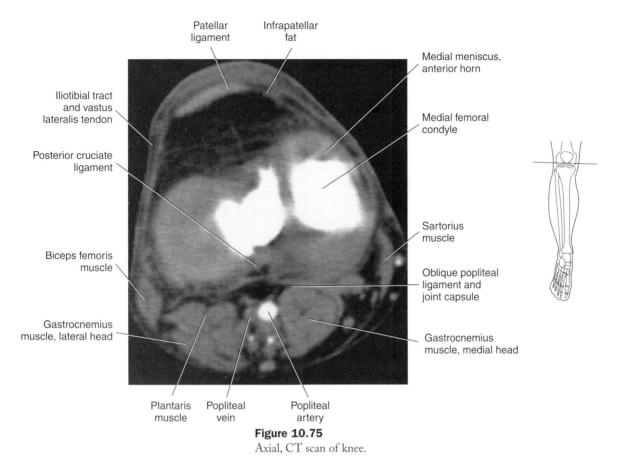

Patellar ligament

Infrapatellar fat

Medial meniscus, anterior horn

Medial femoral condyle

Iliotibial tract and vastus lateralis tendon

Posterior cruciate ligament

Biceps femoris muscle

Gastrocnemius muscle, lateral head

Sartorius muscle

Oblique popliteal ligament and joint capsule

Gastrocnemius muscle, medial head

Plantaris muscle

Popliteal vein

Popliteal artery

Figure 10.75
Axial, CT scan of knee.

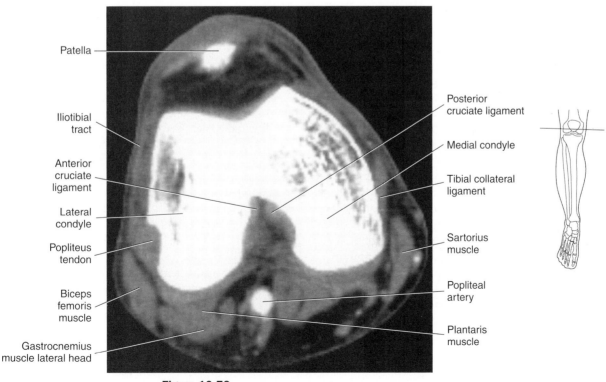

Patella

Iliotibial tract

Anterior cruciate ligament

Lateral condyle

Popliteus tendon

Biceps femoris muscle

Gastrocnemius muscle lateral head

Posterior cruciate ligament

Medial condyle

Tibial collateral ligament

Sartorius muscle

Popliteal artery

Plantaris muscle

Figure 10.76
Axial CT scan of knee with cruciate and collateral ligaments.

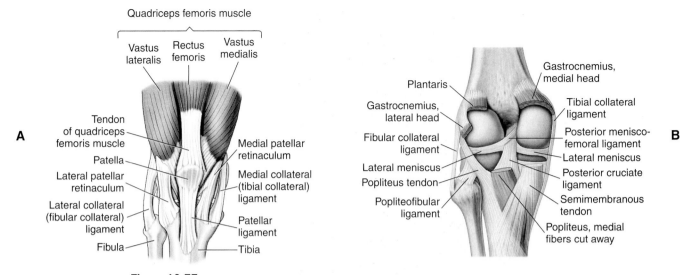

Figure 10.77

A, Anterior view of right knee with retinaculum and ligaments. **B,** Posterior view of right knee with joint capsule and ligaments.

LIGAMENTS The ligaments of the knee are divided into external (extracapsular) and internal (intracapsular) ligaments. The external ligaments are arranged around the knee and serve to strengthen and support the joint capsule. The internal ligaments are found within the joint capsule and serve to provide stability to the tibia and femur.

External ligaments of the knee include the collateral, patellar, and patellar retinaculum; oblique popliteal; and arcuate popliteal ligaments (Figure 10.77). The collateral ligaments provide support for the knee by reinforcing the joint capsule on the medial and lateral sides (Figures 10.66 and 10.68). The **medial collateral (tibial collateral) ligament** is a flattened triangular ligament that originates from the medial femoral epicondyle and extends to the medial tibial condyle, continuing to the medial shaft of the tibia. Along its path it fuses with the medial meniscus. The shorter, **lateral collateral (fibular collateral) ligament** is more of a rounded cord arising from the lateral femoral epicondyle and attaching to the head of the fibula. The anterior joint capsule is strengthened by the patellar ligament and patellar retinaculum. The **patellar ligament** is the strong thick band representing the continuation of the quadriceps tendon and extends from the patella to the tibial tuberosity (Figures 10.77, *A*, through 10.79). The **patellar retinaculum** is formed mainly by fibrous extensions and fascia of various muscles about the knee (Figure 10.70, 10.71, and 10.77, *A*). The **medial patellar retinaculum** is formed mainly by fibers from the vastus medialis muscle and runs distally to attach to the tibia anterior to the medial collateral ligament. The **lateral patellar retinaculum** consists

of fibers from the vastus lateralis and rectus femoris muscles as well as the iliotibial tract and attaches distally to the lateral margin of the tibial tuberosity to increase stability of the lateral joint capsule. The oblique and arcuate popliteal ligaments help reinforce the dorsal surface of the joint capsule. The **oblique popliteal ligament** is an expansion of the semimembranosus tendon that reinforces the central region of the posterior joint capsule. It extends laterally to attach to the intercondylar line of the femur (Figures 10.71 and 10.79). The inferolateral portion of the posterior capsule is strengthened by the **arcuate popliteal ligament** as it passes superiorly from the apex of the fibular head to spread out over the posterior capsule with fibers continuing to the posterior intercondylar area and to the posterior surface of the lateral femoral condyle (Figure 10.70).

INTERNAL LIGAMENTS Cruciate (cross-shaped) ligaments are strong bands of fibers that provide anterior and posterior stability to the knee. The cruciate ligaments are located within the joint capsule but outside the synovial membrane (Figures 10.66 and 10.67). The **anterior cruciate ligament** arises from the anterior part of the tibial spine and extends to attach to the posterior part of the medial surface of the lateral femoral condyle (Figure 10.78). It helps prevent hyperextension and anterior displacement of the tibia. The **posterior cruciate ligament** is the stronger of the two and extends from the posterior tibial spine to the anterior portion of the medial surface of the medial femoral condyle (Figure 10.79). It functions to prevent hyperflexion and posterior displacement of the tibia (Figures 10.68 and 10.72 through 10.76).

KEY: **ACL,** Anterior cruciate ligament; **pl,** patellar ligament; **PCL,** posterior cruciate ligament; **sol,** soleus muscle; **gas,** gastrocnemius muscle; **pop,** popliteus muscle; **qten,** quadriceps tendon.

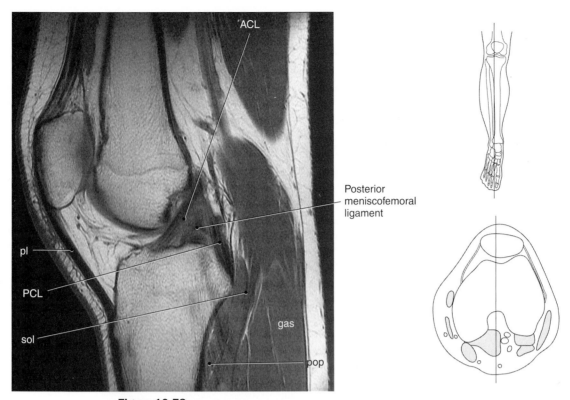

Figure 10.78
Sagittal, T1-weighted MR scan of knee with anterior cruciate ligament.

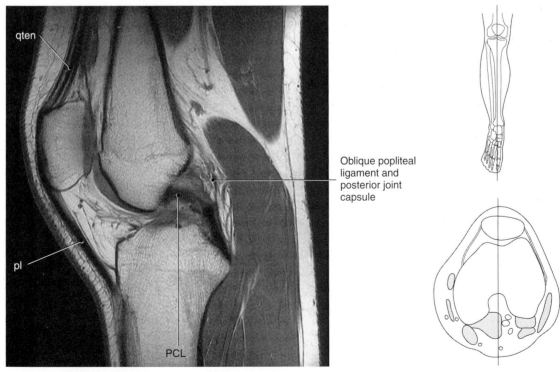

Figure 10.79
Sagittal, T1-weighted MR scan of knee with posterior cruciate ligament.

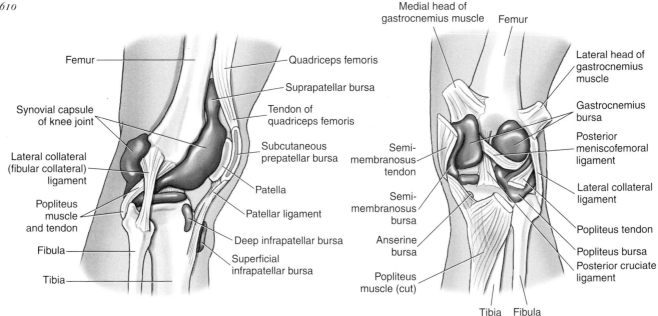

Figure 10.80
Knee bursae. *Left*, Lateral view. *Right*, Posterior view.

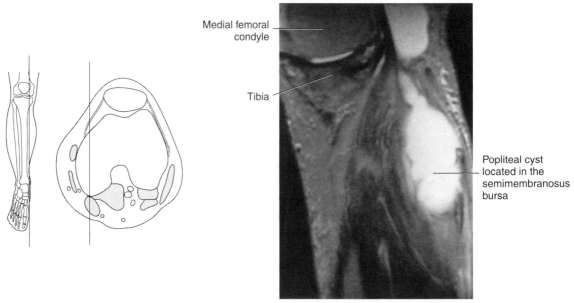

Figure 10.81
Sagittal, T2-weighted MR scan of knee with popliteal cyst.

BURSAE   There are more than 10 bursae located around the knee joint owing to the number of muscles associated with the knee. The major bursa include the suprapatellar, prepatellar, infrapatellar (superficial and deep), gastrocnemius (medial and lateral), semimembranosus, and popliteus bursae (Figures 10.80 and 10.81). The **suprapatellar (quadriceps) bursa** is a large extension of the synovial capsule located between the femur and the quadriceps tendon. The **subcutaneous prepatellar bursa** lies between the anterior surface of the patella and the skin, whereas the **superficial infrapatellar bursa** lies over the patellar ligament between the skin and the tibial tuberosity.

The **deep infrapatellar bursa** is a small bursa located beneath the patellar ligament and anterior to the tibia just above the tibial tuberosity. Behind each femoral condyle is usually a bursa for the respective head of the gastrocnemius muscle. The **gastrocnemius bursae** are located between each muscle head and the joint capsule. The **semimembranosus bursa** is located between the medial head of the gastrocnemius and semimembranosus tendon, and the small **popliteus bursa** lies between the lateral tibial condyle and the popliteus tendon. Bursae are difficult to see on cross-sectional images unless they are abnormal.

Muscles of the Lower Leg

With the exception of the popliteus, all muscles arising from the lower leg are attached to bones of the foot. The muscles of the lower leg can be classified according to their location. They are divided into **anterior** and **posterior groups** by the tibia, fibula, and interosseous membrane. The two main groups are divided again into subgroups or layers. These muscles are demonstrated in Figures 10.82 through 10.99 and described in Table 10.3.

ANTERIOR GROUP   The anterior muscle group can be subdivided into the extensor group located anteriorly and the peroneus group located laterally. The **extensor group** consists of the tibialis anterior, extensor digitorum longus, extensor hallucis longus, and peroneus tertius muscles, and the **peroneus group** includes the peroneus longus and brevis muscles.

EXTENSOR GROUP   The **tibialis anterior muscle** is a long spindle-shaped muscle located just lateral to the anterior surface of the tibia. It arises from the upper two thirds of the lateral surface of the tibia and adjoining interosseous membrane, becoming tendinous over the lower third. The tibialis anterior runs distally and medially over the tibia to insert on the plantar surface of the medial cuneiform and first metatarsal. Its actions include dorsiflexion of the foot at the ankle joint and together with the tibialis posterior muscle it inverts the foot (Figures 10.82 through 10.99).

The **extensor digitorum longus muscle** is located lateral to the tibialis anterior muscle in the anterior aspect of the leg. It arises from the upper two thirds of the fibula and adjoining interosseous membrane and the lateral condyle of the tibia. The tendon of the extensor digitorum longus passes over the front of the ankle joint and gives rise to four separate tendons at the level of the inferior extensor retinaculum that run to the dorsal surface of the second through fifth digits. The extensor digitorum longus muscle is an extensor of the lateral four digits at the metatarso-phalangeal joints (Figures 10.82 through 10.99).

The **extensor hallucis longus muscle** lies posterior to and between the tibialis anterior and extensor digitorum longus muscles. It arises from the middle half of the anterior fibula and interosseous membrane. The tendon of the extensor hallucis longus passes through the inferior extensor retinaculum to the base of the great toe and inserts into the distal phalanx. The extensor hallucis longus muscle extends all the joints of the great toe and provides dorsiflexion of the foot at the ankle joint (Figures 10.82 through 10.99).

The **peroneus tertius muscle** is considered by some to be a distal extension of the extensor digitorum longus muscle. It arises from the anterior surface of the lower fibula, and its tendon inserts on the dorsal aspect of the base of the fifth metatarsal. This muscle functions as a weak evertor and dorsiflexor of the foot at the ankle joint (Figure 10.83).

TABLE 10-3   Muscles of the Lower Leg

MUSCLE	PROXIMAL INSERTION	DISTAL INSERTION	ACTION
Anterior Group			
Extensor Group			
Tibialis anterior	Lateral tibia, upper two thirds	Medial cuneiform, first metatarsal	Dorsiflexion of foot
Extensor digitorum longus	Proximal fibula	Second-fifth digits of foot	Extensor of lateral four digits at the metatarsophalangeal joints
Extensor hallucis longus	Anterior fibula and interosseous membrane	Distal phalanx of first toe	Extends joints of first toe and dorsiflexion of foot
Peroneus Group			
Peroneus tertius	Distal fibula	Fifth metatarsal	Evertor and dorsiflexion of the foot
Peroneus longus	Tibiofibular joint, head of fibula, and lateral condyle of tibia	First metatarsal and medial cuneiform	Plantar flexion and stabilizer of ankle
Peroneus brevis	Lateral surface of distal fibula	Fifth metatarsal	Plantar flexion and stabilizer of ankle
Posterior Group			
Superficial Layer			
Gastrocnemius		Calcaneal tuberosity	Flexor of the foot
Medial head	Supracondylar ridge and adductor tubercle	• Joins soleus tendon at Achilles tendon	
Lateral head	Lateral epicondyle of femur	• Joins soleus tendon at Achilles tendon	
Soleus	Soleal line of tibia and proximal fibula	Achilles tendon	Flexor of the foot
Plantaris	Lateral supracondylar ridge	Achilles tendon	Flexor of the foot
Tibialis posterior	Posterior tibia, interosseous membrane, and posterior fibula	Navicular and medial cuneiform	Flexor of the foot
Deep Layer			
Flexor hallucis longus	Posterior fibula, interosseous membrane, and adjacent fascia	Distal phalanx of first toe	Flexor of the foot
Flexor digitorum longus	Body of tibia below soleal line	Distal phalanges of second-fifth toes	Flexor of the foot
Popliteus	Lateral femoral epicondyle	Posterior, proximal tibia	Flexor of the foot

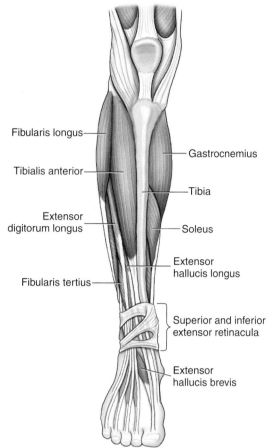

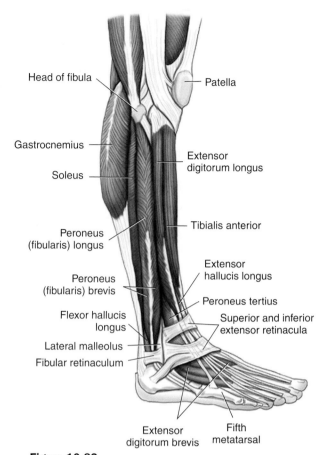

Figure 10.82
Anterior view of right lower leg with retinaculum and ligaments.

Figure 10.83
Lateral view of superficial muscles of the right lower leg.

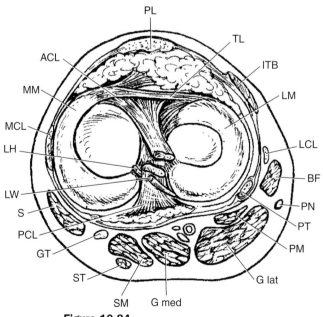

Figure 10.84
Axial view of knee with femoral condyles.

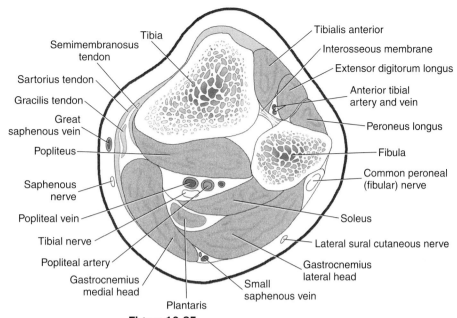

Figure 10.85

Axial view of proximal portion of lower leg.

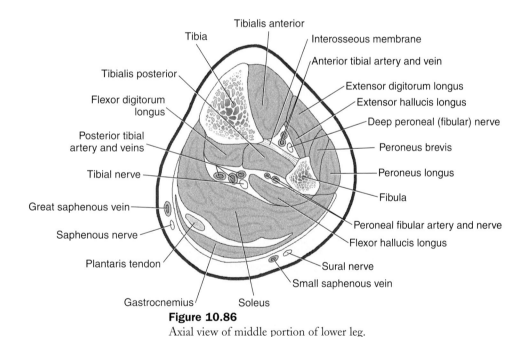

Figure 10.86

Axial view of middle portion of lower leg.

KEY: PL, Patellar ligament; **TL,** transverse ligament; **ITB,** iliotibial band; **LM,** lateral meniscus; **LCL,** lateral collateral ligament; **BF,** biceps femoris; **PN,** peroneal nerve; **PT,** popliteus tendon; **PM,** plantaris muscle; **G lat,** gastrocnemius lateral head; **G med,** gastrocnemius medial head; **SM,** semimembranosus; **ST,** semitendinosus; **GT,** gracilis tendon; **PCL,** posterior cruciate ligament; **S,** sartorius; **LW,** ligaments of Wrisberg; **LH,** ligament of Humphrey; **MCL,** medial collateral ligament; **MM,** medial meniscus; **ACL,** anterior cruciate ligament.

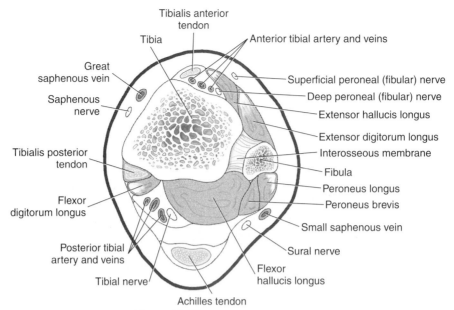

Figure 10.87
Axial view of distal portion of lower leg.

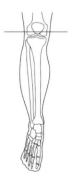

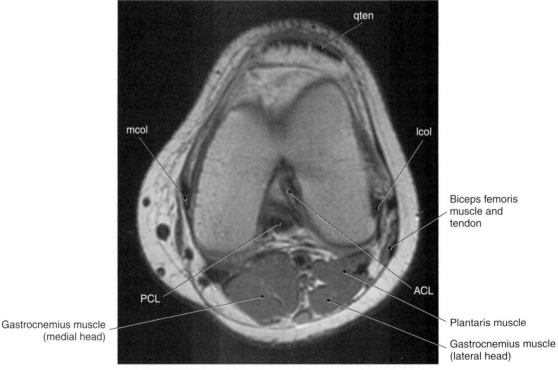

Figure 10.88
Axial, T1-weighted MR scan of distal femur.

KEY: mcol, Medial collateral ligament; **qten,** quadriceps tendon; **lcol,** Lateral collateral ligament; **ACL,** anterior cruciate ligament; **PCL,** posterior cruciate ligament.

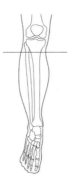

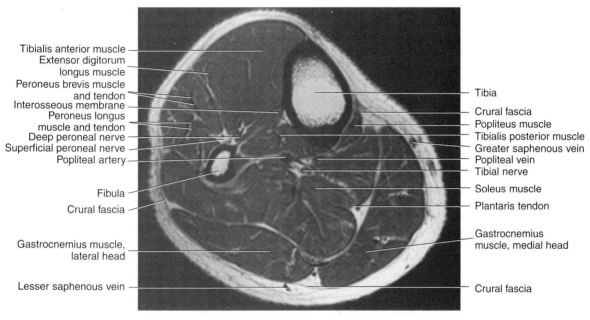

Tibialis anterior muscle

Extensor digitorum
longus muscle

Peroneus brevis muscle
and tendon

Interosseous membrane

Peroneus longus
muscle and tendon

Deep peroneal nerve

Superficial peroneal nerve

Popliteal artery

Fibula

Crural fascia

Gastrocnemius muscle,
lateral head

Lesser saphenous vein

Tibia

Crural fascia

Popliteus muscle

Tibialis posterior muscle

Greater saphenous vein

Popliteal vein

Tibial nerve

Soleus muscle

Plantaris tendon

Gastrocnemius
muscle, medial head

Crural fascia

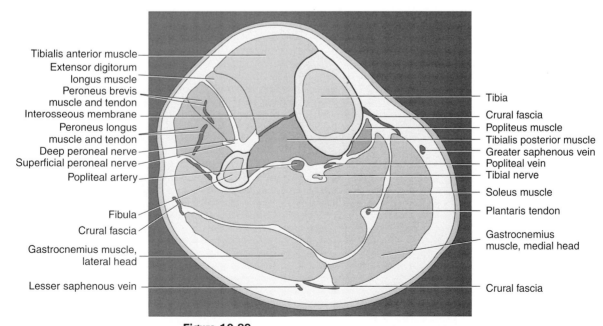

Tibialis anterior muscle

Extensor digitorum
longus muscle

Peroneus brevis
muscle and tendon

Interosseous membrane

Peroneus longus
muscle and tendon

Deep peroneal nerve

Superficial peroneal nerve

Popliteal artery

Fibula

Crural fascia

Gastrocnemius muscle,
lateral head

Lesser saphenous vein

Tibia

Crural fascia

Popliteus muscle

Tibialis posterior muscle

Greater saphenous vein

Popliteal vein

Tibial nerve

Soleus muscle

Plantaris tendon

Gastrocnemius
muscle, medial head

Crural fascia

Figure 10.89
Axial, T1-weighted, MR scan of proximal lower leg.

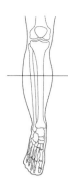

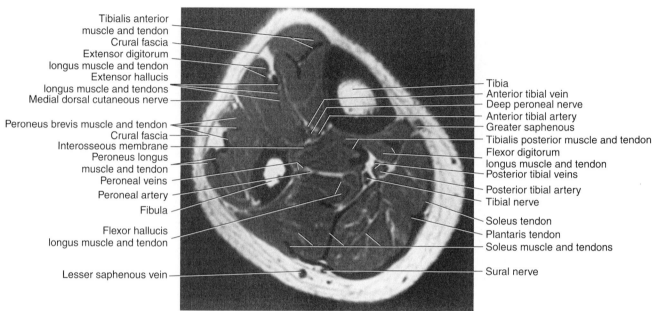

Tibialis anterior
muscle and tendon
Crural fascia
Extensor digitorum
longus muscle and tendon
Extensor hallucis
longus muscle and tendons
Medial dorsal cutaneous nerve

Peroneus brevis muscle and tendon
Crural fascia
Interosseous membrane
Peroneus longus
muscle and tendon
Peroneal veins
Peroneal artery
Fibula

Flexor hallucis
longus muscle and tendon

Lesser saphenous vein

Tibia
Anterior tibial vein
Deep peroneal nerve
Anterior tibial artery
Greater saphenous
Tibialis posterior muscle and tendon
Flexor digitorum
longus muscle and tendon
Posterior tibial veins

Posterior tibial artery
Tibial nerve

Soleus tendon
Plantaris tendon
Soleus muscle and tendons

Sural nerve

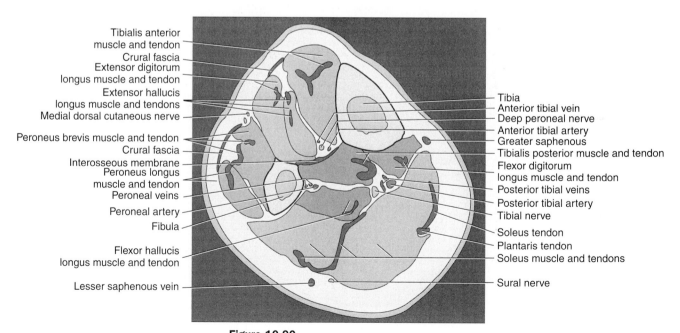

Tibialis anterior
muscle and tendon
Crural fascia
Extensor digitorum
longus muscle and tendon
Extensor hallucis
longus muscle and tendons
Medial dorsal cutaneous nerve

Peroneus brevis muscle and tendon
Crural fascia
Interosseous membrane
Peroneus longus
muscle and tendon
Peroneal veins
Peroneal artery
Fibula

Flexor hallucis
longus muscle and tendon

Lesser saphenous vein

Tibia
Anterior tibial vein
Deep peroneal nerve
Anterior tibial artery
Greater saphenous
Tibialis posterior muscle and tendon
Flexor digitorum
longus muscle and tendon
Posterior tibial veins
Posterior tibial artery
Tibial nerve

Soleus tendon
Plantaris tendon
Soleus muscle and tendons

Sural nerve

Figure 10.90
Axial, T1-weighted MR scan of mid lower leg.

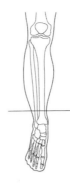

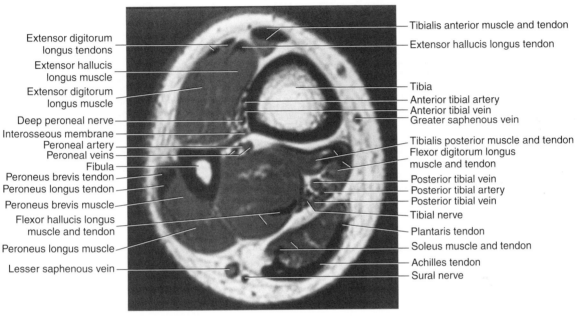

Extensor digitorum
longus tendons

Extensor hallucis
longus muscle

Extensor digitorum
longus muscle

Deep peroneal nerve

Interosseous membrane

Peroneal artery

Peroneal veins

Fibula

Peroneus brevis tendon

Peroneus longus tendon

Peroneus brevis muscle

Flexor hallucis longus
muscle and tendon

Peroneus longus muscle

Lesser saphenous vein

Tibialis anterior muscle and tendon

Extensor hallucis longus tendon

Tibia

Anterior tibial artery

Anterior tibial vein

Greater saphenous vein

Tibialis posterior muscle and tendon

Flexor digitorum longus
muscle and tendon

Posterior tibial vein

Posterior tibial artery

Posterior tibial vein

Tibial nerve

Plantaris tendon

Soleus muscle and tendon

Achilles tendon

Sural nerve

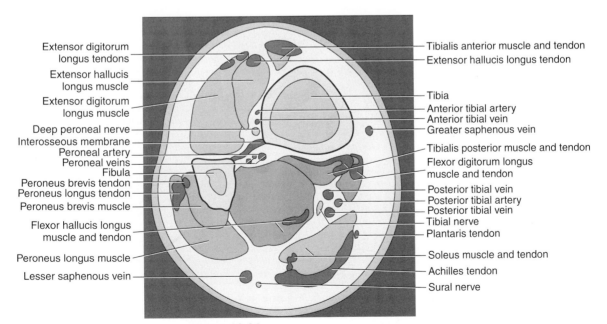

Extensor digitorum
longus tendons

Extensor hallucis
longus muscle

Extensor digitorum
longus muscle

Deep peroneal nerve

Interosseous membrane

Peroneal artery

Peroneal veins

Fibula

Peroneus brevis tendon

Peroneus longus tendon

Peroneus brevis muscle

Flexor hallucis longus
muscle and tendon

Peroneus longus muscle

Lesser saphenous vein

Tibialis anterior muscle and tendon

Extensor hallucis longus tendon

Tibia

Anterior tibial artery

Anterior tibial vein

Greater saphenous vein

Tibialis posterior muscle and tendon

Flexor digitorum longus
muscle and tendon

Posterior tibial vein

Posterior tibial artery

Posterior tibial vein

Tibial nerve

Plantaris tendon

Soleus muscle and tendon

Achilles tendon

Sural nerve

Figure 10.91
Axial, T1-weighted MR scan of distal lower leg.

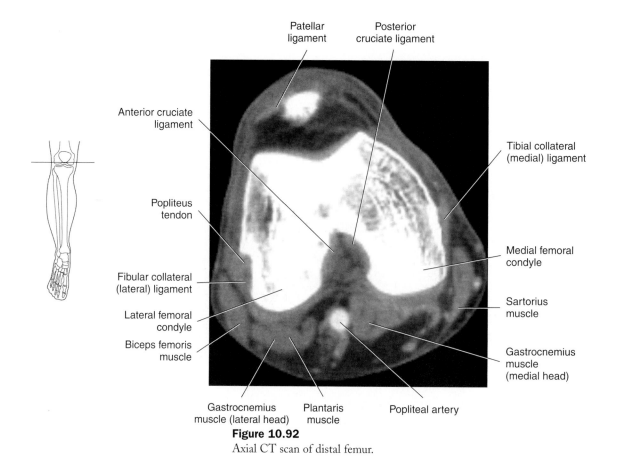

Patellar ligament

Posterior cruciate ligament

Anterior cruciate ligament

Tibial collateral (medial) ligament

Popliteus tendon

Medial femoral condyle

Fibular collateral (lateral) ligament

Lateral femoral condyle

Sartorius muscle

Biceps femoris muscle

Gastrocnemius muscle (medial head)

Gastrocnemius muscle (lateral head)

Plantaris muscle

Popliteal artery

Figure 10.92

Axial CT scan of distal femur.

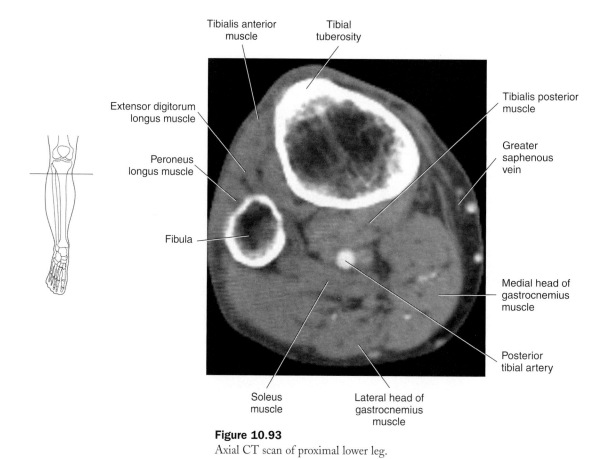

Tibialis anterior muscle

Tibial tuberosity

Extensor digitorum longus muscle

Tibialis posterior muscle

Peroneus longus muscle

Greater saphenous vein

Fibula

Medial head of gastrocnemius muscle

Posterior tibial artery

Soleus muscle

Lateral head of gastrocnemius muscle

Figure 10.93

Axial CT scan of proximal lower leg.

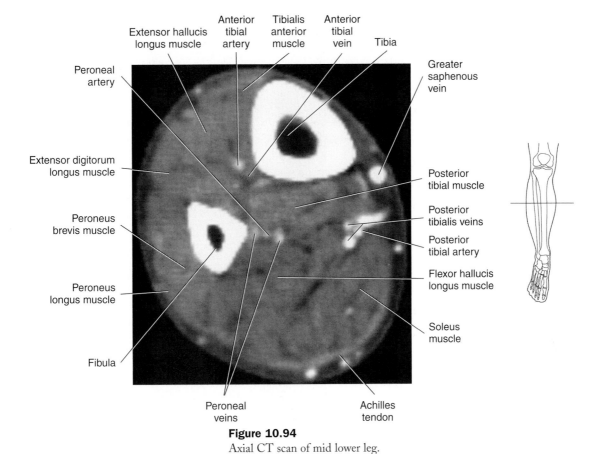

Figure 10.94
Axial CT scan of mid lower leg.

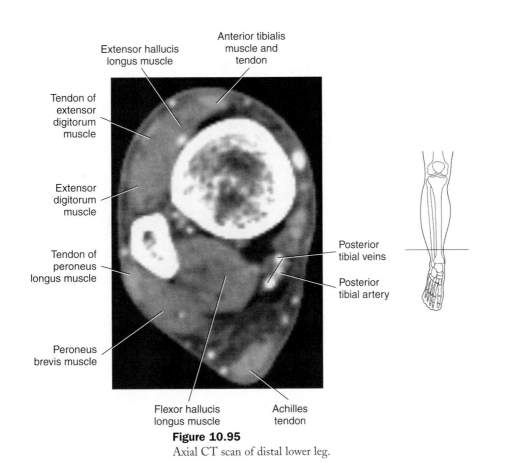

Figure 10.95
Axial CT scan of distal lower leg.

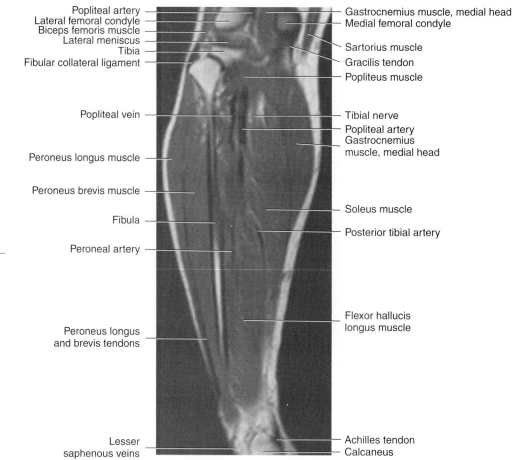

Popliteal artery
Lateral femoral condyle
Biceps femoris muscle
Lateral meniscus
Tibia
Fibular collateral ligament

Gastrocnemius muscle, medial head
Medial femoral condyle
Sartorius muscle
Gracilis tendon
Popliteus muscle

Popliteal vein

Tibial nerve
Popliteal artery
Gastrocnemius muscle, medial head

Peroneus longus muscle

Peroneus brevis muscle

Fibula

Soleus muscle

Peroneal artery

Posterior tibial artery

Peroneus longus and brevis tendons

Flexor hallucis longus muscle

Lesser saphenous veins

Achilles tendon
Calcaneus

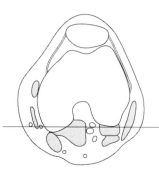

Figure 10.96
Coronal, T1-weighted MR scan of leg.

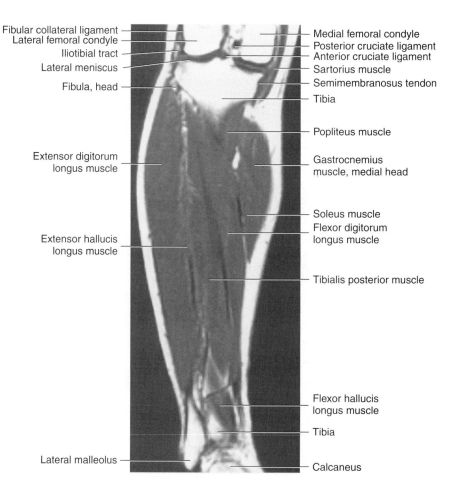

Fibular collateral ligament
Lateral femoral condyle
Iliotibial tract
Lateral meniscus
Fibula, head

Medial femoral condyle
Posterior cruciate ligament
Anterior cruciate ligament
Sartorius muscle
Semimembranosus tendon
Tibia

Popliteus muscle

Extensor digitorum longus muscle

Gastrocnemius muscle, medial head

Soleus muscle
Flexor digitorum longus muscle

Extensor hallucis longus muscle

Tibialis posterior muscle

Flexor hallucis longus muscle

Tibia

Lateral malleolus

Calcaneus

Figure 10.97
Coronal, T1-weighted MR scan of leg.

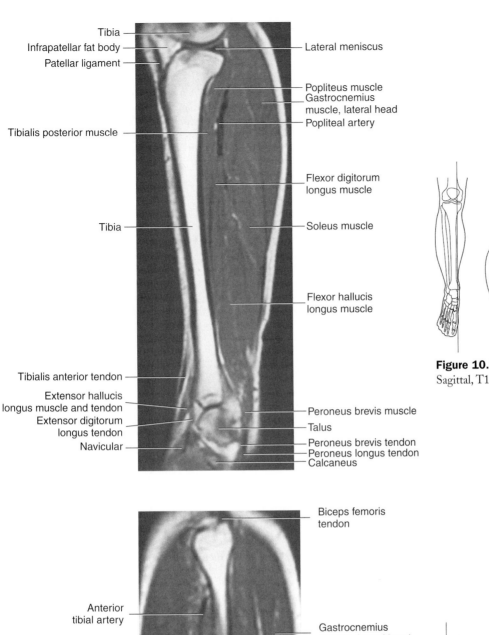

Tibia
Infrapatellar fat body
Patellar ligament

Lateral meniscus

Popliteus muscle
Gastrocnemius muscle, lateral head
Popliteal artery

Tibialis posterior muscle

Flexor digitorum longus muscle

Soleus muscle

Tibia

Flexor hallucis longus muscle

Tibialis anterior tendon

Extensor hallucis longus muscle and tendon
Extensor digitorum longus tendon
Navicular

Peroneus brevis muscle
Talus
Peroneus brevis tendon
Peroneus longus tendon
Calcaneus

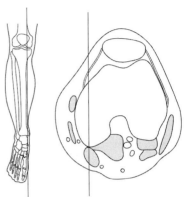

Figure 10.98
Sagittal, T1-weighted MR scan of leg.

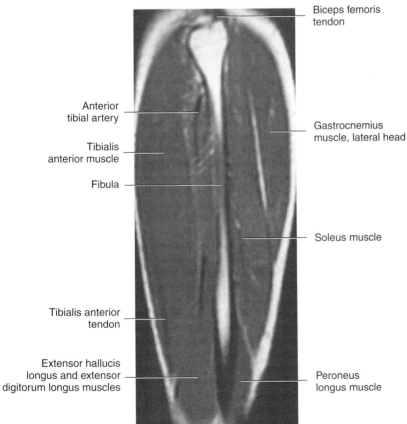

Biceps femoris tendon

Anterior tibial artery

Gastrocnemius muscle, lateral head

Tibialis anterior muscle

Fibula

Soleus muscle

Tibialis anterior tendon

Extensor hallucis longus and extensor digitorum longus muscles

Peroneus longus muscle

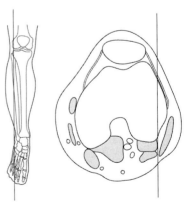

Figure 10.99
Sagittal, T1-weighted MR scan of leg.

PERONEUS GROUP   The two peroneus muscles act as plantar flexors but also stabilize the lateral ankle and longitudinal arch of the foot (Figures 10.82 and 10.83).

The **peroneus (fibularis) longus muscle** is located on the lateral side of the leg arising from the tibiofibular joint, the head of the fibula, and the lateral condyle of the tibia. The peroneus longus has a long belly and an even longer tendon. The tendon of the peroneus longus runs in a shallow groove behind the lateral malleolus, passing below the peroneal tubercle of the calcaneus and across the lateral side of the cuboid. It then runs obliquely across the sole of the foot to insert on the base of the first metatarsal and lateral surface of the medial cuneiform (Figures 10.82, 10.83, 10.94, and 10.95).

The **peroneus (fibularis) brevis muscle** is shorter and smaller than its counterpart. It lies under the peroneus longus, arising from the distal two thirds of the lateral surface of the fibula. The tendon of the peroneus brevis accompanies the tendon of the peroneus longus in a common synovial sheath behind the lateral malleolus, with the peroneus brevis just anterior to the peroneus longus. At approximately the level of the peroneal tubercle of the calcaneus, the tendons separate into their own synovial sheath, with the peroneus brevis tendon attaching to the tuberosity at the base of the fifth metatarsal (Figures 10.82, 10.83, 10.94, and 10.95).

POSTERIOR GROUP   The posterior group is functionally considered the **flexors,** which are responsible for plantar flexion of the foot. This group is subdivided into the superficial layer consisting of the gastrocnemius, soleus, and plantaris muscles and the deep layer with the tibialis posterior, flexor hallucis longus, flexor digitorum longus, and popliteus muscles. These muscles are demonstrated in Figures 10.84 through 10.102 and described in Table 10.3.

SUPERFICIAL LAYER   The **gastrocnemius muscle** is a prominent flexor of the foot and is responsible for giving the calf its shape on the back of the leg. It consists of two heads arising from the medial and lateral femoral condyles. The medial head arises from the medial supracondylar ridge and adductor tubercle on the popliteal surface of the femur. The lateral head arises just behind the lateral epicondyle on the outer surface of the lateral femoral condyle. The two heads form the lower boundaries of the popliteal fossa, and their fibers run distally where they join the tendon of the soleus muscle to form the **Achilles tendon** that inserts on the calcaneal tuberosity (Figures 10.84 through 10.100).

The **soleus muscle** is a broad, flat muscle located beneath the gastrocnemius. It arises from the soleal line on the posterior tibia and the upper third of the fibula. The muscle fibers run distally and merge with the tendon of the gastrocnemius to form the superficial Achilles tendon (Figures 10.84 through 10.101).

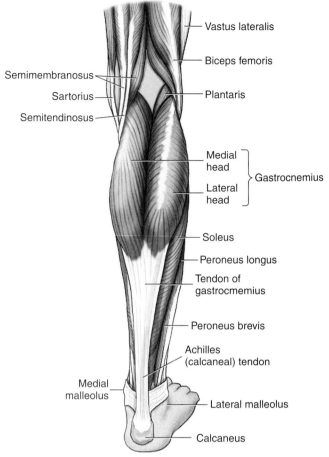

Figure 10.100
Posterior view of superficial muscles of leg.

The **plantaris muscle** is a long, thin muscle that arises from the lowest part of the lateral supracondylar ridge, the adjacent popliteal surface, and joint capsule. The tendon runs inferiorly at an oblique angle between the gastrocnemius and soleus muscles to insert on the medial edge of the Achilles tendon (Figures 10.84 through 10.101).

DEEP LAYER   The **tibialis posterior muscle** is the deepest muscle located on the back of the leg. It arises from the superolateral surface of the posterior tibia just below the soleal line, the interosseous membrane, and the posterior surface of the fibula. The tendon of the tibialis posterior passes through the malleolar groove of the tibia behind the medial malleolus to attach to the tuberosity of the navicular and plantar surface

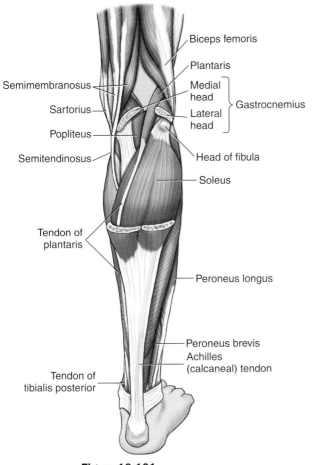

Figure 10.101
Posterior view of soleus muscle.

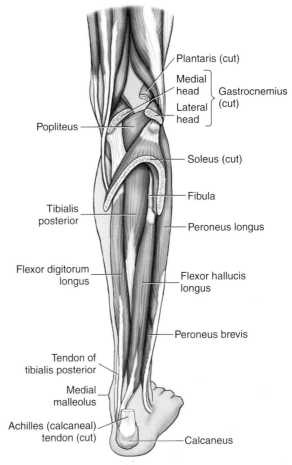

Figure 10.102
Posterior view of deep muscles of leg.

of the medial cuneiform bones (Figures 10.86 and 10.98 and 10.102).

The **flexor hallucis longus muscle** is a powerful muscle located beneath the gastrocnemius and soleus muscles. It arises from the distal two thirds of the posterior fibula, the interosseous membrane, and adjacent fascia. The tendon of the flexor hallucis longus runs distally, crossing over the dorsal aspect of the ankle, through the malleolar groove of the tibia to the sole of the foot, where it inserts into the base of the terminal phalanx of the first toe (Figures 10.86, 10.87, 10.90, 10.91, 10.94, 10.95, and 10.102).

The **flexor digitorum longus muscle** arises from the posterior surface of the body of the tibia immediately below the soleal line. The muscle descends along the tibial side of the leg to become tendinous just above the medial malleolus. The tendon of the flexor digitorum longus passes behind the medial malleolus to the sole of the foot, deep to the flexor hallucis longus, and divides into four individual tendons that insert into the bases of the distal phalanges of the second through fifth digits (Figures 10.86, 10.87, 10.90, 10.91, 10.94, 10.95, and 10.102).

The **popliteus muscle** is a thin triangular muscle that forms the lower floor of the popliteal fossa. It arises just below the lateral femoral epicondyle and extends obliquely to the triangular surface above the soleal (popliteal) line on the posterior tibia (Figures 10.85 and 10.102).

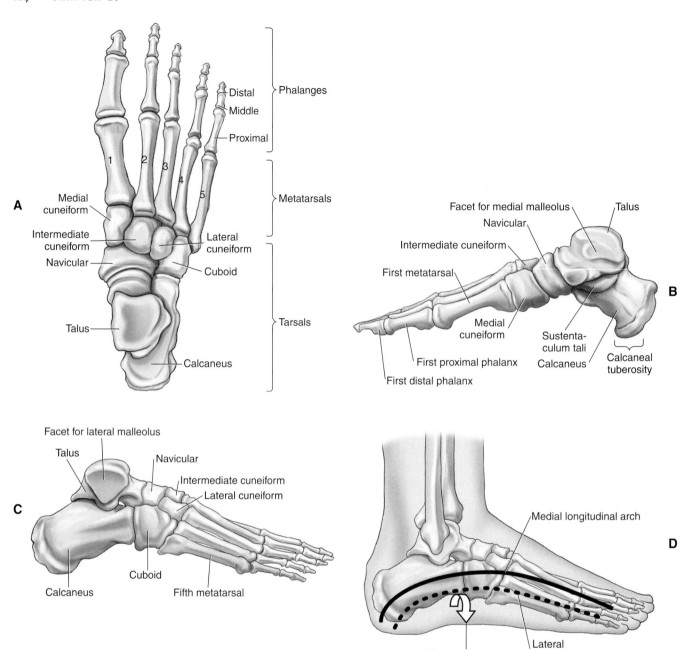

Figure 10.103
Bones of the right foot. **A,** Superior view. **B,** Medial view. **C,** Lateral view. **D,** Arches of foot.

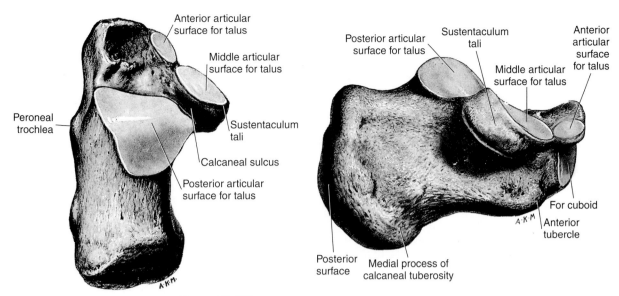

Figure 10.104
Left calcaneus. *Left,* Dorsal aspect. *Right,* Medial aspect.

ANKLE AND FOOT

Bony Anatomy

The bony anatomy of the ankle and foot includes the tarsus, metatarsus, and phalanges. The tarsus consists of seven bones: talus, calcaneus, navicular, cuboid, and three cuneiform bones. Five metatarsals and 14 phalanges make up the toes (Figures 10.103 through 10.125).

TARSUS   The **talus (astragalus)** is the second largest tarsal bone and is responsible, together with the calcaneus, for transmitting the entire weight of the body to the foot. The talus consists of a body, head, and neck. The **body** is wedge shaped with an upper articular surface **(trochlea)** that is wider in front than in back (Figures 10.103, 10.105, and 10.106). The trochlea provides articulation with the tibia (Figures 10.105 through 10.110). The **head** faces anteriorly to articulate with the navicular bone (Figure 10.105). The largest tarsal bone is the **calcaneus,** which lies beneath the talus. It has an elongated cuboid shape with a posterior surface comprising the prominence of the heel. On the medial surface of the calcaneus is a shelflike process termed the **sustentaculum tali,** which provides support for the talus (Figures 10.104 and 10.108 through 10.110). On the plantar surface of the posterior calcaneus is the large **calcaneal tuberosity** for insertion of ligaments and tendons (Figures 10.104 through 10.107). The articulation between the talus and calcaneus is termed the **subtalar joint,** which is composed of three articulations formed by the **anterior, middle,** and **posterior facets** (Figure 10.104). The smallest of the three is the anterior facet, which can be independent of or continuous with the middle facet. The middle facet lies on a

ledge of bone projecting off the medial surface of the calcaneus at the sustentaculum tali (Figures 10.105 and 10.108 through 10.110). This shelf and the entire middle facet joint provide weight-bearing support to the medial side of the ankle. The posterior facet joint is the largest and provides support for most of the body of the talus (Figures 10.104 through 10.107). Separating this facet from the middle and anterior facet joints is the **tarsal canal.** This canal, containing blood vessels, fat, and the interosseous ligament, widens laterally to form the **sinus tarsi** (Figures 10.105 through 10.107). In addition to the talus and calcaneus, the cuboid, navicular, and three cuneiform bones comprise the remaining five tarsal bones of the foot (Figures 10.103 and 10.113 through 10.125). Lateral and anterior to the calcaneus is the **cuboid bone,** which articulates anteriorly with the bases of the fourth and fifth metatarsal bones. The **navicular bone** articulates posteriorly with the talus and anteriorly with the cuneiform bones on the medial side of the foot. The **cuneiform bones** are numbered from medial to lateral or termed *medial, intermediate,* and *lateral* and articulate anteriorly with the first three metatarsal bones.

METATARSALS   The metatarsals are long, slender bones. There are five metatarsals in each foot, with each bone having a distal head, proximal base, and body or shaft in between. The heads articulate with the proximal phalanges of the toes and the bases articulate with the tarsus.

PHALANGES   Each foot has 14 phalanges—3 phalanges for each toe except the great toe, which has just 2. The phalanges of the toes are shorter and stouter than their counterparts in the fingers (Figures 10.103 and 10.113 through 10.125).

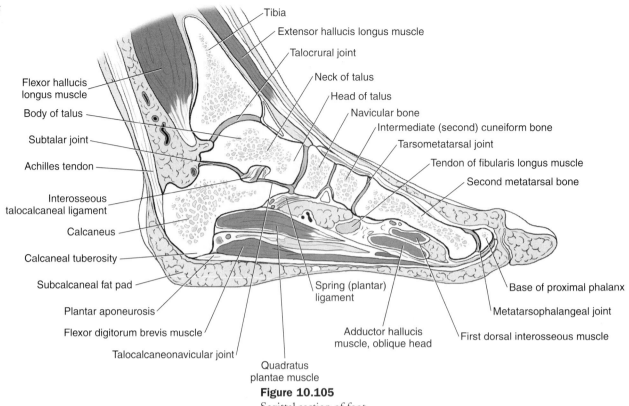

Figure 10.105
Sagittal section of foot.

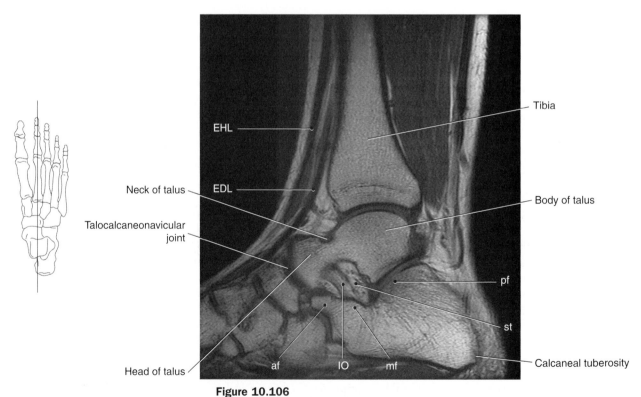

Figure 10.106
Sagittal, T1-weighted MR scan of calcaneus.

KEY: **EHL,** Extensor hallucis longus; **EDL,** extensor digitorum longus; **af,** acetabular fossa;
IO, interosseus ligament; **mf,** medial facet; **st,** sinus tarsi; **pf,** posterior facet.

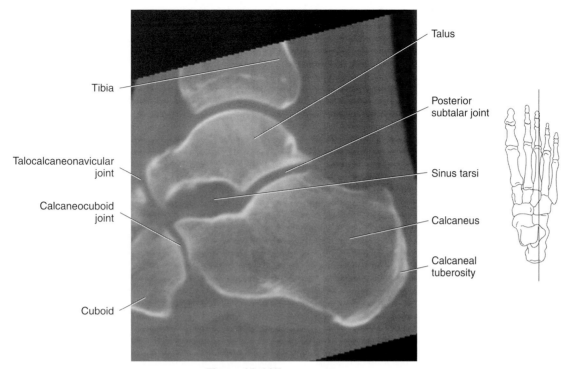

Figure 10.107
Sagittal CT reformat of calcaneus.

Tibia

Talocalcaneonavicular joint

Calcaneocuboid joint

Cuboid

Talus

Posterior subtalar joint

Sinus tarsi

Calcaneus

Calcaneal tuberosity

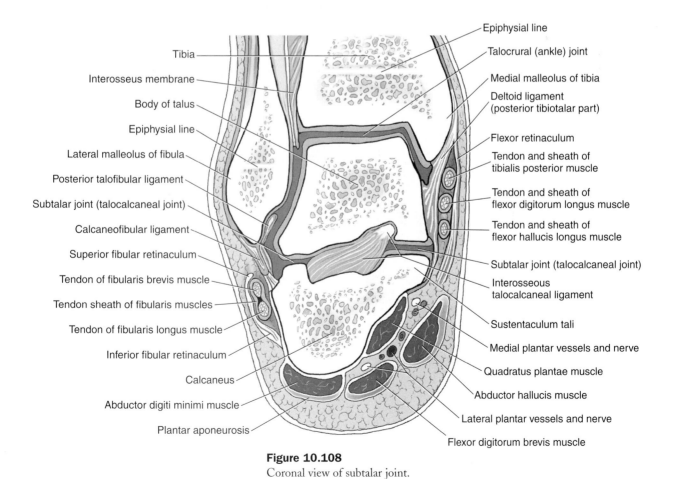

Tibia

Interosseus membrane

Body of talus

Epiphysial line

Lateral malleolus of fibula

Posterior talofibular ligament

Subtalar joint (talocalcaneal joint)

Calcaneofibular ligament

Superior fibular retinaculum

Tendon of fibularis brevis muscle

Tendon sheath of fibularis muscles

Tendon of fibularis longus muscle

Inferior fibular retinaculum

Calcaneus

Abductor digiti minimi muscle

Plantar aponeurosis

Epiphysial line

Talocrural (ankle) joint

Medial malleolus of tibia

Deltoid ligament (posterior tibiotalar part)

Flexor retinaculum

Tendon and sheath of tibialis posterior muscle

Tendon and sheath of flexor digitorum longus muscle

Tendon and sheath of flexor hallucis longus muscle

Subtalar joint (talocalcaneal joint)

Interosseous talocalcaneal ligament

Sustentaculum tali

Medial plantar vessels and nerve

Quadratus plantae muscle

Abductor hallucis muscle

Lateral plantar vessels and nerve

Flexor digitorum brevis muscle

Figure 10.108
Coronal view of subtalar joint.

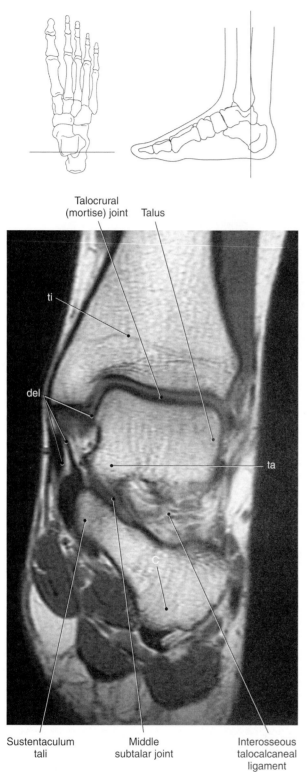

Talocrural
(mortise) joint   Talus

ti

del

ta

C

Sustentaculum   Middle   Interosseous
tali   subtalar joint   talocalcaneal
ligament

Figure 10.109
Coronal, T1-weighted MR scan of subtalar joint.

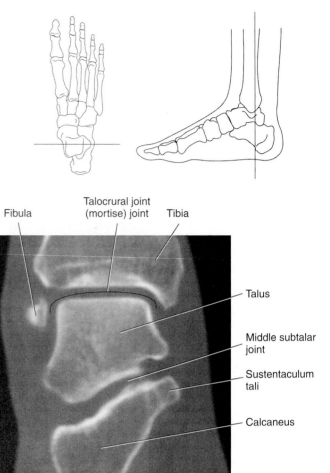

Fibula   Talocrural joint   Tibia
          (mortise) joint

Talus

Middle subtalar
joint

Sustentaculum
tali

Calcaneus

Figure 10.110
Coronal CT reformat of subtalar joint.

KEY: **ti,** Tibia; **del,** deltoid ligament; **ta,** talus; **C,** calcaneus.

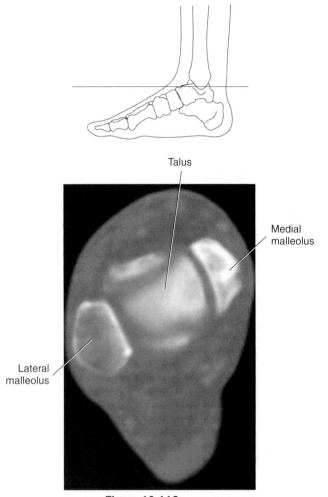

Figure 10.112
Axial CT scan of ankle.

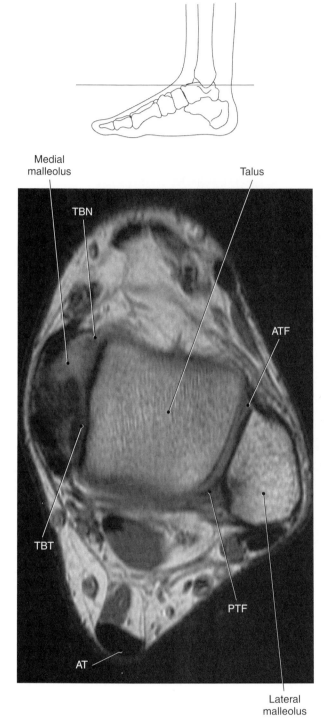

Figure 10.111
Axial, T1-weighted MR scan of ankle.

KEY: TBN, Tibionavicular ligament; **TBT,** tibiotalar ligament; **AT,** Achilles tendon; **PTF,** posterior talofibular ligament; **ATF,** anterior talofibular ligament.

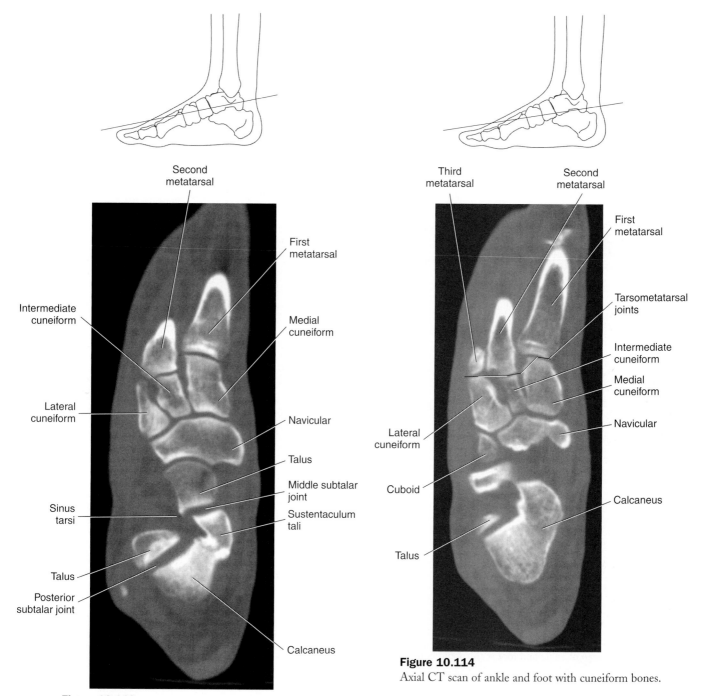

Figure 10.113

Axial CT scan of ankle and foot with navicular bone.

Figure 10.114

Axial CT scan of ankle and foot with cuneiform bones.

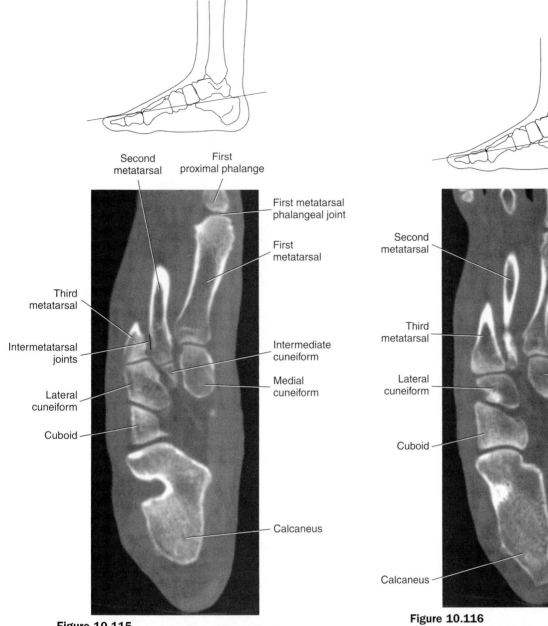

Figure 10.115
Axial CT scan of ankle and foot with cuboid bone.

Figure 10.116
Axial CT scan of ankle and foot with calcaneus.

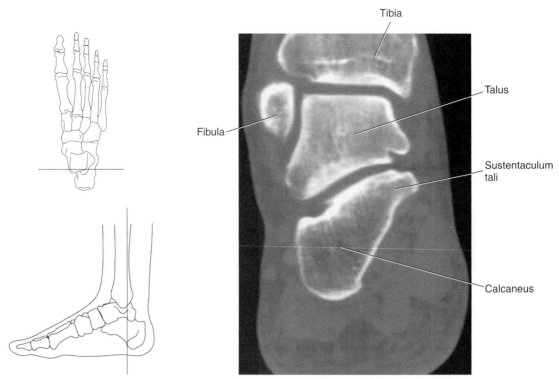

Figure 10.117
Coronal CT reformat of ankle and foot with talus.

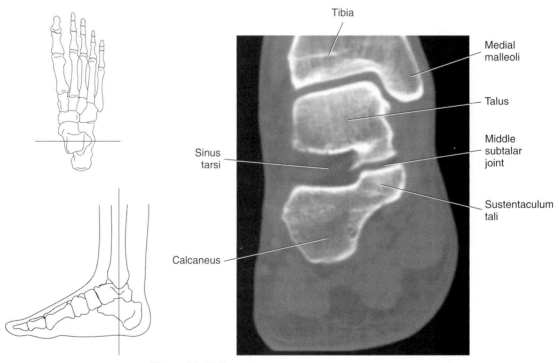

Figure 10.118
Coronal CT reformat of ankle and foot with calcaneus.

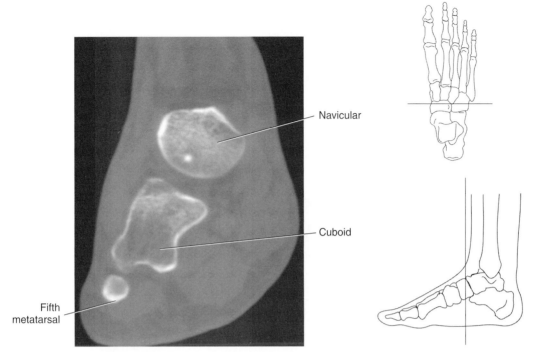

Figure 10.119
Coronal CT reformat of ankle and foot with navicular and cuboid bones.

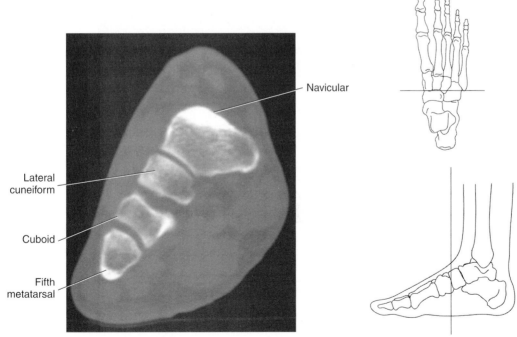

Figure 10.120
Coronal CT reformat of ankle and foot with lateral cuneiform bone.

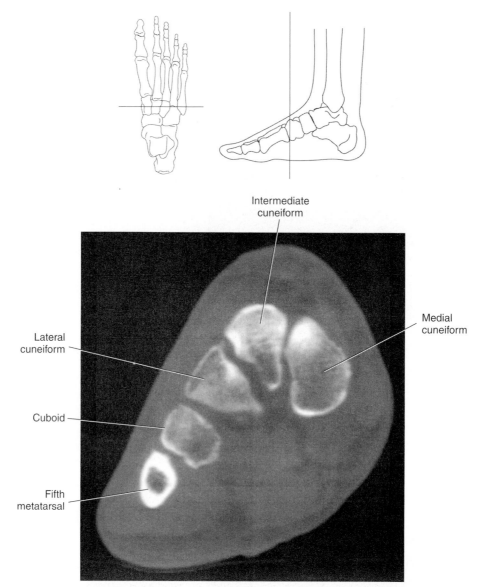

Intermediate
cuneiform

Medial
cuneiform

Lateral
cuneiform

Cuboid

Fifth
metatarsal

Figure 10.121
Coronal CT reformat of ankle and foot with cuneiform bones.

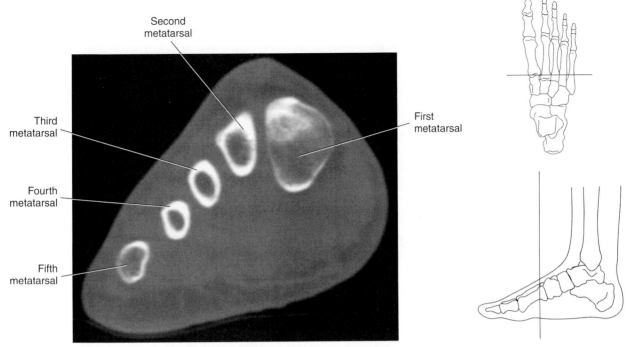

Figure 10.122
Coronal CT reformat of ankle and foot with metatarsals.

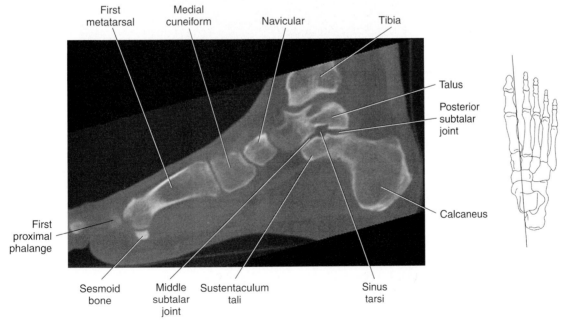

Figure 10.123
Sagittal CT reformat of ankle and foot, medial aspect.

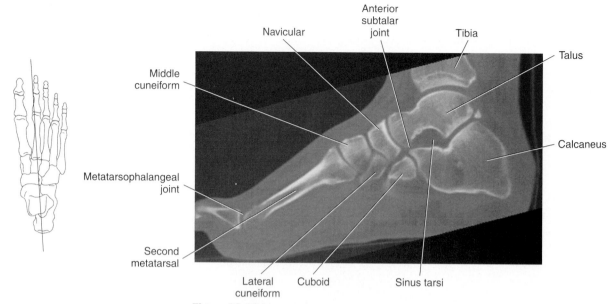

Figure 10.124
Sagittal CT reformat of ankle and foot with talus.

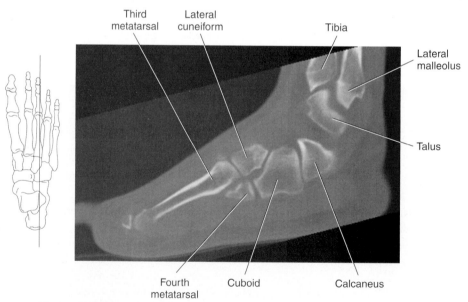

Figure 10.125
Sagittal CT reformat of ankle and foot, lateral aspect.

Joints

The joints of the foot and ankle include the talocrural (ankle joint), intertarsal, tarsometatarsal and intermetatarsal, metatarsophalangeal, and interphalangeal joints.

The **talocrural joint (ankle joint)** is created by the articulations between the tibia, fibula, and talus (astragalus). The tibia and fibula rest on the trochlear surface of the talus to form what is commonly termed the **mortise joint,** which allows for dorsal and plantar flexion. Both the tibia and fibula terminate distally in projections termed *malleoli*, which prevent medial and lateral displacement of the talus (Figures 10.108 through 10.110).

The **intertarsal joints** are created by the articulations between the tarsal bones and include the subtalar, talocalcaneonavicular, calcaneocuboid, transverse (mid-) tarsal, cuneonavicular, intercuneiform, and the cuneocuboid joints. The subtalar joint consists of the articulation between the talus and calcaneus and was discussed earlier (Figures 10.105 and 10.106). The subtalar joint provides the ability to invert and evert the foot. The **talocalcaneonavicular** and **calcaneocuboid** joints combine to form the **transverse** or **midtarsal joint.** This joint provides an irregular plane across the foot extending from side to side, with the talus and calcaneus located posteriorly and the navicular and cuboid located anteriorly (Figures 10.106 and 10.107). The transverse tarsal joint plays an important part in putting the spring in your step by acting as a shock absorber during the push-off phase of walking or running. The cuneonavicular, intercuneiform, and cuneocuboid joints contribute to the flexibility of the foot by providing a slight gliding movement between bones.

The **tarsometatarsal joints** exist between the bases of all five metatarsals and the anterior four tarsal bones (cuboid, three cuneiforms). The articulations between the tarsals and metatarsals permit only limited gliding movement between the bones (Figures 10.105 and 10.113 through 10.116). The **intermetatarsal joints** are the articulations between the bases of the lateral four metatarsals. The intermetatarsal joints permit a small degree of gliding between metatarsals and contribute to eversion and inversion of the foot (Figure 10.115).

METATARSOPHALANGEAL JOINTS   The heads of the metatarsals articulate with the bases of the proximal phalanges at the metatarsophalangeal joints (Figures 10.105, 10.115, and 10.124). This articulation provides flexion and extension of the toes.

INTERPHALANGEAL JOINTS   The heads of the phalanges articulate with the bases of the more distal phalanges to create the interphalangeal joints. The interphalangeal joints are hinge joints that permit plantar and dorsiflexion of the phalanges (Figure 10.103).

ARCHES   The bones of the foot are arranged in transverse and longitudinal arches that provide the flexibility and resiliency of the foot to support the weight of the body, absorb shocks, and provide spring and lift during activity (Figure 10.103, *B* through *D*). The **longitudinal arch (plantar arch)** has two parts: one on the lateral side of the foot **(lateral longitudinal arch)** and one on the medial side of the foot **(medial longi-**

tudinal arch). The bony landmarks for the longitudinal arch on the medial side is the head of the first metatarsal anteriorly and the calcaneal tuberosity posteriorly. On the lateral side the bony landmarks include the head of the fifth metatarsal anteriorly and the calcaneal tuberosity posteriorly. The medial longitudinal arch is more elastic and is associated with greater curvature, whereas the lateral longitudinal arch is flatter and less flexible because it makes contact with the ground. The longitudinal arches provide a firm base for support of the body in the upright position. The **transverse arch** is formed by the distal row of tarsal bones (cuboid, three cuneiforms) and the bases of the metatarsals that create a domed curve across the foot. The transverse arch is the major weight-bearing arch of the foot and helps to distribute body weight over the base of the foot. The integrity of arches is maintained by the tarsal, tarsometatarsal, and intermetatarsal joints and their supporting ligaments (Figure 10.103, *D*).

Fascia, Retinacula, and Ligaments

As in the wrist, fascia in various regions of the ankle will thicken to form retinacula. The retinacula form sheaths for stabilizing tendons crossing over the joints of the ankle. They are called the *flexor, extensor,* and *peroneal retinacula* after the tendons they serve (Figures 10.126 through 10.142). The **flexor retinaculum** is located between the medial malleolus and the medial tubercle of the calcaneus. It forms four tunnels for the passage of the tendons of the tibialis posterior, flexor digitorum longus, flexor hallucis longus muscles, and the posterior tibial vessels and nerve. The **extensor retinaculum** consists of two portions: an upper portion (superior extensor retinacula) and lower portion (inferior extensor retinacula). The **superior extensor retinaculum** runs horizontally between the tibia and fibula just above the ankle joint. It transmits the tendons of the tibialis anterior and extensor hallucis muscles. The **inferior extensor retinaculum** splits into two bands that extend across the dorsum of the foot, originating from the upper surface of the calcaneus and sinus tarsi. The upper band of the inferior extensor retinaculum attaches to the medial malleolus, whereas the lower band extends to the fascia on the medial side of the foot. The tendons of the extensor digitorum longus and peroneus tertius muscles run deep to the inferior extensor retinaculum. The **peroneal retinacula** split into two bands, forming the superior and inferior peroneal retinaculum. The **superior peroneal retinaculum** extends from the lateral side of the calcaneus to the posterior border of the lateral malleolus. The **inferior peroneal retinaculum** extends from the lateral side of the calcaneus to blend with the fibers of the inferior extensor retinaculum. The superior and inferior peroneal retinacula transmit the tendons for the peroneus brevis and peroneus longus muscles.

In addition to the retinacula, another area of thickened fascia is located on the plantar surface of the foot. The **plantar aponeurosis (fascia)** is approximately 80 layers thick, creating some of the thickest fascia within the human body. It begins at the inferior aspect of the calcaneus and spreads anteriorly into

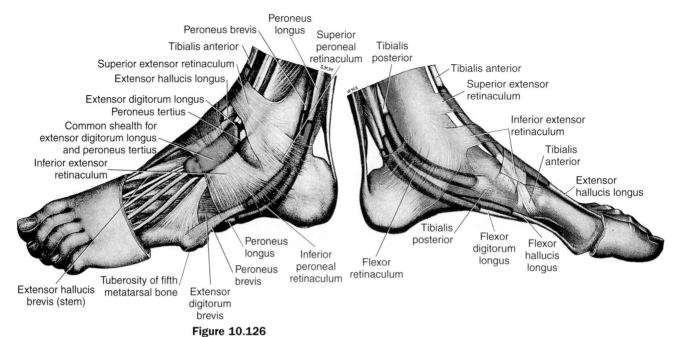

Figure 10.126
Tendons of left foot. *Left,* Lateral aspect. *Right,* Medial aspect.

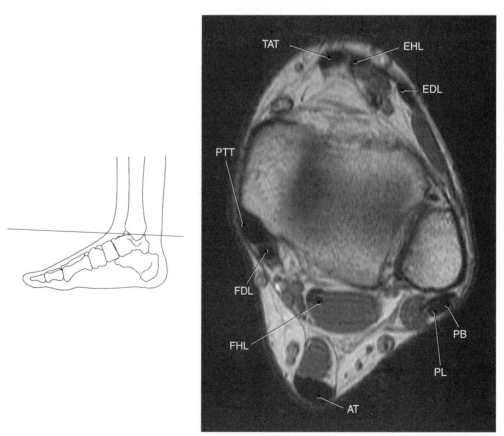

Figure 10.127
Axial, T1-weighted MR scan of ankle ligaments and tendons.

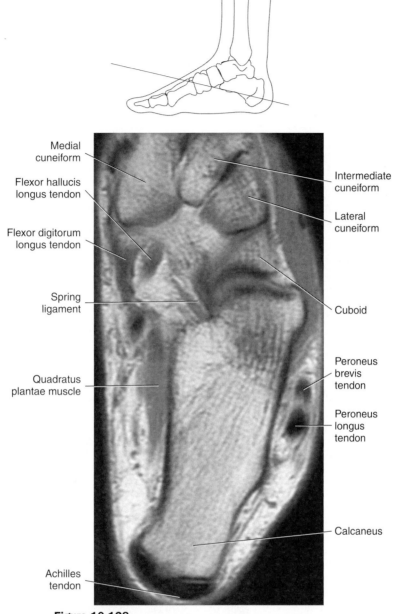

Medial
cuneiform

Flexor hallucis
longus tendon

Flexor digitorum
longus tendon

Spring
ligament

Quadratus
plantae muscle

Achilles
tendon

Intermediate
cuneiform

Lateral
cuneiform

Cuboid

Peroneus
brevis
tendon

Peroneus
longus
tendon

Calcaneus

Figure 10.128
Axial, T1-weighted MR scan of ankle ligaments and tendons.

KEY: TAT, Tibialis anterior tendon; **EHL,** extensor hallucis longus; **EDL,** extensor digitorum longus; **PB,** peroneus brevis; **PL,** peroneus longus; **AT,** Achilles tendon; **FHL,** flexor hallucis longus; **FDL,** flexor digitorum longus; **PTT,** posterior tibialis tendon.

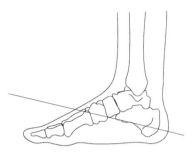

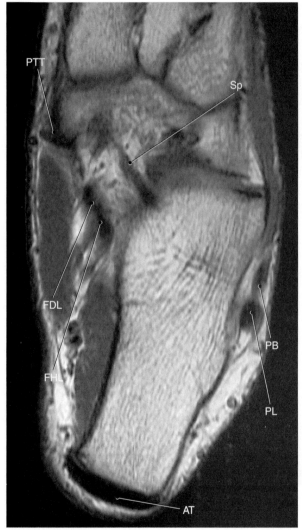

Figure 10.129
Axial, T1-weighted MR scan of ankle ligaments and tendons.

KEY: PTT, Posterior tibialis tendon; **Sp,** spring ligament; **PB,** peroneus brevis; **PL,** peroneus longus; **AT,** Achilles tendon; **FHL,** flexor hallucis longus; **FDL,** flexor digitorum longus.

five separate slips that create the fibrous flexor sheaths of the toes (Figure 10.105). The plantar fascia is extremely important in maintaining the longitudinal arch of the foot. Other support structures of the ankle and foot include a complex architecture of multiple ligaments that provide necessary stability. The main support structures of the ankle include the deltoid ligament, lateral ligaments, spring (plantar) ligament, and interosseous ligament. The **deltoid ligament** provides medial support and is the strongest ligament in the ankle joint. It arises from the medial malleolus and fans out into three bands: **tibiotalar ligament, tibiocalcaneal ligament,** and **tibionavicular ligament** to insert on the talus, calcaneus, and navicular bone, respectively (Figure 10.143). The lateral border of the ankle joint is strengthened by several ligaments termed the **anterior talofibular, calcaneofibular, posterior talofibular, anterior tibiofibular,** and **posterior tibiofibular ligaments** (Figures 10.144 and 10.145). All of these ligaments originate at the fibular malleolus and insert on the adjacent bone structures. The **spring (plantar) ligament** is a triangular band of fibers that arises from the sustentaculum tali and attaches to the posterior surface of the navicular bone (Figure 10.105). It is an important ligament in maintaining the longitudinal arch of the foot. A strong band of tissue binding the talus to the calcaneus is the **interosseous (talocalcaneal) ligament,** which is obliquely oriented in the sinus tarsi (Figures 10.105, 10.106, 10.108, 10.109, and 10.127 through 10.142).

LIGAMENTS OF THE TOES The metatarsophalangeal joint is strengthened laterally by strong collateral ligaments, dorsally from fibers of the extensor tendons, and underneath by the plantar ligament. The **plantar ligament** is a thick fibrocartilaginous plate that attaches to the proximal base of the proximal phalanges, the collateral ligaments, and the deep transverse metatarsal ligaments. The **collateral ligaments** extend from the heads of the metatarsal, fanning out to attach to the bases of the proximal phalanges. The heads of the second through fifth metatarsals are interconnected by the **deep transverse metatarsal ligament.** In a similar manner as the metatarsophalangeal joints, the interphalangeal joints are strengthened laterally by collateral ligaments and on the plantar surface by the plantar ligament.

Tendons

The musculotendinous structures of the ankle can be divided into posterior, anterior, medial, and lateral groups.

POSTERIOR GROUP The posterior group is composed of the single **Achilles tendon (calcaneal),** the largest and most powerful tendon of the body. The Achilles tendon arises from the gastrocnemius and soleus muscles and attaches to the calcaneal tuberosity on the posterior aspect of the calcaneus (Figures 10.101, 10.105, and 10.127 through 10.133).

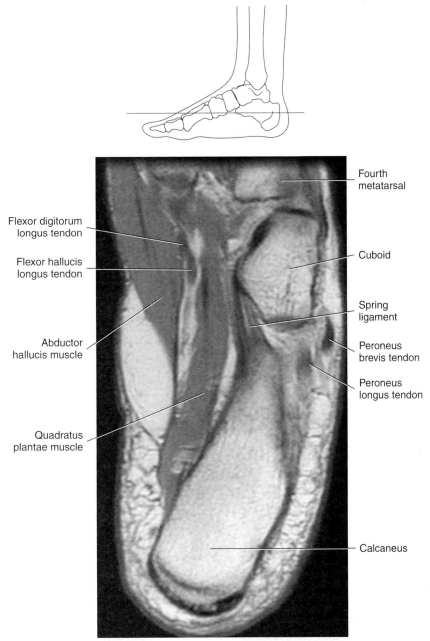

Figure 10.130
Axial, T1-weighted MR scan of ankle ligaments and tendons.

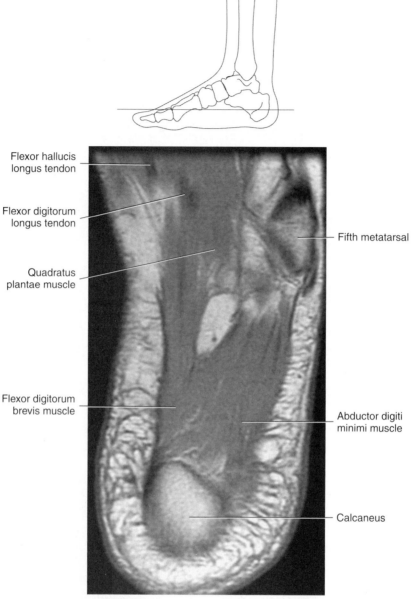

Flexor hallucis
longus tendon

Flexor digitorum
longus tendon

Quadratus
plantae muscle

Flexor digitorum
brevis muscle

Fifth metatarsal

Abductor digiti
minimi muscle

Calcaneus

Figure 10.131
Axial, T1-weighted MR scan of ankle ligaments and tendons.

KEY: TAT, Tibialis anterior tendon; **PTT,** posterior tibialis tendon; **FDL,** flexor digitorum longus;
FHL, flexor hallucis longus; **ti,** tibia; **ta,** talus; **n,** navicular; **c,** calcaneus; **AT,** Achilles tendon;
EHL, extensor hallucis longus; **EDL,** extensor digitorum longus; **sol,** soleus muscle; **IO,** interosseus
ligament; **af,** acetabular fossa; **mf,** medial facet; **pf,** posterior facet.

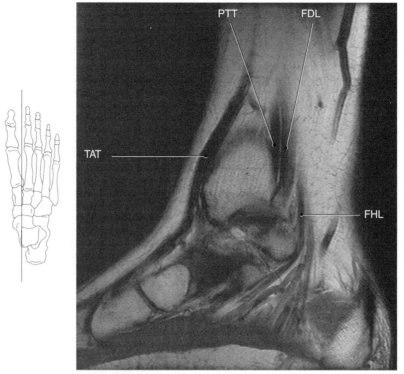

Figure 10.132
Sagittal, T1-weighted MR scan of ankle ligaments and tendons.

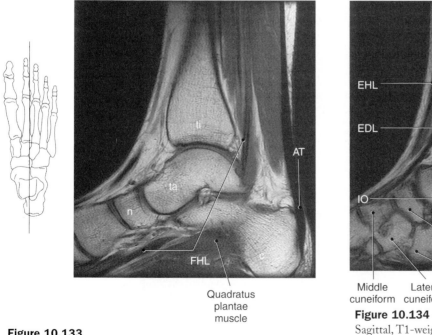

Figure 10.133
Sagittal, T1-weighted MR scan of ankle ligaments and tendons.

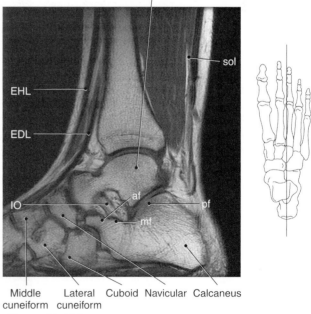

Figure 10.134
Sagittal, T1-weighted MR scan of ankle ligaments and tendons.

KEY: **fi**, Fibula; **PB**, peroneus brevis; **PL**, peroneus longus; **PTBF,** posterior tibiofibular ligament; **PTF,** posterior talofibular ligament; **CF,** calcaneofibular ligament; **PTT,** posterior tibialis tendon; **FDL,** flexor digitorum longus; **FHL,** flexor hallucis longus; **ATF,** anterior talofibular ligament; **ti,** tibia; **del,** deltoid ligaments; **ta,** talus; **C,** calcaneus.

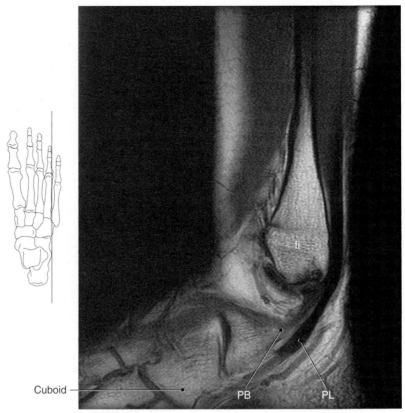

Figure 10.135
Sagittal, T1-weighted MR scan of ankle ligaments and tendons.

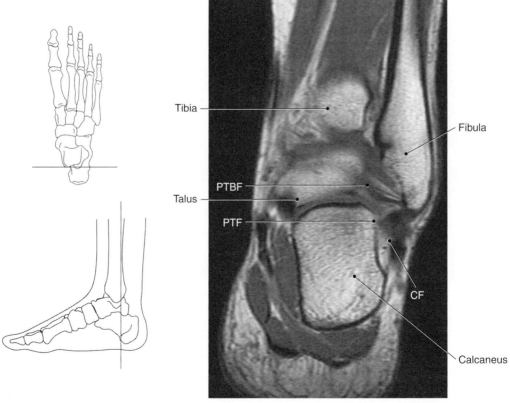

Figure 10.136
Coronal, T1-weighted MR scan of ankle ligaments and tendons.

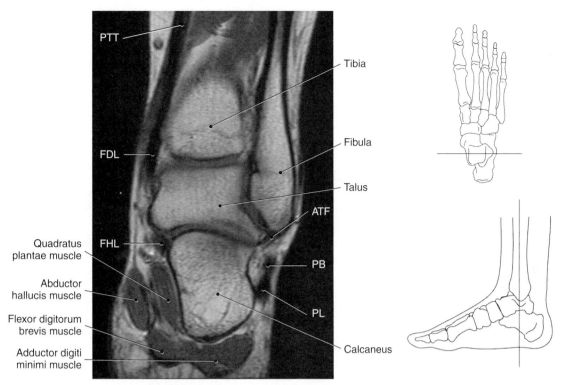

Figure 10.137
Coronal, T1-weighted MR scan of ankle ligaments and tendons.

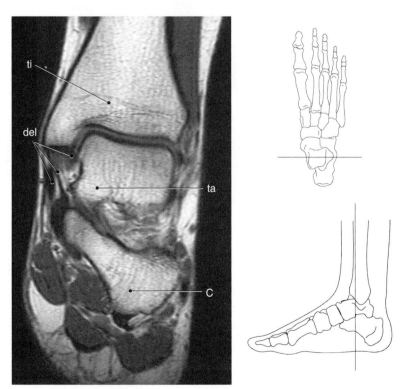

Figure 10.138
Coronal, T1-weighted MR scan of ankle ligaments and tendons.

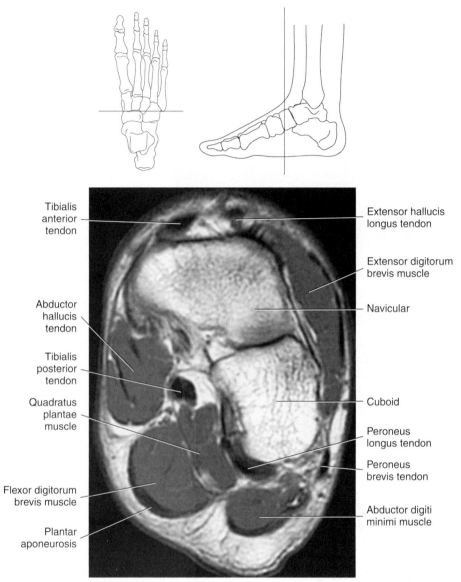

Figure 10.139
Coronal, T1-weighted MR scan of ankle ligaments and tendons.

ANTERIOR GROUP   The anterior group is made up of the tibialis anterior, extensor hallucis longus, and extensor digitorum longus tendons, which are named medial to lateral and act to extend and dorsiflex the foot. The **tibialis anterior** muscle becomes tendinous at the distal tibia and attaches to the plantar and medial aspects of the first cuneiform and metatarsal bones. The tendon of the **extensor hallucis longus** muscle originates from the anterior fibula and inserts on the great toe. The most lateral of this group is the **extensor digitorum longus tendon,** which originates at the level of the lateral malleolus and inserts on the second through the fifth digits (Figures 10.126 through 10.142).

MEDIAL GROUP   The medial group is composed of the posterior tibialis tendons, flexor digitorum longus, and flexor hallucis longus tendons, which as a group act to invert and plantar flex the foot. The **posterior tibialis tendon** fans out in multiple strands that insert on the plantar aspect of the sustentaculum tali, navicular bone, first cuneiform bone, and second through fourth metatarsal bones. Coursing posterior and lateral to the posterior tibialis tendon is the **flexor digitorum longus tendon,** which at its terminal portion inserts on the second through fourth phalanges. The tendon of the **flexor hallucis longus** muscle curves under the sustentaculum tali and then courses along the plantar surface of the foot to insert on the great toe (Figures 10.126 through 10.142).

LATERAL GROUP   The two peroneus tendons, **peroneus longus** and **peroneus brevis,** make up the lateral group and act to evert, weakly plantar flex the foot, and stabilize the ankle joint laterally. These two tendons share a common tendinous sheath behind the lateral malleolus. Below the malleolus they diverge into separate tendon sheaths, with the peroneus brevis tendon inserting on the base of the fifth metatarsal and the peroneus longus tendon curving beneath the calcaneus to insert on the base of the first metatarsal and medial cuneiform bones (Figures 10.126 through 10.142).

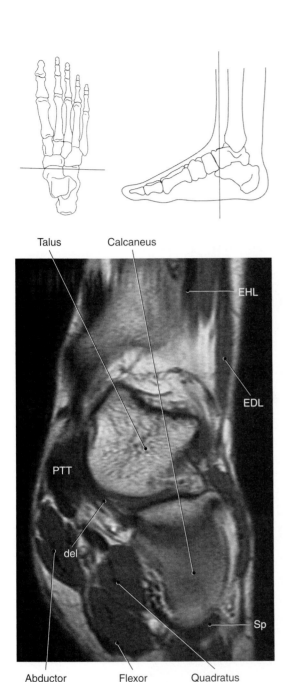

Figure 10.140
Coronal, T1-weighted MR scan of ankle ligaments and tendons.

KEY: **PTT,** Posterior tibialis tendon; **del,** deltoid ligament; **EHL,** extensor hallucis longus; **EDL,** extensor digitorum longus; **Sp,** spring ligament.

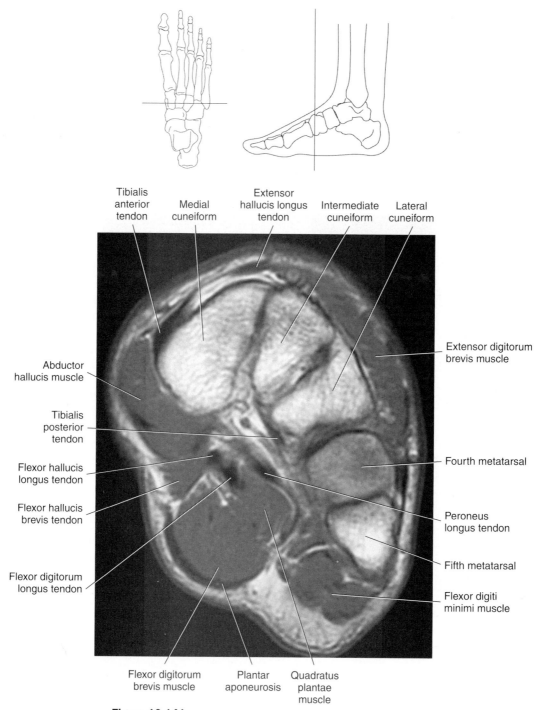

Tibialis anterior tendon

Medial cuneiform

Extensor hallucis longus tendon

Intermediate cuneiform

Lateral cuneiform

Abductor hallucis muscle

Tibialis posterior tendon

Flexor hallucis longus tendon

Flexor hallucis brevis tendon

Flexor digitorum longus tendon

Extensor digitorum brevis muscle

Fourth metatarsal

Peroneus longus tendon

Fifth metatarsal

Flexor digiti minimi muscle

Flexor digitorum brevis muscle

Plantar aponeurosis

Quadratus plantae muscle

Figure 10.141
Coronal, T1-weighted MR scan of ankle ligaments and tendons.

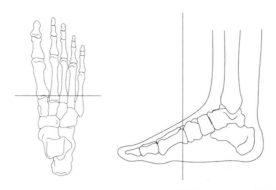

First metatarsal

Abductor hallucis
(oblique head)

Abductor hallucis
muscle

Flexor hallucis
brevis muscle

Flexor hallucis
longus muscle

Plantar
aponeurosis

Flexor digitorum
brevis muscle

Flexor digiti
minimi muscle

Second metatarsal

Third metatarsal

Interosseous
muscles

Fourth metatarsal

Fifth metatarsal

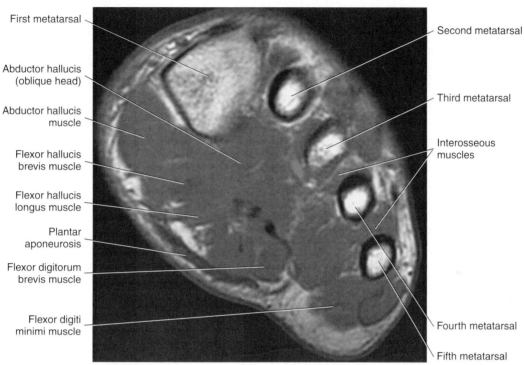

Figure 10.142
Coronal, T1-weighted MR scan of ankle ligaments and tendons.

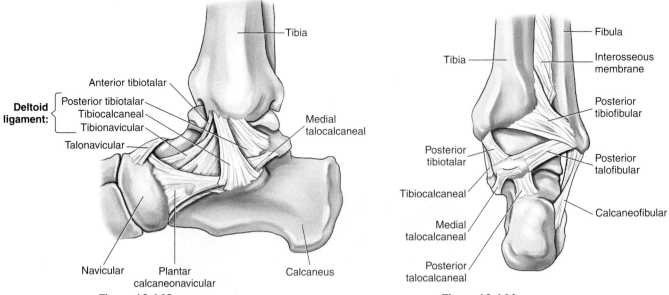

Figure 10.143
Ligaments of right foot, medial view.

Ligaments of right foot, posterior view.
Figure 10.144

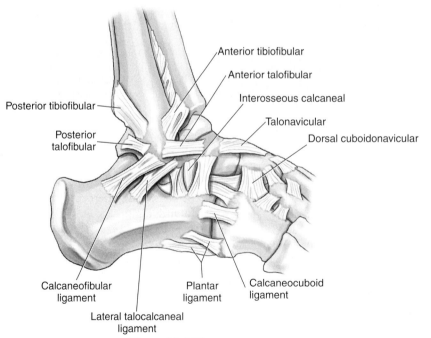

Figure 10.145
Ligaments of right foot, lateral view.

Muscles

The muscles of the foot are divided into the **muscles of the dorsum** and **muscles of the sole of the foot.** These muscles are demonstrated in Figures 10.127 through 10.142 and 10.146 through 10.148 and are described in Table 10.4. The dorsal muscles include the extensor digitorum brevis and the extensor hallucis brevis muscles, which form a fleshy mass on the lateral part of the dorsal foot. The **extensor digitorum brevis** muscle arises from the anterior, upper surface of the calcaneus and passes obliquely across the dorsum to end in three tendons that insert onto the dorsal aponeurosis of the second through fourth digits (Figure 10.146). The extensor digitorum brevis muscle is responsible for dorsiflexion of the second through fourth digits. The **extensor hallucis brevis muscle** splits off of the extensor digitorum brevis muscle to insert on the dorsal aponeurosis of the first toe. It acts to dorsiflex the first digit (Figure 10.147, *A*). The muscles of the sole of the foot can be described by four muscular layers.

FIRST LAYER   The muscles located within the first layer are the most superficial and include the abductor hallucis, flexor digitorum brevis, and abductor digiti minimi muscles (Figure 10.147, *A*). The **abductor hallucis muscle** arises from the medial process of the calcaneal tuberosity and lies along the medial border of the foot to insert on the medial base of the proximal phalanx of the first digit. The **flexor digitorum brevis** muscle also arises from the medial process of the calcaneal tuberosity as well as the plantar aponeurosis to insert on both sides of the middle phalanges of the lateral four digits. The **abductor digiti minimi muscle** arises from the lateral process of the calcaneal tuberosity, the tuberosity of the fifth metatarsal, and the plantar aponeurosis to form the lateral margin of the foot. It inserts on the lateral side of the base of the proximal phalanx of the fifth digit.

SECOND LAYER   This layer is located deep to the first layer and includes the quadratus plantae and lumbrical muscles (Figure 10.147, *B*). The **quadratus plantae muscle** is a small flat muscle that arises as two small slips from the medial and lateral margins of the plantar surface of the calcaneus and joins with the tendon of the flexor digitorum longus that continues to the distal phalanges of the lateral four digits. The four small **lumbrical muscles** arise from the medial surfaces of the individual tendons of the flexor digitorum longus. They insert on the medial margin of the proximal phalanges of the second through fifth digits and extend into the extensor aponeurosis.

THIRD LAYER   The third layer consists of three muscles: the flexor hallucis brevis, adductor hallucis, and flexor digiti minimi brevis muscles (Figure 10.147, *C*). The **flexor hallucis brevis muscle** arises from the medial cuneiform bone and the tibialis posterior tendon. It has two heads that cover the plantar surface of the first metatarsal extending to both sides of the base of the proximal phalanx of the first digit. The **adductor hallucis muscle** has two heads; the oblique head arises from the cuboid and lateral cuneiform bones and the bases of the second and third metatarsals, and the transverse head arises

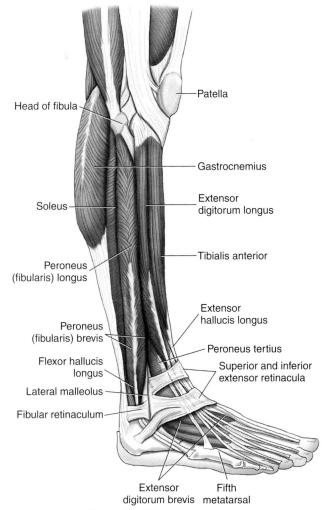

Figure 10.146
Extensor tendons of the lower leg.

from the deep transverse metatarsal ligament and the metatarsal joint capsule. Both heads insert on the lateral side of the base of the proximal phalanx of the first digit. The slender **flexor digiti minimi muscle** arises from the base of the fifth metatarsal and inserts on the base of the proximal phalanx of the fifth digit.

FOURTH LAYER   This layer consists of the interosseous muscles (Figures 10.147, *D* and 10.148). Three plantar and four dorsal interossei muscles are located between the metatarsal bones. The **plantar interosseous muscles** arise from the bases and medial surfaces of the third through fifth metatarsals and insert on the medial sides of the bases of the proximal phalanges of the third through fifth digits. The **dorsal interosseous muscles** are larger than their plantar counterparts, arising from adjacent surfaces of the metatarsal bones and extending to attach to the sides of the proximal phalanx and capsules of the metatarsal phalangeal joints of the second through fourth digits (Figures 10.127 through 10.142 and 10.148).

TABLE 10-4   Muscles of the Foot

MUSCLE	PROXIMAL INSERTION	DISTAL INSERTION	ACTION
Dorsal Surface			
Extensor digitorum brevis	Calcaneus	Second-fourth digits of the foot	Dorsiflexion of second-fourth digits
Extensor hallucis brevis	Extensor digitorum brevis	First toe	Dorsiflexes the first digit
Sole of Foot			
First Layer			
Abductor hallucis	Calcaneal tuberosity	Proximal phalanx of first digit	Abducts first toe from second, flexes metatarsophalangeal joint
Flexor digitorum brevis	Calcaneal tuberosity and plantar aponeurosis	Middle phalanges of second-fifth digits	Flexes metatarsophalangeal and proximal interphalangeal joints of second-fifth digits
Abductor digiti minimi	Calcaneal tuberosity, fifth metatarsal	Proximal phalanx of fifth digit	Abducts fifth toe and flexes metatarsophalangeal joint
Second Layer			
Quadratus plantae	Calcaneus	Distal phalanges of second-fifth digits	Assists the flexor digitorum longus in flexion of toes
Lumbrical	Flexor digitorum longus tendons	Proximal phalanges of second-fifth digits	Flexes metatarsophalangeal joints, extends proximal and distal interphalangeal joints of second-fifth digits
Third Layer			
Flexor hallucis brevis	Medial cuneiform and tibialis posterior tendon	Proximal phalanx of first digit	Flexes metatarsophalangeal joint of first toe
Adductor hallucis		Proximal phalanx of first digit	Adduct first toe toward second and flexes first toe
Oblique head	Cuboid, lateral cuneiform and second and third metatarsals		
Transverse head	Transverse metatarsal ligament and metatarsal joint capsule		
Flexor digiti minimi	Fifth metatarsal	Proximal phalanx of fifth digit	Flexes metatarsophalangeal joint of fifth digit
Fourth Layer			
Plantar interosseous	Third-fifth metatarsals	Proximal phalanges of third-fifth digits	Adducts third-fifth toes, flexes metatarsophalangeal and extends interphalangeal joints of third-fifth digits
Dorsal interosseous	Metatarsals	Proximal phalanx and capsules of metatarsal phalangeal joints of second-fourth digits	Abducts second-fourth digits away from midline, flexes metatarsophalangeal joints, and extends interphalangeal joints of second-fourth digits

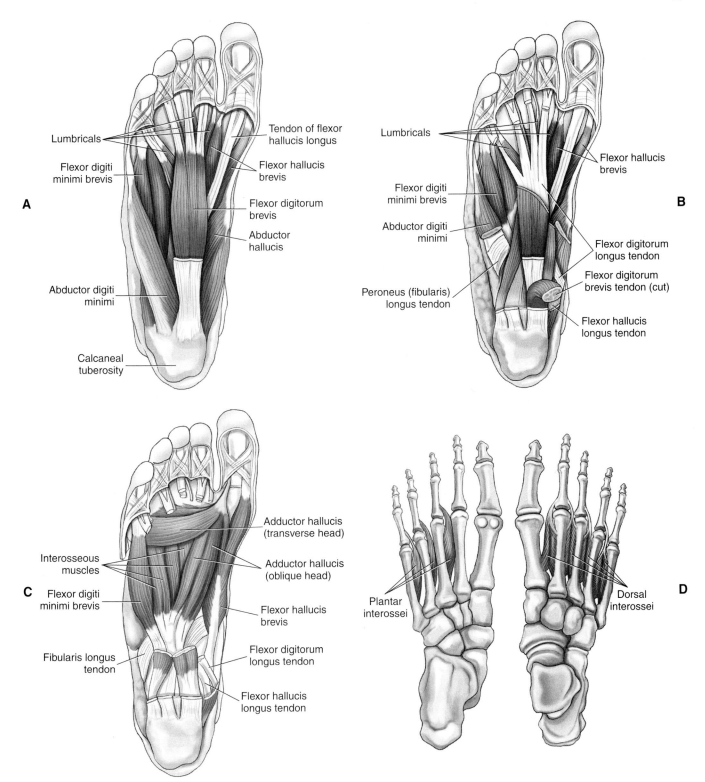

Figure 10.147
Dorsal view of muscles of right foot. **A,** First layer. **B,** Second layer. **C,** Third layer.
D, Fourth layer.

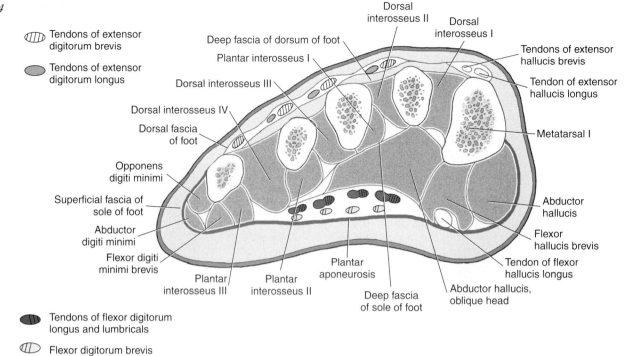

Tendons of extensor digitorum brevis

Tendons of extensor digitorum longus

Tendons of flexor digitorum longus and lumbricals

Flexor digitorum brevis

Dorsal interosseus II

Dorsal interosseus I

Deep fascia of dorsum of foot

Tendons of extensor hallucis brevis

Plantar interosseus I

Tendon of extensor hallucis longus

Dorsal interosseus III

Dorsal interosseus IV

Metatarsal I

Dorsal fascia of foot

Opponens digiti minimi

Abductor hallucis

Superficial fascia of sole of foot

Flexor hallucis brevis

Abductor digiti minimi

Tendon of flexor hallucis longus

Flexor digiti minimi brevis

Abductor hallucis, oblique head

Plantar interosseus III

Plantar interosseus II

Plantar aponeurosis

Deep fascia of sole of foot

Figure 10.148
Coronal view of muscles of foot at metatarsals.

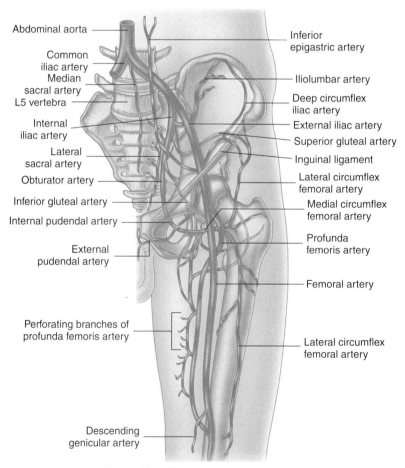

Abdominal aorta

Inferior epigastric artery

Common iliac artery

Iliolumbar artery

Median sacral artery

Deep circumflex iliac artery

L5 vertebra

External iliac artery

Internal iliac artery

Superior gluteal artery

Lateral sacral artery

Inguinal ligament

Obturator artery

Lateral circumflex femoral artery

Inferior gluteal artery

Medial circumflex femoral artery

Internal pudendal artery

Profunda femoris artery

External pudendal artery

Femoral artery

Perforating branches of profunda femoris artery

Lateral circumflex femoral artery

Descending genicular artery

Figure 10.149
Anterior view of iliac and femoral arteries.

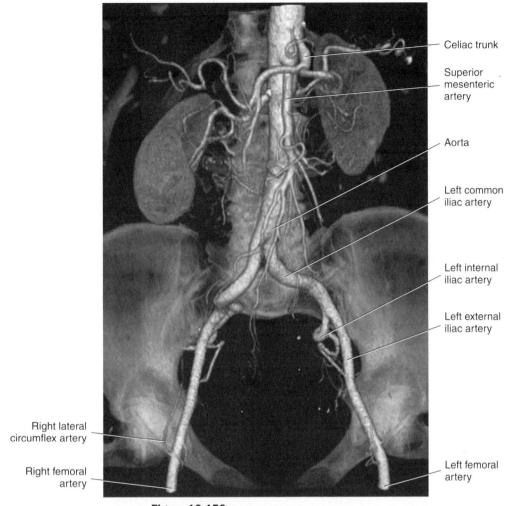

Figure 10.150
3D CT angiography of iliac and femoral arteries.

NEUROVASCULATURE

Arteries

Traveling vertically along the anteromedian aspect of the hip is the femoral artery. The **femoral artery,** an extension of the external iliac artery, enters the anterior compartment of the thigh behind the inguinal ligament, where it is relatively superficial and easily palpable (Figures 10.149 through 10.153). It descends the thigh and continues through the opening in the adductor magnus muscle as the popliteal artery in the knee. The femoral artery and its main branches, superficial and deep, supply all the compartments of the thigh as well as the skin of the anterior abdominal wall, inguinal region, and external genitalia. The superficial branches of the femoral artery accompany the veins of the groin and include the **inferior epigastric, superficial circumflex iliac,** and the **external pudendal arteries.** The largest deep branch of the femoral artery is the **profunda femoris artery,** which arises from the posterolateral aspect of the femoral artery about 4 cm below the inguinal ligament and runs distally behind the femoral artery (Figures 10.151 through 10.153). It passes between the vastus medialis muscle and the muscles of the adductor group. The profundus femoris gives off two large branches: the **medial** and **lateral circumflex femoral arteries** (Figures 10.154 and 10.155). The branches curve around the proximal femur and hip joint to supply the muscles of the adductor group and parts of the gluteal musculature, as well as the extensors and flexors at the thigh. The terminal branches of the profunda femoris artery are the **perforating arteries** (3-5) near the linea aspera that pass through the adductor muscles. One of the perforating arteries gives a large nutrient branch to the head of the femur (Figures 10.154 and 10.155).

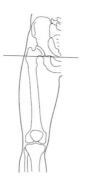

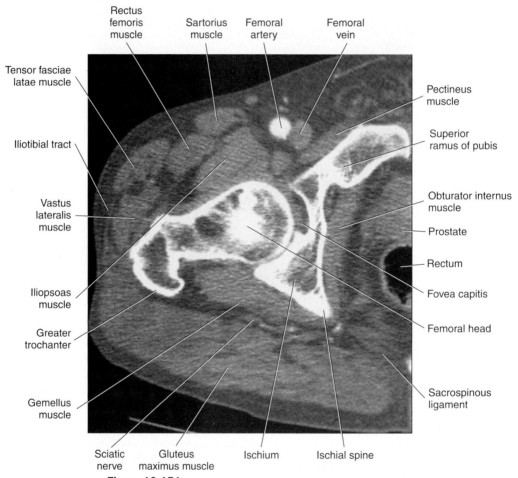

Rectus femoris muscle

Sartorius muscle

Femoral artery

Femoral vein

Tensor fasciae latae muscle

Iliotibial tract

Vastus lateralis muscle

Iliopsoas muscle

Greater trochanter

Gemellus muscle

Pectineus muscle

Superior ramus of pubis

Obturator internus muscle

Prostate

Rectum

Fovea capitis

Femoral head

Sacrospinous ligament

Sciatic nerve

Gluteus maximus muscle

Ischium

Ischial spine

Figure 10.151

Axial, contrast-enhanced CT scan of hip with femoral artery.

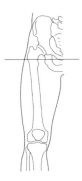

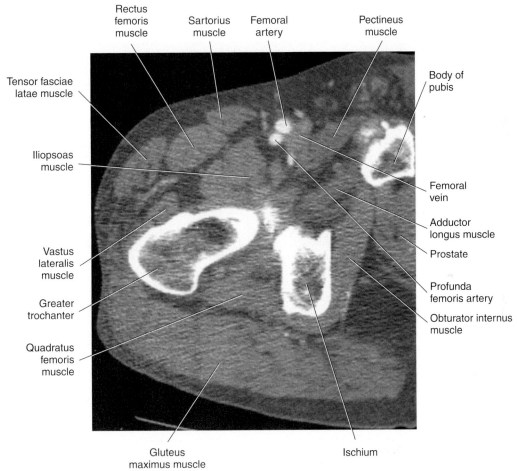

Rectus femoris muscle

Sartorius muscle

Femoral artery

Pectineus muscle

Tensor fasciae latae muscle

Body of pubis

Iliopsoas muscle

Femoral vein

Adductor longus muscle

Vastus lateralis muscle

Prostate

Greater trochanter

Profunda femoris artery

Quadratus femoris muscle

Obturator internus muscle

Gluteus maximus muscle

Ischium

Figure 10.152

Axial, contrast-enhanced CT scan of hip with femoral artery and vein.

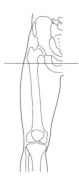

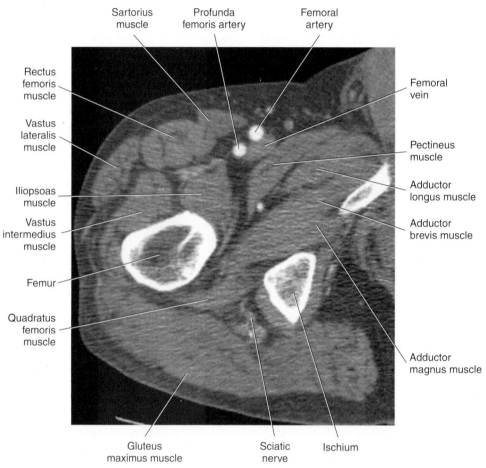

Sartorius muscle

Profunda femoris artery

Femoral artery

Rectus femoris muscle

Vastus lateralis muscle

Iliopsoas muscle

Vastus intermedius muscle

Femur

Quadratus femoris muscle

Femoral vein

Pectineus muscle

Adductor longus muscle

Adductor brevis muscle

Adductor magnus muscle

Gluteus maximus muscle

Sciatic nerve

Ischium

Figure 10.153
Axial, contrast-enhanced CT scan of hip with profundus femoris artery.

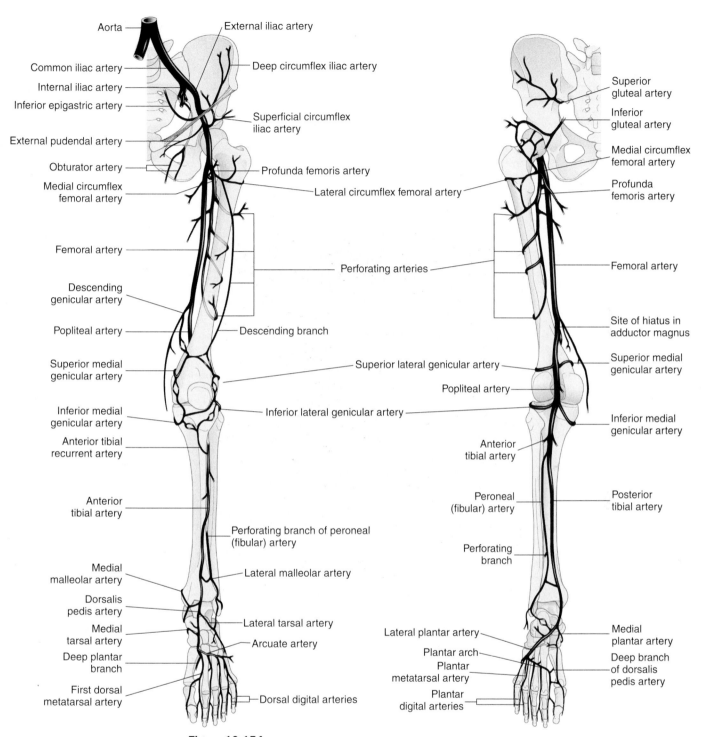

Figure 10.154
Arteries of lower extremity. *Left,* Anterior view. *Right,* Posterior view.

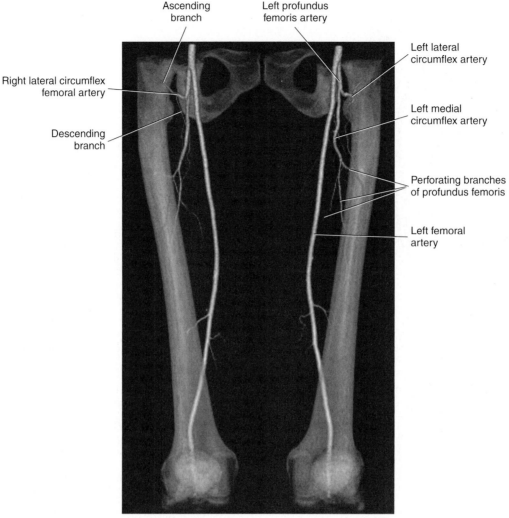

Ascending branch

Left profundus femoris artery

Right lateral circumflex femoral artery

Left lateral circumflex artery

Descending branch

Left medial circumflex artery

Perforating branches of profundus femoris

Left femoral artery

Figure 10.155
3D CT angiography of femoral artery.

POPLITEAL ARTERY   The popliteal artery is the continuation of the femoral artery. It runs deep near the bones of the knee joint during its course through the popliteal fossa. It passes distally over the popliteus muscle and divides into the **anterior** and **posterior tibial arteries** (Figures 10.154 through 10.156). The tibial nerve and popliteal vein accompany the popliteal artery, the tibial nerve being the most superficial of the structures in the popliteal fossa (Figures 10.157 and 10.158). The popliteal artery supplies the surrounding muscles and forms a substantial plexus of articular branches anastomosing around the knee joint. The popliteal artery gives off branches to portions of the thigh muscles near the knee joint, dispatches the **sural arteries** distally to the gastrocnemius muscle, and supplies the knee joint with the anastomosing **genicular arteries** (lateral superior, lateral inferior, medial superior, medial inferior, and descending) (Figure 10.159).

ANTERIOR TIBIAL ARTERY   The anterior tibial artery courses anteriorly at the level of the fibular head into the anterior compartment of the lower leg. It runs distally as far as

the anterior side of the ankle, where it becomes the dorsalis pedis artery. The branches of the anterior tibial artery are the posterior tibial recurrent, the anterior tibial recurrent, the medial anterior malleolar, the lateral anterior malleolar, and numerous muscular branches (Figures 10.154, 10.156, and 10.159).

POSTERIOR TIBIAL ARTERY   The posterior tibial artery is usually larger than the anterior tibial artery. As it passes distally in the posterior compartment, it courses toward the medial side of the leg. The posterior tibial artery terminates by dividing into the medial and lateral plantar arteries in the foot. The **peroneal (fibular) artery** arises from the posterior tibial artery approximately 2 cm below the distal border of the popliteal muscle. It descends posteriorly along the medial aspect of the fibula and terminates on the lateral surface of the calcaneal tuberosity. Branches of the peroneal artery include the fibular nutrient, communicating, perforating, posterior lateral malleolar, and lateral calcaneal, as well as numerous muscular and cutaneous branches (Figures 10.154, 10.156, and 10.159).

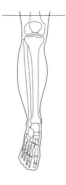

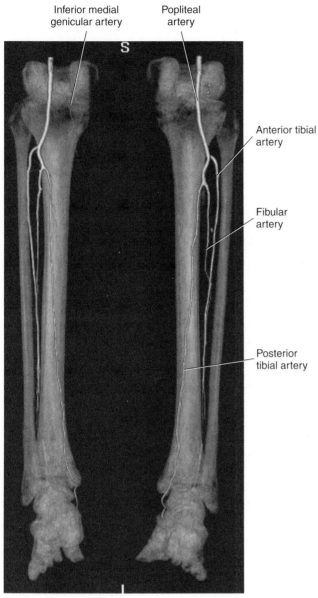

Figure 10.156
3D CT angiography of tibial and fibular arteries.

Figure 10.157
Axial, T1-weighted MR scan of knee with vessels.

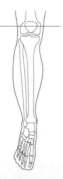

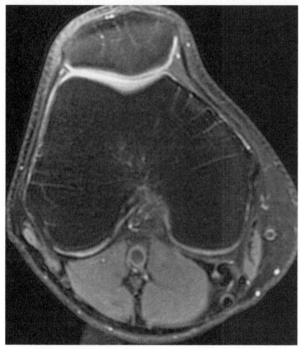

Figure 10.158
Axial, T1-weighted MR scan of knee with vessels.

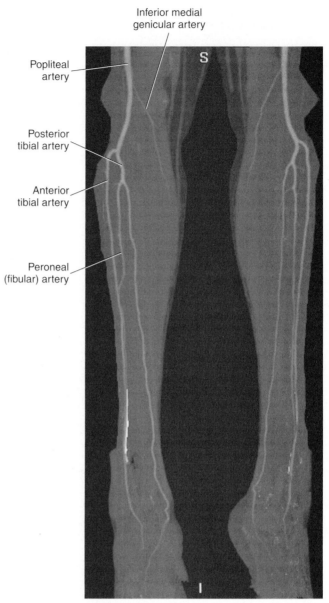

Inferior medial genicular artery

Popliteal artery

Posterior tibial artery

Anterior tibial artery

Peroneal (fibular) artery

S

I

Figure 10.159
CT MIP of lower leg arteries.

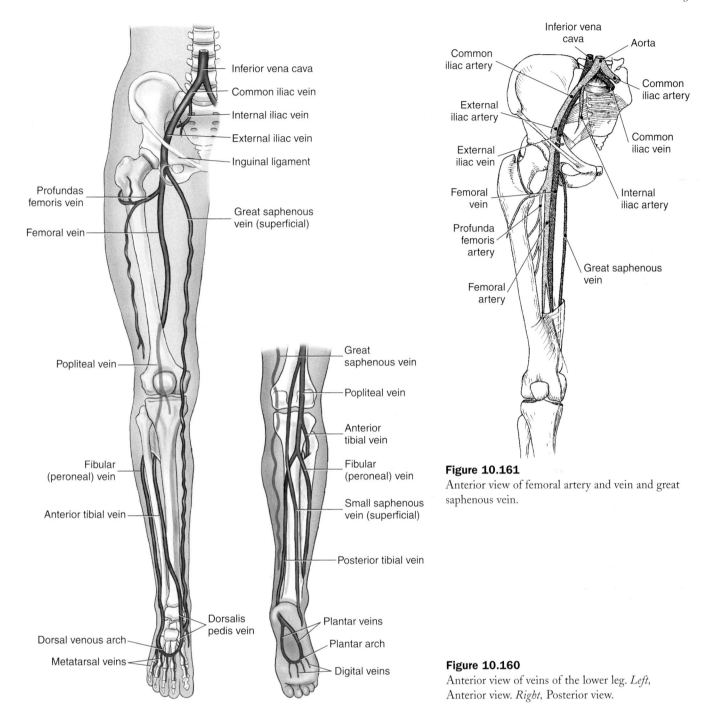

Figure 10.161
Anterior view of femoral artery and vein and great saphenous vein.

Figure 10.160
Anterior view of veins of the lower leg. *Left,* Anterior view. *Right,* Posterior view.

Veins

There are two groups of veins of the lower extremity: superficial and deep. The superficial veins arise in the foot from the dorsal venous arch and merge chiefly into two main trunks, the great saphenous and the small saphenous. The **great saphenous vein** ascends the medial aspect of the leg and thigh to drain into the femoral vein near the hip joint. From the lateral side of the foot, the **small saphenous vein** passes posterolaterally to join the popliteal vein (Figure 10.160).

Between these two superficial veins and the system of the deep veins are numerous deep anastomoses. The deep veins accompany their corresponding arteries. The deep veins begin distally as venae comitantes of the **anterior** and **posterior tibial veins** that unite to form the **popliteal vein.** This becomes the **femoral vein** in the thigh, which courses medial to the femoral artery and continues deep to the inguinal ligament as the **external iliac vein** (Figures 10.151 through 10.153 and 10.160 and 10.161).

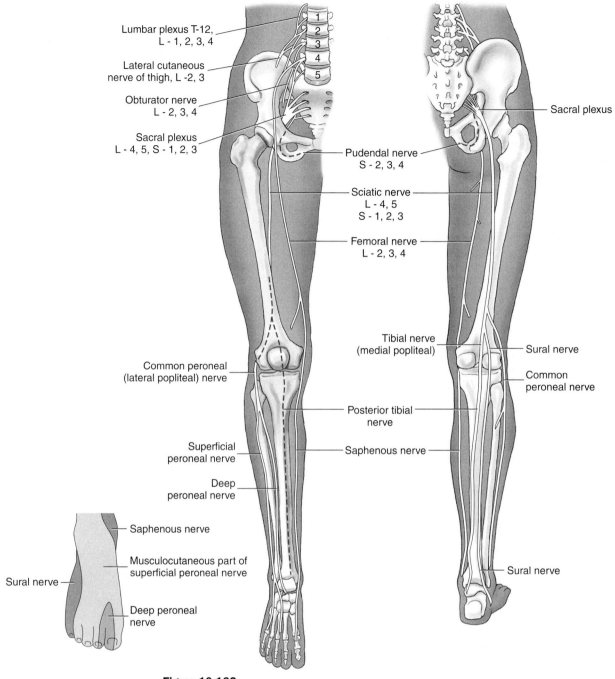

Lumbar plexus T-12,
L - 1, 2, 3, 4

Lateral cutaneous
nerve of thigh, L -2, 3

Obturator nerve
L - 2, 3, 4

Sacral plexus
L - 4, 5, S - 1, 2, 3

Sacral plexus

Pudendal nerve
S - 2, 3, 4

Sciatic nerve
L - 4, 5
S - 1, 2, 3

Femoral nerve
L - 2, 3, 4

Tibial nerve
(medial popliteal)

Sural nerve

Common
peroneal nerve

Common peroneal
(lateral popliteal) nerve

Posterior tibial
nerve

Superficial
peroneal nerve

Saphenous nerve

Deep
peroneal nerve

Saphenous nerve

Musculocutaneous part of
superficial peroneal nerve

Sural nerve

Sural nerve

Deep peroneal
nerve

Figure 10.162
Anterior and posterior views of right leg and foot with nerves.

Nerves

The nerves of the lower extremity are derived from the lumbar and sacral plexuses (see Chapter 4). The **femoral nerve** enters the thigh beneath the inguinal ligament and divides into several superficial and deep branches to supply the anterior compartment of the thigh. The femoral nerve terminates as the **saphenous nerve** to innervate the skin on the medial side of the leg and foot. The **obturator nerve** courses through the obturator canal and immediately divides into anterior and posterior divisions to supply the medial compartment of the thigh. The **sciatic nerve** is the largest peripheral nerve in the body. Its branches supply the posterior compartment of the thigh and all compartments of the distal leg and foot. The sciatic nerve runs deep to the gluteus maximus muscle and descends in the midline of the thigh, where it usually divides into two terminal branches: the **tibial** and **common peroneal (common fibular) nerves** (Figures 10.153, 10.157, 10.158, and 10.162).

ILLUSTRATION CREDITS

Chapter 1

Figure 1.4 from Applegate E: *The sectional anatomy learning system,* ed 2, Philadelphia, 2002, Saunders.

Figures 1.7, 1.9, 1.11 from Ballinger PW: *Merrill's atlas of radiographic positions and radiologic procedures,* ed 10, St. Louis, 2003, Mosby.

Figure 1.8 from Jacobs S: *Atlas of human anatomy,* Philadelphia, 2002, Churchill Livingstone.

Figure 1.12 from Seeram, E: *Computed tomography: Basic principles, clinical applications, and quality control,* ed 2, Philadelphia, 2001, Saunders.

Figure 1.13 from Mitchell DG: *MRI principles,* ed 2, Philadelphia, 2004, Saunders.

Figure 1.15 from Stark DD, Bradley WG: *Magnetic resonance imaging,* ed 3, St. Louis, 1999, Mosby.

Chapter 2

Figures 2.2, 2.3, 2.15, 2.17, 2.24, 2.60, 2.61, 2.73 from Ballinger PW: *Merrill's atlas of radiographic positions and radiologic procedures,* ed 10, St. Louis, 2003, Mosby.

Figure 2.21 from *Mosby's medical, nursing, and allied health dictionary,* ed 6, St. Louis, 2002, Mosby.

Figures 2.37, 2.43, 2.57, 2.58, 2.62, 2.68, 2.72, 2.80, 2.82, 2.99, 2.100, 2.102, 2.113 from Som PM, Curtin HD: *Head and neck imaging,* ed 4, St. Louis, 2003, Mosby.

Chapter 3

Figure 3.9 from Ballinger PW: *Merrill's atlas of radiographic positions and radiologic procedures,* ed 10, St. Louis, 2003, Mosby.

Figures 3.17, 3.35 from Applegate E: *The anatomy and physiology learning system,* ed 2, Philadelphia, 2000, Saunders.

Figures 3.45, 3.85, 3.99 from Standring S: *Gray's anatomy,* ed 39, Philadelphia, 2005, Churchill Livingstone.

Figures 3.60, 3.73, 3.107, 3.108, 3.113, 3.114, 3.128 from Fitzgerald MJT: *Clinical neuroanatomy and related neuroscience,* ed 4, Philadelphia, 2002, Saunders.

Figure 3.88 from Krayenbuhl H, Yasargil M: *Cerebral angiography,* ed 2, London, 1968, Butterworth.

Figure 3.90 from Noback CR, Demarest RJ: *The nervous system: Introduction and review,* New York, 1972, McGraw-Hill.

Figure 3.98 from Langley LL, et al: *Dynamic anatomy and physiology,* ed 4, New York, 1974, McGraw-Hill. Copyright Mosby–Year Book, Inc.

Figure 3.110 from Weir J: *Imaging atlas of human anatomy,* ed 3, St. Louis, 2003, Mosby.

Figure 3.125 from Jacob S: *Atlas of human anatomy,* Philadelphia, 2002, Churchill Livingstone.

Chapter 4

Figure 4.7 from Ballinger PW: *Merrill's atlas of radiographic positions and radiologic procedures,* ed 10, St. Louis, 2003, Mosby.

Figures 4.19, 4.50, 4.51, 4.54, 4.55, 4.58, 4.59B from Larsen WL: *Anatomy development, function, clinical correlations,* Philadelphia, 2002, Saunders.

Figures 4.45, 4.59A, 4.78 from Standring S: *Gray's anatomy,* ed 39, Philadelphia, 2005, Churchill Livingstone.

Figures 4.56, 4.99 from Som PM, Curtin HD: *Head and neck imaging,* ed 4, St. Louis, 2003, Mosby.

Figure 4.62 from *Mosby's medical, nursing, and allied health dictionary,* ed 6, St. Louis, 2002, Mosby.

Figure 4.63 from Jacobs S: *Atlas of human anatomy,* Philadelphia, 2002, Churchill Livingstone.

Figure 4.68 from Weir J: *Imaging atlas of human anatomy,* ed 3, St. Louis, 2003, Mosby.

Figures 4.90, 4.91, 4.94 from Palastanga N, Field D, Soames R, et al: *Anatomy and human movement,* ed 4, Boston, 2002, Butterworth-Heinemann.

Figures 4.105, 4.107, 4.109 from Stark DD, Bradley WG: *Magnetic resonance imaging,* ed 3, St. Louis, 1999, Mosby.

Figure 4.114 Netter illustration used with permission from Icon Learning Systems, a division of MediMedia USA, Inc. All rights reserved.

Chapter 5

Figure 5.2 from Applegate E: *The anatomy and physiology learning system,* ed 2, Philadelphia, 2000, Saunders.

Figures 5.14, 5.45, 5.47, 5.48, 5.49, 5.50, 5.73 from Som PM, Curtin HD: *Head and neck imaging,* ed 4, St. Louis, 2003, Mosby.

Figure 5.17 from *Mosby's medical, nursing, and allied health dictionary,* ed 6, St. Louis, 2002, Mosby.

Figures 5.65, 5.66, 5.67, 5.68, 5.69, 5.70 from Standring S: *Gray's anatomy,* ed 39, Philadelphia, 2005, Churchill Livingstone.

Figure 5.74 from Curry RA, Tempkin BB: *Sonography: Introduction to normal structure and function,* ed 2, Philadelphia, 2004, Saunders.

Chapter 6

Figure 6.3 courtesy Anne Marie Sawyer, Radiologic Sciences Laboratory, Stanford University School of Medicine, Stanford, Calif.

Figure 6.7 from Ballinger PW: *Merrill's atlas of radiographic positions and radiologic procedures,* ed 10, St. Louis, 2003, Mosby.

Figures 6.14, 6.23, 6.69, 6.72 from Standring S: *Gray's anatomy,* ed 39, Philadelphia, 2005, Churchill Livingstone.

Figures 6.15, 6.37, 6.41, 6.43, 6.45, 6.78, 6.80, 6.81, 6.82 from Manning WJ, Pennell DJ: *Cardiovascular magnetic resonance,* Philadelphia, 2002, Churchill Livingstone.

Figures 6.21, 6.109 from Palastanga N, Field D, Soames R, et al: *Anatomy and human movement,* ed 4, Boston, 2002, Butterworth-Heinemann.

Figures 6.25, 6.30 from Haaga JR, Lanzieri CF, Gilkeson RC, et al: *CT and MR imaging of the whole body,* ed 4, St. Louis, 2003, Mosby.

Figure 6.29 from Mountain CF: Revisions in the international system for staging lung cancer, *Chest* 111:1710, 1997.

Figures 6.32, 6.117 from Seidel HM, Ball JW, Dains JE, et al: *Mosby's guide to physical examination,* ed 5, St. Louis, 2003, Mosby.

Figure 6.33 from Applegate E: *The sectional anatomy learning system,* ed 2, Philadelphia, 2002, Saunders.

Figures 6.35, 6.49, 6.52, 6.53, 6.56, 6.58, 6.62, 6.65, 6.67, 6.70, 6.73, 6.87, 6.101 from Weir J: *Imaging atlas of human anatomy,* ed 3, St. Louis, 2003, Mosby.

Figure 6.39 from Applegate E: *The anatomy and physiology learning system,* ed 2, Philadelphia, 2000, Saunders.

Figure 6.61 from Wilson SF, Thompson JM: *Respiratory disorders,* St. Louis, 1990, Mosby.

Figure 6.103 from Jacobs S: *Atlas of human anatomy,* Philadelphia, 2002, Churchill Livingstone.

Figures 6.106, 6.107 from Larsen WL: *Anatomy development, function, clinical correlations,* Philadelphia, 2002, Saunders.

Figure 6.118 from *Mosby's medical, nursing, and allied health dictionary,* ed 6, St. Louis, 2002, Mosby.

Chapter 7

Figures 7.3, 7.23, 7.27, 7.28, 7.60, 7.67, 7.77, 7.83, 7.146, 7.153, 7.161, 7.164, 7.167, 7.176, 7.181, 7.182 from Hagen-Ansert SL: *Textbook of diagnostic ultrasonography,* ed 5, St. Louis, 2001, Mosby.

Figure 7.6 from Larsen WL: *Anatomy development, function, clinical correlations,* Philadelphia, 2002, Saunders.

Figures 7.8, 7.9, 7.13, 7.16, 7.38, 7.41, 7.44, 7.47, 7.74, 7.75, 7.76, 7.85 from Haaga JR, Lanzieri CF, Gilkeson RC, et al: *CT and MR imaging of the whole body,* ed 4, St. Louis, 2003, Mosby.

Figures 7.12, 7.137, 7.162, 7.168 from Standring S: *Gray's anatomy,* ed 39, Philadelphia, 2005, Churchill Livingstone.

Figures 7.29, 7.108, 7.117, 7.173 from Ballinger PW: *Merrill's atlas of radiographic positions and radiologic procedures,* ed 10, St. Louis, 2003, Mosby.

Figures 7.37, 7.40, 7.43, 7.46, 7.98 from Stark DD, Bradley WG: *Magnetic resonance imaging,* ed 3, St. Louis, 1999, Mosby.

Figures 7.174, 7.175 from Webb WR, Brant WE, Helms CA: *Fundamentals of body CT,* ed 2, Philadelphia, 1998, Saunders.

Chapter 8

Figures 8.8, 8.10 from Ballinger PW: *Merrill's atlas of radiographic positions and radiologic procedures,* ed 10, St. Louis, 2003, Mosby.

Figure 8.18 from Larsen WL: *Anatomy development, function, clinical correlations,* Philadelphia, 2002, Saunders.

Figures 8.25, 8.26, 8.31, 8.57, 8.113 from Hagen-Ansert SL: *Textbook of diagnostic ultrasonography,* ed 5, St. Louis, 2001, Mosby.

Figures 8.39, 8.41, 8.50, 8.70, 8.75, 8.93 from Applegate E: *The anatomy and physiology learning system,* ed 2, Philadelphia, 2000, Saunders.

Figure 8.42 courtesy GE Medical Systems, Milwaukee, Wisc.

Figures 8.47, 8.115 from Seidel HM, Ball JW, Dains JE, et al: *Mosby's guide to physical examination,* ed 5, St. Louis, 2003, Mosby.

Figures 8.77, 8.116, 8.117 from Haaga JR, Lanzieri CF, Gilkeson RC, et al: *CT and MR imaging of the whole body,* ed 4, St. Louis, 2003, Mosby.

Figure 8.90 from Standring S: *Gray's anatomy,* ed 39, Philadelphia, 2005, Churchill Livingstone.

Chapter 9

Figures 9.20, 9.21, 9.22, 9.46, 9.47 from Weir J: *Imaging atlas of human anatomy,* ed 3, St. Louis, 2003, Mosby.

Figures 9.23, 9.24, 9.25, 9.26, 9.27 from Stark DD, Bradley WG: *Magnetic resonance imaging,* ed 3, St. Louis, 1999, Mosby.

Figure 9.31 from Seidel HM, Ball JW, Dains JE, et al: *Mosby's guide to physical examination,* ed 5, St. Louis, 2003, Mosby.

Figures 9.80, 9.117 from Miller MD, Cooper DE: *Review of sports medicine and arthroscopy,* ed 2, Philadelphia, 2002, Saunders.

Figure 9.103 from Ballinger PW: *Merrill's atlas of radiographic positions and radiologic procedures,* ed 10, St. Louis, 2003, Mosby.

Figure 9.115 from Palastanga N, Field D, Soames R, et al: *Anatomy and human movement,* ed 4, Boston, 2002, Butterworth-Heinemann.

Figures 9.125, 9.126 from Kang HS, Ahn JM: *MRI of the extremities,* ed 2, Philadelphia, 2002, Saunders.

Chapter 10

Figure 10.2 from Ballinger PW: *Merrill's atlas of radiographic positions and radiologic procedures,* ed 10, St. Louis, 2003, Mosby.

Figure 10.12 from Byrd JWT: Gross anatomy. In Byrd JET (ed): *Operative hip arthroscopy,* New York, Thieme, 1998, pp. 69-82.

Figures 10.31, 10.32, 10.33, 10.77B, 10.104, 10.126, 10.149, 10.154 from Standring S: *Gray's anatomy,* ed 39, Philadelphia, 2005, Churchill Livingstone.

Figure 10.81 from Stark DD, Bradley WG: *Magnetic resonance imaging,* ed 3, St. Louis, 1999, Mosby.

Figure 10.84 from Haaga JR, Lanzieri CF, Gilkeson RC, et al: *CT and MR imaging of the whole body,* ed 4, St. Louis, 2003, Mosby.

Figures 10.89, 10.90, 10.91, 10.96, 10.97, 10.98, 10.99, 10.140 from Kang HS, Ahn JM: *MRI of the extremities,* ed 2, Philadelphia, 2002, Saunders.

INDEX

NOTE: Page numbers followed by f indicate figures; those followed by t indicate tables.

A

Abdomen, 337–428
  abdominal aorta in, 304, 401–417, 401f, 402f
    paired parietal (dorsal) branches of, 403, 403f
    paired visceral branches of, 404f–406f, 405
    unpaired visceral branches of, 407–416, 407f–417f
  abdominal cavity of, 338–350, 338f
    peritoneal spaces in, 345, 345f–347f, 345t
    peritoneum in, 338–341, 338f–344f, 340t
    retroperitoneal spaces in, 345t, 348f, 349, 349f
    retroperitoneum in, 338f–340f, 350
  adrenal glands in, 378, 378f–381f
  gallbladder and biliary system in, 367, 367f–372f
  inferior vena cava and tributaries in, 418–420, 418f
  intestines in, 392–397, 392f–400f
  liver in, 350f, 351–366, 351f
    portal hepatic system of, 359, 359f–361f
    segmental anatomy of, 354, 354f–358f
    surface anatomy of, 352, 353f
    vasculature of, 362f–366f, 363
  lymph nodes in, 422f, 423, 423f
  muscles of, 424–426, 424f–428f, 428t
  pancreas in, 373, 373f–375f
  quadrants and regions of, 8, 8t, 9f
  spleen in, 376, 376f, 377f
  stomach in, 389, 389f–391f
  urinary system in, 382, 382f–388f
Abdominal aorta, 304, 401–417, 401f, 402f, 418f
  paired parietal (dorsal) branches of, 403, 403f
  paired visceral branches of, 404f–406f, 405
  unpaired visceral branches of, 407–416, 407f–417f
Abdominal cavity, 5, 7f, 7t
Abdominal viscera, 351f
Abdominal wall, 424, 424f
  muscles of, 424–426, 424f–428f, 428t
Abdominoaortic nodal groups, 423
Abdominopelvic cavity, 5, 7f, 7t
Abducens nerve, 148f, 148t, 152f, 153f, 154
Abductor digiti minimi tendon, 642f, 646f, 648f, 649f, 651, 652t, 653f, 654f
Abductor hallucis muscle, 641f, 642f, 646f, 648f, 649f, 651, 652t, 654f
Abductor hallucis tendon, 649f
Abductor pollicis brevis muscle, 560, 560f, 561f
Abductor pollicis brevis tendon, 532f
Abductor pollicis longus muscle, 530t, 531f, 532f, 538f, 539
Abductor pollicis longus tendon, 532f, 548f, 556f, 557f
AC (acromioclavicular) joint, 490f–492f, 491, 498f, 503f
AC (acromioclavicular) ligaments, 498, 499f
ACA (anterior cerebral artery), 127f, 128–129, 128f, 130f, 131f, 133f
  in circle of Willis, 135f, 136f, 138f
Accessory collateral ligaments, 548, 550f, 552f
Accessory nerve, 116f, 148f, 148t, 160, 160f
Acetabular foramen, 577
Acetabular fossa, 568, 568f, 569f, 573f, 626f, 643f
Acetabular labrum, 569f, 573, 573f–577f
  anterior, 574f, 575f
  posterior, 574f, 575f, 577f

Acetabular ligament
  transverse, 573f, 575f
Acetabular notch, 568, 568f
Acetabulum, 430f, 433, 433f–435f, 568, 568f, 570f, 572f, 573f
Achilles tendon, 623f, 626f, 638f, 640, 640f
  thickening and edema in, 567f
Acromial angle, 498f
Acromioclavicular (AC) joint, 490f–492f, 491, 498f, 503f
Acromioclavicular (AC) ligaments, 498, 499f
Acromion, 490f–494f, 493, 497f
Adductor brevis muscle, 577f, 583t, 584–592, 587f, 589f, 592f
Adductor hallucis muscle, 626f, 648f, 649f, 651, 652t, 653f
Adductor longus muscle, 583t, 584, 584f, 585f, 587f–589f, 592, 592f
Adductor magnus muscle, 577f–579f, 583t, 584, 584f–589f, 592, 592f
Adductor minimus muscle, 440f
Adductor muscles, 570f
Adductor pollicis muscle, 531f, 560, 560f, 561f
Adductor tubercle, 571f, 572f, 593
Adenohypophysis, 109
Adenoids, 232
Adrenal cortex, 378, 378f
Adrenal glands, 378, 378f–381f
Adrenal mass, 337
Adrenal medulla, 378, 378f
Adrenocortical steroids, 378
AICA (anterior inferior cerebellar artery), 127f, 130f, 132, 133f, 137t, 138f
AIIS, 433f
Ala
  of ilium, 431f, 433, 433f
  of sacrum, 177, 177f, 430, 430f, 431f
Alar ligaments, 179, 181f
Alveolar process
  of mandible, 49f, 56, 56f
  of maxilla, 49f–51f, 50, 53f
Alveoli, 283
Ambient cistern, 95f, 96, 96f
Ampulla
  rectal, 452, 452f
  of vas deferens, 466f, 467
  of Vater, 367, 368f, 373
Amygdala, 99f, 113, 113f, 114f
Amylase, 373
Anal canal, 396f, 452
Anal columns, 452, 452f
Anal sphincter
  external, 396f, 452, 452f
  internal, 452, 452f
Anal triangle, 436, 437f
Anastomotic vein
  inferior, 138f
  superior, 138f
Anatomic neck
  of humerus, 496f, 497, 497f, 522f
Anatomic planes, 2, 2f
Anatomic positions, 2, 2f
Anconeus muscle, 516, 521f, 534f, 538f
Androgens, 378
Angular notch, 389f
Ankle and foot, 625–651
  bony anatomy of, 601f, 624f–636f, 625
  fascia, retinacula, and ligaments of, 637–640, 638f–650f
  joints of, 637

Ankle and foot—cont'd
  muscles of, 561, 651f, 652t, 653f, 654f
  tendons of, 638f–650f, 640–647
Ankle joint, 626f, 627f, 637
Annular ligament, 527, 527f, 529f
Annular pulley(s), 550, 550f, 552f
Annular pulley system, 550, 550f
Annulus fibrosus, 166, 167f, 168f
Anserine bursa, 610f
Antebrachial vein
  intermediate, 564, 565
  median, 564, 565f
Anterior acetabular labrum, 574f, 575f
Anterior arch
  of cervical vertebrae, 169, 169f, 171f
Anterior cardiac veins, 327f, 328
Anterior central vein, 222, 222f
Anterior cerebral artery (ACA), 127f, 128–129, 128f, 130f, 131t, 133f
  in circle of Willis, 135f, 136f, 138f
Anterior cerebral vein, 147f
Anterior choroidal artery, 133f
Anterior circumflex humeral artery, 562f
Anterior clinoid processes, 25, 25f, 27f
Anterior column, 568, 568f, 569f
Anterior commissure, 100, 100f, 102f
Anterior communicating artery, 128, 131f, 133f, 135f, 138f
Anterior compartment
  of globe, 76, 76f, 77f
Anterior cranial fossa, 18, 20f, 20t
Anterior crest, 597f
Anterior cruciate ligament, 603f, 607f, 608, 609f
Anterior external vertebral venous plexuses, 222, 222f, 223f
Anterior fontanel, 48, 48f
Anterior fornix, 461
Anterior horn, 89, 89f, 90f
Anterior inferior cerebellar artery (AICA), 127f, 130f, 132, 133f, 137t, 138f
Anterior inferior iliac spine, 431f, 433f, 573f
Anterior inferior pancreaticoduodenal artery, 410f
Anterior internal vertebral venous plexus, 222, 222f, 223f
Anterior interosseous artery, 562f, 563
Anterior intertransverse muscle, 260f
Anterior jugular vein, 272, 272f
Anterior longitudinal ligament, 179–182, 179f–183f
Anterior median fissure, 122, 122f, 123f
Anterior median (spinal) vein, 222, 222f
Anterior meniscofemoral ligament, 603, 603f
Anterior nasal spine, 49f–51f, 50
Anterior pararenal space, 345t, 348f, 349
Anterior radicular arteries, 219, 220f
Anterior radicular vein, 222, 222f
Anterior scalene muscle, 187f, 264t, 265f, 266
Anterior spinal artery, 133f, 138f, 218f–220f, 219
Anterior spinal branch, 220f
Anterior superior iliac spine, 431f, 572f
Anterior superior pancreaticoduodenal artery, 409
Anterior talofibular ligament, 629f, 640, 645f, 650f
Anterior tibial artery, 659f, 660, 661f, 662f
Anterior tibial recurrent artery, 659f
Anterior tibial vein, 663, 663f

Anterior tibiofibular ligament, 640, 650f
Anterior triangle
    of neck
        muscles within, 250f–259f, 264, 264t, 265f
Anterior ulnar recurrent artery, 562f, 563
Anterior vertebral element, 164, 164f–166f
Anterolateral fontanels, 48, 48f
Antrum of Highmore, 67
Anus, 398f, 452
Aorta, 304, 307f
    abdominal, 304, 401–417, 401f, 402f, 418f
        paired parietal (dorsal) branches of, 403,
            403f
        paired visceral branches of, 404f–406f,
            405
        unpaired visceral branches of, 407–416,
            407f–417f
    ascending, 296f, 304, 306f, 318f, 319f, 322f
    descending, 304, 304f–307f, 318f, 319, 322f
    thoracic, 304
Aortic arch, 296f, 304, 304f–307f, 309f, 322f
    branches of, 318f–320f, 319
Aortic hiatus, 330, 332f
Aortic semilunar valve, 293f, 302f, 303, 303f
Aortic sinus
    left, 323
    right, 323
Apical ligament, 179, 179f, 180f
Apical segmental veins, 404f
Apophyseal joint, 167f, 168f
Appendicular artery, 414f
Appendix, 351f
    vermiform, 392f, 396f, 397, 397f
Aqueduct of Sylvius, 89f, 91, 91f, 93f, 95f
Aqueous humor, 76
Arachnoid granulations, 93f, 94, 94f
Arachnoid mater
    spinal, 193, 194f, 201f
Arachnoid membrane, 86f, 87
Arachnoid villi, 86f, 94
Arcuate arteries, 404f, 659f
Arcuate ligament
    median, 355f
Arcuate line, 430f, 433, 434f, 436f
Arcuate popliteal ligament, 608
Arcuate veins, 404f, 420
Arnold-Chiari malformation, 124
Arterial arcades, 414f
Arteriovenous malformations (AVMs), 133
Artery of Adamkiewicz, 219, 220f
Articular disk, 58f, 60, 60f, 61f
Articular eminence, 58f, 59, 59f
Articular facet(s), 166f, 597f, 600
    inferior, 166f
    superior, 166f
Articular fibular surface, 597
Articular joint capsule
    of shoulder, 503, 503f
Articular processes, 164f–168f, 166
    inferior, 165f–168f, 166
        cervical, 170f, 171f
    superior, 164f–168f, 166
        cervical, 169, 169f–171f
Articular tubercle, 34, 34f
Aryepiglottic folds, 237, 240f
Aryepiglottic muscle, 262
Aryepiglotticus, 262, 262f, 263f, 263t
Arytenoid cartilage, 234f, 237, 238f, 239f
Arytenoid fold, 236f
Arytenoid muscle, 262
    oblique, 263f
    transverse, 263f
Arytenoid transverse oblique muscle, 263t
Ascending colon, 392f, 393f, 396f–398f, 397
Ascending lumbar vein, 418, 419f
ASIS, 430f
Astragalus, 625
Atlanto-occipital joint, 169, 170f, 179f, 180f
Atlanto-occipital membrane(s), 179, 179f, 180f
    anterior, 179, 179f, 180f
    posterior, 179, 179f
Atlas, 169, 171f
Atrioventricular groove, 323
Atrioventricular valves, 303
Atrium(ia)
    of brain, 89, 89f

Atrium(ia)—cont'd
    cardiac
        left, 296, 296f, 298f, 300f, 302f
        right, 296, 296f, 299f, 300f, 302f
Auditory artery
    internal, 138f
Auditory canal
    internal, 30t, 34f, 36, 36f, 39, 44f, 45f, 158f
Auditory tube, 37f, 39, 39f, 42f, 226
Auricle(s)
    cardiac
        left, 296, 296f, 298f, 300f, 302f
        right, 296, 296f, 299f, 300f, 302f
    of ear, 39, 39f
Avascular necrosis (AVN)
    of femoral head, 429f, 569
AVMs (arteriovenous malformations), 133
Axial plane, 2, 2f
Axillary artery, 319, 561, 562f
Axillary nerve, 208
Axillary nodes, 422f
Axillary recess, 503, 503f
Axillary vein, 564, 565f
Axis, 169, 170f, 171f
Azygos veins, 329, 329f
Azygos venous system, 329, 329f

B

Bare area
    of liver, 350f, 351
Basal cisterns, 95, 95f
Basal ganglia, 106, 106f–108f
Basal metacarpal branch, 563f
Basal nuclei, 106, 106f–108f, 148
Basal vein of Rosenthal, 138f, 145, 145f–147f
Basilar artery, 127f–130f, 132, 133f, 137t
    in circle of Willis, 136f, 138f
Basilic vein, 564, 565, 565f
Basivertebral veins, 222, 222f–224f
BBB (blood-brain barrier), 127
Biceps brachii muscle, 515, 515f–518f, 531f
Biceps brachii tendon, 497f, 498f, 503f, 512f,
    537f
Biceps femoris muscle, 579f, 585f, 586f, 588f,
    592
Biceps femoris tendon, 621f
Bicipital aponeurosis, 515, 531f
Bicipital groove, 490f, 493f, 496f, 497, 497f
Bicuspid valve, 293f, 295f, 296f, 302f, 303
Bifid spinous process
    cervical, 169, 171f, 172f
Bile duct(s)
    common, 362f, 367, 367f–369f, 371f, 372f
    intrahepatic, 367, 369f
Biliary system, 367, 367f–372f
    extrahepatic, 367, 368f
Bladder
    urinary, 351f, 447–451, 447f–451f, 454f
Blood-brain barrier (BBB), 127
Blowout fracture, 76
Body cavities, 5, 7f, 7t
Bone window, 11f
Bony labyrinth, 39, 39f–41f, 43f–46f
Bony orbit, 72, 72f–75f
Bony pelvis, 430–437
    ilium in, 433, 433f, 434f
    ischium in, 436
    pelvic inlet and outlet in, 436, 436f
    perineum in, 436, 437f
    pubis in, 435, 435f
    sacrum, coccyx, and os coxae in, 430,
        430f–432f
Bony thorax, 276–278, 276f–278f
Bowman's capsule, 385f
Brachial artery, 561, 562f
Brachial plexus, 206f, 208, 209f–212f, 565, 566f
Brachial veins, 564
Brachialis muscle, 515–516, 515f, 516f, 517t,
    519f
Brachiocephalic artery, 319f, 320f
Brachiocephalic trunk, 318f, 319, 322f
Brachiocephalic veins, 272, 304f, 305f,
    318f–321f, 321
Brachioradialis muscle, 530t, 531f, 532f, 534f,
    538, 538f
Brachioradialis tendon, 534f, 537f

Brain, 85–161
    brainstem of, 110f, 116f, 117–122, 117f
        medulla oblongata in, 122, 122f–124f
        midbrain in, 117, 117f–119f
        pons in, 110f, 120, 121f, 122f
    cerebellum of, 121f, 122f, 124–126,
        124f–126f
    cerebral vascular system of, 127–145
        arterial supply in, 127f, 128–138, 128f
            carotid, 127f–131f, 128–131, 131t
            circle of Willis in, 127f, 135f, 136f, 138,
                138f
            vertebrobasilar, 127f, 132–133,
                132f–137f, 137t
        dural sinuses in, 138–140, 138f–144f
        superficial cortical and deep veins in, 145,
            145f–147f
    cerebrum of, 98–106, 98f, 99f
        basal nuclei of, 106, 106f–108f
        gray and white matter organization of,
            100, 100f–102f
        lobes of, 98f, 103, 103f–105f
    coronal, T1-weighted MR scan of, 85f
    cranial nerves in, 116f, 148–161, 148f, 148t
        abducens, 116f, 148f, 148t, 152f, 153f, 154
        accessory, 116f, 148f, 148t, 160, 160f
        facial, 116f, 148f, 148t, 156, 156f–158f
        glossopharyngeal, 116f, 148f, 148t, 159,
            159f
        hypoglossal, 116f, 148f, 148t, 160f, 161,
            161f
        oculomotor, 116f, 148f, 148t, 152, 152f,
            153f
        olfactory, 116f, 148f, 148t, 149, 149f
        optic, 116f, 148f, 148t, 150, 150f, 151f
        trigeminal, 116f, 148f, 148t, 154, 154f,
            155f
        trochlear, 116f, 148f, 148t, 152, 152f, 153f
        vagus, 116f, 148f, 148t, 159f, 160
        vestibulocochlear, 156, 156f, 157f
    diencephalon of, 109–112
        epithalamus in, 112, 112f
        hypothalamus in, 109, 109f–111f
        thalamus in, 99f, 106f–108f, 109
    limbic system of, 113, 113f–115f
    meninges of, 86–87, 86f–88f
    ventricular system of, 89–96
        cisterns in, 95–96, 95f–97f
        ventricles of, 89–94, 89f–94f
Brainstem, 110f, 116f, 117–122, 117f
    medulla oblongata in, 122, 122f–124f
    midbrain in, 117, 117f–119f
    pons in, 110f, 120, 121f, 122f
Breast, 335, 335f, 336f
Bregma, 48, 48f
Broad ligament, 454f, 456f, 459, 459f
Broca's area, 98f, 103, 103f
Bronchi, 279f–282f, 283, 283t, 284f–286f
    mainstem (primary, principal), 279f–282f,
        283, 284f, 286f, 311f
    secondary or lobar, 279f–281f, 283,
        284f–286f, 311f
    tertiary or segmental, 283, 284f–286f
Bronchioles, 283
Bronchopulmonary segments, 283, 283t, 285f
Buccinator muscle, 260f, 261f, 265f, 267f
Bulb
    of penis, 466f, 473, 474f
Bulbourethral glands, 448f, 462f, 466f, 473,
    473f

C

Calcaneal ligament
    interosseous, 650f
Calcaneal sulcus, 625f
Calcaneal tendon, 601f, 613f, 619f, 622f, 623f,
    640
Calcaneal tuberosity, 624f, 625, 626f, 627f, 653f
Calcaneocuboid joint, 627f, 637
Calcaneocuboid ligament, 650f
Calcaneofibular ligament, 627f, 638f, 640, 644f,
    650f
Calcaneonavicular ligament
    plantar, 639f, 650f
Calcaneus, 620f–624f, 625, 626f–628f,
    630f–632f

Calcarine artery, 130f
Callosomarginal artery, 129, 130f
Calyces
    renal, 382, 383f, 385f–387f
Capitate, 539f–545f, 540
Capitellum, 496f, 522f, 523, 524f, 525f
Cardia, 389f
Cardiac antrum, 389f
Cardiac impression, 281f, 311f, 313f
Cardiac notch, 279, 279f, 281f, 313f, 389f
Cardiac orifice, 389
Cardiac sphincter, 389f
Cardiac valves, 293f, 296f, 298f, 302f, 303, 303f
Cardiac vein(s), 327–328, 327f, 328f
    anterior, 327f, 328
    great, 327, 327f
    middle, 327f, 328
    posterior, 327f, 328
    right, 327f, 328
    small, 327f, 328
Cardinal ligaments, 456, 456f–458f
Cardiophrenic sulcus, 279, 279f
Carditis, 293
Carina, 279f, 283
Carotid artery(ies), 250f–259f, 269, 269f–271f, 270t
    common, 269, 269f–271f, 318f–320f, 319, 322f
        left, 269, 270f, 270t, 271f, 318f–320f, 319, 322f
        right, 269, 270f, 270t, 271f, 318f–320f, 319, 322f
    external, 269, 269f–271f, 270f
    internal, 127f–131f, 128–131, 131t, 269, 269f–271f
        in circle of Willis, 135f, 136f, 138f
Carotid canal, 30t, 35f, 36, 37f
Carotid sheath, 272, 273f
Carotid siphon, 127f, 128, 128f
Carotid space (CS), 268t
Carpal arch
    dorsal, 563
Carpal articular surface, 523f, 524
Carpal bones, 539f–541f, 540
Carpal ligament
    dorsal, 548
    transverse, 546
Carpal tunnel, 546, 548f
Carpal tunnel syndrome, 540
Carpometacarpal compartment, 545f
Carpometacarpal joint, 539f
Carpometacarpal joints, 541f–543f, 545, 545f
Cauda equina, 193f, 196, 196f, 197f, 201f, 202f
Caudal pancreatic artery, 409, 411f
Caudate lobe
    of liver, 352, 352f, 353f, 364f
Caudate nucleus, 106, 106f–108f
Caval hiatus, 330, 332f, 363
Cavernous sinuses, 138f, 140, 142f–144f, 152f, 153f
CBD (common bile duct), 362f, 367, 367f–369f, 371f, 372f
Cecal artery, 414f
    posterior, 414f
Cecum, 392f–398f
Celiac axis, 403f, 407f, 408f, 410f, 415f
Celiac trunk, 401f–403f, 406f–412f, 407, 414f
Central canal, 89f, 196, 198f, 201f
Central sulcus, 98, 98f, 103f
Central tendon, 330, 332f
Central vein
    anterior, 222, 222f
    posterior, 222, 222f
Cephalic vein, 564, 565, 565f
Cerebellar artery
    inferior
        anterior, 127f, 130f, 132, 133f, 137t, 138f
        posterior, 127f, 130f, 132, 133f–135f, 137t, 138f
    superior, 130f, 132, 133f, 134f, 137t, 138f
Cerebellar hemispheres, 124
Cerebellar peduncles, 124f, 125, 126f, 127f
    inferior, 125, 127f
    middle, 125, 126f
    superior, 124f–126f, 125
Cerebellar tonsils, 124, 124f, 125f

Cerebellopontine angle (CPA) cistern, 96, 97f
Cerebellum, 121f, 122f, 124–126, 124f–127f
Cerebral aqueduct, 89f, 91, 91f, 93f, 95f
Cerebral arterial circle, 127f, 135f, 136f, 138, 138f
Cerebral artery
    anterior, 127f, 128–129, 128f, 130f, 131t, 133f
        in circle of Willis, 135f, 136f, 138f
    middle, 127f, 128f, 129–131, 130f, 131f, 131t, 133f
        in circle of Willis, 135f, 136f, 138f
        thalamostriate branches of, 117
    posterior, 127f, 130f, 132–133, 133f–138f, 137f
Cerebral cortex, 100, 100f–102f
Cerebral hemispheres, 98
Cerebral lobes, 98f, 103, 103f–105f
Cerebral peduncles, 116f, 117, 118f–120f
Cerebral vascular system, 127–145
    arterial supply in, 127f, 128–138, 128f
        carotid, 127f–131f, 128–131, 131t
        circle of Willis in, 127f, 135f, 136f, 138, 138f
        vertebrobasilar, 127f, 132–133, 132f–137f, 137t
    dural sinuses in, 138–140, 138f–144f
    superficial cortical and deep veins in, 145, 145f–147f
Cerebral vein(s)
    anterior, 147f
    great, 138f, 140f, 142f, 145, 145f–147f
    internal, 138f, 140f, 145, 145f–147f
    middle
        deep, 138f, 147f
        superficial, 138f, 145f
    superficial, 145f
Cerebral venous system, 138–145, 138f–147f
Cerebrospinal fluid (CSF)
    flow through ventricular system of, 93f, 94
Cerebrum, 98–106, 98f, 99f
    basal nuclei of, 106, 106f–108f
    gray and white matter organization of, 100, 100f–102f
    lobes of, 98f, 103, 103f–105f
Cervical artery
    transverse, 562f
Cervical canal, 454, 454f
Cervical enlargement, 204
Cervical ligament(s)
    lateral, 456, 456f–458f
    transverse, 459f
Cervical lymph nodes, 248–249, 248f, 249t, 250f–259f
Cervical lymphadenopathy, 225f, 291f
Cervical nerves, 201f
Cervical plexus, 206f–209f, 207
Cervical space
    posterior, 268t
Cervical spinal cord
    axial, T1-weighted MR scan of, 203f, 204f
Cervical vertebrae, 164f, 167f, 169, 169f–173f
Cervix, 447f, 453f, 454
Chest mass, 275f
Chiasmatic cistern, 93f, 95f, 96, 96f
Cholesteatomas, 41
Chordae tendineae, 296f, 300f, 303
Choroid plexus, 93f, 94, 94f
Choroidal artery
    anterior, 133f
Choroidal vein, 138f, 145f, 147f
Cingulate gyrus, 99f, 100f, 113, 113f, 115f
Circle of Willis, 127f, 135f, 136f, 138, 138f
Circular muscle, 263f
Circumflex artery, 322f, 323, 325f, 326f, 477f
    lateral, 477f, 655f, 660f
    medial, 477f, 650f
Circumflex femoral artery
    lateral, 654f, 655, 659f, 660f
    medial, 578f, 654f, 655, 659f
Circumflex humeral artery
    anterior, 562f
    posterior, 562f
Circumflex iliac artery
    deep, 475, 482t, 654f, 659f
    superficial, 655, 659f

Cistern(s), 95–96, 95f–97f
Cisterna magna, 91f–93f, 95f, 96
Claustrum, 106, 107f, 108f
Clavicle, 490f, 491, 494f, 495f, 503f
    fracture of, 489f
Clavicular head muscle, 264t
Clavicular notch, 490f
Clinoid processes
    anterior, 25, 25f, 27f
    posterior, 25, 25f
Clitoris, 447f, 453f
Clivus, 32, 32f, 33f
Coccygeal nerves, 201f
Coccygeus muscles, 440t, 443, 443f–445f
Coccyx, 175f, 177, 177f, 430, 430f, 432f, 433f
Cochlea, 39, 39f, 40f, 46f
Cochlear branch, 156
Colic artery(ies)
    left, 416, 417f, 477f
        lower, 416f
        superior, 416f
    middle, 413, 414f, 415f
    right, 413, 414f
Colic flexure
    left, 392f, 393f, 396f, 397, 398f, 399f
    right, 392f, 393f, 396f, 397, 398f, 399f
Colic impression, 350f
Collateral ligament(s)
    of fingers, 550f
    lateral
        of elbow, 527, 528f, 529f
        of knee, 603f, 604f, 608, 608f, 610f, 612f
    medial
        of elbow, 527, 527f, 528f
        of knee, 603f, 604f, 608, 608f
    radial, 527, 528f, 529f, 545f, 546, 546f, 548
    of toes, 640
    ulnar, 527, 527f, 528f, 545f, 546, 546f, 548
Collecting duct, 385f
Colliculi, 116f, 117, 118f–120f
Colon, 397, 397f, 398f
    ascending, 392f, 393f, 396f–398f, 397
    descending, 392f, 396f–398f, 397
    transverse, 392f, 393f, 396f–399f, 397
Common bile duct (CBD), 362f, 367, 367f–369f, 371f, 372f
Common carotid artery, 269, 269f–271f, 318f–320f, 319, 322f
    left, 269, 270f, 270t, 271f, 318f–320f, 319, 322f
    right, 269, 270f, 270t, 271f, 318f–320f, 319, 322f
Common fibular nerve, 664
Common hepatic artery, 362f, 363, 364f, 401f, 402f, 407, 407f–411f
Common hepatic duct (CHD), 362f, 367, 367f–370f
Common iliac artery(ies), 401, 402f, 405f, 475, 476f, 480f, 483f
    left, 402f, 476f, 477f, 481f, 482f
    right, 401f, 475f–477f, 482f
Common iliac lymph nodes, 422f, 486f, 487
    lateral, 487
    median, 487
Common iliac vein, 483, 483f, 484f, 485f
    left, 477f
Common interosseous artery, 562f, 563
Common peroneal nerve, 586f, 613f, 664, 664f
Communicating artery
    posterior, 135f, 136f, 138f
Condyle(s)
    lateral
        of femur, 593, 593f–595f
        of humerus, 522f, 523
        of occipital bone, 30, 31f
        of tibia, 595, 595f
    medial
        of femur, 593, 593f, 595f
        of humerus, 522f, 523
        of tibia, 597, 597f
    occipital, 30, 31f
Condyloid process, 56, 56f–58f
Confluence of sinuses, 140, 141f, 142f, 147f
Constrictor muscle(s), 260, 260f, 261t, 263f
    inferior, 260, 260f, 261t, 262f

Constrictor muscle(s)—cont'd
middle, 260, 260f, 261t
superior, 260, 260f, 261t, 263f
Conus medullaris, 193f, 194f, 196, 196f–198f, 201f
Convoluted tubules, 382
Cooper's ligaments, 335, 335f
Coracoacromial arch, 498
Coracoacromial ligament, 498, 498f, 499f, 503f, 513f
Coracobrachialis muscle, 512f, 515f, 516, 516f, 517t
Coracoclavicular ligaments, 498, 499f, 500f, 513f
Coracohumeral ligament, 498, 499f, 500f, 502f, 503f
Coracoid process, 490f, 492f–495f, 493, 497f, 498f
Cornea, 76
Corniculate cartilages, 234f, 237, 240f
Cornu
of coccyx, 177
Cornua
of uterus, 454
Coronal plane, 2, 2f
Coronal suture, 47, 47f
Coronary artery(ies), 322f–326f, 323
left, 322f, 323, 323f, 325f, 326f
right, 322f–325f, 323
Coronary groove, 323
Coronary ligaments, 340f, 340t, 341, 344f
Coronary sinus, 327, 327f, 328f
Coronoid fossa, 496f, 522f, 523, 524f
Coronoid process, 56, 56f, 57f, 522f, 524, 524f–526f
Corpora cavernosa, 466f, 468f–470f, 473, 473f, 474f
Corpus callosum, 99f–102f, 100
Corpus spongiosum, 466f, 468f–470f, 473, 473f, 474f
Cortical veins
superficial, 138f, 145, 145f
Corticosteroids, 378
Costal cartilages, 276, 276f, 278f
Costal facet(s), 165f, 174, 174f
inferior, 165f
superior, 165f
Costocervical trunk, 562f
Costodiaphragmatic recess, 279f, 283
Costomediastinal recess, 279f, 283
Costophrenic sulcus, 279, 279f, 280f
Costotransverse joints, 174, 174f, 276, 278f
Costovertebral joints, 174, 174f, 276, 278f
Cotyloid ligament, 573
Cowper's glands, 448f, 462f, 466f, 473, 473f
CPA (cerebellopontine angle) cistern, 96, 97f
CPR (curved planar reformation), 13–14, 13f, 14f
Cranial fossae, 18, 20f, 20t
Cranial nerves, 116f, 148–161, 148f, 148t
abducens, 116f, 148f, 148t, 152f, 153f, 154
accessory, 116f, 148f, 148t, 160, 160f
facial, 116f, 148f, 148t, 156, 156f–158f
glossopharyngeal, 116f, 148f, 148t, 159, 159f
hypoglossal, 116f, 148f, 148t, 160f, 161, 161f
oculomotor, 116f, 148f, 148t, 152, 152f, 153f
olfactory, 116f, 148f, 148t, 149, 149f
optic, 116f, 148f, 148t, 150, 150f, 151f
trigeminal, 116f, 148f, 148t, 154, 154f, 155f
trochlear, 116f, 148f, 148t, 152, 152f, 153f
vagus, 116f, 148f, 148t, 159f, 160
vestibulocochlear, 156, 156f, 157f
Cranial root, 160
Cranium, 17–48, 18f, 19f
anterior view of, 18f, 19f
ear structures in, 39, 39f–46f
ethmoid bone in, 18f, 19f, 23–24, 23f, 24f
fetal, 48, 48f
fontanels of, 48, 48f
foramina and fissures of, 25–29, 30t
frontal bone in, 18f, 19f, 22, 22f
inner, 21f
lateral, 19f, 21f
occipital bone in, 18f, 19f, 30–32, 30f–33f
parietal bone in, 18f, 19f, 20, 21f
sagittal view of, 18f

Cranium—cont'd
sphenoid bone in, 18f, 19f, 25–29, 25f–29f, 30t
sutures of, 47, 47f
temporal bone in, 18f, 19f, 34–38, 34f–38f
trauma to, 17f
Cremaster muscle, 463f
Cribriform plate, 20f, 23, 23f, 30t
Cricoarytenoid muscle
lateral, 262, 262f, 263t
posterior, 262, 262f, 263f, 263t
Cricoid cartilage, 234f–236f, 237, 240f
Cricothyroid muscle, 260f, 262f, 263t, 265f
Crista galli, 23, 24f
Critical zone
of shoulder, 504
Cruciate ligament
anterior, 603f, 607f, 608, 609f
posterior, 603f, 604f, 607f–610f, 608
Cruciate pulleys, 550, 550f
Cruciform ligament, 179, 179f, 180f
Crura
of diaphragm, 330, 332f
of penis, 466f, 473
Crural fascia, 615f, 616f
CS (carotid space), 268t
CSF (cerebrospinal fluid)
flow through ventricular system of, 93f, 94
CT numbers, 11, 11f
Cubital lymph nodes, 565f
Cubital tunnel, 527f, 528f
Cubital vein
median, 564, 565f
Cuboid bone, 624f, 625, 627f
Cuboideonavicular ligament
dorsal, 646f, 650f
Cuneiform bone(s), 624f, 625, 630f, 631f
intermediate, 624f, 626f, 639f, 648f
lateral, 624f, 639f, 648f
medial, 624f, 639f, 648f
Cuneiform cartilage, 237, 240f
Curved planar reformation (CPR), 13–14, 13f, 14f
Cutaneous nerve
dorsal
intermediate, 616f
medial, 616f
lateral, 566, 566f, 664f
posterior femoral, 585f, 586f
sural
lateral, 613f
medial, 615f
Cyst
follicular, 453f, 460
popliteal, 610f
Cystic artery, 362f, 407
Cystic duct, 350f, 362f, 367, 367f–369f

D
da Vinci, Leonardo, 1
Danger space (DS), 267f, 268t
Dartos muscle, 463f
Dartos tunica, 463
Deep artery of thigh, 477f
Deep circumflex iliac artery, 475, 482t, 654f, 659f
Deep circumflex iliac vein, 485f
Deep dorsal vein of penis, 485f
Deep femoral artery, 578f, 587f
Deep femoral vein, 578f
Deep fibular nerve, 613f–615f
Deep infrapatellar bursa, 610, 610f
Deep inguinal nodes, 422f, 486f
Deep middle cerebral vein, 138f, 147f
Deep palmar arch, 562f, 563, 565
Deep peroneal nerve, 613f–617f, 664f
Deep plantar branch, 659f
Deep transverse intermetacarpal ligament, 551f
Deep transverse metacarpal ligament (DTML), 548, 552f
Deep transverse metatarsal ligament, 640
Deep veins
of cerebrum, 138f, 145, 145f–147f
of upper extremity, 565f
Deltoid ligament, 627f, 640, 645f, 647f, 650f

Deltoid muscle, 503f, 504f, 506f–508f, 511, 511f, 511t, 512f
Deltoid tuberosity, 496f, 497, 522f
Deltopectoral lymph nodes, 565f
Demifacets, 166f, 174, 174f
Dens, 169, 169f, 170f
Dentate nucleus, 124f, 125f, 126
Denticulate ligaments, 195, 195f, 201f
Depressor anguli oris muscle, 265f
Depressor labii inferioris muscle, 265f
Dermatomes, 199, 203f
Descending colon, 392f, 396f–398f, 397
Descending genicular artery, 586f, 654f, 659f
Diagonal branch, 325f
Diaphragm, 330, 330t, 332f
Diencephalon, 109–112
epithalamus in, 112, 112f
hypothalamus in, 109, 109f–111f
thalamus in, 99f, 106f–108f, 109
Digastric muscle, 264, 264t, 265f
anterior belly of, 261f
Digital arteries
dorsal, 659f
plantar, 659f
Digital cube, 12f, 13
Digital veins, 663f
Directional terminology, 3, 3t
Display orientation, 2, 3f
Distal interphalangeal (DIP) joint, 539f, 540, 550f
Distal phalanges
of foot, 624f
of hand, 539f, 540, 550f
Distal radioulnar articulation, 543f, 545, 545f
Distal radioulnar joint (DRUJ), 523f, 543f, 545, 545f
Distal tibiofibular joint, 597f
Dorsal arch, 565
Dorsal branches
of abdominal aorta, 401, 403
Dorsal carpal arch, 563
Dorsal carpal ligament, 548
Dorsal cavity, 5, 7f, 7t
Dorsal cuboideonavicular ligament, 646f, 650f
Dorsal cutaneous nerve
intermediate, 616f
medial, 616f
Dorsal digital arteries, 659f
Dorsal horns, 199, 201f
Dorsal intercarpal arch, 563f
Dorsal intercarpal ligament, 547f, 556f
Dorsal interosseous muscles
of foot, 626f, 651, 652t, 653f, 654f
of hand, 557, 559f–561f
Dorsal metatarsal artery
first, 659f
Dorsal pancreatic artery, 409, 410f, 411f
Dorsal radiocarpal arch, 563f
Dorsal radiocarpal ligament, 546, 547f
Dorsal radiotriquetral ligament, 547f
Dorsal rami, 204, 206f
Dorsal root, 194f, 196, 198f, 200f, 203f, 206f
Dorsal root ganglion, 168f, 194f, 198f–200f, 199
Dorsal scapular artery, 562f
Dorsal talonavicular ligament, 646f
Dorsal tendons
or wrist, 554, 554f–559f
Dorsal venous arch, 578f
Dorsal venous network, 565
Dorsalis pedis artery, 659f
Dorsum sellae, 25, 25f, 26f
DRUJ (distal radioulnar joint), 523f, 543f, 545, 545f
DS (danger space), 267f, 268t
DTML (deep transverse metacarpal ligament), 548, 552f
Duct of Wirsung, 367, 373
Ductus deferens, 448f, 449f, 462f–464f, 466f, 467, 469f
Duodenal bulb, 389f, 392, 393f
Duodenojejunal flexure, 392, 393f, 414f
Duodenojejunal junction, 394f
Duodenum, 392, 393f, 394f, 399f
Dura mater
cerebral, 86, 86f

Dura mater—cont'd
  spinal, 193, 193f, 201f
Dural sheath
  spinal, 193, 193f, 194f
Dural sinuses, 138–140, 138f–144f
Dural sleeve, 200f

E
EAM (external auditory meatus), 30t, 39, 39f, 42f, 46f
  and temporal bone, 34, 34f, 35f, 37f
Ear, 39, 39f–46f
  external, 39, 39f, 40f, 42f, 46f
  inner, 39, 39f–41f, 43f–46f
  middle, 39, 39f, 42f, 43f, 45f
  petrous portion of, 40f
Ejaculatory duct, 448f, 462f, 467, 472f
Elbow, 523–539
  bony anatomy of, 522f–526f, 523–526
  forearm muscles of, 530–539, 530t, 531f–538f
  joint capsule and fat pads of, 526, 526f
  ligaments of, 527, 527f–529f
Embolism
  pulmonary, 314
Endocardium, 296, 296f, 302f
Endolymph, 39
Endolymphatic duct, 39, 41f
Endolymphatic sac, 39, 41f
Endometrium, 454, 454f
Epicardial fat, 294f, 295f
Epicardium, 294, 294f, 296, 302f
Epicondyle
  lateral
    of femur, 571f, 572f, 593, 593f, 595f
    of humerus, 496f, 522f, 523, 524f, 525f
  medial
    of femur, 571f, 593, 593f, 595f
    of humerus, 496f, 522f, 523, 524f, 525f
Epididymis, 448f, 462f–466f, 463, 469f
Epidural hematoma, 87
Epidural space
  spinal, 168f, 193, 193f, 194f
Epigastric artery
  inferior, 475, 477f, 479f, 482t, 654f, 659f
  superficial, 655
Epigastric vein
  inferior, 485f
Epiglottis, 234–237, 234f–238f, 240f, 255f, 256f
Epiglottitis
  acute, 237
Epinephrine, 378
Epiphyseal line, 627f
Epiploic appendages, 392f, 396f, 397
Epiploic foramen (of Winslow), 338, 342f
Epithalamus, 112, 112f
Erector spinae muscles, 186t, 188, 188f, 191f
Esophageal hiatus, 330, 332f
Esophagogastric junction, 389, 390f
Esophagus, 241, 241f, 289, 289f
Estrogens, 378, 460
Ethmoid air cells, 23–24, 24f
Ethmoid bone, 18f, 19f, 23–24, 23f, 24f
Ethmoid bulla, 23f, 24
Ethmoid notch, 22
Ethmoid sinuses, 23–24, 24f, 64f–66f, 65, 65t
Eustachian tube, 37f, 39, 39f, 42f, 226
Extensor carpi radialis brevis muscle, 530t, 532f, 534f, 538, 538f
Extensor carpi radialis brevis tendon, 532f, 535f, 537f, 548f, 556f, 557f
Extensor carpi radialis longus muscle, 530t, 532f, 534f, 538, 538f
Extensor carpi radialis longus tendon, 532f, 535f, 537f, 548f, 556f, 557f
Extensor carpi ulnaris muscle, 530t, 531f, 532f, 534f, 538f, 539
Extensor carpi ulnaris tendon, 532f, 548f, 556f, 557f
Extensor digiti minimi muscle, 530t, 531f, 532f, 538f, 539
Extensor digiti minimi tendons, 532f, 535f, 548f, 555f–557f
Extensor digitorum brevis muscle, 638f, 639f, 646f, 651, 651f, 652t
Extensor digitorum brevis tendon, 649f

Extensor digitorum longus muscle, 611, 611t, 612f–621f, 626f
Extensor digitorum longus tendon, 646f, 647, 648f, 649f
Extensor digitorum muscle, 530t, 531f, 532f, 534f, 538, 538f
Extensor digitorum tendons, 532f, 535f, 537f, 548f, 553f, 555f–557f
Extensor hallucis brevis muscle, 638f, 646f, 648f, 651, 652t
Extensor hallucis brevis tendon, 649f, 654f
Extensor hallucis longus muscle, 611, 611t, 612f–614f, 616f, 617f, 619f–621f
Extensor hallucis longus tendon, 646f, 647, 648f, 649f, 654f
Extensor hood, 550, 551f
Extensor indicis muscle, 530t, 532f, 538f, 539
Extensor indicis tendon, 535f, 548f
Extensor mechanism, 550, 551f
Extensor muscles
  of leg, 611, 611t
Extensor pollicis brevis muscle, 530t, 532f, 538f, 539
Extensor pollicis brevis tendon, 532f, 535f, 548f, 556f, 557f
Extensor pollicis longus muscle, 538f
Extensor pollicis longus tendon, 532f, 535f, 548f, 556f
Extensor retinaculum
  of ankle, 637
    inferior, 612f, 637, 638f, 651f
    superior, 612f, 637, 638f, 651f
  of wrist, 548, 548f, 549f
Extensor tendons
  of wrist and hand, 548f, 549f, 554f
External anal sphincter, 396f, 452, 452f
External auditory meatus (EAM), 30t, 39, 39f, 42f, 46f
  and temporal bone, 34, 34f, 35f, 37f
External capsule, 106, 107f, 108f
External carotid artery, 269, 269f–271f, 270f
External iliac artery, 475, 475f–477f, 479f–483f
  right, 401f, 475f
External iliac lymph nodes, 486f, 487
External iliac veins, 483, 483f, 485f, 663, 663f
External intercostal muscles, 330, 330f, 424f, 427f
External jugular veins, 272, 272f, 273t, 321
External landmarks, 3, 4f, 5f
External os, 454, 454f
External pudendal arteries, 654f, 655, 659f
External urethral orifice, 451, 473f
External venous plexuses, 222
Extrahepatic biliary system, 367, 368f
Extrapelvic muscles, 438, 438f, 439f
Extreme capsule, 106, 107f, 108f
Extrinsic ligaments
  of wrist, 545f–547f, 546
Eye. *See* Orbit.

F
Facet(s)
  on vertebral bodies, 166f
Facet joints, 166, 166f–168f
Facial bone(s), 49–58, 49f
  inferior nasal conchae as, 49f, 55, 55f
  lacrimal bone as, 49f–51f, 50
  mandible as, 49f, 56, 56f–58f
  maxilla as, 49f, 50, 51f, 53
  nasal bone as, 49f–51f, 50, 52f
  palatine bone as, 50, 50f, 52f
  trauma to, 17f
  vomer as, 49f, 55
  zygoma as, 49f–52f, 50, 54f
Facial nerve, 116f, 148f, 148t, 156, 156f–158f
Facial nerve canal, 30t, 34f, 38
Facial planes
  of neck, 250f–259f, 266, 267f, 268t
Falciform ligament, 338f, 341, 344f, 350f–352f, 352, 354f
Fallopian tubes, 447f, 453f, 454f, 456f, 460
False pelvis, 436, 436f
False vocal cords, 234f, 237
Falx cerebelli, 87, 88f
Falx cerebri, 86, 86f–88f

Fascia lata, 587f
Female pelvis, 447f
Female reproductive organs, 453–461, 453f–461f
Femoral artery, 654f–660f, 655, 663f
  deep, 578f, 587f
Femoral cutaneous nerve
  posterior, 585f, 586f
Femoral head, 568, 568f–572f, 575f, 577f, 578f
  avascular necrosis of, 429f, 569
Femoral ligament, 577
Femoral neck, 430f, 568, 569f, 570f, 572f, 595f
Femoral nerve, 213, 213f, 664, 664f
Femoral shaft, 570f, 572f, 595f, 600f
Femoral vein, 656f–658f, 663, 663f
  deep, 578f
Femorotibial articular, 602
Femur, 568, 571f, 585f
  distal, 593, 594f–596f
Fetus
  cranium of, 48, 48f
Fibrous pericardium, 294
Fibula, 593, 595f, 597f–599f, 600, 601f
Fibular artery, 659f, 660, 661f, 662f
  peroneal, 613f
Fibular collateral ligament, 603f, 604f, 608, 608f, 610f, 612f
Fibular nerve
  common, 664
  deep, 613f–615f
  peroneal, 613f
  superficial, 614f, 615f
Fibular notch, 597, 597f
Fibular retinaculum, 612f, 651f
  inferior, 627f
  superior, 627f
Fibular vein, 663f
Fibularis brevis muscle, 611t, 612f–617f, 619f–623f, 622, 651f
Fibularis brevis tendon, 638f, 641f, 646f, 647
Fibularis longus muscle, 611t, 612f–623f, 622
Fibularis longus tendon, 638f, 641f, 646f, 647, 648f, 653f
Fibularis tertius muscle, 611, 611f, 612f
Filum terminale, 193–195, 193f
Fimbriae, 454f, 460
First dorsal metatarsal artery, 659f
First lumbar vein, 419f
Fissure(s), 98
Fissure for the gallbladder, 351, 351f
Flexor accessorius muscle, 653f
Flexor carpi radialis muscle, 530t, 531, 531f, 532f, 534f, 535f
Flexor carpi radialis tendon, 537f, 548f, 556f, 557f, 560f
Flexor carpi ulnaris muscle, 530t, 531, 531f, 532f, 534f, 535f, 538f
Flexor carpi ulnaris tendon, 532f, 535f, 537f, 557f, 560f
Flexor digiti minimi brevis muscle, 560, 560f, 561f, 648f, 653f, 654f
Flexor digiti minimi brevis tendon, 649f
Flexor digiti minimi muscle, 560f, 651, 652t
Flexor digitorum brevis muscle, 642f, 646f, 648f, 651, 652t, 653f
Flexor digitorum brevis tendon, 649f, 653f
Flexor digitorum longus muscle, 620f, 621f, 623, 623f
Flexor digitorum longus tendon, 646f, 647, 648f, 649f, 653f
Flexor digitorum profundus muscle, 530t, 531f, 532f, 534f, 537
Flexor digitorum profundus tendon, 537f, 548f, 552f, 560f, 561f
Flexor digitorum superficialis muscle, 530t, 531, 531f, 532f
Flexor digitorum superficialis tendon, 537f, 548f, 556f, 560f, 561f
Flexor hallucis brevis muscle, 641f, 648f, 649f, 651, 652t, 653f, 654f
Flexor hallucis longus muscle, 611t, 612f–614f, 616f, 617f, 619f–621f, 623, 623f, 626f
Flexor hallucis longus tendon, 646f, 647, 648f, 649f, 653f, 654f
Flexor muscles
  of leg, 611t, 622–623

Flexor pollicis brevis muscle, 531f, 560, 560f, 561f
Flexor pollicis longus muscle, 530t, 532f, 537, 537f
Flexor pollicis longus tendon, 532f, 537f, 548f, 555f, 556f, 560f, 561f
Flexor retinaculum
    of ankle, 627f, 637
    of wrist, 531f, 546, 548f, 549f, 560f
Flexor tendons
    of wrist and hand, 548f, 549f, 554f
Follicular cyst, 453f, 460
Fontanels, 48, 48f
Foot. See Ankle and foot.
Foramen lacerum, 30t, 37f, 38
Foramen magnum, 30, 30f, 30t
Foramen of Luschka, 89f, 91
Foramen of Magendie, 89f, 91
Foramen of Monro, 89f, 90f, 91
Foramen of Winslow, 338, 342f
Foramen ovale, 25, 25f, 28f, 30t, 296
Foramen rotundum, 25, 25f, 30t
Foramen spinosum, 25, 25f, 28f, 30t
Forearm muscles, 530–539, 530t, 531f–538f
    dorsal
        deep, 530t, 538f, 539
        superficial, 530t, 538–539, 538f
    ventral
        deep, 530t, 537, 537f
        superficial, 530–531, 530t, 531f–536f
Fornix, 113, 113f, 115f, 461
Fossa ovalis, 296, 296f
Fourth lumbar vein, 419f
Fourth ventricle, 89f–93f, 91
Fovea capitis, 568, 568f–571f, 573f
Fracture(s)
    blowout, 76
    of clavicle, 489f
    femoral head
        avascular necrosis after, 569
    Le Fort, 50
    of spine, 163f
Frontal bone, 18f, 19f, 22, 22f
Frontal foramen, 30t
Frontal fossa, 18, 20f, 20t
Frontal gyrus
    inferior, 103f
Frontal horn, 89, 89f, 90f
Frontal lobe, 98f, 99f, 103, 103f
Frontal notch, 30t
Frontal process
    of maxilla, 50, 50f–52f
Frontal sinuses, 64f, 65t, 66f, 69, 69f
Frontopolar artery, 130f
Fundus
    of stomach, 389, 389f, 390f
    of uterus, 454

G
Gallbladder, 351f, 367, 367f–372f
Gallbladder fossa, 351, 367
Gastric artery, 408f
    left, 401f, 402f, 407, 407f, 410f, 411f
    right, 362f, 407–409, 407f, 410f
Gastric impression, 350f
Gastric vein, 361f, 366f
    left, 484f
    right, 484f
Gastrocnemius bursae, 610, 610f
Gastrocnemius muscle, 608f, 610f, 611f, 612f, 613f, 615f, 618f, 620f–623f, 622
Gastrocnemius tendon, 622f
Gastrocolic ligaments, 340t, 341
Gastroduodenal artery, 402f, 407, 407f, 409, 410f
    right, 409f, 410f
Gastroepiploic artery
    left, 362f, 407f, 409, 411f
    right, 362f, 407f, 409
Gastrohepatic ligament, 342f
Gastrolienal ligament, 340t
Gastro-omental artery
    left, 409
    right, 409
Gastrophrenic ligaments, 341
Gastrosplenic ligaments, 338f, 340t, 341, 343f, 376

Gemellus muscle(s), 575f, 577f, 578f, 579t, 580f, 582f, 583
    inferior, 575f, 577f, 578f, 579t, 580f, 583
    superior, 569f, 577f, 578f, 579t, 580f, 583
Genicular artery(ies), 660
    descending, 586f, 654f, 659f
    inferior
        lateral, 659f
        medial, 605f, 659f, 661f, 662f
        superior medial, 659f
Genioglossus muscle, 260, 260f, 261f, 261t
Geniohyoid muscle, 260f, 261f, 264, 264t
Genitofemoral nerve, 463f
Genu
    of corpus callosum, 100, 100f
Gerota's fascia, 348f, 349, 378, 379f, 382, 383f, 386f, 387f
Glans penis, 466f, 473, 473f, 474f
Glenohumeral joint, 490f, 493, 493f, 495f
Glenohumeral ligament(s), 497f–499f, 498, 502f
    inferior, 498f–500f
    middle, 497f, 497f–499f, 501f, 502f, 513f
    superior, 498f, 499f, 513f
Glenoid cavity, 492f, 493, 498f
Glenoid fossa, 492f–494f, 493, 497f, 503f
Glenoid labrum, 497f, 498, 498f, 503f
Glenoid lip, 497f, 498, 498f
Glenoid muscle, 494f
Glenoid process, 490f, 492f, 493
Glisson's capsule, 351
Globe, 76, 76f–79f
    trauma to, 76
Globus pallidus, 106, 107f
Glomerulus, 382
Glossopharyngeal nerve, 116f, 148f, 148t, 159, 159f
Glottis, 237, 238f–240f
Glucagon, 373
Glucocorticoids, 378
Gluteal artery, 481f
    inferior, 475, 475f, 477f–480f, 482f, 482t
    superior, 475, 477f, 482f, 482t, 654f, 659f
Gluteal tuberosity, 569, 571f, 572f
Gluteal vein
    inferior, 478f, 485f
    superior, 484f, 485f
Gluteus maximus muscle, 438, 438f, 439f, 579, 579f–582f, 579t
Gluteus medius muscles, 438, 438f, 439f, 577f, 578f, 579–580, 579f–582f, 579t
Gluteus medius tendon, 574f
Gluteus minimus muscles, 438, 438f, 439f, 577f, 578f, 579t, 580, 580f–582f
Gluteus minimus tendon, 574f, 575f
Gluteus muscles, 438, 438f, 439f, 579–583
Gnostic area, 103f
Gonadal artery(ies), 401f, 403f, 405, 406f, 407f, 477f
    left, 401f, 475f
    right, 401f, 475f
Gonadal vein(s), 406f, 407f, 418f, 419, 483
    left, 419
    right, 419, 419f
Gonion, 56, 56f
Gracilis muscle, 579f, 583t, 584, 584f, 585f, 587f–589f
Gracilis tendon, 586f, 612f, 620f
Gray matter
    cerebral, 99f–102f, 100
    periaqueductal, 117, 117f, 118f
    of spinal cord, 196
Gray scale, 10f–12f, 11
Great anterior radicular artery, 219, 220f
Great cardiac vein, 327, 327f
Great cerebral vein, 138f, 140f, 142f, 145, 145f–147f
Great pancreatic artery, 373f, 409, 410f, 411f
Great saphenous vein, 613f, 614f, 663f, 663f
Great vessels, 304–314, 304f–315f, 318f
Greater curvature
    of stomach, 389, 389f, 390f
Greater multiangular bone, 539f–541f, 540
Greater omentum, 340f, 341, 342f, 343f
Greater sac, 338, 338f, 340f
Greater saphenous vein, 615f–619f, 646f

Greater trochanter, 430f, 433f, 435f, 568, 569f–575f
Greater tubercle
    of humerus, 490f, 493f, 494f, 496f, 497, 497f
Greater wings
    of sphenoid bone, 25, 25f, 28f
Gustatory area, 103f
Guyton's canal, 546, 549f
Gyri, 98

H
Hamate, 539f–545f, 540
Hamate hook, 539f, 541f, 542f
Hamstrings, 579f, 583t, 585f–591f, 592
Hand, 540–566
    bony anatomy of, 540, 540f–544f
    joints of, 545, 545f
    ligaments and fascia of, 546–550, 546f–553f
    muscles and tendons of, 554–560, 554f–561f
Hard palate, 50, 52f, 53f
Hartmann's pouch, 368f
Haustra, 392f, 396f, 397
Heart, 293–303
    apex of, 293, 293f, 296f
    base (posterior aspect) of, 293, 293f, 296f
    chambers of, 296, 296f–302f
    circulation of blood through, 302f, 316
    diaphragmatic (inferior) surface of, 293, 293f
    inferior border of, 293, 293f
    left border of, 293, 293f
    off-axis imaging of, 316–317, 316f, 317f
    pericardium of, 294, 294f, 295f
    pulmonary (left) surface of, 293
    right border of, 293, 293f
    sternocostal (anterior) surface of, 293
    superficial landmarks of, 293, 293f, 294f
    superior border of, 293, 293f
    valves of, 293f, 296f, 298f, 302f, 303, 303f
    wall of, 296, 296f
Hematoma
    epidural, 87
Hemiazygos veins, 329, 329f, 419f
Hepatic artery, 354f, 362f–364f, 367f, 410f, 483f
    common, 362f, 363, 364f, 401f, 402f, 407, 407f–411f
    left, 362f, 363, 364f, 402f, 407f, 410f
    proper, 362f, 363, 407, 410f
    right, 363, 364f, 402f, 410f
Hepatic duct, 350f, 369f
    common, 362f, 367, 367f–370f
    left, 367, 367f, 368f
    right, 367, 367f, 368f
Hepatic flexure, 392f, 393f, 396f, 397, 398f, 399f
Hepatic vein(s), 354f, 359f, 361f, 363, 364f–367f, 418f, 419f, 420
    left, 354f, 355f, 359f, 363, 364f, 365f, 420
    middle, 354f–356f, 359f, 363, 364f–366f, 420
    right, 354f, 359f, 361f, 364f–366f, 420
Hepatoduodenal ligaments, 341, 342f
Hepatogastric ligaments, 341
Hernias
    indirect inguinal, 438
Herniated intervertebral disks, 208
Herniation
    tonsillar, 124
Herpes zoster virus, 195
Heschl's gyrus, 103, 103f
Hilum, 279f, 282, 282f
Hip(s), 568–592
    articular capsule of, 579
    bony anatomy of, 568–569, 568f–572f
    cross-section image of, 2f
    labrum and ligaments of, 573–578, 573f–578f
    muscles of, 579–583, 579f–582f, 579t
Hippocampus, 113, 113f–115f
    damage to, 113
Horizontal long axis (HLA) view, 316f, 317, 317f
Hounsfield unit (HU), 11, 11f
Humeral artery
    circumflex
        anterior, 562f
        posterior, 562f
Humeral head, 493f, 494f, 496f, 497, 522f

Humeral ligament
  transverse, 498, 499f, 502f
Humerus, 490f, 494f, 496f, 497, 503f, 504f
  distal, 519f, 523
  proximal, 518f
Hyoglossus muscle, 260, 261f, 261t
Hyoid bone, 256f, 257f
Hypoglossal canals, 21f, 30, 30f, 30t, 31f
Hypoglossal nerve, 116f, 148f, 148t, 160f, 161, 161f
Hypoglossus muscle, 265f
Hypophysis, 109, 110f, 111f
Hypothalamic nuclei, 109f
Hypothalamus, 109, 109f–111f
Hypothenar muscle group, 555f, 556f, 560, 560f, 561f

I

IAC (internal auditory canal), 30t, 34f, 36, 36f, 39, 44f, 45f, 158f
Ileal artery, 413, 414f
Ileocecal valve, 392, 392f–395f
Ileocolic artery, 413, 414f, 415f
Ileum, 351f, 392, 392f–398f
Iliac artery(ies)
  circumflex
    deep, 475, 482t, 654f, 659f
    superficial, 655, 659f
  common, 401, 402f, 405f, 475, 476f, 480f, 483f
    left, 402f, 476f, 477f, 481f, 482f
    right, 401f, 475f–477f, 482f
  external, 475, 475f–477f, 479f–483f
    right, 401f, 475f
  internal, 475, 475f–481f
    left, 401f, 475f
    right, 401f, 475f
Iliac crest, 431f, 433, 433f, 434f, 572f
Iliac fossa, 430f, 431f, 433, 433f, 434f, 572f
Iliac lymph nodes
  common, 422f, 486f, 487
    lateral, 487
    median, 487
  external, 486f, 487
  internal, 486f, 487
Iliac spine
  inferior, 433
    anterior, 431f, 433f, 573f
    posterior, 432f, 433f
  superior, 433
    anterior, 431f, 572f
    posterior, 432f, 433f
Iliac vein(s)
  common, 483, 483f, 484f, 485f
    left, 477f
  deep circumflex, 485f
  external, 483, 483f, 485f, 663, 663f
Iliac veins
  internal, 476f, 478f, 479f, 483, 484f, 485f
Iliacus muscle, 440, 440f, 440t, 441f, 583, 583t, 584f
Iliocostalis cervicis muscle, 186t
Iliocostalis lumborum muscle, 186t, 188f
Iliocostalis muscles, 186t, 187f, 188, 188f, 192f
Iliocostalis thoracis muscle, 186t
Iliofemoral ligament, 569f, 573f–575f, 577–578
Iliolumbar artery, 475, 477f, 482t, 654f
Iliolumbar veins, 419f, 484f
Iliopsoas muscle, 438f–440f, 440, 442f, 444f
Iliopsoas tendon, 574f, 575f, 577f, 578f
Iliotibial (IT) band, 574f, 575f, 579f, 584, 584f, 588f
Iliotibial tract, 574f, 575f, 579f, 584, 584f, 588f
Ilium, 431f–434f, 433, 568, 568f, 569f
Image display, 10f, 11–15
  gray scale in, 10f–12f, 11
  MPR and 3D, 12f–15f, 13–15
Incus, 39, 39f, 43f, 45f
Inferior anastomotic vein, 138f
Inferior aperture
  of pelvis, 436
Inferior articular facet, 166f
Inferior articular processes, 165f–168f, 166
  cervical, 170f, 171f

Inferior cerebellar peduncles, 125, 127f
Inferior colliculi, 116f, 117, 118f, 119f
Inferior constrictor muscle, 260, 260f, 261t, 262f
Inferior costal facet, 165f
Inferior epigastric artery, 475, 477f, 479f, 482t, 654f, 659f
Inferior epigastric vein, 485f
Inferior extensor retinaculum, 612f, 637, 638f, 651f
Inferior fibular retinaculum, 627f
Inferior frontal gyrus, 103f
Inferior gemellus muscle, 575f, 577f, 578f, 579t, 580f, 583
Inferior glenohumeral ligament, 498f–500f
Inferior gluteal artery, 475, 475f, 477f–480f, 482f, 482t
Inferior gluteal vein, 478f, 485f
Inferior horn, 89, 89f–92f
Inferior iliac spine, 433
  anterior, 431f, 433f, 573f
  posterior, 432f, 433f
Inferior ischial ramus, 436
Inferior lateral genicular artery, 659f
Inferior medullary velum, 91, 91f
Inferior mesenteric artery, 401f, 403f, 414f–417f, 416
Inferior mesenteric vein, 359f, 414f, 484f
Inferior nasal conchae, 49f, 51f, 55, 55f
Inferior nasal meatus, 55, 55f
Inferior oblique muscle, 81, 81f, 84f
Inferior orbital fissure, 30t, 72, 72f, 75f
Inferior pancreaticoduodenal artery, 413, 414f
Inferior peroneal retinaculum, 637, 638f
Inferior phrenic artery(ies), 401f, 403, 403f, 475f, 483f
  left, 403
  right, 402f, 403
Inferior phrenic suprarenal artery, 403f
Inferior phrenic vein(s), 418, 419f
  left, 418, 418f
  right, 418, 418f
Inferior pubic ramus, 430f, 435, 435f, 572f
  right, 436f
Inferior pudendal vein, 485f
Inferior pulmonary vein
  left, 304f, 305f, 307f, 310, 310f, 311f, 314f
  right, 304f, 307f, 309f, 310, 310f, 311f
Inferior rectus muscle, 81, 81f–84f
Inferior root
  of orbit, 72, 72f
Inferior sagittal sinus, 138–140, 138f, 140f
Inferior suprarenal arteries, 405
Inferior thyroid artery, 562f
Inferior trunk, 565
Inferior ulnar collateral artery, 562f
Inferior vena cava (IVC)
  in abdomen, 354f, 418–420, 418f–421f
  in pelvis, 477f, 483, 483f, 484f
  in thorax, 304f, 305f, 314, 315f, 322f
Inferior vertebral notch, 165f, 166f
Inferior vesical artery, 475, 482t
Inferior vesical vein, 485f
Infracolic compartment, 345, 345f, 345t
Infracolic spaces, 345, 345f, 345t, 347f
Infraglenoid tubercle, 492f, 493, 495f
Infrahyoid muscles, 264, 264t, 265f, 333f
Infrahyoid region, 266, 268t
Infraorbital canal, 72, 73f
Infraorbital foramen, 30t, 49f, 50, 51f, 72, 72f
Infraorbital groove, 71f, 72, 72f
Infrapatellar bursa
  deep, 610, 610f
  subcutaneous, 610f
  superficial, 610
Infrapatellar fat body, 607f, 621f
Infraspinatus muscle, 504f, 506f–508f, 511f, 511t, 512f, 513, 513f
Infraspinous fossa, 492f, 493
Infratentorial fossa, 18, 20f, 20t
Infundibulopelvic ligament, 456f
Infundibulum
  of ethmoid bone, 24, 24f
  of osteomeatal complex, 70, 70f, 71f
  of pituitary gland, 109, 109f–111f
  of uterine tubes, 460

Inguinal canal, 463f
Inguinal hernias
  indirect, 438
Inguinal ligament, 426, 438, 463f, 654f
Inguinal lymph nodes, 487, 487f
  deep, 422f, 486f
  superficial, 422f, 486f
Inguinal ring
  superficial, 463f
  external, 427f
Inner inguinal ring, 456f
Innermost intercostal muscles, 330
Innominate trunk, 318f, 319
Insula, 99f, 103, 103f–105f
Insulin, 373
Interatrial septum, 296, 296f, 300f
Intercarpal arch
  dorsal, 563f
Intercarpal compartment, 545f
Intercarpal joints, 543f, 545
Intercarpal ligament(s), 545f, 546, 546f
  dorsal, 547f, 556f
Intercondylar eminence, 593f, 597, 597f, 604f
Intercondylar fossa, 593, 594f, 595f
Intercondylar line, 593
Intercondylar notch, 571f, 602f
Intercondylar tubercles
  lateral, 597
Intercostal muscles, 330, 330f–332f, 330t, 334f
  external, 330, 330f, 424f, 427f
  innermost, 330
  internal, 330, 330f, 424f, 427f
Intercostal spaces, 276
Intercostalis intimi muscle, 330f
Intercuneiform ligament
  interosseous, 639f
Interlobar arteries, 404f
Interlobar fissure, 351, 351f, 352
Interlobar veins, 404f, 420
Interlobular arteries, 404f
Interlobular veins, 404f, 420
Intermediate antebrachial vein, 564, 565
Intermediate cuneiform bone, 624f, 626f, 639f, 648f
Intermediate dorsal cutaneous nerve, 616f
Intermetacarpal articulation, 545
Intermetacarpal joint, 543f, 545
Intermetacarpal ligament
  deep transverse, 551f
Intermetatarsal joints, 631f, 637
Intermuscular septum
  posterior, 615f
Internal anal sphincter, 452, 452f
Internal auditory artery, 138f
Internal auditory canal (IAC), 30t, 34f, 36, 36f, 39, 44f, 45f, 158f
Internal capsule, 106, 106f–108f
Internal carotid artery, 127f–131f, 128–131, 131t, 269, 269f–271f
  in circle of Willis, 135f, 136f, 138f
Internal cerebral veins, 138f, 140f, 145, 145f–147f
Internal iliac artery, 475, 475f–481f
  left, 401f, 475f
  right, 401f, 475f
Internal iliac lymph nodes, 486f, 487
Internal iliac veins, 476f, 478f, 479f, 483, 484f, 485f
Internal intercostal muscles, 330, 330f, 424f, 427f
Internal jugular veins
  in brain, 138, 145f
  in neck, 269f, 272, 272f, 273t
  in thorax, 318f, 321
Internal landmarks, 5, 5t, 6f
Internal oblique muscles, 424f, 425f, 426, 427f, 428t, 438
Internal occipital protuberance, 32, 33f
Internal os, 454, 454f
Internal pudendal artery, 475, 477f, 479f, 481f, 482f, 654f
Internal pudendal vein, 485f
Internal thoracic arteries, 320f, 321
Internal thoracic vein, 320f
Internal urethral sphincter, 450
Internal venous plexus, 222, 223f

Interosseous artery(ies), 563
  anterior, 562f, 563
  common, 562f, 563
  posterior, 562f, 563
Interosseous calcaneal ligament, 650f
Interosseous intercuneiform ligament, 639f
Interosseous ligament, 545f, 626f, 640, 643f
Interosseous membrane, 524f, 526, 598f,
    615f–617f, 650f
Interosseous muscles
  of foot, 653f
    dorsal, 626f, 651, 652t, 653f, 654f
    plantar, 651, 652f–654f
  of hand, 557, 559f–561f, 653f
    dorsal, 557, 559f–561f
Interosseous talocalcaneal ligament, 639f
Interosseous tendon, 552f
Interpeduncular cistern, 95f, 96, 96f
Interphalangeal joint(s)
  of foot, 637
  of hand
    distal, 539f, 540, 550f
    proximal, 539f, 540, 550f
Interspinous ligament, 179f, 182f, 183f
Intertarsal joints, 637
Intertransverse muscle
  anterior, 260f
Intertrochanteric crest, 568, 571f, 572f
Intertrochanteric line, 568, 571f, 572f
Intertubercular groove, 493f, 496f, 497, 497f,
    522f
Interventricular artery
  posterior, 322f
Interventricular branch
  posterior, 323
Interventricular foramen, 89f, 90f, 91
Interventricular groove, 304f
  posterior, 323
Interventricular septum, 296, 300f–302f
Intervertebral disks, 166, 166f–168f
  herniated, 208
Intervertebral foramina, 164–166, 166f, 167f
Intervertebral veins, 222, 222f
Intestines, 392–397, 392f–400f
Intrahepatic bile ducts, 367, 369f
Intrinsic ligaments
  of wrist, 545f, 546, 546f
Iris, 76
Ischial ramus, 432f, 433f
  inferior, 436
  superior, 436
Ischial spine, 432f, 433f, 435f, 436, 436f
Ischial tuberosity, 430f, 432f, 433f, 435f, 436,
    436f
Ischioacetabular ligament, 577
Ischiocavernous muscle, 463f
Ischiofemoral ligament, 573f–575f
Ischium, 430f, 432f–435f, 436, 568, 568f, 570f,
    572f–575f
Island of Reil, 99f, 103, 103f–105f
Isthmus
  of thyroid gland, 246, 246f
IT (iliotibial) band, 574f, 575f, 579f, 584, 584f,
    588f
IVC. See Inferior vena cava (IVC).

J
Jejunal artery, 413
Jejunum, 392, 392f–395f, 397f–399f
Jugular foramen, 30t, 36, 36f
Jugular fossa, 35f, 36, 37f
Jugular notch, 276, 276f
Jugular vein(s), 250f–259f, 269f–271f, 272,
    273f, 321
  anterior, 272, 272f
  external, 272, 272f, 273t, 321
  internal
    in brain, 138, 145f
    in neck, 269f, 272, 272f, 273t
    in thorax, 318f, 321

K
Kidneys, 382, 382f
Knee and lower leg, 593–623
  bony anatomy of, 593–602, 593f–602f
  bursae of, 610, 610f

Knee and lower leg—cont'd
  ligaments of, 608, 608f, 609f
  menisci of, 603, 603f–607f
  muscles of, 611–623, 611t, 612f–623f
Kohlrausch's fold, 452, 452f
Kyphotic curves, 164, 164f

L
Labia majora, 447f, 453f
Labia minora, 447f, 453f
Labrum, 497f, 498, 498f
Labyrinth(s)
  bony, 39, 39f–41f, 43f–46f
  of ethmoid bone, 23, 24f, 65
  membranous, 39, 41f
Lacrimal apparatus, 80, 80f, 81f
Lacrimal bones, 49f–51f, 50
Lacrimal canaliculi, 80, 80f
Lacrimal fossa, 72, 72f
Lacrimal gland, 76, 78f, 79f, 80, 84f
Lacrimal groove, 30t, 49f, 50, 50f, 72, 72f
Lacrimal sac, 50, 80, 80f
Lactiferous ducts, 335, 335f
LAD (left anterior descending) artery, 319,
    322f, 323, 323f, 325f, 326f
Lambda, 48
Lambdoidal suture, 47, 47f
Lamina(e)
  vertebral, 164, 164f, 165f
Lamina terminalis, 89f, 91
Landmarks
  external (surface), 3, 4f, 5f
  internal, 5, 5t, 6f
Large bowel, 396f–400f, 397
Large intestine, 396f–400f, 397
Laryngeal muscles, 262, 262f, 263f, 263t
Laryngopharynx, 226f–228f, 232, 232f, 233f
Larynx, 234–237, 234f–240f
Lateral aperture, 89f, 91
Lateral cervical ligaments, 456, 456f–458f
Lateral circumflex artery, 477f, 655f, 660f
Lateral circumflex femoral artery, 654f, 655,
    659f, 660f
Lateral collateral ligament
  of elbow, 527, 528f, 529f
  of knee, 603f, 604f, 608, 608f, 610f, 612f
Lateral common iliac lymph nodes, 487
Lateral condyle(s)
  of femur, 593, 593f–595f
  of humerus, 522f, 523
  of occipital bone, 30, 31f
  of tibia, 595, 595f
Lateral cricoarytenoid muscle, 262, 262f, 263t
Lateral cuneiform, 624f, 639f, 648f
Lateral cutaneous nerve, 566, 566f, 664f
Lateral epicondyle
  of femur, 571f, 572f, 593, 593f, 595f
  of humerus, 496f, 522f, 523, 524f, 525f
Lateral fissure, 98, 98f, 99f, 104f, 105f
Lateral horn, 201f
Lateral intercondylar tubercles, 597
Lateral lenticulostriate arteries, 131
Lateral ligament
  of TMJ, 60, 60f, 61f
Lateral longitudinal arch, 624f, 637
Lateral malleolar artery, 659f
Lateral malleolus, 597f, 600, 612f, 620f, 622f
Lateral masses
  of cervical vertebrae, 169, 169f, 170f
  of ethmoid bone, 23, 24f, 65
  of sacrum, 177, 177f, 178f, 430, 430f, 431f
Lateral meniscus, 603, 603f–605f, 608f, 612f,
    620f, 621f
Lateral patellar retinaculum, 608, 608f
Lateral plantar artery, 641f, 646f, 648f, 659f
Lateral plantar nerve, 627f, 639f, 641f, 646f,
    648f
Lateral popliteal nerve, 586f, 613f, 664f
Lateral pterygoid muscle, 62, 62f, 63f
Lateral rectus muscle, 81, 82f, 83f
Lateral sacral artery, 475, 477f, 482f, 482t, 654f
Lateral sacral veins, 485f
Lateral supracondylar line, 572f, 593
Lateral supracondylar ridge, 496f, 522f
Lateral sural cutaneous nerve, 613f
Lateral talocalcaneal ligament, 650f

Lateral tarsal artery, 659f
Lateral thoracic artery, 562f
Lateral tibial plateau, 595f, 597f, 598f
Lateral umbilical ligaments, 449f, 450, 456f
Lateral ventricles, 89, 90f, 92f–94f
Latissimus dorsi muscle, 504, 504f, 510t
Le Fort fractures, 50
Left anterior descending (LAD) artery, 319,
    322f, 323, 323f, 325f, 326f
Left aortic sinus, 323
Left colic artery, 416, 417f, 477f
  superior, 416f
Left colic flexure, 392f, 393f, 396f, 397, 398f,
    399f
Left common carotid artery, 269, 270f, 270t,
    271f, 318f–320f, 319, 322f
Left common iliac artery, 402f, 476f, 477f, 481f,
    482f
Left common iliac vein, 477f
Left coronary artery, 322f, 323, 323f, 325f, 326f
Left gastric artery, 401f, 402f, 407, 407f, 410f,
    411f
Left gastric vein, 484f
Left gastroepiploic artery, 362f, 407f, 409, 411f
Left gastro-omental artery, 409
Left gonadal artery, 401f, 475f
Left gonadal vein, 419
Left hepatic artery, 362f, 363, 364f, 402f, 407f,
    410f
Left hepatic duct, 367, 367f, 368f
Left hepatic vein, 354f, 355f, 359f, 363, 364f,
    365f, 420
Left inferior phrenic artery, 403
Left inferior phrenic vein, 418, 418f
Left inferior pulmonary vein, 304f, 305f, 307f,
    310, 310f, 311f, 314f
Left internal iliac artery, 401f, 475f
Left main portal vein, 359
Left marginal artery, 323
Left portal vein, 356f–358f, 484f
Left posterior ventricular vein, 328
Left pulmonary artery, 304, 304f, 305f, 307f,
    309f
Left pulmonary veins, 322f, 323f, 326f
Left renal artery, 405f, 406f, 417f, 483f
Left renal vein, 405f, 420, 421f
Left superior pulmonary vein, 304f, 305f, 307f,
    309f–311f, 310, 314f
Left suprarenal vein, 420
Left testicular vein, 484f
Lens, 76, 76f
Lenticulostriate arteries
  lateral, 131
  medial, 128
Lentiform nucleus, 106, 106f–108f
Lesser curvature
  of stomach, 389, 389f, 390f
Lesser multiangular bone, 539f–541f, 540
Lesser omentum, 338f, 341, 342f
Lesser sac, 338–341, 338f, 340f, 341f
Lesser saphenous veins, 615f–617f, 620f
Lesser trochanter, 430f, 568, 569f–572f
Lesser tubercle
  of humerus, 490f, 493f, 496f, 497, 497f
Lesser wings
  of sphenoid bone, 25, 25f, 28f
Levator anguli oris muscle, 265f
Levator ani muscles, 440t, 443, 443f–446f, 452f
Levator glandulae thyroideae muscle, 265f
Levator labii superioris alaeque nasi muscle,
    265f
Levator labii superioris muscle, 265f
Levator scapulae muscle, 264t, 265f, 266, 266f,
    504, 504f, 506f, 510t
Levator veli palatini muscle, 260f, 263f
Levatores costarum muscle, 331f
Lienal artery, 409
Lienorenal ligaments, 338f, 340t, 376, 376f
Ligament(s)
  of spine, 179–182, 179f–185f
Ligament of Humphrey, 603, 612f
Ligament of the head of the femur, 568, 569f
Ligament of Treitz, 392, 393f
Ligament of Wrisberg, 603, 612f
Ligamentum arteriosum, 304, 304f, 307f, 322f
Ligamentum flava, 182, 182f–185f

Ligamentum nuchae, 179, 179f–181f, 184f
Ligamentum teres, 341, 350f, 352, 568, 569f, 573f, 574f, 578f
  fissure for, 351, 351f
Ligamentum venosum, 352, 352f, 356f, 357f
  fissure for, 351, 351f
Limbic system, 113, 113f–115f
Linea alba, 426, 427f, 431f
Linea aspera, 568–569, 571f, 572f, 588f
Lingual tonsils, 226, 226f, 227f
Lingula, 279, 279f, 281f, 313f
Lipase, 373
Lister's tubercle, 523f, 524, 539f
Liver, 350f, 351–366, 351f
  portal hepatic system of, 359, 359f–361f
  segmental anatomy of, 354, 354f–358f
  surface anatomy of, 352, 353f
  vasculature of, 362f–366f, 363
Lobar fissure
  main, 351, 351f
Long plantar ligament, 641f
Long radiolunate ligament, 547f
Long saphenous vein, 585f, 586f
Longissimus capitis muscle, 186t, 188f
Longissimus cervicis, 186t
Longissimus muscles, 186t, 187f, 188, 188f, 192f, 425f
Longissimus thoracis, 186t
Longitudinal arch, 637
  lateral, 624f, 637
  medial, 624f, 637
Longitudinal fissure, 98, 99f, 103f
Longitudinal ligament
  anterior, 179–182, 179f–183f
  posterior, 179f–185f, 182
Longitudinal muscle, 263f
Longus capitis muscle, 264t, 265f
Longus colli muscle, 264t
Loops of Henle, 382, 385f
Lordotic curves, 164, 164f
Lower extremity, 567–664
  ankle and foot in, 625–651
    bony anatomy of, 624f–636f, 625
    fascia, retinacula, and ligaments of, 637–640, 638f–650f
    joints of, 637
    muscles of, 561, 651f, 652t, 653f, 654f
    tendons of, 638f–650f, 640–647
    arteries of, 654f–662f, 655–660
  hip in, 568–592
    articular capsule of, 579
    bony anatomy of, 568–569, 568f–572f
    labrum and ligaments of, 573–578, 573f–578f
    muscles of, 579–583, 579f–582f, 579t
  knee and lower leg of, 593–623
    bony anatomy of, 593–602, 593f–602f
    bursae of, 610, 610f
    ligaments of, 608, 608f, 609f
    menisci of, 603, 603f–607f
    muscles of, 611–623, 611t, 612f–623f
  nerves of, 664, 664f
  thigh muscles of, 583–592, 583t, 584f–592f
  veins of, 663, 663f, 664f
Lower left colic arteries, 416f
Lower leg. *See* Knee and lower leg.
Lower segmental artery, 404f
Lumbar arteries, 401f, 402f, 403, 475f, 477f
Lumbar azygos vein, 419f
Lumbar nerves, 201f
Lumbar nodes, 422f
Lumbar plexus, 206f, 213, 213f, 214f, 664f
Lumbar vein(s), 418, 419f, 420f
  ascending, 418, 419f
  first, 419f
  second, 419f
  third, 419f
Lumbar vertebrae, 164f–168f, 175, 175f, 176f
Lumbosacral enlargement, 204
Lumbosacral plexus, 206f
Lumbrical muscles, 557–560, 559f, 560f, 651, 653f
Lunate, 539f–545f, 540
Lung(s), 279–282, 279f–282f
  anterior border of, 279, 280f, 281f, 311f
  apex of, 279, 279f, 281f, 311f, 312f

Lung(s)—cont'd
  bases (diaphragmatic surfaces) of, 279, 279f, 281f, 311f
  costal surface of, 279, 279f
  cystic disease of, 282
  hilum of, 279f, 282, 282f
  horizontal fissure of, 279, 279f, 281f, 311
  inferior border of, 279, 279f, 281f, 312f
  lateral angle of, 279, 279f, 280f
  lingula of, 279, 279f, 281f
  lobes of, 279, 279f, 280f
  medial angle of, 279, 279f
  mediastinal or medial surface of, 279, 279f, 311f, 312f
  oblique fissure of, 279, 279f–281f, 311f
  posterior border of, 279, 281f, 312f
Lung cancer, 283
  staging of, 291t
Lung window, 11f
Lymph nodes
  abdominal, 422f, 423, 423f
  cervical, 225f, 248–249, 248f, 249t, 250f–259f, 422f
  iliac
    common, 422f, 486f, 487
      lateral, 487
      median, 487
    external, 486f, 487
    internal, 486f, 487
  inguinal, 487, 487f
    deep, 422f, 486f
    superficial, 422f, 486f
  lumbar, 422f
  mediastinal, 290, 290f, 291f, 291t
  obturator, 486f, 487
  pelvic, 486f, 487, 487f
  preaortic, 486f
  sacral, 486f, 487
  supraclavicular (sentinel), 290
  visceral, 423
Lymph vessels, 292, 292f
Lymphatic duct
  right, 292, 292f
Lymphatic system, 290–292, 290f–292f, 291t, 422f

M
Magnetic resonance (MR) imaging, 11, 12f
Main lobar fissure, 351, 351f
Main pancreatic duct, 367
Main portal vein, 357f–359f, 410f
  left, 359
  right, 359
Major calyces, 382, 385f
Malar bone, 49f–52f, 50, 54f
Male pelvis, 448f
Male reproductive organs, 462–473, 462f–474f
Malleolar artery
  lateral, 659f
  medial, 659f
Malleolar fossa, 597f, 600
Malleolar groove, 600
Malleolus(i), 601f
  lateral, 597f, 600, 612f, 620f, 622f
  medial, 597, 597f, 622f, 623f
Malleus, 39, 39f, 43f, 45f
Mamillary bodies, 99f, 113, 113f
Mammary gland, 335, 335f, 336f
Mammary layer, 335, 336f
Mandible, 49f, 56, 56f–58f
Mandibular branch, 154, 154f
Mandibular condyle, 56, 56f–58f
Mandibular fossa, 34, 34f, 58f, 59, 59f
Mandibular notch, 56, 56f
Mandibular rami, 56, 57f
Manubrium, 276, 276f, 277f, 490f
Marginal artery, 416f
  left, 323
Marginal branch
  right, 322f, 323
Massa intermedia, 100f, 107f, 109
Masseter muscle, 62, 62f, 63f, 265f, 267f
Mastication
  muscles of, 62, 62f, 63f
Masticator space (MS), 267f, 268t
Mastoid antrum, 35f, 36, 36f

Mastoid fontanels, 48, 48f
Mastoid process, 34f, 36, 36f
Maxilla, 49f–51f, 50, 53f
Maxillary branch, 154, 154f
Maxillary region, 50f, 73f
Maxillary sinuses, 50, 50f, 64f, 65t, 66f, 67, 67f
Maximum intensity projection (MIP), 15, 15f
MCA (middle cerebral artery), 127f, 128f, 129–131, 130f, 131f, 131t, 133f
  in circle of Willis, 135f, 136f, 138f
  thalamostriate branches of, 117
MCP (metacarpophalangeal) joint, 539f, 540, 552f
Meckel's cave, 37f, 38, 155f
Medial circumflex artery, 477f, 650f
Medial circumflex femoral artery, 578f, 654f, 655, 659f
Medial collateral ligament
  of elbow, 527, 527f, 528f
  of knee, 603f, 604f, 608, 608f
Medial condyle(s)
  of femur, 593, 593f, 595f
  of humerus, 522f, 523
  of tibia, 597, 597f
Medial cuneiform, 624f, 639f, 648f
Medial dorsal cutaneous nerve, 616f
Medial epicondyle
  of femur, 571f, 593, 593f, 595f
  of humerus, 496f, 522f, 523, 524f, 525f
Medial genicular artery
  superior, 659f
Medial longitudinal arch, 624f, 637
Medial malleolar artery, 659f
Medial malleolus, 597, 597f, 622f, 623f
Medial meniscus, 596f, 598f, 603, 603f–605f, 607f, 612f
Medial patellar retinaculum, 605f, 608, 608f
Medial plantar artery, 641f, 659f
Medial plantar nerve, 627f, 639f, 641f, 646f, 648f
Medial popliteal nerve, 664f
Medial pterygoid muscle, 62, 62f, 63f
Medial rectus muscle, 81, 82f, 83f
Medial supracondylar line, 593
Medial supracondylar ridge, 522f
Medial sural cutaneous nerve, 615f
Medial talocalcaneal ligament, 650f
Medial tarsal artery, 659f
Medial tibial plateau, 593f, 597f, 598f
Medial umbilical ligaments, 449f, 450, 456f
Median antebrachial vein, 564, 565f
Median aperture, 89f, 91
Median arcuate ligament, 355f
Median common iliac lymph nodes, 487
Median cubital vein, 564, 565f
Median fissure
  anterior, 122, 122f, 123f
  posterior, 122
Median nerve, 208, 209f, 565, 566f
Median raphe, 463
Median sacral artery, 403, 654f
Median sacral vein, 419f, 483, 484f
Median umbilical ligament, 449f, 450, 456f
Mediastinal compartments, 286, 287f
Mediastinal lymph nodes, 290, 290f, 291f, 291t
Mediastinal window, 11f
Mediastinum, 5, 7f, 7t, 279f, 286–289, 287f
  and diaphragm, 312f
  and pulmonary vessels, 312f
  thymus gland in, 286, 287f, 288f
  trachea and esophagus in, 289, 289f
Mediocarpal compartment, 545f
Medulla oblongata, 116f, 122, 122f–124f
Medullary pyramids, 117f, 122, 122f
Medullary velum
  inferior, 91, 91f
  superior, 91, 91f
Membranous labyrinth, 39, 41f
Membranous urethra, 448f, 449f, 451, 462f, 467f, 470f
Meniere's disease, 41
Meninges
  cranial, 86–87, 86f–88f
  spinal, 193–195, 193f–195f, 201f
Meniscofemoral ligament
  anterior, 603, 603f

Meniscofemoral ligament—cont'd
  posterior, 603, 603f, 604f, 608f, 610f
Meniscus(i), 603, 603f–607f
  lateral, 603, 603f–605f, 608f, 612f, 620f, 621f
  medial, 596f, 598f, 603, 603f–605f, 607f, 612f
  of TMJ, 58f, 60, 60f, 61f
Mental foramen, 30t, 56, 56f
Mesencephalon, 116f–119f, 117
Mesenteric artery
  inferior, 401f, 403f, 414f–417f, 416
  superior, 401f–403f, 410f, 411f, 413, 413f–416f
Mesenteric vein
  inferior, 359f, 414f, 484f
  superior, 350f, 358f, 361f, 410f, 484f
Mesentery, 340f, 341, 342f
Mesocolon, 396f
Metacarpal(s), 539f, 540, 541f–545f, 550f
Metacarpal base, 539f
Metacarpal compartment ligament, 545f
Metacarpal head, 539f
Metacarpal ligament(s), 545
  deep transverse, 548, 552f
Metacarpal muscle group, 557–560, 559f, 560f
Metacarpophalangeal (MCP) joint, 539f, 540, 552f
Metatarsal artery
  first dorsal, 659f
  plantar, 659f
Metatarsal bones, 624f, 625, 626f
Metatarsal ligament
  deep transverse, 640
Metatarsal veins, 663f
Metatarsophalangeal joints, 626f, 631f, 636f, 637
Midbrain, 116f–119f, 117
Midcarpal joints, 543f, 545, 545f
Middle cardiac vein, 327f, 328
Middle cerebellar peduncles, 125, 126f
Middle cerebral artery (MCA), 127f, 128f, 129–131, 130f, 131f, 131t, 133f
  in circle of Willis, 135f, 136f, 138f
  thalamostriate branches of, 117
Middle cerebral vein
  superficial, 138f, 145f
Middle colic artery, 413, 414f, 415f
Middle constrictor muscle, 260, 260f, 261t
Middle cranial fossa, 18, 20f, 20t
Middle glenohumeral ligament, 495f, 497f–499f, 501f, 502f, 513f
Middle hepatic vein, 354f–356f, 359f, 363, 364f–366f, 420
Middle nasal conchae, 24, 24f, 55f
Middle nasal meatus, 55, 55f
  drainage into, 65, 65t, 69
Middle phalanges
  of foot, 624f
  of hand, 539f, 540, 550f
Middle rectal artery, 475, 477f, 482t
Middle rectal veins, 484f, 485f
Middle sacral artery, 477f, 483f
Middle sacral vein, 418f, 483f
Middle scalene muscle, 264t, 265f, 266
Middle segmental artery, 404f
Middle suprarenal arteries, 378f, 403f, 405
Middle trunk, 565
Midtarsal joint, 637
Mineralocorticoids, 378
Minor calyces, 382, 385f
MIP (maximum intensity projection), 15, 15f
Mitral valve, 293f, 295f, 296f, 302f, 303
Modiolus muscle, 265f
Mons pubis, 447f, 453f
Morison's pouch, 345, 346f, 347f
Mortise joint, 626f–628f, 637
MPR (multiplanar reformation), 13, 13f
MR (magnetic resonance) imaging, 11, 12f
MS (masticator space), 267f, 268t
Multiangular bone
  greater, 539f–541f, 540
  lesser, 539f–541f, 540
Multifidus muscle, 186, 186f–188f, 186t, 190, 190f
Multiplanar reformation (MPR), 13, 13f
Mumps virus
  and parotid gland, 245

Muscles of mastication, 62, 62f, 63f
Musculocutaneous nerve, 208, 209f, 565, 566, 566f
Musculus uvulae, 263f
Mylohyoid muscle, 261f, 264, 264t, 265f
Myocardium, 295f, 296, 296f, 302f
Myometrium, 453f–455f, 454

N

Nasal bones, 49f–52f, 50
Nasal conchae
  inferior, 49f, 51f, 55, 55f
  middle, 24, 24f, 55f
  superior, 24, 24f, 55f
Nasal meatus(i), 55, 55f
  drainage into, 65, 65t, 67, 68, 69
  inferior, 55, 55f
  middle, 55, 55f
    drainage into, 65, 65t, 69
  superior, 55, 55f
    drainage into, 65, 65t, 68
Nasal septum, 54f, 55
Nasal spine
  anterior, 49f–51f, 50
Nasal turbinates, 24, 24f
Nasolacrimal canal, 30t
Nasolacrimal duct, 80, 80f, 81f
Nasopharynx, 226, 226f, 228f, 229f
Navicular bone
  of foot, 624f, 625, 626f, 630f, 633f
  of hand, 539f, 540, 540f
Neck, 225–273
  cervical lymph nodes in, 225f, 248–249, 248f, 249t, 250f–259f
  esophagus and trachea in, 241, 241f
  facial planes and spaces of, 250f–259f, 266, 267f, 268t
  larynx in, 234–237, 234f–240f
  muscles of, 260–266
    within anterior triangle, 250f–259f, 264, 264t, 265f
    laryngeal, 262, 262f, 263f, 263t
    pharyngeal, 260, 260f, 261f, 261t
    within posterior triangle, 250f–259f, 266, 266f, 267f
  pharynx in, 226–232, 226f–233f
  salivary glands in, 242–245, 242f–245f
  sequential scans of, 250f–259f
  thyroid gland in, 246, 246f, 247f
  vascular structures of, 269–272
    carotid arteries in, 250f–259f, 269, 269f–271f, 270t
    carotid sheath in, 272, 273f
    jugular veins as, 250f–259f, 269f–271f, 272, 273t
    vertebral arteries in, 250f–259f, 270f, 270t, 271f, 272
Nephron, 382, 385f
Nerve plexuses, 204–217, 206f
  brachial, 206f, 208, 209f–212f
  cervical, 206f–209f, 207
  lumbar, 206f, 213, 213f, 214f
  sacral, 206f, 213f, 215, 215f–217f
Nerve root sleeve, 200f
Neurohypophysis, 109
Norepinephrine, 378
Nucleus pulposus, 166, 167f, 168f

O

Oblique arytenoid muscle, 263f
Oblique muscle(s), 81, 81f–84f
  external, 424f, 425f, 426, 427f, 428t, 438
  inferior, 81, 81f, 84f
  internal, 424f, 425f, 426, 427f, 428t, 438
  superior, 81, 82f–84f, 260f
Oblique plane, 2, 2f
Oblique popliteal ligament, 607f, 608
Oblique retinacular ligament, 551f
Oblique vein of left atrium, 328
Obturator artery, 475, 477, 480f, 482t, 654f, 659f
Obturator externus muscle, 440, 440t, 442f, 577f, 578f, 579t, 580f, 583
Obturator foramen, 430f, 431f, 433f, 436, 436f, 572f
Obturator internus muscle, 440, 440f, 440t, 442f, 574f, 575f, 579t, 580–583, 580f

Obturator internus tendon, 574f, 577f, 578f
Obturator nerve, 585f, 664, 664f
Obturator nodes, 486f, 487
Obturator veins, 485f
Obtuse marginal branch, 325f
Occipital bone, 18f, 19f, 30–32, 30f–33f
Occipital condyle, 30, 31f
Occipital horn, 89, 89f, 90f
Occipital lobe, 98f, 103, 103f
Occipital protuberance
  internal, 32, 33f
Occipital sinus, 138f
Occipitofrontalis muscle, 265f
Oculomotor nerve, 116f, 148f, 148t, 152, 152f, 153f
Odontoid process, 169, 169f–171f
Olecranon bursa, 526f
Olecranon fossa, 522f, 523, 525f
Olecranon process, 524, 524f
Olfactory bulb, 149, 149f
Olfactory nerve, 116f, 148f, 148t, 149, 149f
Olfactory tracts, 113, 115f, 149, 149f
Olives, 122, 122f–124f
OMC (osteomeatal complex), 70, 70f, 71f
Omental bursae, 338–341, 338f
Omentum, 341
  greater, 340f, 341, 342f, 343f
  lesser, 338f, 341, 342f
Omohyoid muscle, 264, 264t, 265f
Ophthalmic artery, 127f, 128, 131t
Ophthalmic branch, 154, 154f
Ophthalmic vein(s), 140
  superior, 78f, 79f, 82
Opponens digiti minimi muscle, 560, 560f, 561f, 654f
Opponens pollicis muscle, 560, 560f, 561f
Optic canal, 25, 27f, 30t, 72, 72f–74f
Optic chiasm, 110f, 150, 150f, 151f
  damage to, 98
Optic nerve, 76f, 82, 83f, 116f, 148f, 148t, 150, 150f, 151f
  damage to, 98
Optic radiations, 150, 151f
Optic strut, 72, 72f
Optic tracts, 99f, 150, 150f, 151f
Orbicular zone, 579
Orbicularis oculi muscle, 265f, 267f
Orbicularis oris muscle, 267f
Orbit, 72–84
  blowout fracture of, 76
  bony, 72, 72f–75f
  lacrimal apparatus of, 80, 80f, 81f
  muscles of, 81, 81f–84f
  optic nerve of, 76f, 77f, 82
  retroorbital fat of, 81f–83f, 82
  sagittal view of, 50f
  soft tissue structures of, 76, 76f–79f
Orbital artery, 130f
Orbital fissure
  inferior, 30t, 72, 72f, 75f
  superior, 18f, 28f, 29, 30t, 72, 72f, 74f
Orbital plates
  of ethmoid bone, 20f, 23, 24f
  of frontal bone, 22, 22f, 24f
Orbitofrontal artery, 129
Oropharynx, 226, 228f–232f, 253f, 254f
Os calcis, 600f
Os coxae, 430–436, 432f–435f
Os magnum, 539f, 540, 540f
Ossicles, 39, 39f, 43f, 45f
Osteomeatal complex (OMC), 70, 70f, 71f
Ostia, 70
Oval window, 39, 39f
Ovarian arteries, 405, 477f, 483f
Ovarian ligament, 454f, 456f, 460
Ovarian vein, 418f, 483f
  right, 484f
Ovaries, 453f, 454f, 456f, 460, 460f
Ovum(a), 460

P

PAG (periaqueductal gray matter), 117, 117f, 118f
Palatine bones, 50, 50f, 52f
Palatine process
  of maxilla, 50, 51f, 52f

Palatine tonsils, 226, 226f, 227f, 229f
Palatoglossus muscle, 260, 261t
Palatopharyngeus muscle, 260, 261t, 263f
Palmar aponeurosis, 531f
Palmar arch
    deep, 562f, 563, 565
    superficial, 562f, 563, 563f, 565
Palmar carpal arch, 563
Palmar interossei, 559f, 561f
Palmar ligament, 546, 548
Palmar longus tendon, 556f
Palmar plate, 550f, 552f, 553f
Palmar radiocarpal arch, 563
Palmar radioulnar ligament, 547f
Palmar tendons, 548f, 549f, 554, 554f
Palmaris brevis muscle, 531f
Palmaris longus muscle, 530t, 531, 531f, 532f
Palmaris longus tendon, 532f, 557f, 560f
Pampiniform plexus, 463f, 465f
Pancreas, 351f, 373, 373f–375f
Pancreatic artery
    caudal, 409, 411f
    dorsal, 409, 410f, 411f
    great, 373f, 409, 410f, 411f
Pancreatic branches, 409
Pancreatic duct(s), 367f–369f, 375f
    main, 367
Pancreatic tail, 373
Pancreaticoduodenal artery
    inferior, 413, 414f
        anterior, 410f
    superior, 362f, 410f
        anterior, 409
        posterior, 409, 410f
Pancreaticoduodenal vein, 484f
Pancreatitis
    acute, 373
Papillary muscles, 296, 296f, 300f
Paracolic gutters, 345, 345f, 345t, 347f
Parahippocampal gyrus, 99f, 103, 113f, 115f
Paranasal sinuses, 64–71, 64f
    drainage locations of, 65t
    ethmoid, 64f–66f, 65t
    frontal, 64f, 65t, 69, 69f
    maxillary, 64f, 65t, 66f, 67, 67f
    and osteomeatal complex, 70, 70f, 71f
    sphenoid, 64f–66f, 65t, 68, 68f
Parapharyngeal space (PPS), 267f, 268t
Paraplegia, 213
Pararenal fat, 383f
Pararenal space(s), 345t, 348f, 349, 349f
    anterior, 345t, 348f, 349
    posterior, 345t, 348f, 349
Parathyroid glands, 246, 246f
Paravertebral gutters, 382
Parietal bone, 18f, 19f, 20, 21f
Parietal branches
    of abdominal aorta, 401, 403
Parietal eminence, 20, 21f
Parietal lobe, 98f, 103, 103f
Parietal pericardium, 294, 294f
Parietal peritoneum, 338, 338f, 340f
Parietal pleura, 279f, 283, 283f
Parietooccipital artery, 130f
Parotid duct, 242, 242f
Parotid glands, 242, 242f–244f, 252f, 253f
    mumps virus and, 245
Parotid space (PS), 268t
Patella, 592f, 602, 602f, 603f
    apex of, 593f, 602f
    base of, 593f, 602f
Patellar ligament, 584, 592f, 599f, 603f,
    607f–610f, 608
Patellar retinaculum, 608
    lateral, 608, 608f
    medial, 605f, 608, 608f
Patellar surface
    of femur, 571f, 593, 594f
Patellofemoral articulation, 602
Patellofemoral joint, 594f, 602, 602f
PCA (posterior cerebral artery), 127f, 130f,
    132–133, 133f–138f, 137t
PCS (posterior cervical space), 268t
Pectineal line, 430f, 434f, 435, 436f, 569,
    572f
Pectineus muscle, 583t, 584, 584f, 589f

Pectoralis major muscle, 333, 333f, 333t, 334f,
    514f, 514t, 515
Pectoralis minor muscle, 333, 333f, 333t, 334f,
    514f, 514t, 515
Pectoralis muscles, 333, 333f, 333t, 334f, 514f
Pedicles, 164, 164f–166f
Pelvic brim, 434f, 436, 436f
Pelvic cavity, 5, 7f, 7t
Pelvic diaphragm muscles, 440t, 443, 443f–446f
Pelvic inlet, 436, 436f
Pelvic lymph nodes, 486f, 487, 487f
Pelvic outlet, 436, 436f
Pelvic spaces, 459, 459f
Pelvic wall muscles, 440, 440f–442f, 440t
Pelvis, 429–487
    bony, 430–437
        ilium in, 433, 433f, 434f
        ischium in, 436
        pelvic inlet and outlet in, 436, 436f
        perineum in, 436, 437f
        pubis in, 435, 435f
        sacrum, coccyx, and os coxae in, 430–436,
            430f–435f
    false, 436, 436f
    female, 447f
    lymph nodes of, 486f, 487, 487f
    male, 448f
    muscles of, 438–446
        extrapelvic, 438, 438f, 439f
        of pelvic diaphragm, 440t, 443, 443f–446f
        pelvic wall, 440, 440f–442f, 440t
    true, 436, 436f
    vasculature of, 475–485
        arteries in, 475, 475f–482f, 482t
        venous drainage in, 483, 483f–485f
    viscera of, 447–474
        female reproductive organs as, 453–461,
            453f–461f
        male reproductive organs as, 462–473,
            462f–474f
        rectum as, 452, 452f
        urinary bladder as, 447–451, 447f–451f
Penile urethra, 451
Penis, 448f, 462f, 463f, 473, 473f, 474f
Peptidases, 373
Perforating arteries, 654f, 655, 659f, 660f
Perforating veins, 565f
Periaqueductal gray matter (PAG), 117, 117f,
    118f
Pericallosal artery, 129, 130f
Pericardial cavity, 279f, 294, 294f
Pericardium, 294, 294f, 295f
    parietal, 294, 294f
    serous, 294
    visceral, 294, 294f
Perimetrium, 454, 454f
Perineal flexure, 452
Perineum, 436, 437f
Perirenal fat, 378, 380f, 382, 383f, 386f, 387f
Perirenal spaces, 345t, 348f, 349, 349f
Peritoneal cavity, 338, 338f, 340f
Peritoneal ligaments, 341, 456f
Peritoneal spaces, 341f–343f, 345, 345f–347f,
    345t
Peritoneum, 338–341, 338f–344f, 340t
    parietal, 338, 338f, 340f
    visceral, 338, 338f
Peritonitis, 341
Peroneal artery, 659f, 660, 662f
Peroneal fibular artery, 613f
Peroneal fibular nerve, 613f
Peroneal nerve, 213f, 215, 612f
    common, 586f, 613f, 664, 664f
    deep, 613f–617f, 664f
    superficial, 614f, 615f, 664f
Peroneal retinaculum, 637
    inferior, 637, 638f
    superior, 637, 638f
Peroneal trochlea, 625, 625f
Peroneal veins, 616f, 617f, 619f, 663f
Peroneus brevis muscle, 611t, 613f, 619f, 622
Peroneus brevis tendon, 638f, 641f, 646f, 647
Peroneus longus muscle, 611t, 613f, 619f, 622
Peroneus longus tendon, 638f, 641f, 646f, 647,
    648f, 653f
Peroneus muscles, 611t, 622

Peroneus tertius muscle, 611, 611t, 612f, 638f,
    651f
Peroneus tertius tendon, 641f, 646f, 648f
Perpendicular plate, 23, 24f
Petrosal sinuses, 138f, 140, 142f
Phalanges
    of foot, 624f, 625
        distal, 624f
        middle, 624f
        proximal, 624f, 626f, 631f, 635f
    of hand, 539f, 540, 541f
        distal, 539f, 540, 550f
        middle, 539f, 540, 550f
        proximal, 539f, 540, 541f, 542f, 550f
Pharyngeal mucosal space (PMS), 268t
Pharyngeal muscles, 260, 260f, 261f, 261t
Pharyngeal tonsils, 226, 226f, 227f, 232
Pharynx, 226–232, 226f–233f
Phrenic artery(ies), 403
    inferior, 401f, 403, 403f, 475f, 483f
    left, 403
    right, 402f, 403
Phrenic nerve, 207, 208f
Phrenic suprarenal artery
    inferior, 403f
Phrenic vein(s), 483f
    inferior, 418, 419f
    left, 418, 418f
    right, 418, 418f
Phrenocolic ligament, 340t
Pia mater, 86f, 87
    spinal, 193, 194f
PICA (posterior inferior cerebellar artery), 127f,
    130f, 132, 133f–135f, 137t, 138f
Pineal gland, 100f, 112, 112f, 116f
Pinna, 39, 39f
PIP (proximal interphalangeal joint, 539f, 540,
    550f
Piriform sinuses (recesses), 227f, 232, 232f,
    233f, 236f, 237
Piriformis muscle, 438f–440f, 440, 440t, 580,
    580f–582f
Pisiform, 539f–543f, 540
Pisohamate ligament, 547f
Pituitary gland, 109, 110f, 111f
Pituitary stalk, 109, 109f–111f
Pixels, 10f, 11
Plantar aponeurosis, 626f, 627f, 637–640
Plantar arch, 637, 659f, 663f
Plantar artery
    lateral, 641f, 646f, 648f, 659f
    medial, 641f, 659f
Plantar branch
    deep, 659f
Plantar calcaneonavicular ligament, 639f, 650f
Plantar digital arteries, 659f
Plantar fascia, 626f, 637–640
Plantar interosseous muscles, 651, 652f–654f
Plantar ligament, 626f, 640, 649f, 650f
    long, 641f
Plantar metatarsal artery, 659f
Plantar nerve
    lateral, 627f, 639f, 641f, 646f, 648f
    medial, 627f, 639f, 641f, 646f, 648f
Plantar veins, 663f
Plantaris muscle, 608f, 611t, 622, 622f, 623f
Plantaris tendon, 615f–617f, 623f
Platysma muscle, 261f, 264t, 265f, 267f
Pleura, 279f, 283, 283f
    parietal, 279f, 283, 283f
    visceral, 279f, 283, 283f
Pleural cavities, 5, 7f, 7t, 279f–283f, 283
Pleural effusion, 283f
Plexuses, 204–217, 206f
    brachial, 206f, 208, 209f–212f
    cervical, 206f–209f, 207
    lumbar, 206f, 213, 213f, 214f
    sacral, 206f, 213f, 215, 215f–217f
PMS (pharyngeal mucosal space), 268t
Pons, 110f, 116f, 117f, 120, 121f, 122f
Pontine cistern, 93f, 96
Pontine vessels, 132, 133f, 137t, 138f
Popliteal artery, 659f, 660, 661f, 662f
Popliteal cyst, 610f
Popliteal ligament
    arcuate, 608

Popliteal ligament—cont'd
oblique, 607f, 608
Popliteal line, 597, 597f
Popliteal nerve
lateral, 586f, 613f, 664f
medial, 664f
Popliteal surface, 593
Popliteal vein, 663, 663f
Popliteofibular ligament, 608f
Popliteus bursa, 610, 610f
Popliteus muscle, 613f, 615f, 620f, 621f, 623, 623f
Popliteus tendon, 607f, 608f, 610f, 612f, 618f
Porta hepatis, 351, 359
Portal fissure, 351
Portal hepatic system, 359, 359f–361f
Portal hypertension, 359
Portal splenic confluence, 373
Portal vein(s), 359, 359f–362f
left, 356f–358f, 484f
main, 357f–359f, 410f
left, 359
right, 359
right, 356f–358f, 361f, 484f
Portocaval anastomosis, 484f
Postcentral gyrus, 98, 98f, 103f
Posterior acetabular labrum, 574f, 575f, 577f
Posterior arch
of cervical vertebrae, 169, 169f, 171f
Posterior atlanto-occipital membrane, 179, 179f
Posterior cardiac vein, 327f, 328
Posterior cecal artery, 414f
Posterior central vein, 222, 222f
Posterior cerebral artery (PCA), 127f, 130f, 132–133, 133f–138f, 137f
Posterior cervical space (PCS), 268t
Posterior circumflex humeral artery, 562f
Posterior clinoid processes, 25, 25f
Posterior column, 568, 568f, 569f
Posterior commissure, 100, 100f, 102f, 104f
Posterior communicating artery, 135f, 136f, 138f
Posterior compartment
of globe, 76, 76f, 77f
Posterior cranial fossa, 18, 20f, 20t
Posterior cricoarytenoid muscle, 262, 262f, 263f, 263t
Posterior cruciate ligament, 603f, 604f, 607f–610f, 608
Posterior descending artery, 323
Posterior external venous plexuses, 222, 222f, 223f
Posterior femoral cutaneous nerve, 585f, 586f
Posterior fontanel, 48, 48f
Posterior fornix, 461
Posterior horn, 89, 89f, 90f
Posterior inferior cerebellar artery (PICA), 127f, 130f, 132, 133f–135f, 137t, 138f
Posterior inferior iliac spine, 432f, 433f
Posterior intermuscular septum, 615f
Posterior internal vertebral venous plexus, 222, 222f, 223f
Posterior interosseous artery, 562f, 563
Posterior interventricular artery, 322f
Posterior interventricular branch, 323
Posterior interventricular groove, 323
Posterior longitudinal ligament, 179f–185f, 182
Posterior median (spinal) veins, 222, 222f
Posterior meniscofemoral ligament, 603, 603f, 604f, 608f, 610f
Posterior pararenal space, 345t, 348f, 349
Posterior radicular arteries, 219, 220f
Posterior radicular vein, 222, 222f
Posterior scalene muscle, 187f, 264t, 265f, 266
Posterior spinal arteries, 219, 220f
Posterior spinal branch, 220f
Posterior subtalar joint, 627f
Posterior superior iliac spine, 432f, 433f
Posterior superior pancreaticoduodenal artery, 409, 410f
Posterior talocalcaneal ligament, 650f
Posterior talofibular ligament, 627f, 629f, 640, 650f
Posterior tibial artery, 659f, 660, 661f, 662f
Posterior tibial nerve, 664f
Posterior tibial veins, 663, 663f

Posterior tibialis tendon, 601f, 640f, 643f, 644f, 647f, 647f
Posterior tibiofibular ligament, 640, 644f, 650f
Posterior tibiotalar ligament, 650f
Posterior triangle
of neck
muscles within, 250f–259f, 264t, 266, 266f, 267f
Posterior ulnar recurrent artery, 562f, 563
Posterior vertebral element, 164, 164f, 165f
Posterolateral fontanels, 48, 48f
Pouch of Douglas, 459
PPS (parapharyngeal space), 267f, 268t
Preaortic nodes, 486f
Precentral gyrus, 98, 98f, 103f
Prepatellar bursa
subcutaneous, 610, 610f
Prepuce, 473f
Prevertebral muscles, 264t
Prevertebral space (PVS), 267f, 268t
Primary visual area, 103
Profunda brachii artery, 562f
Profunda femoris artery, 654f, 655, 657f–660f, 663f
Profunda femoris vein, 585f, 663f
Progesterone, 460
Pronator quadratus muscle, 530t, 532f537f, 537
Pronator teres muscle, 530t, 531, 531f, 532f, 534f
Proper hepatic artery, 362f, 363, 407, 410f
Prostate cancer, 472
Prostate gland, 462f, 466f, 470f–473f, 471–472
Prostatic urethra, 448f, 451, 451f, 462f, 471f–473f
Prostatic venous plexus, 485f
Proximal interphalangeal (PIP) joint, 539f, 540, 550f
Proximal phalanges
of foot, 624f, 626f, 631f, 635f
of hand, 539f, 540, 541f, 542f, 550f
Proximal tibiofibular joint, 597f
PS (parotid space), 268t
Psoas major muscle, 440f, 583, 583t, 584f
Psoas minor muscle, 584f
Psoas muscles, 190, 191f, 192f, 424, 424f, 425f, 428f
Pterygoid canal, 28f, 29, 29f, 30t
Pterygoid hamulus, 26f, 28f, 29, 29f
Pterygoid muscle(s), 62, 62f, 63f
lateral, 62, 62f, 63f
medial, 62, 62f, 63f
Pterygoid plates, 28f, 29
Pterygoid process, 29
Pubic branch, 477f
Pubic ramus
inferior, 430f, 435, 435f, 572f
right, 436f
superior, 430f, 435, 435f, 572f
right, 436f
Pubic symphysis, 430f, 434f–436f, 435, 572f
female, 447f, 453, 453f
male, 462f
Pubis, 432f, 433f, 435, 435f, 568, 568f, 570f, 572f–574f
Pubofemoral ligament, 573f, 578
Puboprostatic ligament, 451
Pubovesical ligament, 451, 459f
Pudendal artery(ies), 475f
external, 654f, 655, 659f
internal, 475, 477f, 479f, 481f, 482t, 654f
Pudendal nerve, 664f
Pudendal vein
inferior, 485f
internal, 485f
Pulmonary arteries, 304, 304f, 307f, 309f
Pulmonary branch, 304f, 305f
Pulmonary embolism, 314
Pulmonary ligament, 311f
Pulmonary semilunar valve, 293f, 302f, 303
Pulmonary trunk, 296f, 304, 307f, 308f, 314f
Pulmonary vein(s), 304–310, 304f, 307f, 309f–311f
left, 322f, 323f, 326f
inferior, 304f, 305f, 307f, 310, 310f, 311f, 314f

Pulmonary vein(s)—cont'd
superior, 304f, 305f, 307f, 309f–311f, 310, 314f
right
inferior, 304f, 307f, 309f, 310, 310f, 311f
superior, 304f, 307f, 309f–311f, 310, 322f, 326f
Putamen, 106, 107f
PVS (prevertebral space), 267f, 268t
Pyloric antrum, 389, 389f, 391f
Pyloric canal, 389f
Pyloric orifice, 389f
Pyloric sphincter, 389, 389f, 391f, 393f
Pyramidalis muscle, 427f

Q
Quadrate ligament, 527
Quadrate lobe
of liver, 352, 353f
Quadratus femoris muscle, 444f, 577f, 578f, 579t, 580f–582f, 583
Quadratus lumborum muscle, 190, 191f, 192f, 424, 424f–426f, 428t
Quadratus plantae muscle, 626f, 627f, 641f, 646f, 648f, 651, 652t
Quadriceps bursa, 610
Quadriceps femoris muscle, 583t, 584, 584f, 608f, 610f
Quadriceps femoris tendon, 584f, 586f, 608f, 610f
Quadriceps ligament, 584
Quadriceps tendon, 587f, 594f, 599f, 603f, 605f, 609f, 614f
Quadrigeminal cistern, 95f, 96, 96f
Quadrigeminal plate, 116f, 117, 118f, 119f
Quadriplegia, 213

R
Radial artery, 562f, 563, 563f
Radial collateral ligament, 527, 528f, 529f, 545f, 546, 546f, 548
Radial dorsal tubercle, 523f, 524
Radial fossa, 496f
Radial groove, 522f
Radial head, 522f–525f, 524
Radial neck, 523f, 524, 525f
Radial nerve, 208, 209f, 565, 566, 566f
Radial notch, 522f–524f, 524
Radial recurrent artery, 562f, 563
Radial tuberosity, 522f–524f, 524
Radial veins, 222, 564, 565
Radicular artery(ies)
anterior, 219, 220f
great, 219, 220f
posterior, 219, 220f
Radicular vein
anterior, 222, 222f
posterior, 222, 222f
Radiocarpal arch
dorsal, 563f
palmar, 563
Radiocarpal articulation, 545
Radiocarpal joint, 543f–545f
Radiocarpal ligament
dorsal, 546, 547f
Radiohumeral articulations, 522f, 523
Radiolunate ligament
long, 547f
short, 547f
Radioscaphocapitate ligament, 547f
Radioscapholunate ligament, 547f
Radiotriquetral ligament
dorsal, 547f
Radioulnar articulation(s), 523
distal, 543f, 545, 545f
Radioulnar joint
distal, 523f, 543f, 545, 545f
Radioulnar ligament
palmar, 547f
Radius, 523f, 524, 524f, 539f, 541f, 542f
distal, 524, 524f
proximal, 524, 524f
styloid process of, 539f, 541f, 542f
Ray tracing, 14, 14f
Rectal ampulla, 452, 452f
Rectal artery, 479f

Rectal artery—cont'd
    middle, 475, 477f, 482t
    superior, 416, 416f, 417f, 477f
Rectal columns, 452, 452f
Rectal fold
    transverse, 452, 452f
Rectal vein(s)
    middle, 484f, 485f
    superior, 483, 484f
Rectal venous plexus, 485f
Rectouterine pouch, 453f, 456f, 457f, 459, 459f
Rectum, 392f, 398f, 452, 452f
Rectus abdominis muscles, 424f, 426, 428t, 438, 442f
Rectus capitis lateralis muscle, 260f
Rectus femoris muscle, 583t, 584, 584f, 585f
Rectus femoris tendon, 574f, 575f
Rectus muscle(s), 81, 81f–84f
    inferior, 81, 81f–84f
    lateral, 81, 82f, 83f
    medial, 81, 82f, 83f
    superior, 81, 81f–84f
Red nucleus, 117, 118f, 119f
Red pulp, 376
Regional terminology, 3, 3t, 4f
Renal artery(ies), 402f–406f, 405
    left, 405f, 406f, 409f, 417f, 483f
    right, 401f, 402f, 405f, 406f, 409f, 417f
Renal artery stenosis, 405
Renal calyces, 382, 383f, 385f–387f
Renal columns, 385f
Renal cortex, 382, 383f–386f
Renal fascia, 348f, 349, 378, 382, 383f, 386f, 387f
Renal hilum, 386f, 387f
Renal impression, 350f
Renal medulla, 382, 383f–385f
Renal papilla, 385f
Renal pelvis, 382, 383f–387f
Renal pyramids, 382, 383f–386f
Renal sinus, 382, 385f
Renal vein(s), 402f, 404f, 405f, 419f, 420, 421f, 484f
    left, 405f, 420, 421f
    right, 418f, 420, 421f, 483f, 484f
Reproductive organs
    female, 453–461, 453f–461f
    male, 462–473, 462f–474f
Rete testis, 463, 464f
Reticular formation, 117, 117f
Retina, 76
Retinacula
    of hip joint, 579
Retinacular ligament
    oblique, 551f
    transverse, 551f
Retromammary layer, 335, 336f
Retromandibular vein, 272, 272f
Retroorbital fat, 81f–83f, 82
Retroperitoneal spaces, 345t, 348f, 349, 349f
Retroperitoneum, 338f–340f, 350
Retropharyngeal space (RPS), 268t
Retropubic space, 453f, 459, 459f, 462f, 470f
Rhomboid muscles, 266f, 331f, 334f, 504, 504f, 510t
Ribs, 276, 276f, 277f
Right anterior branch, 322f
Right aortic sinus, 323
Right cardiac vein, 327f, 328
Right colic artery, 413, 414f
Right colic flexure, 392f, 393f, 396f, 397, 398f, 399f
Right common carotid artery, 269, 270f, 270t, 271f, 318f–320f, 319, 322f
Right common iliac artery, 401f, 475f–477f, 482f
Right coronary artery, 322f–325f, 323
Right external iliac artery, 401f, 475f
Right gastric artery, 362f, 407–409, 407f, 410f
Right gastric vein, 484f
Right gastroduodenal artery, 409f, 410f
Right gastroepiploic artery, 362f, 407f, 409
Right gastro-omental artery, 409
Right gonadal artery, 401f, 475f
Right gonadal vein, 419, 419f

Right hepatic artery, 363, 364f, 402f, 410f
Right hepatic duct, 367, 367f, 368f
Right hepatic vein, 354f, 359f, 361f, 364f–366f, 420
Right inferior accessory fissure, 351f
Right inferior phrenic artery, 402f, 403
Right inferior phrenic vein, 418, 418f
Right inferior pubic ramus, 436f
Right inferior pulmonary vein, 304f, 307f, 309f, 310, 310f, 311f
Right internal iliac artery, 401f, 475f
Right main portal vein, 359
Right marginal branch, 322f, 323
Right ovarian vein, 484f
Right portal vein, 356f–358f, 361f, 484f
Right pulmonary artery, 304, 304f, 305f, 307f, 309f, 311f, 322f
Right renal artery, 401f, 402f, 405f, 406f, 409f, 417f
Right renal vein, 418f, 420, 421f, 483f, 484f
Right superior pubic ramus, 436f
Right superior pulmonary veins, 304f, 307f, 309f–311f, 310, 322f, 326f
Right suprarenal artery, 401f, 475f
Right suprarenal vein, 419f, 420
Right testicular vein, 484f
Rima glottidis, 237, 238f–240f
Rivinus's ducts, 242f.245
Roentgen, Wilhelm Conrad, 1
Rostrum
    of corpus callosum, 100, 100f
Rotator cuff, 511f–513f, 513
Rotator cuff lesions, 504
Rotatores muscle, 186, 186t, 188f, 190, 190f
Round ligament
    of liver, 341
    of uterus, 455f, 456, 456f
Round window, 39, 39f, 41f
RPS (retropharyngeal space), 268t
Rugae, 389, 389f, 390f

S
SA (short axis) view, 316f, 317, 317f
Sacral artery
    lateral, 475, 477f, 482f, 482t, 654f
    median, 403, 654f
    middle, 477f, 483f
Sacral cornu, 177
Sacral flexure, 452
Sacral foramina, 175f, 177, 177f, 430, 431f
Sacral hiatus, 164f, 177
Sacral lymph nodes, 486f, 487
Sacral nerve, 201f
Sacral plexus, 206f, 213f, 215, 215f–217f, 664f
Sacral promontory, 175f, 177, 177f, 178f, 430, 431f, 436f
Sacral vein(s)
    lateral, 485f
    median, 419f, 483, 484f
    middle, 418f, 483f
Sacroiliac (SI) joints, 177, 177f, 178f, 430, 430f, 431f
Sacrotuberous ligament, 574f, 575f
Sacrum, 164f, 175f, 177, 177f, 178f, 430, 430f–433f
Sagittal plane, 2, 2f
Sagittal sinus
    inferior, 138–140, 138f, 140f
    superior, 138, 138f, 139f
Sagittal suture, 47, 47f
Salivary glands, 242–245, 242f–245f
Salpingopharyngeus muscle, 260, 261t, 263f
Saphenous nerve, 213, 213f, 664, 664f
Saphenous vein(s)
    great, 613f, 614f, 663, 663f
    greater, 615f–619f, 646f
    lesser, 615f–617f, 620f
    long, 585f, 586f
    short, 586f
    small, 613f, 614f, 663, 663f
Sartorius muscle, 580f–582f, 583–584, 583t, 584f–589f
SASD (subacromial-subdeltoid) bursa, 497f, 502f, 503, 503f
SC (sternoclavicular) joints, 276, 276f, 277f, 490f, 491, 491f

SCA (superior cerebellar artery), 130f, 132, 133f, 134f, 137t, 138f
Scalene muscle(s), 264t, 265f, 266, 333f, 334f
    anterior, 187f, 264t, 265f, 266
    middle, 264t, 265f, 266
    posterior, 187f, 264t, 265f, 266
Scalenus anterior muscle, 187f, 264t, 265f, 266
Scalenus medius muscle, 264t, 265f, 266
Scalenus posterior muscle, 187f, 264t, 265f, 266
Scaphocapitate ligament, 547f
Scaphoid, 539f–545f, 540
Scaphotrapezium trapezoid ligament, 547f
Scapula, 490f, 492f–495f, 493
Scapular artery
    dorsal, 562f
Scapular fossa, 493f
Scapular muscles, 511–513, 511f–513f, 511t
Scapular notch, 490f, 492f, 493
Scapular spine, 490f, 492f, 493, 493f, 504f
Sciatic nerve, 215, 215f–217f, 664, 664f
Sciatic notch
    greater, 432f, 433f, 436
    lesser, 432f, 433f, 436
SCM (sternocleidomastoid muscle), 187f, 264, 264t, 265f, 267f, 333f
Scrotal septum, 463f
Scrotum, 448f, 462f, 463
Second lumbar vein, 419f
Sectional anatomy
    history of, 1
Segmental artery(ies), 404f, 406f
    lower, 404f
    middle, 404f
    upper, 404f
Sella turcica, 25, 25f, 68
Semicircular canals, 38f, 39, 39f, 44f
Semilunar, 539f–541f, 540
Semilunar hiatus, 70, 70f
Semilunar notch, 524f
Semilunar valves, 303, 303f
Semimembranosus bursa, 610, 610f
Semimembranosus muscle, 579f, 583t, 592, 605f, 622f, 623f
Semimembranosus tendon, 577f, 608f, 610f, 620f
Seminal vesicles, 448f, 462f, 466f, 467, 470f
Seminiferous tubules, 464f
Semispinalis capitis muscle, 186, 186f–188f, 186t, 190f
Semispinalis cervicis muscle, 186, 186t, 190f
Semispinalis muscles, 186, 186t, 187f, 188f, 190
Semispinalis thoracis muscle, 186, 186t, 190f
Semitendinosus muscle, 579f, 583t, 592, 605f, 622f, 623f
Semitendinosus tendon, 586f
Sentinel lymph nodes, 290
Septal vein, 145, 147f
Septum
    of frontal sinuses, 69, 69f
Septum pellucidum, 89, 90f, 91
Serous pericardium, 294
Serratus anterior muscles, 333, 333f, 333t, 512f, 514f, 514t, 515
Serratus posterior inferior muscle, 330, 330t, 331f
Serratus posterior superior muscle, 330, 330t, 331f
Sesamoid bones
    in foot, 635f
    in hand, 541f, 542f
Shaded surface display (SSD), 14, 14f
Shin bone, 593f, 596, 596f–601f
Shingles, 195
Short axis (SA) view, 316f, 317, 317f
Short radiolunate ligament, 547f
Short saphenous vein, 586f
Shoulder, 491–522
    articular joint capsule of, 503, 503f
    body anatomy of, 490f–497f, 491–497
    bursae of, 503, 503f
    critical zone of, 504
    labrum and ligaments of, 498, 498f–502f
    MR arthrogram of, 517f, 518f, 520f
    muscles and tendons of, 504–522, 504f–521f
SI (sacroiliac) joints, 177, 177f, 178f, 430, 430f, 431f

Sigmoid arteries, 416f, 417f
Sigmoid branches, 416
Sigmoid colon, 396f, 397, 398f, 400f
Sigmoid sinuses, 138f, 140, 141f, 142f
Sigmoid veins, 484f
Sinus tarsi, 600f, 625, 626f, 627f
Skull. *See* Cranium.
Small bowel, 351f, 392, 392f–394f
Small cardiac vein, 327f, 328
Small intestine, 351f, 392, 392f–394f
Small saphenous vein, 613f, 614f, 663, 663f
Sodium bicarbonate, 373
Soft palate, 226, 226f–229f
Soleal line, 597, 597f
Soleus muscle, 611t, 612f, 615f–623f, 622
Soleus tendon, 616f, 617f
Somatomotor cortex, 103f
Somatosensory cortex, 103f
Spermatic cords, 463f, 464f, 467, 467f–469f
Sphenoethmoidal recess, 66f, 68
Sphenoid bone, 18f, 19f, 25–29, 25f–29f, 30t
Sphenoid fontanels, 48, 48f
Sphenoid sinuses, 25, 25f, 64f–66f, 65t, 68, 68f
Sphincter of Oddi, 367, 367f
Spin density—weighted image, 11, 12f
Spinal artery(ies), 218f–221f, 219
    anterior, 133f, 138f, 218f–220f, 219
    posterior, 219, 220f
Spinal branch(es), 219, 220f
    anterior, 220f
    posterior, 220f
Spinal cord, 196–199, 196f–203f
    veins of, 222, 222f
Spinal ganglion, 201f
Spinal meninges, 193–195, 193f–195f, 201f
Spinal nerve(s), 198f–203f, 199
Spinal nerve root, 160, 168f
Spinal veins, 222, 222f–224f
Spinalis capitis muscle, 186, 186f, 187f, 188f
Spinalis cervicis muscle, 186, 186f, 186t
Spinalis muscles, 186t, 188
Spinalis thoracis muscle, 186, 186t, 188f
Spine, 163–224
    fracture of, 163f
    ligaments of, 179–182, 179f–185f
    muscles of, 186–192, 186t
        deep, 190, 190f–192f
        intermediate, 188, 188f, 189f
        superficial, 186, 186f, 187f
    plexuses of, 204–217, 206f
        brachial, 206f, 208, 209f–212f
        cervical, 206f–209f, 207
        lumbar, 206f, 213, 213f, 214f
        sacral, 206f, 213f, 215, 215f–217f
    spinal cord and nerve roots of, 196–199, 196f–203f
    spinal meninges in, 193–195, 193f–195f
    vasculature of, 219–222
        arterial, 218f–221f, 219
        venous, 222, 222f–224f
    vertebral column of, 164–178, 164f–168f
        cervical vertebrae in, 164f, 169, 169f–173f
        lumbar vertebrae in, 164f, 175, 175f, 176f
        sacrum and coccyx in, 164f, 177, 177f, 178f
        thoracic vertebrae in, 164f, 174, 174f
Spinous process(es), 164, 164f, 165f, 167f, 168f
    cervical, 169, 171f, 173f
        bifid, 169, 171f, 172f
    thoracic, 174, 174f
Spiral valves of Heister, 367, 368f
Spleen, 351f, 376, 376f, 377f
Splenial artery, 129
Splenic artery, 362f, 364f, 401f, 402f, 405f, 407f–412f, 409
Splenic flexure, 392f, 393f, 396f, 397, 398f, 399f
Splenic vein, 359f–361f, 410f, 484f
Splenium
    of corpus callosum, 100, 100f
Splenius capitis muscle, 186, 186f, 186t, 187f, 264t, 265f, 266
Splenius cervicis muscle, 186, 186t, 187f, 264t
Splenius muscles, 186, 186f, 186t, 187f
Splenorenal ligament, 340t
Spongy urethra, 448f, 462f, 473f
Spring ligament, 626f, 640, 640f, 647f
Squamous suture, 47, 47f

SSD (shaded surface display), 14, 14f
Stacking
    of transverse images, 12f, 13
Stapes, 39, 39f, 45f
Stensen's duct, 242, 242f
Sternal angle, 276, 276f, 277f
Sternal head muscle, 264t
Sternoclavicular (SC) joints, 276, 276f, 277f, 490f, 491, 491f
Sternocleidomastoid (SCM) muscle, 187f, 264, 264t, 265f, 267f, 333f
Sternohyoid muscle, 264, 264t, 265f
Sternothyroid muscle, 264, 264t, 265f
Sternum, 276, 277f, 278f
Stomach, 351f, 389, 389f–391f
Straight sinus, 138f, 140, 140f–142f
Striate arteries, 133f
Striate veins, 147f
Styloglossus muscle, 260, 261f, 261t, 265f
Stylohyoid muscle, 260f, 264, 264t, 265f
Styloid process
    of radius, 523f, 524, 524f
    of temporal bone, 31f, 34f, 38, 38f
    of ulna, 523f, 524f
Stylomastoid foramen, 30t, 38, 38f
Stylopharyngeus muscle, 260, 260f, 261t
Subacromial bursa, 503f, 512f
Subacromial-subdeltoid (SASD) bursa, 497f, 502f, 503, 503f
Subarachnoid cisterns, 95, 95f
Subarachnoid space
    cranial, 86f, 87, 93f, 95
    spinal, 193, 193f, 194f, 201f
Subcalcaneal fat pad, 626f
Subclavian artery, 305f, 318f–320f, 319, 322f, 562f
Subclavian veins, 269f, 272, 318f, 320f, 321, 564
Subclavius muscle, 333, 333t, 334f, 507f, 514f, 514t, 515
Subcostal vein, 419f
Subcutaneous infrapatellar bursa, 610f
Subcutaneous prepatellar bursa, 610, 610f
Subdeltoid bursa, 503f, 512f
Subdural space
    cranial, 87
    spinal, 193, 194f, 201f
Subhepatic spaces, 345, 345f–347f, 345t
Sublingual ducts, 242f, 245
Sublingual glands, 242–245, 242f, 245f
Submandibular duct, 242, 242f
Submandibular glands, 242, 242f, 244f, 245f
Submandibular space, 267f
Subphrenic spaces, 345, 345f, 345t, 346f
Subscapular artery, 562f
Subscapular bursa, 503, 503f, 512f
Subscapular fossa, 493
Subscapularis muscle, 508f, 511t, 512f, 513, 513f
Subscapularis tendon, 495f, 497f, 498f
Substantia nigra, 117, 118f, 119f
    damage to, 117
Subtalar joint, 625, 626f–628f, 630f, 631f, 635f, 636f
    posterior, 627f
Sulci, 98
Superficial cerebral veins, 145f
Superficial circumflex iliac artery, 655, 659f
Superficial cortical veins, 138f, 145, 145f
Superficial epigastric artery, 655
Superficial external inguinal ring, 427f
Superficial fibular nerve, 614f, 615f
Superficial infrapatellar bursa, 610
Superficial inguinal nodes, 422f, 486f
Superficial inguinal ring, 463f
Superficial middle cerebral vein, 138f, 145f
Superficial palmar arch, 562f, 563, 563f, 565
Superficial peroneal nerve, 614f, 615f, 664f
Superior anastomotic vein, 138f
Superior aperture
    of pelvis, 436
Superior articular facet, 166f
Superior articular processes, 164f–168f, 166
    cervical, 169, 169f–171f
Superior cerebellar artery (SCA), 130f, 132, 133f, 134f, 137t, 138f
Superior cerebellar peduncles, 124f–126f, 125

Superior colliculi, 116f, 117, 118f, 120f
Superior constrictor muscle, 260, 260f, 261t, 263f
Superior costal facet, 165f
Superior extensor retinaculum, 612f, 637, 638f, 651f
Superior fibular retinaculum, 627f
Superior gemellus muscle, 569f, 577f, 578f, 579t, 580f, 583
Superior glenohumeral ligament, 498f, 499f, 513f
Superior gluteal artery, 475, 477f, 482f, 482t, 654f, 659f
Superior gluteal vein, 484f, 485f
Superior iliac spine, 433
    anterior, 431f, 572f
    posterior, 432f, 433f
Superior ischial ramus, 436
Superior left colic artery, 416f
Superior medial genicular artery, 659f
Superior medullary velum, 91, 91f
Superior mesenteric artery, 401f–403f, 410f, 411f, 413, 413f–416f
Superior mesenteric vein, 350f, 358f, 361f, 410f, 484f
Superior nasal conchae, 24, 24f, 55f, 68
Superior nasal meatus, 55, 55f
    drainage into, 65, 65t, 68
Superior oblique muscle, 81, 82f–84f, 260f
Superior ophthalmic vein, 78f, 79f, 82
Superior orbital fissure, 18f, 28f, 29, 30t, 72, 72f, 74f
Superior pancreaticoduodenal artery, 362f, 410f
Superior peroneal retinaculum, 637, 638f
Superior pubic ramus, 430f, 435, 435f, 572f
    right, 436f
Superior rectal artery, 416, 416f, 417f, 477f
Superior rectal vein, 483, 484f
Superior rectus muscle, 81, 81f–84f
Superior sagittal sinus, 138, 138f, 139f
Superior suprarenal arteries, 378f, 403, 403f, 405
Superior temporal gyrus, 103
Superior thoracic artery, 562f
Superior thyroarytenoid muscle, 262f
Superior trunk, 565
Superior ulnar collateral artery, 562f
Superior vena cava, 304f, 307f, 311f, 314, 318, 322f
    tributaries of, 321, 321f
Superior venous palmar arch, 565f
Superior vertebral notch, 166f
Supinator muscle, 530t, 531f, 534f, 538f, 539
Supraclavicular lymph nodes, 290
Supracolic compartment, 345, 345f, 345t
Supracondylar line
    lateral, 572f, 593
    medial, 593
Supracondylar ridge
    lateral, 496f, 522f
    medial, 522f
Supraglenoid tubercle, 492f, 493, 495f
Suprahyoid muscles, 264, 264t, 265f
Suprahyoid region, 266, 268t
Supraorbital foramen, 18f, 22, 22f, 30t
Supraorbital notch, 18f, 22, 22f, 30t
Suprapatellar bursa, 586f, 610, 610f
Suprapatellar fat body, 605f
Suprarenal artery(ies), 404f, 405, 483f
    inferior, 405
        phrenic, 403f
    middle, 378f, 403f, 405
        right, 401f, 475f
    superior, 378f, 403, 403f, 405
Suprarenal glands, 378, 378f–381f
Suprarenal vein(s), 418f, 420, 483f
    left, 420
    right, 419f, 420
Suprasellar cistern, 93f, 95f, 96, 96f
Supraspinatus muscle, 503f, 504f, 506f, 507f, 511f, 511t, 513, 513f
Supraspinatus tendon, 497f, 498f
Supraspinous fossa, 492f, 493
Supraspinous ligament, 179, 180f, 182f–185f
Sural arteries, 660

Sural cutaneous nerve
  lateral, 613f
  medial, 615f
Sural nerve, 613f, 614f, 616f, 617f, 664f
Surface landmarks, 3, 4f, 5f
Surgical neck
  of humerus, 496f, 497, 497f, 522f
Suspensory ligament(s)
  of breast, 335, 335f
  of ovaries, 454f, 456f, 460
  of penis, 471f
  of uterus, 456, 456f
Sustentaculum tali, 624f, 625, 625f
Sutures, 47, 47f
Sylvian fissure, 98, 98f, 99f
Symphysis pubis, 430f, 434f–436f, 435
  female, 447f, 453, 453f
  male, 462f

T
T1-weighted image, 11, 12f
T2-weighted image, 11, 12f
Taenia coli, 396f, 397
Tail of Spence, 335, 335f
Talocalcaneal joint, 627f
Talocalcaneal ligament, 626f, 627f, 638f, 640
  interosseous, 639f
  lateral, 650f
  medial, 650f
  posterior, 650f
Talocalcaneonavicular joint, 626f, 627f, 637
Talocrural joint, 626f–628f, 637
Talofibular ligament
  anterior, 629f, 640, 645f, 650f
  posterior, 627f, 629f, 640, 650f
Talonavicular ligament, 650f
  dorsal, 646f
Talus, 624f, 625, 632f, 635f, 636f
Tarsal(s), 624f
Tarsal artery, 659f
Tarsal canal, 625
Tarsometatarsal joints, 626f, 630f, 637
Tarsus, 625
Tectorial membrane, 179, 179f, 180f
Tectum, 117, 118f, 119f
Tegmentum, 117, 117f, 118f
Temporal bone, 18f, 19f, 34–38, 34f–38f
Temporal fossa, 18, 20f, 20t
Temporal gyrus, superior, 103
Temporal horn, 89, 89f–92f
Temporal lobe, 98f, 103, 103f
Temporalis muscle, 62, 62f, 63f, 265f, 267f
Temporomandibular joint (TMJ), 56, 59–63
  articular disk and ligaments of, 58f, 60, 60f,
    61f
  bony anatomy of, 58f, 59, 59f
  lateral view of, 58f
  muscles of, 62, 62f, 63f
Temporomandibular ligament, 60, 60f, 61f
Tendo calcaneus, 617f, 639f, 641f
Tensor fascia latae muscle, 581f, 582f, 583t,
  584, 584f, 589f
Tensor veli palatini muscle, 260f, 263f
Tentorium cerebelli, 86, 86f–88f
Teres major muscle, 504f, 508f, 511, 511f, 511t
Teres minor muscle, 504f, 508f, 511f, 511t, 513,
  513f
Testicular arteries, 405, 463f, 483f
Testicular vein, 462f, 483f, 484f
Testis(es), 448f, 462f–465f, 464, 469f
TFCC (triangular fibrocartilage complex), 543f,
  545, 545f, 546, 546f
Thalamostriate vein, 138f, 145, 145f–147f
Thalamus, 99f, 106f–108f, 109, 110f
Thecal sac, 193, 193f, 194f, 201f
Thenar muscle of thumb, 537f
Thenar muscle group, 560, 561f
Thick ascending limb, 385f
Thigh muscles, 583–592, 583t, 584f–592f
  anterior, 583–584, 583t, 584f–591f
  medial, 583t, 584–592, 584f–591f
  posterior, 583t, 584f–591f, 592
Thin descending limb, 385f
Third lumbar vein, 419f
Third ventricle, 89f, 90f, 91, 92f
Thoracic apertures, 276f–278f, 278

Thoracic artery(ies)
  internal, 320f, 321
  lateral, 562f
  superior, 562f
Thoracic cage, 276–278, 276f–278f
Thoracic cavity, 5, 7f, 7t
Thoracic duct, 292, 292f, 422f, 423
Thoracic inlet, 276f, 278
Thoracic nerves, 201f
Thoracic outlet, 276f, 278, 278f
Thoracic spinal cord
  axial, T1-weighted MR scan of, 204f–206f
Thoracic vein, internal, 320f
Thoracic vertebrae, 164f–166f, 174, 174f, 276
Thoracic walls, anterior and lateral, muscles
    connecting upper extremity to, 514f,
    514t, 515
Thoracoacromial artery, 562f
Thoracoacromial trunk, 562f
Thorax, 275–336
  azygos venous system in, 329, 329f
  bony, 276–278, 276f–278f
  branches of aortic arch in, 318f–320f, 319
  breast in, 335, 335f, 336f
  bronchi in, 283, 283t, 284f–286f
  with chest mass, 275f
  coronary circulation in, 323–328
    cardiac veins in, 327–328, 327f, 328f
    coronary arteries in, 322f–326f, 323
  great vessels of, 304–314, 304f–315f
  heart in, 293–303
    chambers of, 296, 296f–302f
    circulation of blood through, 302f, 316
    off-axis imaging of, 316–317, 316f, 317f
    pericardium of, 294, 294f, 295f
    superficial landmarks of, 293, 293f, 294f
    valves of, 296f, 298f, 302f, 303, 303f
    wall of, 296, 296f
  lungs in, 279–282, 279f–282f
  lymphatic system in, 290–292, 290f–292f,
    291t
  mediastinum of, 286–289, 287f
    thymus gland in, 286, 287f, 288f
    trachea and esophagus in, 289, 289f
  muscles of, 330–333, 330f–332f, 330t
    connecting upper extremity to anterior and
      lateral thoracic walls, 333, 333f, 333t,
      334f
  pleural cavities in, 279f–283f, 283
  tributaries of superior vena cava in, 321, 321f
Three-dimensional imaging, 12f–15f, 13–15
Thymosin, 286
Thymus gland, 286, 287f, 288f
Thyroarytenoid muscle(s), 262, 262f, 263t
  superior, 262f
Thyrocervical trunk, 562f
Thyrohyoid muscle, 264, 264t, 265f
Thyroid artery, inferior, 562f
Thyroid cartilage, 234, 234f–236f, 238f, 239f,
  257f, 258f
Thyroid gland, 246, 246f, 247f, 259f
Tibia, 593f, 596, 596f–601f
Tibial artery, 661f
Tibial collateral ligament, 603f, 604f, 608, 608f
Tibial nerve, 213f, 215, 664, 664f
  posterior, 664f
Tibial plateau(s), 593f, 595f, 597, 597f, 598f
  lateral, 595f, 597f, 598f
  medial, 593f, 597f, 598f
Tibial recurrent artery
  anterior, 659f
Tibial spine, 593f, 595f, 597, 597f
Tibial tuberosity, 593f, 597, 597f, 600f, 618f
Tibial vein(s)
  anterior, 663f, 663f
  posterior, 663f, 663f
Tibialis anterior muscle, 611, 611t, 612f–619f,
  621f
Tibialis anterior tendon, 638f, 643f, 646f, 647,
  648f
Tibialis muscle, 619f
Tibialis posterior muscle, 611t, 613f–621f,
  622, 623f, 638f
Tibialis posterior tendon, 622–623, 623f, 640f,
  643f, 644f, 647, 647f
Tibialis tendon, 619f

Tibiocalcaneal ligament, 640, 650f
Tibiofibular articulation, 598f, 599f
Tibiofibular joint
  distal, 597f
  proximal, 597f
Tibiofibular ligament
  anterior, 640, 650f
  posterior, 640, 644f, 650f
Tibiofibular syndesmosis, 627f
Tibionavicular ligament, 629f, 640, 650f
Tibiotalar ligament, 629f, 640
  posterior, 650f
Tic douloureux, 86
Tissue relaxation, 11, 12f
TMJ. *See* Temporomandibular joint (TMJ).
Tongue muscles, 261f
Tonsillar herniation, 124
Torcular herophili, 140, 141f, 142f, 147f
Trachea, 241, 241f, 279f, 283, 285f, 289, 289f
Tracheal cartilage, 234f
Transversalis fascia, 424f
Transverse acetabular ligament, 573f, 575f
Transverse arch, 624f, 637
Transverse arytenoid muscle, 263f
Transverse carpal ligament, 546
Transverse cervical artery, 562f
Transverse cervical ligament, 459f
Transverse colon, 392f, 393f, 396f–399f, 397
Transverse fissure, 351
Transverse foramen, 169, 169f
Transverse humeral ligament, 498, 499f, 502f
Transverse images
  stacks of, 12f, 13
Transverse joint, 637
Transverse ligament
  of hip, 573–577
  of knee, 603, 603f, 612f
  of spine, 179, 179f–182f
Transverse plane, 2, 2f
Transverse process(es), 164, 164f, 165f
  cervical, 169f–172f
  thoracic, 174, 174f
Transverse rectal fold, 452, 452f
Transverse retinacular ligament, 551f
Transverse sinuses, 138f, 140, 141f, 142f
Transversospinal muscles, 186, 186t, 190, 190f,
  192f
Transversus abdominis muscle, 424f, 425f, 426,
  427f, 428f, 428t
Trapezium, 539f–543f, 540, 545f
Trapezius muscle, 264t, 265f–267f, 266, 333f,
  504, 504f, 510t
Trapezoid, 539f–545f, 540
Trauma to skull and facial bones, 17f
Triangular fibrocartilage complex (TFCC),
  543f, 545, 545f, 546, 546f
Triangular ligament(s)
  of finger, 551f
  peritoneal, 340t
Triceps brachii muscle, 516, 516f, 517f, 518f,
  519f, 521f
Tricuspid valve, 293f, 295f, 296f, 302f, 303
Trigeminal cave, 37f, 38
Trigeminal cistern, 154, 154f
Trigeminal nerve, 116f, 148f, 148t, 154, 154f,
  155f
Trigeminal neuralgia, 86
Trigone, 89, 89f, 451
Triquetral, 539f–543f, 540, 545f
Triquetrohamate ligament, 547f
Triquetrum, 539f–543f, 540, 545f
Trochanter
  greater, 430f, 433f, 435f, 568, 569f–575f
  lesser, 430f, 568, 569f–572f
Trochlea, 496f, 522f, 523, 524f–526f
  peroneal, 625, 625f
Trochlear nerve, 116f, 148f, 148t, 152, 152f,
  153f
Trochlear notch, 524, 524f
True pelvis, 436, 436f
True vocal cords, 234f–236f, 237, 238f–240f
Tuberculum sellae, 25, 25f
Tunica albuginea, 463, 464f
Tunica vaginalis, 463f
Tympanic cavity, 39, 39f, 42f, 43f, 45f
Tympanic membrane, 39, 39f, 42f

U

Ulna, 523f, 524–526, 539f, 541f, 542f
  distal, 524f, 526
  proximal, 524, 524f, 525f
  styloid process of, 539f, 541f, 542f
Ulnar artery, 562f, 563, 563f
Ulnar collateral artery
  inferior, 562f
  superior, 562f
Ulnar collateral ligament, 527, 527f, 528f, 545f, 546, 546f, 548
Ulnar head, 523f, 524f
Ulnar nerve, 208, 209f, 524, 565–566, 566f
Ulnar notch, 523f, 524
Ulnar recurrent artery
  anterior, 562f, 563
  posterior, 562f, 563
Ulnar tuberosity, 524, 524f
Ulnar vein, 564, 565
Ulnocapitate ligament, 547f
Ulnohumeral articulations, 522f, 523
Ulnolunate ligament, 547f
Ulnotriquetral ligament, 547f
Umbilical artery, 475, 475f, 477f, 482t
Umbilical fissure, 351, 351f
Umbilical ligament(s)
  lateral, 449f, 450, 456f
  medial, 449f, 450, 456f
  median, 449f, 450, 456f
Umbilical vein, 484f
Umbilicus, 449f
Unciform bone, 539f, 540, 540f
Uncinate process
  of pancreas, 373, 373f
  of paranasal sinuses, 24, 24f, 70, 70f, 71f
Upper arm muscles, 515–516, 515f–521f, 517t
Upper extremity, 489–566
  elbow in, 523–539
    bony anatomy of, 522f–526f, 523–526
    forearm muscles of, 530–539, 530t, 531f–538f
    ligaments of, 527, 527f–529f
  muscles connecting anterior and lateral thoracic walls to, 514f, 514t, 515
  muscles connecting vertebral column to, 504, 504f–510f, 510t
  neurovasculature of, 561–566, 562f–566f
  shoulder in, 491–522
    articular joint capsule of, 503, 503f
    body anatomy of, 490f–497f, 491–497
    bursae of, 503, 503f
    labrum and ligaments of, 498, 498f–502f
    muscles and tendons of, 504–522, 504f–521f
  wrist and hand of, 540–566
    bony anatomy of, 540, 540f–544f
    joints of, 545, 545f
    ligaments and fascia of, 546–550, 546f–553f
    muscles and tendons of, 554–560, 554f–561f
Upper segmental artery, 404f
Ureters, 382, 382f, 385f, 387f, 388f
Urethra, 451
  female, 447f, 451, 453f
  male, 448f–451f, 451, 462f, 466f, 471f–473f
  membranous, 448f, 449f, 451, 462f, 467f, 470f
  prostatic, 448f, 451, 451f, 462f, 471f–473f
Urethral orifice
  external, 451, 473f
Urethral sphincter
  internal, 450
Urethral sphincter muscle, 451
Urinary bladder, 351f, 447–451, 447f–451f, 454f
Urinary system, 382, 382f–388f
Urogenital diaphragm, 445f, 473f
Urogenital triangle, 436, 437f
Uterine artery, 475, 477f, 482t
Uterine cavity, 453f–455f
Uterine ligament, 457f
Uterine tubes, 447f, 453f, 454f, 456f, 460
Uterine vein, 484f, 485f
Uterine venous plexus, 485f
Uterosacral ligaments, 456, 456f, 457f
Uterus, 447f, 453, 453f–457f
  suspensory ligaments of, 456, 456f
Uvula, 226, 226f–229f, 255f

V

Vagina, 447f, 453f, 454f, 459f, 461, 461f
Vaginal artery, 475, 477f, 482t
Vaginal vault, 461
Vaginal venous plexus, 485f
Vagus nerve, 116f, 148f, 148t, 159f, 160
Valleculae, 226, 227f, 230f, 231f
Vas deferens, 448f, 449f, 462f–464f, 466f, 467, 469f
Vastus intermedius muscle, 583t, 584, 585f, 587f–589f, 592f
Vastus lateralis muscle, 570f, 581f, 583t, 584, 584f–589f, 592f
Vastus lateralis tendon, 607f
Vastus medialis muscle, 583t, 584, 584f–589f, 592f
Vastus medialis tendon, 605f
Vein of Galen, 138f, 140f, 142f, 145, 145f–147f
Vena cava
  inferior
    in abdomen, 354f, 418–420, 418f–421f
    in pelvis, 477f, 483, 483f, 484f
    in thorax, 304f, 305f, 314, 315f, 322f
  superior, 304f, 307f, 311f, 314, 318, 322f
    tributaries of, 321, 321f
Venous palmar arch
  superior, 565f
Venous plexus(es), 483
  external, 222
  internal, 222, 223f
  prostatic, 485f
  rectal, 485f
  uterine, 485f
  vaginal, 485f
  vertebral, 222, 222f, 223f
    anterior internal, 222, 222f, 223f
    posterior internal, 222, 222f, 223f
  vesical, 485f
Ventral branches of abdominal aorta, 401, 405, 407
Ventral cavity, 5, 7f, 7t
Ventral horns, 199, 201f
Ventral median fissure, 201f
Ventral rami, 204, 206f
Ventral root, 194f, 196f, 198f, 200f, 203f, 206
Ventricle(s)
  of brain, 89–94, 89f–94f
    lateral, 89, 90f, 92f–94f
    third, 89f, 90f, 91, 92f
  cardiac
    left, 296, 296f, 300f–302f
    right, 296, 296f, 297f, 300f–302f
Ventricular system, 89–96
  cisterns in, 95–96, 95f–97f
  ventricles of, 89–94, 89f–94f
Ventricular vein
  left posterior, 328
Vermiform appendix, 392f, 396f, 397, 397f
Vertebra(e)
  cervical, 164f, 167f, 169, 169f–173f
  lumbar, 164f–168f, 175, 175f, 176f
  structure of, 164–166, 164f–168f
  thoracic, 164f–166f, 174, 174f
Vertebra prominens, 169, 172f
Vertebral arch, 164, 164f, 165f
Vertebral arteries
  in cranium, 127f, 128f, 130f, 132, 132f–138f, 137t
  in neck, 250f–259f, 270f, 270t, 271f, 272
Vertebral body, 164, 164f–166f
Vertebral canal, 164
Vertebral column, 164–178, 164f–168f
  cervical vertebrae in, 164f, 169, 169f–173f
  curvatures of, 164, 164f
  lumbar vertebrae in, 164f, 175, 175f, 176f
  muscles connecting upper limb to, 504, 504f–510f, 510t
  sacrum and coccyx in, 164f, 177, 177f, 178f
  structure of, 164–166, 164f–168f
  thoracic vertebrae in, 164f, 174, 174f
  veins of, 222, 222f–224f

Vertebral element
  anterior, 164, 164f–166f
  posterior, 164, 164f, 165f
Vertebral end plates, 164, 165f
Vertebral foramen, 164, 164f, 165f
Vertebral notch, 164, 165f, 165f
Vertebral veins, 222f, 272, 273t
Vertebral venous plexuses, 222, 222f, 223f
  anterior external, 222, 222f, 223f
  posterior internal, 222, 222f, 223f
Vertebrobasilar system, 127f, 132–133, 132f–137f, 137t
Vertex, 20, 21f
Vertical long axis (VLA) view, 316, 316f
Verumontanum, 471, 473f
Vesical artery
  inferior, 475, 482t
Vesical fascia, 459f
Vesical vein(s), 485f
  inferior, 485f
Vesical venous plexus, 485f
Vesicouterine ligament, 456f
Vesicouterine pouch, 453f, 457f, 459f
Vestibular aqueduct, 39, 41f
Vestibular branch, 156
Vestibular folds, 234f, 237
Vestibule of ear, 39, 39f
Vestibulocochlear nerve, 156, 156f, 157f
Villi, 393
Visceral branches
  of abdominal aorta, 401, 405, 407
Visceral lymph nodes, 423
Visceral pericardium, 294, 294f
Visceral peritoneum, 338, 338f
Visceral pleura, 279f, 283, 283f
Visceral space (VS), 267f, 268t
Visual area, primary, 103
Vitreous humor, 76
VLA (vertical long axis) view, 316, 316f
Vocal cords
  false, 234f, 237
  true, 234f–236f, 237, 238f–240f
Vocal folds, 240f
Vocalis muscle, 262, 263t
Volar ligament, 546, 548
Volar plate, 550f, 552f, 553f
Volume rendering (VR), 15, 15f
Vomer, 49f, 51f, 55
Voxels, 10f, 11
VS (visceral space), 267f, 268t

W

Wernicke's area, 103, 103f
Wharton's duct, 242, 242f
White matter
  cerebral, 99f–102f, 100
  of spinal cord, 196
White pulp, 376
Window level (WL), 11
Window width (WW), 11
Windowing, 11, 11f
Wrist, 540–566
  bony anatomy of, 540, 540f–544f
  joints of, 545, 545f
  ligaments and fascia of, 546–550, 546f–553f
  muscles and tendons of, 554–560, 554f–561f
WW (window width), 11

X

Xiphoid process, 276, 276f, 277f

Z

Zona orbicularis, 579
Zygapophyseal joints, 166, 166f–168f
Zygoma, 49f–52f, 50, 54f
Zygomatic arch, 29f, 34, 35f, 49f, 50, 52f, 54f
Zygomatic process
  of mandible, 49f
  of maxilla, 49f, 50, 51f
  of temporal bone, 32f, 34, 34f, 35f
Zygomaticus major muscle, 265f
Zygomaticus muscle, 267f